Tuberculosis

LUNG BIOLOGY IN HEALTH AND DISEASE

Executive Editor

Claude Lenfant

Former Director, National Heart, Lung, and Blood Institute
National Institute of Health
Bethesda, Maryland

Tuberculosis
Fourth Edition
The Essentials

Edited by

Mario C. Raviglione
World Health Organization
Geneva, Switzerland

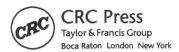

CRC Press
Taylor & Francis Group
Boca Raton London New York

CRC Press is an imprint of the
Taylor & Francis Group, an **Informa** business

Cover photo by Riccardo Venturi. TB patient in Borama, Somalia, March 2006. Annalena Tonelli Hospital, founded by the social and health promoter Ms. Annalena Tonelli, murdered in 2003, for the assistance to poor TB patients.

CRC Press
Taylor & Francis Group
6000 Broken Sound Parkway NW, Suite 300
Boca Raton, FL 33487-2742

First issued in paperback 2017

© 2010 by Taylor & Francis Group, LLC
CRC Press is an imprint of Taylor & Francis Group, an Informa business

No claim to original U.S. Government works

ISBN-13: 978-1-4200-9021-5 (hbk)
ISBN-13: 978-1-138-11766-2 (pbk)

Library of Congress Cataloging-in-Publication Data

Tuberculosis : the essentials. – 4th ed. / edited by Mario C. Raviglione.
     p. ; cm. – (Lung biology in health and disease ; 237)
   Rev. ed. of: Reichman and Hershfield's tuberculosis. 3rd ed. / edited by Mario C. Raviglione. c2006.
   Includes bibliographical references and index.
   ISBN-13: 978-1-4200-9021-5 (hb : alk. paper)
   ISBN-10: 1-4200-9021-6 (hb : alk. paper)   1. Tuberculosis.   I. Raviglione, Mario C.   II. Reichman and Hershfield's tuberculosis.   III. Series: Lung biology in health and disease ; v. 237.
   [DNLM: 1. Tuberculosis.   W1 LU62 v.237 2009 / WF 200 T88253 2009]
   RC311.T826 2009
   362.196 '995–dc22
                           2009028283

Visit the Taylor & Francis Web site at
http://www.taylorandfrancis.com

and the CRC Press Web site at
http://www.crcpress.com

Introduction

The readership of the series of monographs Lung Biology in Health and Disease have surely noted that this volume, edited by Dr. Mario C. Raviglione and titled *Tuberculosis: The Essentials,* is the fourth edition of a "subseries on tuberculosis" that began in 1993. In addition, a number of other volumes in the series, which may not include the word tuberculosis in the title, have chapters relevant to this lung disease.

Thus, one may ask "why is the series presenting so many editions and so much information on the same subject?" The answer to this question is largely to be found in the Preface written by Dr. Raviglione. He describes, in the Preface, how and why decisions were made to publish these four editions, and he further explains why the time elapsed between each edition has decreased by stating "the field of tuberculosis is moving faster and faster."

One can interpret this statement in many ways. For example, although the rate of tuberculosis has peaked, the number of cases worldwide has further increased as the world population increases. At the same time, fundamental and clinical research has markedly increased worldwide in order to address emerging problems such as drug resistance and the association of tuberculosis with HIV. Yes, indeed, all aspects of tuberculosis are going faster and faster!

The goal of the series of monographs Lung Biology in Health and Disease is to transfer new information to physicians caring for patients and to fundamental research scientists to seek answers to emerging questions and to pursue new avenues of research. Well over a thousand publications about pulmonary tuberculosis appear each year and this new edition of *Tuberculosis, Fourth Edition: The Essentials,* with chapters authored by leading world authorities, is a vehicle to transfer this new information. It will undoubtedly help physicians provide better care to their patients and meet the important goal of stimulating new research.

As the Executive Editor of this series, I am very grateful to Dr. Raviglione and to the authors for adding to the series such a landmark contribution.

Claude Lenfant, MD
Vancouver, Washington, U.S.A.

Preface

The third edition of *Tuberculosis—A Comprehensive International Approach* was published just three years ago with the aim to provide health workers, students, scientists, and all interested in the field with a textbook featuring the "state-of-the-art" knowledge in tuberculosis control and research. Judging from the success of the book, we succeeded in disseminating the most up-to-date understandings in the field, thanks to the over 100 scientific authorities and colleagues who contributed their expertise and knowledge.

However, the field of tuberculosis is moving faster and faster, with information becoming available very rapidly in all aspects of the disease. For instance, by the time of publication of the third edition, the international health community became acutely aware of the existence of extensively drug-resistant tuberculosis (XDR-TB)—a form of multidrug-resistant tuberculosis (MDR-TB) resistant to the most powerful first- and second-line antituberculosis drugs. This recognition has caused great concern internationally, not only because XDR-TB has been found in most places where second-line drugs have been used, but also because XDR-TB has started affecting people living with HIV/AIDS, resulting in extremely high case fatality. The fear generated by XDR-TB is without precedents in the tuberculosis world, as the specter of an incurable disease, like in the preantibiotic era, has reappeared. Almost simultaneously with the recognition of XDR-TB, the World Health Organization has announced that global tuberculosis rates per capita might have reached a peak in 2004. This is also unprecedented, as rates had been increasing annually for decades, at least globally. This is largely the result of a changing direction of the HIV/AIDS incidence curve in Africa. In this region, the HIV/AIDS factor had determined the dramatic increases of tuberculosis rates starting in the 1980s until very recently. Peaking of the HIV epidemic has meant finally also a decrease of tuberculosis in many countries. At the same time, the interaction between tuberculosis and HIV has been recognized also outside of the tuberculosis community, and combined approaches between national HIV/AIDS and tuberculosis programs have started to produce results.

In the field of tuberculosis research, the recent demonstration that molecular diagnostics, such as the line-probe assays, may reduce dramatically the time of detection of multidrug-resistant tuberculosis and be applicable also to resource-limited settings has spurred a sense of hope that was not felt for decades. At last, the first products of the recent investments in tuberculosis research and development after many years of neglect have become available. This is unprecedented too. Similarly, advances are evident in various research fields, with new drugs in the pipeline and a dozen vaccine candidates getting ready for large clinical trials.

These new developments prompted the decision to update the third edition of our book very rapidly. While the first (1993) and second (2000) editions, edited by L. B. Reichman and E. S. Hershfield, were separated by seven years and the second and third (2006) editions by six years, this time, the publishers have decided to pursue a rapid update to keep the pace of the new discoveries and observations in the field of tuberculosis. However, not all chapters of the 2006 third edition are in need of an update. Thus, we have decided to focus only on those topics that are constantly and frequently changing. Hence, we have selected fifteen essential areas, which were updated to provide the reader with the best information available today. To begin, tuberculosis epidemiology, both descriptive and general, is changing constantly, as is the complex field of pathogenesis. We have therefore asked prominent scientists in these fields to present the latest information. The clinical chapters of diagnosis and treatment of the various forms of tuberculosis, including those associated with HIV and those due to drug-resistant organisms, are fundamental for the clinician and in need of regular update. This has been achieved by asking expert authorities to take a new look at the case management of tuberculosis, including its variants of HIV-associated tuberculosis and MDR-TB. Control-related issues of paramount importance include the status of drug resistance in the world, on which new important information has become available in 2008; the programmatic approach to drug-resistant tuberculosis, which has required quick strategic adjustments during 2008 to cope with the emerging threat of XDR-TB; and the approach against HIV-associated tuberculosis with the clearer recognition of the interventions necessary from both the HIV/AIDS and tuberculosis programs. All these are also part of the comprehensive Stop TB Strategy launched in 2006, which in itself needs some refining after the first years of implementation. For this reason, we are presenting in this edition the latest updates of the strategy that, today, covers comprehensively all major thematic areas of control and research. In addition, the issue of case detection has become very prominent since we have witnessed a slowing down in the growth of cases detected by programs world-wide: this requires a specific chapter assessing what can be done to increase and accelerate detection of cases while maintaining high treatment success rates. Finally, the field of research is ever evolving and new information needs to be disseminated rapidly for a better knowledge of the area. Thus, the three chapters devoted to development of new diagnostics, drugs, and vaccines present the latest information available from some of the key scientists involved in research toward new tools.

These topics constitute our fifteen essential chapters that form this fourth edition. We have entitled it *Tuberculosis, Fourth Edition: The Essentials*. In our intention, most chapters are the updated versions of those in the third edition, while the remaining ones in that edition remain valid and constitute a source of additional knowledge for those who will approach the complex and fascinating field of tuberculosis starting with the "Essentials."

Mario C. Raviglione, MD

Contributors

Nicholas A. Be   Center for Tuberculosis Research, Division of Infectious Diseases, Department of Medicine, Johns Hopkins University School of Medicine, Baltimore, Maryland, U.S.A.

William R. Bishai   Center for Tuberculosis Research, Division of Infectious Diseases, Department of Medicine, Johns Hopkins University School of Medicine, Baltimore, Maryland, U.S.A.

Léopold Blanc   Stop TB Department, World Health Organization, Geneva, Switzerland

Antonino Catanzaro   University of California, San Diego, School of Medicine, San Diego, California, U.S.A.

Christopher Dye   Stop TB Department, World Health Organization, Geneva, Switzerland

Haileyesus Getahun   Stop TB Department, World Health Organization, Geneva, Switzerland

Ann Ginsberg   Global Alliance for TB Drug Development, New York, New York, U.S.A.

Enrico Girardi   Clinical Epidemiology Unit, National Institute for Infectious Diseases "L. Spallanzani," Rome, Italy

Philippe Glaziou   Stop TB Department, World Health Organization, Geneva, Switzerland

Ruth Griffin   CMMI, Department of Infectious Diseases and Microbiology, Imperial College London, London, U.K.

Anthony D. Harries   International Union against Tuberculosis and Lung Disease, Paris, France, and London School of Hygiene and Tropical Medicine, London, U.K.

Philip C. Hopewell   Division of Pulmonary and Critical Care Medicine, San Francisco General Hospital, Francis J. Curry National Tuberculosis Center, Department of Medicine, University of California, San Francisco, California, U.S.A.

Sanjay K. Jain   Center for Tuberculosis Research, Division of Infectious Diseases, Department of Medicine, Johns Hopkins University School of Medicine; Department of Pediatrics, Division of Pediatric Infectious Diseases, Johns Hopkins University School of Medicine, Baltimore, Maryland, U.S.A.

Ernesto Jaramillo   Stop TB Department, World Health Organization, Geneva, Switzerland

Michael E. Kimerling   The Bill and Melinda Gates Foundation, Seattle, Washington, U.S.A.

Knut Lönnroth   Stop TB Department, World Health Organization, Geneva, Switzerland

Phung K. Lam   University of California, San Diego, School of Medicine, San Diego, California, U.S.A.

Kitty Lambregts-Van Weezenbeek   KNCV Tuberculosis Foundation, The Hague, The Netherlands

Megan Murray   Harvard School of Public Health and Brigham and Women's Hospital, Boston, Massachusetts, U.S.A.

Paul P. Nunn   Stop TB Department, World Health Organization, Geneva, Switzerland

Richard J. O'Brien   Foundation for Innovative New Diagnostics (FIND), Geneva, Switzerland

Salah Ottmani   Stop TB Department, World Health Organization, Geneva, Switzerland

Mark D. Perkins   Foundation for Innovative New Diagnostics (FIND), Geneva, Switzerland

Sharon Perry   Stanford University School of Medicine, Division of Geographic Medicine and Infectious Diseases, Stanford, California, U.S.A.

Mario C. Raviglione   Stop TB Department, World Health Organization, Geneva, Switzerland

Alasdair Reid   Joint United Nations Programme on HIV/AIDS (UNAIDS), Geneva, Switzerland

Michael L. Rich   Partners In Health and Brigham and Women's Hospital, Division of Global Health Equity, Boston, Massachusetts, U.S.A.

Kwonjune Seung   Partners In Health and Brigham and Women's Hospital, Division of Global Health Equity, Boston, Massachusetts, U.S.A.

Melvin Spigelman   Global Alliance for TB Drug Development, New York, New York, U.S.A.

Jelle Thole   TuBerculosis Vaccine Initiative, Lelystad, The Netherlands

Mukund Uplekar   Stop TB Department, World Health Organization, Geneva, Switzerland

Diana Weil   Stop TB Department, World Health Organization, Geneva, Switzerland

Abigail Wright   Stop TB Department, World Health Organization, Geneva, Switzerland

Douglas Young   CMMI, Department of Infectious Diseases and Microbiology, Imperial College London, London, U.K.

Matteo Zignol   Stop TB Department, World Health Organization, Geneva, Switzerland

Contents

1

The Global Tuberculosis Epidemic: Scale, Dynamics, and Prospects for Control

CHRISTOPHER DYE and PHILIPPE GLAZIOU

Stop TB Department, World Health Organization, Geneva, Switzerland

I. Introduction

Drugs that can cure most tuberculosis (TB) patients have been available since the 1950s, yet TB remains the world's most important cause of death from an infectious agent, besides the human immunodeficiency virus (HIV) with which it is intimately linked (1). TB control is high on the international public health agenda, not just because of the enormous burden of the disease, but also because short-course chemotherapy is recognized to be among the most cost-effective of all health interventions (2,3). The evidence from studies of the burden on health and cost-effectiveness have been central to promotion of the World Health Organization's DOTS strategy, and the enhanced Stop TB Strategy, which combine best practices in the diagnosis and treatment of patients with active TB (4–6).

Against that background, we describe the scale and direction of the TB epidemic, the documented and potential impact of DOTS and the Stop TB Strategy and, finally, offer some insights into how TB could be eliminated during the 21st century.

II. Global and Regional Tuberculosis Epidemics: Scale and Dynamics

A. Methods to Estimate Tuberculosis Incidence, Prevalence, and Mortality

The quality of epidemiological evaluation rests on the methods used to collect and analyze TB data. The number of new TB cases arising per capita each year (incidence) is the central measure of progress toward elimination, which is the principal long-term goal of TB control (Table 1) (7). Incidence is also the overarching indicator of Millennium Development Goal 6, target 8 (7,8), and incidence estimates (for sputum smear–positive cases) form the denominator of the WHO "case detection rate," with notified cases as the numerator (9).

Because TB is a rare disease (usually measured as cases per 100,000 population), it is not practically feasible to measure incidence by counting cases arising in cohorts under continuous observation. A better alternative is to improve routine surveillance so that case reports are more or less complete as, for example, in the Netherlands, the United Kingdom, and the United States of America, where there is a long tradition of reporting TB morbidity and mortality (10,11). In most countries with a relatively high incidence of TB, surveillance is far from complete, as reflected in estimates of case detection (section V).

Table 1   Goals, Target, and Indicators for Tuberculosis Control

---

Millennium Development Goal 6

Combat HIV/AIDS, malaria, and other diseases

Target 8: To have halted by 2015 and begun to reverse the incidence of malaria and other major diseases

Indicator 23: Prevalence and death rates associated with TB

Indicator 24: Proportion of TB cases detected and cured under DOTS (the basis of the WHO recommended Stop TB Strategy)

Stop TB Partnership targets

By 2005: At least 70% of people with sputum smear–positive TB will be diagnosed, and at least 85% cured. These are targets set by the World Health Assembly of WHO.

By 2015: TB prevalence and death rates will be cut by 50% relative to 1990 levels. This means reducing prevalence to approximately 150 per 100,000 or lower and deaths to approximately 15 per 100,000 per year or lower by 2015, including TB cases coinfected with HIV. The number of people dying from TB in 2015 would be less than approximately one million, including those coinfected with HIV.

By 2050: TB will be "eliminated," i.e., global incidence will be less than one case per million population per year.

Abbreviations: TB, tuberculosis; AIDS, acquired immune deficiency syndrome; HIV, human immunodeficiency virus; WHO, World Health Organization.
Source: From Ref. 7.

Clearly, low case detection partly explains why incidence is still high: no diagnosis or late diagnosis allows persistent transmission.

Unlike incidence, TB prevalence can be measured in a single population-based survey (12,13). The drawback of such surveys is that they are costly and laborious, mainly because there are usually few cases of active TB in a community at any one time (typically between 0.1% and 1% in countries regarded as highly endemic). Since 2000, however, national surveys have successfully been carried out in Cambodia (14), China (15), Eritrea (16), and Indonesia (17), and more are planned.

TB is ranked among the top 10 causes of death worldwide (1), and most of the burden of TB, measured in terms of disability-adjusted life years (DALYs, the common currency of morbidity and mortality), is due to premature deaths of young adults. TB deaths are not comprehensively reported in the majority of highly endemic countries, especially in Africa and Asia, because these countries do not yet have reliable death registration systems (18). Verbal autopsy, which has been used in surveys that investigate all causes of death, is an alternative, interim method of evaluating TB mortality, but needs further validation. Deaths are counted in cohorts of patients treated under the Stop TB Strategy, but these cohorts do not usually include the majority of TB patients in any country, and a variable proportion of patients are lost through default and transfer between health centers (10). Indirect estimates of mortality can easily be calculated from the product of incidence and case fatality rates, but these depend on accurate measures of both quantities.

Although the prevalence of *Mycobacterium tuberculosis* infection, and the annual risk of infection derived from it, are not direct measures of disease burden, tuberculin skin-test (TST) surveys have long been used to measure both (19–23). There are numerous practical difficulties in the application of TST, concerning both the measurement of infection and its interpretation with respect to transmission and disease incidence (24–27). Although several new assays (interferon gamma release assays) for *M. tuberculosis* infection have recently been devised (28–30), TST is still the only practical method of evaluating infection in large populations. The main problem with TST is its low specificity (false positives are common); for this reason the test is best used comparatively, to evaluate geographical and temporal variation in risk of infection (11,31).

B. Tuberculosis Burden and Trends

Based on data gathered and analyzed by the methods described above, there were an estimated 9.3 million new cases of TB in 2007, of which 5.6 million were reported to public health authorities and WHO (4). Approximately 4.1 million cases were sputum smear–positive, the most infectious form of the disease. The WHO African region has the highest estimated incidence rate (363 per 100,000 population per year), but the majority of TB patients live in the most populous countries of Asia: Bangladesh, China, India, Indonesia, and Pakistan together account for roughly half the new cases arising each year (Fig. 1). About 80% of new cases arising each year live in the 22 top-ranking ("high-burden") countries.

In 2007, countries reported 1.7 million sputum-smear TB cases among men, but only 904,000 among women. In some instances, women have poorer access to diagnosis and treatment (32), but the broader pattern also reflects real epidemiological differences between the sexes. Although there is some evidence that young adult women (15–44 years) are more likely than men to develop active TB following infection (23), this effect is typically outweighed by the much higher exposure and infection rates among adult men (33,34).

The estimate of 9.3 million new TB cases in 2007 is an increase of 40% on 6.6 million in 1990, the MDG reference year. The growth rate of the epidemic slowed from the mid 1990s onward so that, between 2006 and 2007, the total number of cases increased by 0.4% but the incidence per capita fell by 0.8%. The global increase during the 1990s was attributable mainly to the proliferation of cases in countries of Eastern Europe (mainly the former Soviet Union) and in sub-Saharan Africa. Trends in case reports suggest that the incidence per capita in both regions was stable or in slow decline by 2007 (4). Annual case reports also indicate that incidence rates have been steady or falling for at least two decades in the Southeast Asia and Western Pacific Regions, and in Western and Central Europe, North and Latin America, and the Middle East (Fig. 2).

The resurgence of TB in Eastern European countries (mainly the former Soviet republics) can be explained by economic decline and the failure of TB control and other health services since 1991 (35,36). Based on periodic surveys, around 10% or more of new TB cases in the Baltic states of Estonia, Latvia, and Lithuania, and some parts of Russia are multidrug resistant (MDR-TB), that is, resistant to at least isoniazid and rifampicin, the two most effective antituberculosis drugs (37). Drug resistance is likely to be a by-product of the events that led to TB resurgence in these countries, not the primary cause of it, but is clearly now a major impediment to control in that region. While parts of Eastern Europe are clearly hotspots for drug resistance, reporting a high prevalence of MDR among TB cases (estimated 18–22% of all TB, or 80,000 cases in 2006), MDR cases are more numerous in the heavily populated Southeast Asia (150,000 cases) and

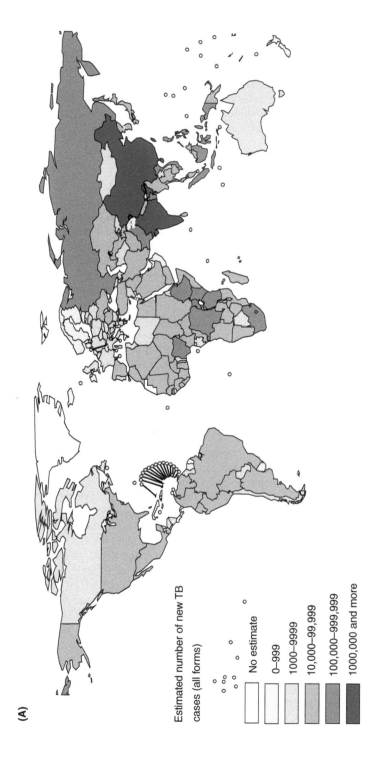

(A)

Estimated number of new TB
cases (all forms)

No estimate

0–999

1000–9999

10,000–99,999

100,000–999,999

1000,000 and more

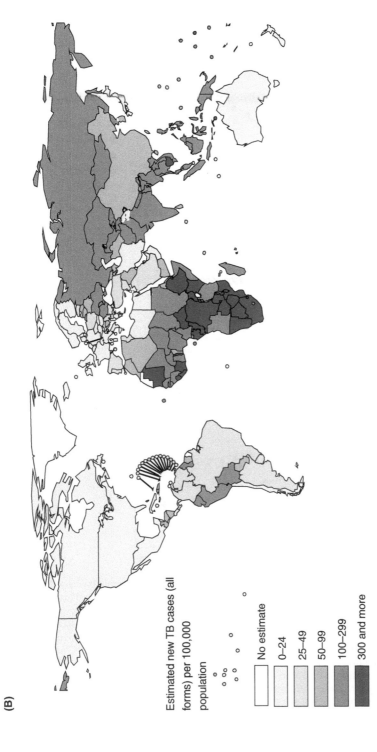

Figure 1 Distribution of tuberculosis (TB) in the world in 2007. Maps show (**A**) the estimated numbers of new TB cases (all forms) by country and (**B**) the incidence per 100,000 population. *Source:* From Ref. 10.

(A)

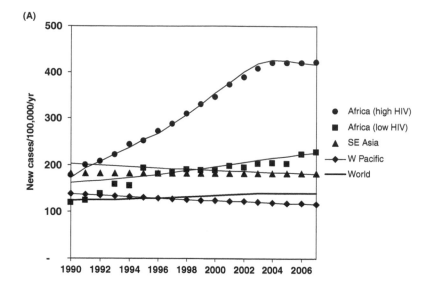

(B)

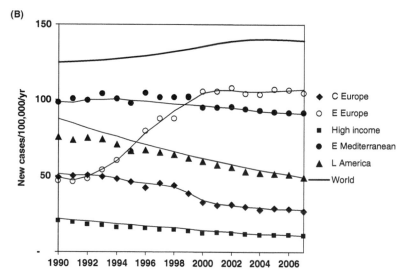

Figure 2 Trajectories of the tuberculosis epidemic for nine epidemiologically different regions of the world. Points mark trends in incidence rates, derived from case notifications for 1990 to 2007. The two panels separate regions with estimated incidence rates (**A**) above or (**B**) below the global average in 1990 (heavy line). Groupings of countries are based on the WHO regions of Africa (subdivided into two regions comprising those countries with high HIV-infection rates, more than or equal to 4% of patients (all ages), in 2007, and those with low rates of HIV infection, less then 4%), Central Europe, Eastern Europe (former Soviet countries plus Bulgaria and Romania), Eastern Mediterranean, Established Market Economies (all 30 OECD countries, except Mexico, Slovakia, and Turkey, plus Singapore), Latin America, Southeast Asia, and Western Pacific. The countries in each region are listed in full elsewhere (10).

Western Pacific Regions (153,000 cases). Globally, 3% to 4% of new TB cases were estimated to be MDR in 2006, while the prevalence among previously treated cases was much higher, at 18% to 21% (37). Exacerbating the problem of resistance, 50 countries that use second-line TB drugs had reported extensively drug resistant strains by 2008; these are refractory, not only to isoniazid and rifampicin (MDR), but also to one or more fluoroquinolones (such as ciprofloxacin, levofloxacin, moxifloxacin, and ofloxacin) and to one or more injectables (the polypeptide capreomycin, or the aminoglycosides kanamycin and amikacin).

Among the 2.7 million additional cases arising in 2007, as compared with 1990, 2 million were living in the WHO African Region. This increase in Africa is attributable principally to the spread of HIV infection (10,38). Globally, an estimated 12% of new tuberculosis cases were infected with HIV in 2007, but there was marked variation among regions—from 33% in the African Region to 1.4% in the Western Pacific Region. HIV infection rates in TB patients have so far remained below 1% in Bangladesh, China, and Pakistan. Across Africa, the rise in the number of TB cases is slowing (though this may not be true in every country), probably because HIV infection rates are also beginning to stabilize or fall (39), although some national TB surveillance systems may have been overloaded by patients. With limited access to antiretroviral therapy (ART), HIV has probably had a smaller effect on TB prevalence than on incidence because the duration of TB among HIV-infected patients is relatively short: for people with advanced HIV infection, the progression to severe tuberculosis is rapid, with a marked reduction in life expectancy (40). In places where HIV infection rates are high in the general population, they are even higher among TB patients; estimates for 2007 exceeded 50% in Botswana, Malawi, South Africa, Zambia, and Zimbabwe, among other countries.

An estimated 1.7 million people died of tuberculosis in 2007, including 381,000 patients who were coinfected with HIV (10). Although mortality trends have not been measured directly in most countries, mathematical modeling suggests that the global TB mortality rate per capita began to fall around year 2000, three to four years before the fall in per capita incidence (10,41).

III. Tuberculosis Control

There are essentially three ways to control TB: prevent infection, stop progression from infection to active disease, and treat active disease. In principle, infection can be prevented by treating or isolating patients with active infectious disease, or by vaccination. The recent expansion of TB control in some areas of high HIV prevalence has exposed a neglect of the basic principles of infection control, where immunosuppressed patients have been exposed to patients with active TB in clinics and hospitals (42,43).

Regarding vaccination, roughly 100 million infants (more than 80% of the annual cohort) are vaccinated each year with bacille Calmette–Guérin (BCG), and the effect of this vaccine is mainly to prevent serious forms of disease in children—meningitis and miliary TB. The most complete analysis of effectiveness to date suggests that BCG given to children worldwide in 2002 prevented approximately 30,000 cases of childhood meningitis and about 11,500 cases of miliary TB during their first five years, or one case for every 3400 and 9300 vaccinations, respectively (44). The protective efficacy against pulmonary tuberculosis in adults is highly variable, and often very low (45). BCG is cheap and cost-effective, but far from being the ideal vaccine.

To stop the progression from latent to active TB, individuals at high risk of TB who have a positive TST but not active disease (e.g., associates of active cases, especially children, and immigrants to low-incidence countries) can be offered preventive therapy, most commonly with the relatively safe and inexpensive drug, isoniazid [isoniazid preventive therapy (IPT)]. Randomized, controlled, clinical trials have shown that 12 months of daily isoniazid gives 25% to 92% protection against developing active TB, but toward the upper end of this range when patients adhere fully to the treatment regimen (46,47). However, IPT is not widely used, mainly because compliance with long-term daily treatment is generally poor among healthy people. A relatively high risk of TB among people carrying latent infections is usually still a low risk in absolute terms. Isoniazid is a relatively safe drug, but hepatitis arises as a side effect of IPT in around 1% of patients. The exceptionally high risk of TB among people coinfected with *M. tuberculosis* and HIV is a reason for encouraging wider use of IPT, especially in Africa (48–51).

Among the control methods that are possible with current technology, only BCG vaccination and the treatment of active TB have so far been implemented on a large scale. Because drug treatment is the dominant form of TB control worldwide, section IV gives an overview of the efficacy, historical effectiveness, and goals of combination chemotherapy, and section V describes its implementation from the 1990s onward as DOTS and the Stop TB Strategy.

IV. Combination Chemotherapy, DOTS, and the Stop TB Strategy

The treatment of patients with active TB is central to DOTS strategy, and to the more comprehensive Stop TB Strategy. Apart from standardized, combination drug therapy, DOTS also requires bacteriological diagnosis, patient supervision and support, and a monitoring and evaluation system to assess implementation and epidemiological impact. The broader Stop TB Strategy explicitly addresses the problems of TB/HIV and MDR-TB, describes how TB control can engage all care providers and contribute to health-system strengthening, how to empower people and communities with TB, and promotes research (5).

Combination chemotherapy for patients carrying drug-susceptible strains of *M. tuberculosis*, when carried out to the highest standards, gives cure rates of 95% or more with a low risk of relapse (52) and can delay the spread of resistance, perhaps for decades. At case detection rates of at least 70% and cure rates of 85% or more, and in the absence of HIV infection, TB incidence per capita rate should fall at around 5% to 10% per year, and TB prevalence and mortality more quickly (53–55).

The known efficacy of treatment and the practicalities of case finding have led to the internationally agreed targets for TB control, framed in terms of the treatment of active TB and embraced by the Millennium Development Goals. These are to detect 70% of sputum smear–positive cases and successfully treat 85% of such cases. As a result, TB incidence per capita should be falling by 2015, and prevalence and mortality rates should be halved in comparison with 1990 levels (Table 1) (7).

These predictions hold for both drug-resistant and drug-susceptible TB; the distinct challenge in treating drug-resistant strains is in achieving high cure rates. These expectations do not, however, allow for the complications associated with HIV coinfection and drug resistance. For example, the impact of treatment will be less than that suggested above when HIV is spreading through a population (56,57). Nor do the anticipated reductions in TB incidence account for changes in risk due to factors such as air pollution (58,59), tobacco smoke (59–62), diabetes (63–65), malnutrition and undernutrition (66,67), and alcohol misuse (68).

The best results in the control of endemic TB have been achieved in native communities (Inuit and others) of Alaska, Canada, and Greenland, where the incidence per capita was reduced by 13% to 18% annually from the early 1950s (21). This decline was probably caused mainly by the treatment of active disease, though the effect was enhanced by IPT. Over a much wider area in Western Europe, TB declined at 7% to 10% per year after drugs became available during the 1950s, though the incidence rate was already falling at 4% to 5% per year before chemotherapy.

In principle, TB incidence could be forced down more quickly than seen in Europe and North America, by as much as 30% per year, if new cases could be found soon enough to eliminate transmission (69). In general, the decline is faster when a larger fraction of cases arises from recent infection (i.e., in areas where transmission rates have recently been high) and slower where there is a large backlog of asymptomatic (latent) infection, and where rates of reactivation are higher among latently infected people. These facts explain why it should be easier to control epidemic than endemic disease: during an outbreak in an area that previously had little TB, the reservoir of latent infection is small, and most new cases come from recent infection. Aggressive intervention during an outbreak of MDR-TB in New York City, where most cases were probably due to recent transmission, cut the number of MDR-TB cases by over 40% per year (70,71).

The long-term aim of TB control is to eliminate new cases, but cutting prevalence and death rates is arguably more important in the short-term. About 90% of the burden of TB, as measured in terms of DALYs lost, is due to premature death rather than illness (1), and prevalence and mortality can be reduced faster than incidence in chemotherapy programs. For example, the TB death rate among the Alaskan Inuit population dropped by an average of 30% per year in the period 1950 to 1970 (72).

V. Implementation and Impact of DOTS and the Stop TB Strategy

A. Case Detection

More than 37 million TB patients were diagnosed and treated in DOTS programs between 1994 and 2007. Despite this mounting total, only 62% of all estimated new smear-positive cases were reported by DOTS programs to WHO in 2007, with much variation between regions of the world [Fig. 3(A)]. The case detection rate in DOTS programs has been accelerating globally. The recent improvement in case finding has been due mostly to rapid implementation in India, where detection increased from 1.6% in 1998 to 68% in 2007, and in China, where detection increased from 30% in 2002 to 79% in 2007. In 2007, almost all (98%) TB cases reported to WHO were reported by DOTS programs.

B. Treatment Success

Many of the 178 national DOTS programs in existence by the end of 2007 have shown that they can treat a high proportion of patients successfully. The average treatment success among 2.5 million smear-positive patients in the 2006 DOTS cohort was very nearly 85%, close to achieving the international target (Fig. 4). Concealed by this high proportion of successful treatments are poorer results in Africa, Eastern Europe, and in the established

(A)

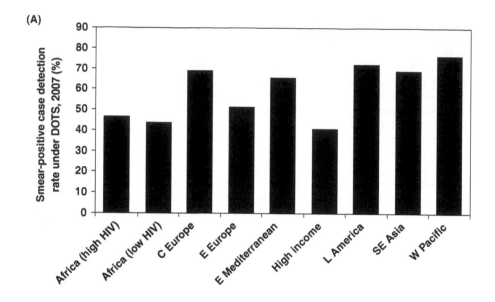

(B)

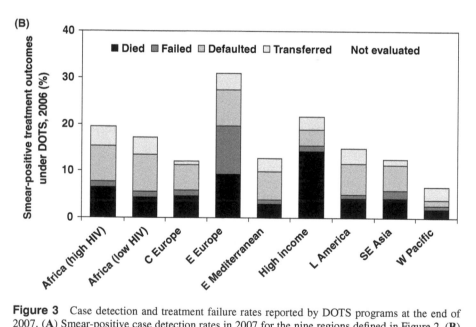

Figure 3 Case detection and treatment failure rates reported by DOTS programs at the end of 2007. (**A**) Smear-positive case detection rates in 2007 for the nine regions defined in Figure 2. (**B**) Adverse outcomes of treatment in the 2006 DOTS cohort, for each of the nine regions defined in Figure 2. *Source*: From Ref. 10.

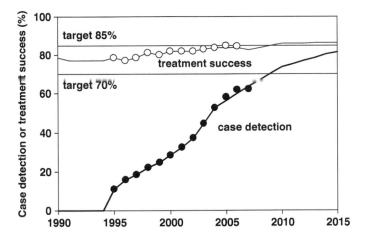

Figure 4 Progress toward the targets of 70% smear-positive case detection by DOTS programs (filled points, heavy lines) and 85% treatment success (open points, light lines). Points show the measured progress in smear-positive case detection from 1995 to 2007 and treatment success for the 1994 to 2006 cohorts. Lines project changes to 2015, as proposed in the Global Plan to Stop TB.

market economies (Fig. 3). In the African countries most affected by HIV [Africa (high HIV], 6.2% of patients died during treatment, and 18.4% were lost to follow-up (defaulted, transferred to other treatment centers, or not evaluated). In the high-income countries, the death rate was higher than in any other region (14.2%), because a large proportion of patients are elderly. In Eastern Europe, where rates of drug resistance are relatively high, 10.4% of patients failed to respond to treatment and 9.2% died during treatment.

C. Incidence, Prevalence, and Mortality

Although the decline in TB has almost certainly been accelerated by good chemotherapy programs since the 1950s (section IV), there have been few recent, unequivocal demonstrations of impact in high-burden countries. Three examples come, with qualifications, from Morocco, Peru, and Vietnam. Between 1996 and 2005, the incidence of pulmonary TB among Moroccan children up to four years of age fell by more than 8% per year, suggesting that the risk of infection was falling at least as quickly (73). This is consistent with the observation that the average age of TB cases has been rising for over 20 years in Morocco. And yet the overall reduction in pulmonary TB per capita has been only 3% to 4% per year. While the reason for the slow decline in Morocco is not fully understood, it is clear that TB incidence (case numbers and rates) is higher in urban than in rural areas and higher in adult men than in women. TB incidence has been falling more slowly than average among men, but the decline has also been unexpectedly slow among women. DOTS was launched in Peru in 1991, and high rates of case detection and cure pushed down the per capita incidence of pulmonary TB by 6% per year from 1992 to 2000 (74). Vietnam apparently exceeded the targets for case detection and treatment success since 1997, and yet the case notification rate remained approximately stable over that period (31). Closer inspection of surveillance data shows that, while case notification rates have

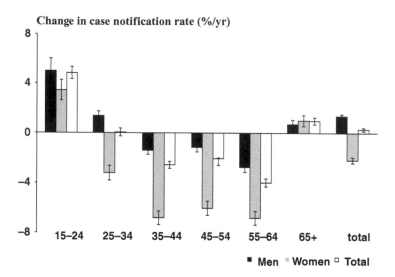

Change in case notification rate (%/yr)

■ Men ▨ Women ▢ Total

Figure 5 Average annual change in TB case notification rates for men (black), women (gray) and both together (white) in different age classes in Vietnam, 1997 to 2004. Error bars are 95% confidence limits. *Source*: Data From Ref. 75.

been falling among adults aged 35 to 64 years (especially women), they are increasing among 15- to 24-year-olds (especially men; Fig. 5) (75). These increases and decreases in different age groups, and for men and women, are almost equal in magnitude.

Indirect assessments of the effect of DOTS suggest that 70% of the TB deaths expected in the absence of DOTS were averted in Peru between 1991 and 2000, and more than half the TB deaths expected in the absence of DOTS are prevented each year in DOTS-served provinces of China (74,76). There have been few direct measures of the reduction in TB prevalence over time, but surveys done in China in 1990 and 2000 showed a 32% (95% confidence limits, 9–51%) reduction in the prevalence per capita of all forms of TB in DOTS areas, as compared with the change in the prevalence in other parts of the country (15). The findings of a 2004 national survey in Indonesia indicate that the per capita prevalence of smear-positive TB was threefold lower than in surveys carried out around 1979 and 1982 (17). But not all of this reduction can be attributed to the DOTS program, or even to the direct effects of chemotherapy.

VI. The Future of Tuberculosis Control

A. The Global Plan to Stop TB, 2006–2015

To generate greater momentum and TB control, and to align research, development, and implementation, the Global Plan to Stop TB was launched in 2006 (77). The Global Plan is the blueprint for implementation of the Stop TB Strategy, which should meet the Millennium Development Goals for TB by 2015. The Plan also lays out the process and budget needed to develop the new diagnostics, drugs, and vaccines required to eliminate TB by mid-century.

The Global Plan proposes that 50 million patients would be treated between 2006 and 2015. Mathematical modelling suggests that the impact will be sufficient to satisfy MDG target 8 "to have halted and begun to reverse incidence," globally and in each of the seven regions. The annual incidence of new cases per capita is already in decline, and the total number of new cases is expected to fall well before 2015. Ambitious plans for TB control in the Southeast Asia and Western Pacific regions are reflected in the relatively rapid declines in incidence per capita expected by 2015 (7–9% per year). Even with these rates of decline in Asia, TB incidence would still exceed 10 per 100,000 globally in 2050, which is 100 times greater than the target for TB elimination (<1 case per million population).

The targets of halving prevalence and death rates between 1990 and 2015 are more challenging. Projections suggest that these targets can be met globally with full implementation of the Global Plan, but not in Africa or Eastern Europe [Fig. 6(A)]. Based on the calculated rate of decline in mortality from 2006 to 2015 in the African countries most affected by HIV [Africa (high HIV)], the target death rate would not be reached before 2025.

In Eastern Europe, but not in Africa, prevalence rates are also expected to remain high compared with 1990 levels. In Eastern Europe, a relatively high proportion of patients have chronic TB, which is commonly MDR. In Africa, patients who are infected with HIV do not suffer from TB for long; their illness typically progresses quickly, and they either are cured or die. This bleak outlook for TB control in Africa and Eastern Europe arises in large part from the choice of 1990 as the MDG reference year. In that year, TB incidence rates in these two regions were close to their lowest levels for at least half a century, and most of the recent rise in incidence happened during the 1990s. The same projections also show that, over the 10 years from 2006 to 2015, the impact of the enhanced DOTS strategy, assuming full implementation, would be almost as great in Africa and Eastern Europe as in other regions of the world: a reasonable goal in all regions would be to halve prevalence and death rates between 2005 and 2015 [Fig. 6(B)].

The incidence of MDR-TB cases has fallen faster than the incidence of all TB in Hong Kong, Republic of Korea, and Mexico, but it is not yet known whether treatment with second-line drugs can disproportionately reduce MDR-TB deaths on a large scale (78).

B. New Methods of Control and the Prospects for TB Elimination

This discussion of the Stop TB Strategy has focused on the chemotherapy of active disease because drug treatment is likely to remain the principal method of TB control for the next decade or longer. In the longer term, TB elimination might be achieved through a combination of measures to prevent infection, to stop progression from infection to active disease, and to treat active disease. Multimillion dollar initiatives, operating under the umbrella of the Stop TB Partnership, were launched around the turn of the millennium to develop better diagnostics, drugs, and vaccines (77). An examination of the principles of TB elimination shows how the products of this new research could radically change the approach to TB control (79–81).

To eliminate TB by 2050 (outside sub-Saharan Africa), the incidence rate must fall at an average of 16% annually from 2007 onward. This rate of decline might be achieved for a few years, but is unlikely to be sustainable. The reason is that when transmission

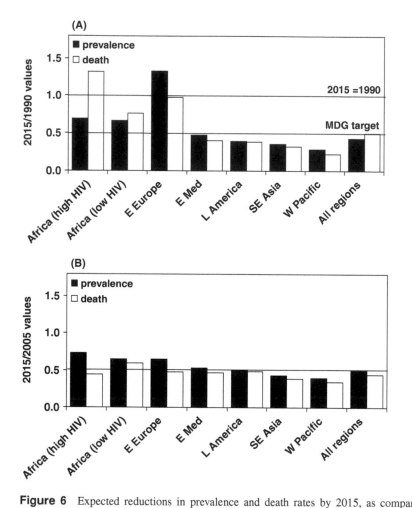

Figure 6 Expected reductions in prevalence and death rates by 2015, as compared with the estimated rates in (**A**) Millennium Development Goals baseline year 1990 or (**B**) with the rates in 2005. Although targets for halving prevalence and death rates between 1990 and 2015 (bars <0.5) are unlikely to be reached in Africa and Eastern Europe (**A**), the impact of the Global Plan to Stop TB (2006–2015) is not expected to be much less in these two regions during the period 2006 to 2015 (**B**).

and incidence fall, a growing proportion of cases arise from the slow reactivation of long-standing latent infections, rather than from the rapid progression of recent infections. The initial rate of decline in incidence is controlled by primary progression, but the long-term rate of decline is governed by reactivation.

Combinations of interventions can, in principle, push TB closer to elimination, but some combinations are more effective than others. Beginning with an incidence of approximately 1000 per million in 2007 (similar to the Southeast Asia Region), Figure 7(A) shows the expected incidence in 2050 when preexposure vaccination (to prevent infection) is combined, at various levels of coverage, with the treatment of patients with active TB. The effects of the two approaches are similar when used alone: the two curved edges of the surface running from the back corner decline to approximately 10 cases per million in 2050. Intensifying either control method yields sharply diminishing returns. The two methods are more effective in combination, but the additional impact is small; that is, the surface in Figure 7(A) is flat for most combinations of vaccination and treatment. This is because drug treatment to stop transmission at source has effects that are similar to vaccination, which protects those who are exposed to infection. One intervention partly substitutes for the other; they act neither independently nor synergistically. Therefore, a preexposure vaccine will be most useful in addition to treatment when the detection rate of active TB cases is low, and vice versa.

The effect of two interventions in combination will be greater if each attacks a different etiological pathway. One intervention should stop the fast route to active TB (infection and progressive primary disease) and the other should prevent the reactivation of latent infection. The treatment of latent TB, either by preventive drug therapy or postexposure vaccination, is relatively ineffective when used alone [approximately 100 cases per million in 2050; Fig. 7(B) and 7(C)], but powerful in combination with the treatment of active TB [Fig. 7(B) and 7(D)] or with preexposure vaccination [Fig. 7(C)]. When these combined approaches are implemented intensively, TB incidence can be forced close to or below the elimination threshold by 2050. In the examples shown in Figures 7(B) and (C), incidence is reduced to 0.14 per million by 2050, about seven times lower than expected if effects were independent. The proportional effect on TB mortality is still greater [cf Figs. 7(B) and (D)].

VII. Conclusion

The total number of TB cases in the world increased during the 1990s for two main reasons: the spread of HIV/AIDS in sub-Saharan Africa and the collapse of the Soviet Union. TB incidence in sub-Saharan Africa appears to have stabilized or begun to fall, mainly because HIV incidence started to fall prior to year 2000. Annual case reports from countries of the former Soviet Union indicate that incidence has stabilized, or began falling again, in that region too. In other regions of the world, most importantly in Asia where the majority of new TB patients are found each year, TB continued to decline throughout the 1990s, albeit slowly. In aggregate, the number of new TB cases per capita arising each year was, according to best estimates, falling slowly in 2007, while the number of deaths began falling sooner. The central challenge in TB control today is to accelerate the slow decline in incidence that is seen in most high-burden countries.

These epidemiological trends have undoubtedly been influenced by chemotherapy, which has existed in most countries in some form since the 1950s. But drug treatment delivered via DOTS and the Stop TB Strategy will have had a measurable impact only in countries that achieved high coverage by the mid-1990s. Although there is a great deal of circumstantial evidence that chemotherapy programs can drive TB incidence downwards, more direct, recent demonstrations of impact are restricted to a few countries such as Morocco (reduced infection), Peru (reduced incidence), Vietnam (reduced incidence in women aged 25–64 years) and China (reduced prevalence). There is also strong evidence—from Estonia, Hong Kong, and the United States of America—that the incidence of MDR-TB can be reduced where drug sensitivity testing is used to select

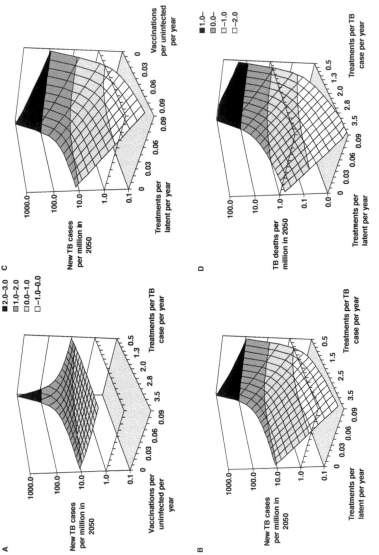

Figure 7 Pairwise combinations of three control methods to eliminate TB, starting from an annual incidence of approximately 1000 per million population in 2007. Surfaces show the expected incidence rates in 2050 with (**A**) preexposure vaccination and treatment of active TB, (**B**) treatment of latent infection and active TB, (**C**) treatment of latent infection and preexposure vaccination. (**D**), as for (**B**), but with TB death rate as the outcome. Shading in (**A**)–(**C**) indicates ranges of incidence rates per million population reached by 2050: <1 (white, below elimination threshold), <10 (light gray), <100 (dark gray), ≥ 100 (black). Because there are fewer TB deaths than cases, the grayscale in (**D**) is shifted by a factor of 10. *Source:* From Ref. 82.

effective combinations of first- and second-line drugs. Modelling studies suggest that chemotherapy programs are likely to be effective in populations with high rates of HIV infection, but the evidence remains equivocal. In short, DOTS and the Stop TB Strategy have had demonstrable effects in some countries, but have not yet become the dominant force in TB epidemiology worldwide (36).

To boost TB control, the Global Plan to Stop TB attempted to define what interventions would be needed, and at what rate they must be implemented, to ensure that incidence is falling by 2015, and to halve TB prevalence and death rates between 1990 and 2015. The fully implemented Plan will, according to calculations, bring down TB incidence long before 2015 (satisfying MDG target 8). It will also, by 2015, halve prevalence and death rates worldwide, and in all major endemic regions except Africa and Eastern Europe. It will not reduce incidence fast enough to reach the 2050 target for elimination (<1 case per million population).

The forecasting models used to make these predictions are strongly influenced by the experiences of Europe and North America since the 1950s, and may omit some important features of TB epidemiology that now apply in Asia, Africa, or the Americas. These include the changing risks associated with tobacco smoking, air pollution, diabetes and other nutritional disorders, aging populations, migration, and urban crowding.

Knowing that epidemiological forecasts are uncertain, much more effort must be given to measurement and evaluation. The effects of large-scale public health programs, such as DOTS, can never be assessed under experimental conditions, but periodic population-based surveys of the prevalence of active disease and infection will show trends, which will in some countries be attributable to TB control. TB deaths need to be counted more comprehensively and more accurately, either as a component of general cause-of-death surveys or through systems of routine death registration. The evidence from surveys of prevalence and mortality should be supplemented by fuller analyses of the vast body of surveillance data that is routinely collected by national control programs. One purpose of measurement is to evaluate the effects of the Stop TB Strategy; another is to quantify the counter-effects of diabetes, tobacco use, and other risk factors.

To do as much as planned by 2015, the Stop TB Strategy must push the basic DOTS package of care beyond the limits of public notification systems. This means forging better links between DOTS programs and other, nonparticipating public clinics and hospitals. It also means engaging medical services in prisons and the armed forces, private clinicians, nongovernmental organizations, mission hospitals, and clinics in the corporate sector (83–86). Continuing collaboration is needed with HIV/AIDS programs, to find a higher proportion of TB cases, and sooner, among HIV-positive people, to offer IPT to those who are eligible, to follow best practice in infection control, and to provide ART to HIV-positive patients with and without active TB (87–89). Beyond the specific problem of tuberculosis control, the Stop TB Strategy has a wider role in helping to expand and strengthen national health services (90,91).

To eliminate TB will require the successful development and deployment of at least some of the new tools described in the Global Plan. Improved TB diagnostics, both to shorten diagnostic delays for patients with active TB and perhaps to improve the feasibility of treating latent infection, are under active development, and some are reaching field application (80,92–96). The possibilities for preventive therapy may also increase with the development of shorter, safer regimens (97,98). New drugs for active TB could improve cure rates by reducing the duration of treatment to four months or less, by increasing treatment success among patients with MDR-TB, or by reducing the frequency of relapse among patients coinfected with HIV (99,100). There is no guarantee that a new vaccine will be available before 2015, or that it will have high efficacy against pulmonary TB (81,101,102). But if such a vaccine can be made, mass immunization could change the approach to TB control, shifting the emphasis from cure to prevention. Whatever the technological developments, they need to find field application urgently, not just to accelerate progress toward the MDGs, but to provide any hope that TB can be eliminated during the 21st century.

References

1. World Health Organization. The Global Burden Of Disease: 2004 Update. Geneva, Switzerland: World Health Organization, 2008.
2. Murray CJL, Dejonghe E, Chum HJ, et al. Cost-effectiveness of chemotherapy for pulmonary tuberculosis in 3 sub-Saharan African Countries. Lancet 1991; 338:1305–1308.
3. Dye C, Floyd K. Tuberculosis. In: Jamison DT, Alleyne GAO, Breman JG, et al., eds. Disease Control Priorities in Developing Countries, 2nd ed. Washington, DC: Oxford University Press, 2006:289–309.
4. World Health Organization. Global Tuberculosis Control 2009: Surveillance, Planning, Financing. Geneva, Switzerland: World Health Organization, 2009.
5. Raviglione MC, Uplekar MW. WHO's new Stop TB Strategy. Lancet 2006; 367:952–955.
6. World Health Organization. Implementing the WHO Stop TB Strategy: A Handbook for National Tuberculosis Programmes. Geneva, Switzerland: World Health Organization, 2008.
7. Dye C, Maher D, Weil D, et al. Targets for global tuberculosis control. Int J Tuberc Lung Dis 2006; 10:460–462.
8. United Nations Statistics Division. Millennium Indicators Database. 2007. Available at: mdgs.un.org/unsd/mdg/Default.aspx. Accessed December 10, 2008.
9. World Health Organization. Global Tuberculosis Control: Surveillance, Planning, Financing. Geneva, Switzerland: World Health Organization, 2007.
10. World Health Organization. Global Tuberculosis Control 2008: Surveillance, Planning, Financing. Geneva, Switzerland: World Health Organization, 2008.
11. Dye C, Bassili A, Bierrenbach AL, et al. Measuring tuberculosis burden, trends and the impact of control programmes [published online ahead of print January 16, 2008]. Lancet Infect Dis 2008; 8:233–243.
12. World Health Organization (17 authors). Assessing Tuberculosis Prevalence Through Population-Based Surveys. Manila, Philippines: World Health Organization, 2007.
13. Glaziou P, van der Werf MJ, Onozaki I, et al. Tuberculosis prevalence surveys: Rationale and cost. Int J Tuberc Lung Dis 2008; 12:1003–1008.
14. National Center for Tuberculosis and Leprosy Control. National tuberculosis prevalence survey, 2002, Cambodia. Phnom Penh, Cambodia: National Center for Tuberculosis and Leprosy Control, Ministry of Health, Royal Government of Cambodia, 2005.
15. China Tuberculosis Control Collaboration. The effect of tuberculosis control in China. Lancet 2004; 364:417–422.
16. Sebhatu M, Kiflom B, Seyoum M, et al. Determining the burden of tuberculosis in Eritrea: A new approach. Bull World Health Organ 2007; 85:593–599.
17. Soemantri S, Senewe FP, Tjandrarini DH, et al. Three-fold reduction in the prevalence of tuberculosis over 25 years in Indonesia. Int J Tuberc Lung Dis 2007; 11:398–404.
18. Korenromp EL, Bierrenbach AL, Williams BG, et al. The measurement and estimation of tuberculosis mortality. Int J Tuberc Lung Dis 2009; 13:283–303.

19. Odhiambo JA, Borgdorff MW, Kiambih FM, et al. Tuberculosis and the HIV epidemic: Increasing annual risk of tuberculous infection in Kenya, 1986–1996. Am J Public Health 1999; 89:1078–1082.

20. Egwaga SM, Cobelens FG, Muwinge H, et al. The impact of the HIV epidemic on tuberculosis transmission in Tanzania. AIDS 2006; 20:915–921.

21. Styblo K. Epidemiology of Tuberculosis, 2nd ed. The Hague, The Netherlands: KNCV Tuberculosis Foundation, 1991.

22. Cauthen GM, Pio A, ten Dam HG. Annual risk of tuberculous infection (reprinted). Bull World Health Organ 2002; 80:503–511.

23. Rieder HL. Epidemiologic Basis of Tuberculosis Control, 1st ed. Paris, France: International Union Against Tuberculosis and Lung Disease, 1999.

24. Rieder HL. Methodological issues in the estimation of the tuberculosis problem from tuberculin surveys. Tuber Lung Dis 1995; 76:114–121.

25. Rieder H. Annual risk of infection with *Mycobacterium tuberculosis*. Eur Respir J 2005; 25:181–185.

26. van Leth F, van der Werf MJ, Borgdorff MW. Prevalence of tuberculous infection and incidence of tuberculosis: A re-assessment of the Styblo rule. Bull World Health Organ 2008; 86:20–26.

27. Dye C. Breaking a law: Tuberculosis disobeys Styblo's rule. Bull World Health Organ 2008; 86:4.

28. Pai M, Zwerling A, Menzies D. Systematic review: T-cell-based assays for the diagnosis of latent tuberculosis infection: An update. Ann Intern Med 2008; 149:177–184.

29. Connell TG, Rangaka MX, Curtis N, et al. QuantiFERON-TB Gold: State of the art for the diagnosis of tuberculosis infection? Expert Rev Mol Diagn 2006; 6:663–677.

30. Bakir M, Dosanjh DPS, Deeks J, et al. Use of T cell-based diagnosis of tuberculosis infection to optimise interpretation of tuberculin skin testing in child tuberculosis contacts. Clin Infect Dis 2009; 48:302–312.

31. Huong NT, Duong BD, Co NV, et al. Tuberculosis epidemiology in six provinces of Vietnam after the introduction of the DOTS strategy. Int J Tuberc Lung Dis 2006; 10:963–969.

32. Hudelson P. Gender differentials in tuberculosis: The role of socio-economic and cultural factors. Tuber Lung Dis 1996; 77:391–400.

33. Borgdorff MW, Nagelkerke NJ, Dye C, et al. Gender and tuberculosis: A comparison of prevalence surveys with notification data to explore sex differences in case detection. Int J Tuberc Lung Dis 2000; 4:123–132.

34. Hamid Salim MA, Declercq E, Van Deun A, et al. Gender differences in tuberculosis: A prevalence survey done in Bangladesh. Int J Tuberc Lung Dis 2004; 8:952–957.

35. Shilova MV, Dye C. The resurgence of tuberculosis in Russia. Philos Trans R Soc Lond B Biol Sci 2001; 356:1069–1075.

36. Dye C, Lonnroth K, Jaramillo E, et al. Trends in tuberculosis and their determinants: An overview of 134 countries [published online ahead of print July 2009]. Bull World Health Organ.

37. World Health Organization. Anti-Tuberculosis Drug Resistance in the World. Fourth Global Report. Geneva, Switzerland: World Health Organization, 2008.

38. Corbett EL, Watt CJ, Walker N, et al. The growing burden of tuberculosis: Global trends and interactions with the HIV epidemic. Arch Intern Med 2003; 163:1009–1021.

39. UNAIDS, Joint United Nations Programme on HIV/AIDS. Report on the Global HIV/AIDS Epidemic 2008. Geneva; 2008.

40. Corbett EL, Charalambous S, Moloi VM, et al. Human immunodeficiency virus and the prevalence of undiagnosed tuberculosis in African gold miners. Am J Respir Crit Care Med 2004; 170:673–679.

41. Dye C, Watt CJ, Bleed DM, et al. Evolution of tuberculosis control and prospects for reducing tuberculosis incidence, prevalence, and deaths globally. J Am Med Assoc 2005; 293: 2767–2775.

42. Bock NN, Jensen PA, Miller B, et al. Tuberculosis infection control in resource-limited settings in the era of expanding HIV care and treatment. J Infect Dis 2007; 196(suppl 1): S108–S113.

43. World Health Organization. Tuberculosis Infection Control in the Era of Expanding Care and Treatment. Geneva, Switzerland: World Health Organization, 2007.

44. Trunz BB, Fine P, Dye C. Effect of BCG vaccination on childhood tuberculous meningitis and miliary tuberculosis worldwide: A meta-analysis and assessment of cost-effectiveness. Lancet 2006; 367:1173–1180.

45. Fanning A, FitzGerald JM. BCG vaccines: History, efficacy, and policies. In: Raviglione M, ed. Reichman and Hershfield's Tuberculosis: A Comprehensive International Approach, 3rd ed. New York: Informa Healthcare USA, Inc., 2006:541–554.

46. Cohn DL, El-Sadr WM. Treatment of latent tuberculosis infection. In: Raviglione MC, ed. Reichman and Hershfield's Tuberculosis: A Comprehensive International Approach. New York: Informa Healthcare USA, Inc., 2006:265–306.

47. Sterling TR. New approaches to the treatment of latent tuberculosis. Semin Respir Crit Care Med 2008; 29:532–541.

48. Woldehanna S, Volmink J. Treatment of latent tuberculosis infection in HIV infected persons. Cochrane Database Syst Rev 2004:CD000171.

49. World Health Organization. Interim Policy on Collaborative TB/HIV Activities. Geneva, Switzerland: World Health Organization, 2004.

50. Churchyard GJ, Scano F, Grant AD, et al. Tuberculosis preventive therapy in the era of HIV infection: Overview and research priorities. J Infect Dis 2007; 196:S52–S62.

51. Grant AD, Charalambous S, Fielding KL, et al. Effect of routine isoniazid preventive therapy on tuberculosis incidence among HIV-infected men in South Africa: A novel randomized incremental recruitment study. J Am Med Assoc 2005; 293:2719–2725.

52. Nunn AJ, Phillips PP, Gillespie SH. Design issues in pivotal drug trials for drug sensitive tuberculosis (TB). Tuberculosis (Edinb) 2008; 88(suppl 1):S85–S92.

53. Dye C, Garnett GP, Sleeman K, et al. Prospects for worldwide tuberculosis control under the WHO DOTS strategy. Directly observed short-course therapy. Lancet 1998; 352:1886–1891.

54. Borgdorff MW, Floyd K, Broekmans JF. Interventions to reduce tuberculosis mortality and transmission in low- and middle-income countries. Bull World Health Organ 2002; 80: 217–227.

55. Styblo K, Bumgarner JR. Tuberculosis Can Be Controlled with Existing Technologies: Evidence. Paris, France: Tuberculosis Surveillance Research Unit, International Union Against Tuberculosis and Lung Disease, 1991.

56. Currie CS, Williams BG, Cheng RC, et al. Tuberculosis epidemics driven by HIV: Is prevention better than cure? AIDS 2003; 17:2501–2508.

57. Williams BG, Granich R, Chauhan LS, et al. The impact of HIV/AIDS on the control of tuberculosis in India. Proc Natl Acad Sci U S A 2005; 102:9619–9624.

58. Baris E, Ezzati M. Should interventions to reduce respirable pollutants be linked to tuberculosis control programmes? BMJ 2004; 329:1090–1093.

59. Lin H, Ezzat M, Murray M. Tobacco smoke, indoor air pollution and tuberculosis: A systematic review and meta-analysis. PLoS Med 2007:e4.

60. Slama K, Chiang C-Y, Enarson DA, et al. Tobacco and tuberculosis: A qualitative systematic review and meta-analysis. Int J Tuberc Lung Dis 2007; 10:1049–1061.

61. Bates MN, Khalakdina A, Pai M, et al. Risk of tuberculosis from exposure to tobacco smoke: A systematic review and meta-analysis. Arch Intern Med 2007; 167:335–342.

62. Lin HH, Murray M, Cohen T, et al. Effects of smoking and solid-fuel use on COPD, lung cancer, and tuberculosis in China: A time-based, multiple risk factor, modelling study. Lancet 2008; 372:1473–1483.
63. Stevenson CR, Forouhi NG, Roglic G, et al. Diabetes and tuberculosis: The impact of the diabetes epidemic on tuberculosis incidence. BMC Public Health 2007; 7:234.
64. Stevenson CR, Critchley JA, Forouhi NGR, et al. Diabetes and the risk of tuberculosis: A neglected threat to public health? Chronic Illness 2007; 3:228–245.
65. Jeon CY, Murray MB. Diabetes mellitus increases the risk of active tuberculosis: A systematic review of 13 observational studies. PLoS Med 2008; 5:e152.
66. Cegielski JP, McMurray DN. The relationship between malnutrition and tuberculosis: Evidence from studies in humans and experimental animals. Int J Tuberc Lung Dis 2004; 8:286–298.
67. Lönnroth K, Williams BG, Dye C. A consistent log-linear relationship between tuberculosis incidence and body-mass index. Int J Epidemiol. In press.
68. Lonnroth K, Williams BG, Stadlin S, et al. Alcohol use as a risk factor for tuberculosis – a systematic review. BMC Public Health 2008; 8:289.
69. Dye C. Tuberculosis 2000–2010: Control, but not elimination. Int J Tuberc Lung Dis 2000; 4:S146–S152.
70. Frieden TR, Fujiwara PI, Washko RM, et al. Tuberculosis in New York City – turning the tide. N Engl J Med 1995; 333:229–233.
71. Paolo WF Jr, Nosanchuk JD. Tuberculosis in New York City: Recent lessons and a look ahead. Lancet Infect Dis 2004; 4:287–293.
72. Grzybowski S, Styblo K, Dorken E. Tuberculosis in Eskimos. Tubercle 1976; 57(suppl): S1–S58.
73. Dye C, Ottmani S, Laasri L, et al. The decline of tuberculosis epidemics under chemotherapy: A case study in Morocco. Int J Tuberc Lung Dis 2007; 11:1225–1231.
74. Suarez PG, Watt CJ, Alarcon E, et al. The dynamics of tuberculosis in response to 10 years of intensive control effort in Peru. J Infect Dis 2001; 184:473–478.
75. Vree M, Duong BD, Sy DN, et al. Tuberculosis trends, Vietnam. Emerg Infect Dis 2007; 13:332–333.
76. Dye C, Fengzeng Z, Scheele S, et al. Evaluating the impact of tuberculosis control: Number of deaths prevented by short-course chemotherapy in China. Int J Epidemiol 2000; 29: 558–564.
77. Stop TB Partnership and World Health Organization. The Global Plan to Stop TB, 2006–2015. Geneva, Switzerland: Stop TB Partnership, 2006. Report No.: WHO/HTM/STB/2006.35.
78. Dye C. Doomsday postponed? Preventing and reversing epidemics of drug-resistant tuberculosis. Nat Rev Microbiol 2009; 10:81–87.
79. Salomon JA, Lloyd-Smith JO, Getz WM, et al. Prospects for advancing tuberculosis control efforts through novel therapies. PLoS Med 2006; 3:e273.
80. Keeler E, Perkins M, Small PM, et al. Reducing the global burden of tuberculosis: The contribution of improved diagnosis. Nature 2006; 444(suppl 1):49–57.
81. Young DB, Dye C. The development and impact of tuberculosis vaccines. Cell 2006; 124: 683–687.
82. Dye C, Williams BG. Eliminating human tuberculosis in the 21st century. J R Soc Interface 2008; 5:653–662.
83. World Health Organization. Engaging all health care providers in TB control: Guidance on implementing public-private mix approaches. Geneva, Switzerland: World Health Organization, 2006.
84. Malmborg R, Mann G, Thomson R, et al. Can public-private collaboration promote tuberculosis case detection among the poor and vulnerable? Bull World Health Organ 2006; 84:752–758.

85. World Health Organization. Public-Private Mix for DOTS: Towards Scaling Up. Geneva, Switzerland: World Health Organization, 2005. Report No.: WHO/HTM/TB/2005.356.

86. Dewan PK, Lal SS, Lonnroth K, et al. Improving tuberculosis control through public-private collaboration in India: Literature review. BMJ 2006; 332:574–578.

87. Havlir DV, Getahun H, Sanne I, et al. Opportunities and challenges for HIV care in overlapping HIV and TB epidemics. J Am Med Assoc 2008; 300:423–430.

88. Granich RM, Gilks CF, Dye C, et al. Universal voluntary HIV testing with immediate antiretroviral therapy as a strategy for eliminating HIV transmission: A mathematical model [published online ahead of print November 26, 2008]. Lancet 2008; 373:48–57.

89. Williams BG, Dye C. Antiretroviral drugs for tuberculosis control in the era of HIV/AIDS. Science 2003; 301:1535–1537.

90. Atun RA, Lennox-Chhugani N, Drobniewski F, et al. A framework and toolkit for capturing the communicable disease programmes within health systems: Tuberculosis control as an illustrative example. Eur J Public Health 2004; 14:267–273.

91. World Health Organization. Stop TB Policy Paper: Contributing to health system strengthening. Guiding principles for national tuberculosis programmes. Geneva, Switzerland: World Health Organization, 2008.

92. Dinnes J, Deeks J, Kunst H, et al. A systematic review of rapid diagnostic tests for the detection of tuberculosis infection. Health Technol Assess 2007; 11:1–196.

93. Pai M, Dheda K, Cunningham J, et al. T-cell assays for the diagnosis of latent tuberculosis infection: Moving the research agenda forward. Lancet Infect Dis 2007; 7:428–438.

94. Grandjean L, Moore DA. Tuberculosis in the developing world: Recent advances in diagnosis with special consideration of extensively drug-resistant tuberculosis. Curr Opin Infect Dis 2008; 21:454–461.

95. Dosanjh DP, Hinks TS, Innes JA, et al. Improved diagnostic evaluation of suspected tuberculosis. Ann Intern Med 2008; 148:325–336.

96. Lalvani A. Diagnosing tuberculosis infection in the 21st century: New tools to tackle an old enemy. Chest 2007; 131:1898–1906.

97. Gao XF, Wang L, Liu GJ, et al. Rifampicin plus pyrazinamide versus isoniazid for treating latent tuberculosis infection: A meta-analysis. Int J Tuberc Lung Dis 2006; 10:1080–1090.

98. Menzies D, Long R, Trajman A, et al. Adverse events with 4 months of rifampin therapy or 9 months of isoniazid therapy for latent tuberculosis infection: A randomized trial. Ann Intern Med 2008; 149:689–697.

99. Spigelman MK. New tuberculosis therapeutics: A growing pipeline. J Infect Dis 2007; 196(suppl 1):S28–S34.

100. Global Alliance for TB Drug Development. TB Alliance Portfolio. Available at: www .tballiance.org/home/home.php. cited August 2008. Accessed December 10, 2008.

101. Kaufmann SH. Envisioning future strategies for vaccination against tuberculosis. Nat Rev Immunol 2006; 6:699–704.

102. Ly LH, McMurray DN. Tuberculosis: Vaccines in the pipeline. Expert Rev Vaccines 2008; 7:635–650.

2
The Epidemiology of Tuberculosis

MEGAN MURRAY
Harvard School of Public Health and Brigham and Women's Hospital, Boston, Massachusetts, U.S.A.

I. Introduction

Tuberculosis (TB) is an ancient and widespread infectious disease that has been identified both in ancient human remains (1–4) and in almost every geographical setting. Despite its ubiquity, the risk of acquiring TB has varied markedly over both time and place as well as among members of specific populations. This chapter focuses on understanding the community and individual determinants of TB both across and within specific populations. Such an understanding is essential to reach a full appreciation of the pathogenesis of the disease as well as to design and implement effective TB interventions and control programs.

Studies of the determinants of TB are complicated by the natural history of the disease, which involves multiple steps including exposure to infection, infection, disease and, finally, death in those who eventually succumb. Specific risk factors for each of these steps have been identified. In some cases, these determinants are risk factors for several different stages while, in others, they are distinct or even work in different directions, increasing risk for some steps while protecting against others. Studying these risks requires a set of methodological tools, each of which has its own limitations that contribute to the level of certainty or uncertainty in our estimates of the strengths of association between risk factors and TB.

This chapter first presents a model of the process through which determinants affect each step in the pathogenesis of TB; then describes the range of diagnostic and epidemiologic tools and approaches that have been used to elucidate the contribution of specific risk factors to this process. The subsequent sections focus on the etiologic epidemiology of TB, reviewing the evidence for risk factors associated with exposure, infection, disease, and death, respectively.

II. A Model of TB Pathogenesis and Epidemiology

Rieder proposed a conceptual model for TB epidemiology based on a TB classification scheme put forward by the American Thoracic Society and the U.S. Centers for Disease Control and Prevention (5,6). This model incorporates four steps in the pathogenesis of TB: exposure, subclinical infection, active TB, and death, and it denotes the transitions between each of these stages as steps with their own sets of determinants. In this chapter, the original model has been modified to encompass several additional steps that may also have distinct determinants and which could contribute to the dynamics of TB epidemics;

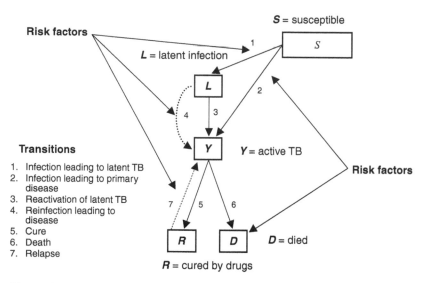

Figure 1   Pathogenesis model of TB progression.

these include reactivation of latent TB, relapse after cure, and reinfection of individuals with latent infection. Figure 1 presents this modified model, adding to the original model the additional transitions cited above.

Since these transitions mark distinct steps on the route to clinical TB, it makes epidemiologic sense to identify etiologic determinants for each and to assess these risk factors individually. While this approach may provide some clarity and precision in identifying the causal mechanisms that lead to each stage of the disease process, it may also obscure the ultimate quantitative contribution of each risk factor to the occurrence of clinical disease in individuals and the dynamics of TB within a population. If a specific risk factor acts to increase risk at multiple steps in the pathway to disease, its ultimate effect on increasing the likelihood that an affected person will have clinical TB may be amplified to a degree, which is not itself measured by any of the specific studies that focus on individual transitions. For example, residence in a prison may increase an individual's chance of being exposed to TB by placing him or her in contact with other individuals with infectious TB. It may also increase the chance of infection conditional on such an exposure or the chance of early progression to TB disease since prisoners may be more likely than civilians to have other risk factors for TB such as alcoholism, smoking, low body mass index, and/or HIV infection. Furthermore, prisoners might be more likely to relapse after cure since they may receive suboptimal care more often than their civilian counterparts. Ideally, assessment of incarceration as a risk factor would yield an estimate of the number of cases of TB that occurred in a specific setting that would not have occurred had none of the prisoners been incarcerated. Such an estimate is referred to as a counterfactual (7) since it refers to what would have happened if, contrary to fact, a specific risk had not been present while all others were. In such situations where specific risk factors affect multiple transitions, studies that assess determinants in those who have never been infected with those with disease may be the best way to capture the full impact of the risk factor, even if they do not elucidate the exact mechanism through which these risk factors work.

Determinants may also act on TB epidemics in ways that do not involve changes in an affected individual's risk of exposure, infection, or disease but rather affect community level variables that alter the efficacy of control measures. For example, a high prevalence of HIV in a community might contribute to the occurrence of TB in an HIV-negative individual who lives in that community in two ways. Given the increased risk of active TB in persons coinfected with HIV and TB, regions with a high burden of HIV might be expected to have high numbers of infectious coinfected patients. In this case, HIV could have the indirect effect of increasing the risk of TB in those who are not affected [although the role of coinfected patients in spreading disease to non–HIV-infected persons is complex and controversial (8–10)]. In the context of a communicable infectious disease, the term "indirect effect" refers to the effect of a risk factor or intervention on modifying risk in a person who does not have that risk factor or did not receive the intervention but is exposed to a person who does (11).

The community burden of HIV may also lead to a diversion of resources from other public health and treatment programs which could undermine TB control and lead to excess cases among individuals who do not have HIV. This is another form of indirect effect, in which individuals are put at increased risk when the number of infectious cases in a population increases but, in this case, the indirect effect is mediated by determinants specific to a population rather than the presence of an individual level risk factor in another person. Such effects cannot be assessed in routine epidemiologic studies that examine individual risk factors but require the comparison of populations that experience different levels of health burdens or interventions.

In summary, risk factors for TB can be categorized by the specific step in the pathogenesis of TB in affected individuals including exposure to infection, infection, primary disease, reactivation, relapse, reinfection, and death. Although delineation of the determinants of each of these steps will help elucidate the mechanisms responsible for the progression of TB, it may misestimate the actual contribution of risk factors that affect more than one step. Risk factors can also modify TB risk in unaffected individuals indirectly when they increase the number of cases to which an unaffected person is exposed or when they affect a community's ability to implement infection control measures that reduce epidemic disease.

III. Exposure to TB/Infection

A. Organism

As suggested by the pathway in Figure 1, the risk of being infected with TB can be divided into two different steps in pathogenesis. Individuals cannot become infected unless they have been exposed to some source of infectious bacilli of one of the three main species of the *M. tuberculosis* complex. The vast majority of TB cases occur after exposure to the organism, *M. tuberculosis*, but infection can also occur after exposure to *M. bovis* and *M. africanum*. *M. tuberculosis* and *M. africanum* bacilli are transmitted when people with active pulmonary TB cough, speak, sing, or otherwise aerosolize bacilli present in their respiratory tracts, and when these organisms are inhaled by susceptible hosts. *M. bovis* can also be transmitted from person to person through the airborne route although it was more often transmitted from animals to humans through the consumption of milk from infected cows in the era prior to pasteurization and programs to identify and remove infected cattle from herds (12–14).

B.   Prevalence of Infectious Cases

The risk of exposure to *M. tuberculosis* and *M. africanum* varies directly with the number of infectious cases with which a susceptible individual comes into contact, that is, close enough to permit airborne transmission. Since it is not usually possible to accurately enumerate such contacts on an individual basis, the number of smear-positive TB cases in a specific population, that is, the prevalence, can serve as a rough indicator of the average risk of exposure incurred by members of that community. Prevalence reflects both the incidence and duration of a disease and thus, the average risk of exposure increases with both incidence and the duration of infectiousness of incident infectious cases. In turn, the average duration of infectiousness of a TB case within a specific population reflects the availability and efficacy of control programs that ensure rapid diagnosis and prompt treatment of infectious cases. The risk of exposure to *M. bovis* also varies with the number of infectious cases to which an individual is exposed although these infectious cases can include both infectious humans and animals that infect humans either through contaminated milk or close contact.

Prevalence studies of infectious TB typically involve screening a population for smear-positive disease. Two recent reviews describe procedures to sample the population, screen using symptoms, chest X-ray or both, and identify a high probability sample for further screening with sputum smear microscopy and culture (15,16). Such studies are complicated by the need for large sample sizes to accurately assess prevalence and to detect trends over time and by the expense of mass chest radiography and sputum microscopy. In the absence of actual data on the number of prevalent cases, prevalence can be estimated from incidence data if one assumes that there is a fixed duration of infectiousness (17). A series of prevalence studies conducted at the national and subnational level have shown that the prevalence of infectious TB varies over time and across geographical settings both between and within national boundaries. In six national surveys conducted since 1995, prevalence ranged from 50 per 100,000 in Eritrea to a high of 310 per 100,000 in the Philippines (18–23). Similarly, recent estimates from the World Health Organization show heterogeneity in TB prevalence over time with prevalence declining or remaining stable in seven of nine epidemiologically distinct regions of the world between 1990 and 2003 but increasing in two African areas (reviewed in Ref. 24).

IV.   Risk Factors for Exposure

Although exposure probability varies with the number of prevalent cases on a population level, there is also considerable heterogeneity in the risk of exposure to TB among different members of a specific country or population. This heterogeneity reflects both migration and social mixing patterns within these communities. Studies on the risk of exposure within specific subpopulations have compared the risk of infection in different groups characterized by presence or absence of a specific risk factor. Although these studies do not allow investigators to distinguish between risk of exposure to an infectious case and risk of infection conditional on such an exposure, many of the risk factors involved are more likely to represent different social mixing patterns than biological differences in the probability of infection. Other factors, such as age, gender, and comorbidities, may modify the risk of TB at either or both steps and thus studies of TB infection do not provide clear guidance as to which transition has been affected.

TB infection has typically been ascertained using the tuberculin skin test (TST). Tuberculin refers to a mixture of *M. tuberculosis* protein antigens that elicit a delayed hypersensitivity response in humans. Rieder has reviewed the historical development and test characteristics of the TST in detail (5); characteristics of this test are also described in chapter 4 of this text. Briefly, TST involves injecting a standardized dose of purified protein derivatives (PPD) from killed tubercle bacilli intradermally and observing the size of the resulting induration. Since some of the antigens in PPD cross-react with proteins specific to environmental mycobacteria as well as the live vaccine strain of *M. bovis*, BCG, interpretation of the TST can be complicated by false-positive results. Similarly, false-negative tests can occur among those with impaired immune responses to these antigens. Thus, the sensitivity and specificity of TST often depend on regional differences in the prevalence of environmental mycobacteria or HIV and other forms of immunosuppression. Other limitations of this test have been reviewed by Menzies and colleagues (25); these include random variability in test results due to errors in administration or reading, false-positive tests due to "boosting" of preexisting immunity to other mycobacteria on re-administration of TST, and reversion of a positive skin test to negative over time. Newer tests for TB infection have recently been licensed. These use an enzyme-linked immunosorbent assay to quantify the production of interferon-γ by circulating T cells in whole blood after exposure to tubercle antigens (26). While such tests have been shown to be more specific than TST in those who have been vaccinated with BCG, they appear to be no more sensitive than TST, and their utility for etiologic studies of TB infection has not been well studied. All of these considerations suggest a need for caution in the interpretation of the results of TSTs and in the results of studies of etiologic factors involved in TB infection. Despite the potential pitfalls inherent in measuring TB infection, numerous studies have examined risk factors for TST positivity and for conversion of the TST. We first review those that are most likely to be associated with an increased risk of exposure, considering characteristics of the exposed host as well as of the infectious host. We then review risk factors that may reflect either an increased risk of exposure or an increased risk of infection given an exposure.

A. Population Density

Even within communities with a given prevalence of infectious TB, there is substantial variation in the number of infectious cases to which specific individuals are exposed. Living in densely populated areas increases the probability of being exposed to a contact with infectious disease. In a large study among white male U.S. navy recruits, lifelong residents of urban areas were 1.5 times more likely to be positive skin test reactors than those who were lifetime residents of farms (27). A similar urban–rural differential has been reported in subsequent studies in multiple other countries including the island of Zanzibar in Tanzania in 1961 (28), Korea in 1965 (29), Orissa State of Eastern India in 2002 to 2003 (30) and India in 2005 (31).

B. Congregate Settings

On a finer scale, dwelling within congregate settings in contrast to household environments has frequently been shown to be a determinant of TB infection, with increasing likelihood of TB infection in increasingly crowded living environments. Although numerous studies have demonstrated a higher proportion of skin test reactors among residents of mines (32), nursing homes (33,34), homeless shelters (35,36), and prisons (37–39), skin test positivity only indicates previous TB infection and does not provide information as to when or where an infection took place. Individuals entering institutional settings are often highly vulnerable—either because of age, the concurrence of other comorbidities or social and behavioral characteristics that may have increased their risk of previous TB exposure and infection prior to dwelling in a congregate setting. Thus, the assessment of the contribution of congregate settings to the risk of TB exposure and infection requires the demonstration of skin test conversion rather than simple TST positivity.

Stead and colleagues assessed the rate of skin test conversion among elderly people who were skin test negative on admission to nursing homes in Arkansas, U.S.A. (40). Among those who lived in homes in which there was a known case of infectious TB, 5% converted per year. More significantly, in those homes in which no TB case had been recognized over the previous three years, 3.5% converted per year, leading Stead to conclude that nosocomial transmission of TB could pose a substantial threat to elderly institutionalized people.

Several studies have also demonstrated rates of skin test conversion as high as 6.3% (41) and 9% per year (42) among inmates of U.S. prisons which were not selected on the basis of harboring a known case. In one of these studies, conducted in a sample of state prisons in Maryland in the 1990s (41), residents of prisons of higher population density had a relative risk of conversion of 2.4% in comparison with prisoners housed in lower density facilities. In another study conducted in Singapore (38), prisoners with a known TB contact were compared to residents of households in which there was a known TB case. Interestingly, even after conditioning on level of exposure, prisoners were twice as likely to convert their TST, suggesting either that they were more vulnerable to infection after exposure or that the intensity of exposure within the prison setting was higher than in households. Among employees of New York State prisons in 1992, those with low and high numbers of prisoner cases had relative risks of conversion of 1.7% and 2.2%, respectively, compared to employees who did not contact prisoners (39).

In other congregate settings such as homeless shelters and hospitals, where the risk of TB exposure seems likely to be high and where molecular epidemiologic tools have documented TB transmission, the transient nature of the exposure makes it difficult to follow-up persons who are initially skin test negative for evidence of skin test conversion and to therefore quantify the relative risk of infection among the exposed. Nonetheless, since TB screening studies in shelters and hospitals have documented high prevalences of smear-positive cases, it follows that in the absence of rigorous infection control measures, residents of these facilities are more heavily exposed to TB than those who dwell in the community (43).

Within households of infectious TB patients, the closeness of contact is a more reliable indicator of risk of infection than the number of people who live in the home. Contacts who share a bedroom (44) or report closer physical proximity (45,46) were more likely to be skin test positive that other household members. Several studies, however, showed that within households in which there was an infectious case, household crowding did not increase the risk of infection (47) and in some cases, the risk of infection fell as the number of persons living in the household rose (48), suggesting that, on average, there might be less close contact between individual household members as the number of potential pairwise contacts increased.

C. Factors Associated with Infectious Source Case

Among those exposed to a person with active TB, the risk of becoming infected and converting a TST varies with a number of characteristics of the infectious source case. Multiple studies conducted over the past 60 years have shown that the proportion of household contacts of an infectious case who are skin test positive is higher among those exposed to a smear-positive case compared to an index case who is smear negative (49–58). Those who were exposed to cases classified as both smear and culture negative were at even lower risk of positivity (59–66). Within each of these categories, prevalence in household contacts fell over calendar time, presumably reflecting declining background rates of TB prevalence (Fig. 2). Contacts exposed to index patients with higher numbers of acid-fast bacilli on sputum smears are also more likely to be TST positive (67,68). Similarly, a contact with infectious source cases who have cavitary disease is more likely to be associated with TST positivity than those with other forms of pulmonary disease (52,69,70). Treatment of the index case rapidly reduces the number of bacilli expectorated in sputum and reduces subsequent infections in contacts (71–75). In a recent study of household TB transmission in the Yunnan Province of China, contacts of patients who received TB treatment within 30 days of the onset of symptoms were significantly less likely to be TST positive than were contacts of those who delayed treatment, and their risk increased with the duration of the treatment delay. (69). Other studies have documented

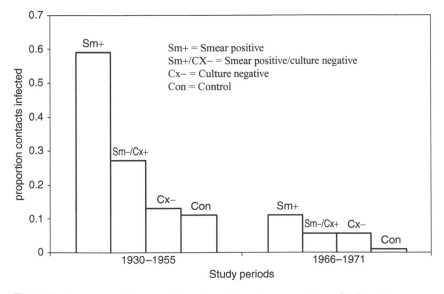

Figure 2 Proportion of household contacts infected by smear status of index case.

the role of coughing in transmission of TB infection. Loudon and Spohn found that TST positivity in contacts of patients who coughed >48 times per night was 1.63 times higher than in contacts of those who coughed <12 times per night (76). Singing has also been associated with TB transmission; in an analysis of a boarding school outbreak, contacts exposed to the index case in the choir were five times as likely to be skin test positive as those exposed by sharing a dormitory room or meals (77).

Given the growing importance of HIV in the dynamics of TB epidemics, numerous investigators have sought to assess the contribution of HIV to the relative infectiousness of coinfected patients. Cruciani and colleagues conducted a meta-analysis of the impact of HIV on infectiousness (78); this study included 4 cohort studies (79–82) and 13 case-control or cross-sectional studies of which 5 reported disease, skin test positivity, or conversion among exposed health care workers (83–87) and 8 reported disease or skin test positivity among exposed household contacts (88–95). Pooled estimates from studies of conversion among health care workers did not differ among those exposed to HIV-positive and -negative index cases although health care workers exposed to HIV-infected TB patients in a 1992 study in Puerto Rico were more likely to be skin test positive than those exposed to HIV-negatives [OR 6.4 (95% CI 2.2–18)]. Among household contacts, the odds of being skin test positive were significantly lower among contacts of HIV-infected compared to HIV-negative index cases (pooled OR 0.66, CI 0.2–0.72) although this difference failed to meet statistical significance when that analysis was confined to HIV negative contacts. While the authors of this study contend that these pooled estimates support the hypothesis that HIV-infected TB cases are no more infectious than HIV negative cases (78), others have noted the marked heterogeneity present in the results of the included studies and have argued against the pooling of these data.

D. Strains

In addition to the personal characteristics of infectious cases, it is possible that transmission also varies depending on the specific strain or lineage of the organism. Among the three main *M. tuberculosis* complex organisms that cause TB in humans, it is well documented that *M. bovis* is much less transmissible from human to human than *M. tuberculosis* (96,97), but no difference in transmission was noted in the single study that compared skin test reactivity after exposure to *M. africanum* and *M. tuberculosis* (98). The recent recognition that the Beijing lineage of *M. tuberculosis* may be an "epidemic" strain has also raised the question of whether exposure to Beijing or other high prevalence lineages might be more likely to lead to infection than other strains (99,100). While many field and laboratory studies have investigated the virulence of Beijing (101–103), only one to date has measured skin test positivity within exposed households; in this study, exposure to different lineages had no impact on transmission although there was a higher rate of progression to disease after exposure to Beijing (98). Such studies may be compromised by problems with the TST, which may detect infection with some strains more readily than others.

E. Drug Resistance

Another potential source of biological differences in infecting strains has been the drug resistance profile of the isolate. Early work in animal models suggested that isoniazid resistant strains of *M. tuberculosis* were less virulent to guinea pigs and mice than were sensitive strains (104). Subsequent studies found that growth rates of isoniazid resistant strains varied depending on the specific mutations conferring resistance, with some high fitness resistant mutants having near normal growth in animals (105–107). Within studies of household contacts of cases with sensitive and resistant *M. tuberculosis*, there were no differences in the proportion of patients with TB infection as diagnosed by TST positivity (108,109). To date, household studies comparing resistant and sensitive strains of *M. tuberculosis* have not stratified on specific mutations conferring resistance.

F. Factors Associated with Exposed Host

The risk of TB infection can be assessed, not only in terms of characteristics of the infecting source case, but also in terms of risk factors specific to the potentially exposed host. In some cases, it is impossible to ascertain whether these characteristics are risk factors for exposure or for infection conditional on exposure. For example, the annual risk of skin test conversion increases with age from infancy to early adulthood (110). Since social mixing is more common between people of similar ages than across age groups (111,112), one would expect that skin test conversion would be most common in the age groups in which the prevalence of active TB is highest. However, it is also true that immune responses vary dramatically with age and thus it is not possible to attribute age-associated trends with risk of exposure rather than risk of infection. Gender differentials pose a similar problem; it is clear that men are more likely to be skin test positive than women in almost all studied populations but this is likely to reflect the fact that men have more social contacts than women (113). When risk of infection is measured in household studies that assess skin test conversion after an exposure rather than just skin test positivity, that is, those that condition on an exposure, female gender does not emerge as a predictor of infection.

In some studies, ethnicity has been associated with prevalent TB infection. For example, in a study of patients recently admitted to a city hospital, African-Americans were five times more likely to be tuberculin positive than whites (114). Stead et al. found similar results when they followed nursing home residents for skin test conversion; in that setting, African-Americans were more likely to convert than whites even when both groups were living in a home with an infectious patient (115). Nonetheless, as was suggested by the household studies cited above which showed that even within households, proximity to the infectious case was an important predictor of infection, these data may be explained by differentials in exposure within a congregate setting. When investigators studied infection among schoolchildren uniformly exposed to a physical education teacher with infectious TB, they found no racial differences in susceptibility to infection (116).

Relatively few studies have examined other host characteristics as risk factors for TB exposure or infection in distinction from TB disease. Several of these have shown that some host risk factors for disease, such as alcoholism, silicosis, and smoking (117), are also modest risk factors for TST positivity. Although such risk factors are likely to be biological determinants of TB disease, they may also be indicators of social mixing patterns that put those with such vulnerabilities in contact with people likely to have infectious TB. For example, multiple studies conducted in different countries have identified bars as sites of TB transmission (118–124). Since drinkers are also likely to frequent bars, their alcohol use may contribute to the occurrence of TB both by increasing their exposure and later in the pathway of pathogenesis, and by increasing their likelihood of progressing to disease once exposed (125).

V. Risk of TB Progression After Infection

Among those infected with the tubercle bacilli, only a small minority will actually progress to overt disease. Studies that follow those who have converted their skin test for the occurrence of disease suggest that 5% to 20% of those infected will develop active TB over the course of their lives, with the majority of those cases occurring within the first two to five years after initial infection. Although some risk factors have been clearly identified as determinants of progression, many of these are rare conditions that account for only a small fraction of the actual incident cases of TB while some, such as HIV/AIDS are both common and associated with a high risk of progression. Other determinants of progression have a relatively modest effect but may account for a substantial portion of the burden of disease since they occur so frequently in infected populations. Here we consider the evidence for the impact of specific risk factors in mediating disease progression among those known to be infected with the tubercle bacilli.

A. Time Since Infection

Several longitudinal cohort studies have found that the risk of disease progression after infection is highest in the first two years after skin test conversion, then declines over the subsequent three years, and remains level thereafter (126,127). Figure 3 provides pooled data on the incidence of TB among exposed household contacts as a function of time since either infection or study start. Although these data demonstrate a consistent trend in the occurrence of disease after infection, they also show significant variability in absolute rates in different settings; these differences may reflect variations in the distribution of other risk factors for progression in diverse populations including differences in age

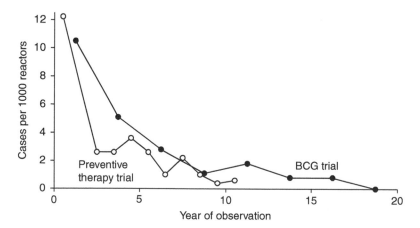

Figure 3 Incidence of TB in exposed persons receiving placebo as a function of time since infection in a preventive therapy trial and time from enrollment in a BCG vaccine trial. *Source*: From Refs. 5, 127, 128.

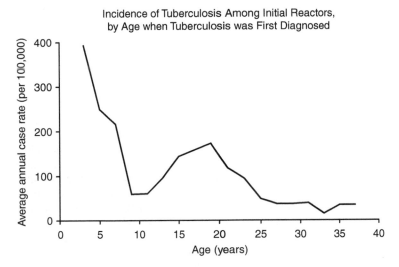

Figure 4   TB incidence among infected persons by age of diagnosis. *Source*: From Ref. 129.

distribution, innate susceptibility, or the predominant infecting lineage of *M. tuberculosis*. Importantly, they may also reflect the fact that some incident disease that occurs after an initial infection may be due to a recently acquired reinfection rather than to the infection that led to the initial skin test conversion.

B.   Age

The occurrence of TB disease in skin test reactors varies with age. Comstock and colleagues followed more than 82,000 children in Puerto Rico with positive TSTs for two decades (129). TB incidence was highest in the youngest children, fell consistently over mid-childhood years and then began to rise in early adolescence reaching a peak before a subsequent decline in late adolescence (Fig. 4). This surge in TB incidence in adolescence has been so consistent in other populations (130) that it has led some investigators to propose that an unidentified sexually transmitted disease might play some role in disease progression (131).

C.   Gender

Holmes and colleagues reviewed seven studies which compared rates of progression in infected men and women (113,132–137); this analysis showed that risk was equivalent among male and female children until early adolescence and then increased for women through age 30 to 40, depending on the specific study. While most of these studies followed patients who were tuberculin positive at study onset, Gedde-Dahl in Norway enrolled skin test negatives and followed them first for skin test conversion and then for disease. In this study, conducted in the 1930s and 1940s, nearly half of the converters developed TB within eight years and women aged 20 to 29 had rates that were 25% to 30% higher than men while men over 30 experienced higher rates than women (135). Although these findings raise the question of the role of pregnancy and the postpartum period in altering the risk of progression, several previous reviews have found no clear association between pregnancy and risk of TB progression (138,139). Studies on postpartum risk are conflicting with some citing no increased risk and others suggesting a higher risk in the postpartum period than during pregnancy (140–144).

D. Body Mass Index

Low body mass index (BMI) has been consistently associated with increased risk of progression to TB among those infected. When tuberculin positive navy recruits were followed for the occurrence of active TB, those who were 10% or more under ideal body weight had a relative risk of TB of 3.4 (145,146). Multiple subsequent studies have confirmed this link in geographical settings as diverse as Norway (147), South India (148), the United Kingdom (149), Rwanda (150), and the United States (reviewed in Ref. 151). Surprisingly, the inverse trend in TB incidence as a function of BMI continues even as individuals become obese; a recent study in Hong Kong (152) found that after controlling for other risk factors, obese (BMI > 30) and overweight (BMI 25 to <30) individuals were protected from developing active TB with hazard ratios of 0.36 and 0.55, respectively, compared to those of normal weight. The authors of this study note recent scientific work suggesting that adipose tissue may have endocrine functions that mediate host immune response and T-cell activity (153).

E. HIV Status

Among risk factors that increase the risk of progression to TB, HIV is the one that has had the most impact on altering TB incidence rates over the past several decades. Despite the many studies that demonstrate that HIV is a strong determinant of disease, relatively few studies have documented the incidence of TB among HIV patients who are skin test positive or who have been observed to convert. Such studies have been difficult to carry out since current evidence and guidelines support the use of TB preventive therapy for newly diagnosed HIV patients, regardless of skin test status (154). Selwyn and colleagues conducted the first study comparing TB risk in HIV-positive and -negative intravenous drug users in New York City. Of those who converted their skin test in both groups, 7 of 49 HIV-positive patients progressed to TB during an average of 22 months of follow-up, yielding a rate of approximately 8 per 100 person-years (155). None of the 26 HIV-negative converters developed active tuberculosis during that period. These data may underestimate the real incidence of TB among HIV-infected patients since HIV often renders patients anergic to tuberculin, and those coinfected patients who were most immunocompromised would not have been included in this calculation. Furthermore, half this group received INH chemoprophylaxis. Other studies have documented the incidence of TB disease among HIV-infected patients who were either skin test positive at baseline or converted but have not enrolled a comparison group of HIV negative TB-infected patients (156–158). These studies have found similar rates of disease progression to that reported by Selwyn, with one study among Ugandan HIV positive TST reactors reporting approximately 6.4 cases per 100 person-years while another reported a rate of 5.42 cases per 100 person-years (158). In subsequent studies, low CD4 and high viral loads were further risk factors for disease while treatment with highly active antiretroviral therapy reduced risk (159,160).

Importantly, few studies have followed people who were infected with *M. tuberculosis* after having been infected with HIV and in the absence of preventive therapy. Presumably, these people are especially at high risk conferred both by the increased probability of disease during the immediate postinfection period and by the immunosuppressive effects of HIV.

F. Smoking and Indoor Air Pollution

Among studies on smoking and the risk of active tuberculosis reviewed in a recent meta-analysis (148,161–183), only two compared cases to skin test positive controls; these studies showed that smokers had 3.6 times the risk of TB (178) while those exposed to passive smoke were 5.4 times as likely to progress to TB as nonexposed counterparts (183). Other studies did not specifically choose controls that had been TB infected; most of these also reported a positive association between TB disease and smoke exposure although the relative risks ranged from 0.95 to 4.6 (184). This study also cited three studies (161,184,185), which showed an association between indoor air pollution and TB disease although two others found no effect (148,171).

G. Silicosis

Although many studies have identified silicosis in miners as a strong risk factor for active TB, these have not directly followed those who are skin test positive for progression of disease, that is, they have not conditioned on exposure and infection. Nonetheless, since these studies have usually been conducted in high-risk settings such as mines where the risk of TB exposure among those with and without silicosis would be expected to be similar, it is reasonable to assume that the relative risk of TB disease in silicotics reported in these studies reflects differences in the rates of infection or progression rather than in exposure. Two studies conducted prior to the HIV epidemic estimated the relative risk in active TB among occupationally exposed silicotics to be 26 and 30 times greater than in controls (186,187). Increased risk has also been observed among those exposed to silica and dust but who have not met the case definition for silicosis (188–191). teWaternaude noted a prevalence of odds of 1.4 for each one interquartile increase in the level of silica and dust exposure even in the absence of overt silicosis. This study of active miners estimated a prevalence of current TB disease of 32.5% (188). Among South African gold miners at risk for both HIV and silicosis, Corbett and colleagues reported a multiplicative effect of the two risk factors (192).

H. Diabetes

Several recent systematic reviews have pooled data on the risk of TB disease among diabetics to estimate a summary effect (193,194). In one of these (193), results from prospective cohort studies (195–197) suggested that diabetics were three times more likely than controls to develop TB disease while results from case control and cross-sectional studies were more heterogeneous with relative risks ranging from 1.2 to 7.8 (150,167,198–205). Since none of these studies restricted or adjusted for TB infection, the hypothesis that diabetes increases risk of exposure or infection, rather than progression, could not be excluded. Investigators from Hong Kong followed household contacts of index cases for the occurrence of active TB; this study found that diabetics were nine times more likely to be diagnosed with TB within three months of the diagnosis of the index case and 3.4 times as likely over the subsequent five years (206). Although this study did not record tuberculin sensitivity, it both conditioned on a household exposure and adjusted for potential confounders and thus provides support for the contention that diabetes affects either infection or progression rather than exposure. Despite these data, it remains possible that diabetics who seek medical care or are frequently hospitalized might be more likely to encounter persons with infectious TB than those without medical conditions. The role of diabetes in TB may be complicated by two other possible associations. Since type 2 diabetes is more likely to occur in overweight or obese individuals and since high BMI appears to protect against TB progression, there may be complex biological interactions between weight and diabetes and their impacts on TB. Even more challenging to disentangle are the possible interactions between socioeconomic status and diabetes. In some regions such as India, diabetics are more often of high socioeconomic status (207) while in others, such as the Europe, there is an inverse association between diabetes and indicators of socioeconomic position (208). Since poverty operates to increase TB through multiple routes (crowding, low BMI, indoor air pollution), the effect of these sometime unmeasured confounders may vary in different geographical and social settings.

I. Other Medical Conditions

A variety of other medical and surgical conditions have been associated with high rates of TB disease although few studies have been able to definitely link these risk factors to disease progression rather than exposure and infection (209–212). Medical conditions that have been reported to increase TB risk include a variety of malignancies, especially hematologic malignancies (209) and carcinoma of the head and neck (210). Kamboj and Sepkowitz reviewed TB diagnoses among cancer patients admitted to the Sloan Kettering Cancer Center in New York City between 1980 and 2004, estimated disease-specific incidence rates and compared these to rates reported in the general population (211). Rates were highest in patients admitted for hematologic malignancies, especially stem cell transplant recipients as well as for those with head and neck carcinomas. Rates in patients with other solid tumors were consistent with those reported in New York City residents. Patients with end-stage renal disease have also consistently been shown to be at high risk from TB, a risk exacerbated by the use of peritoneal or hemodialysis (213–218). One recent study showed that even among cancer patients, those with coexisting renal failure had an incidence 20-fold higher than those without renal disease (211). More recently, TB risk has been observed to increase in patients with autoimmune disorders such as rheumatoid arthritis who have received TNF-α inhibitors (219). A review of these therapies cited evidence for the association between infliximab use and subsequent TB; this included the temporal association, a higher rate in those receiving therapy than in the general U.S. population and the occurrence of forms of TB usually associated with immunosuppression (219). While corticosteroid use has also long been considered a risk factor for TB, there is little evidence to support this association. (220–223). Surgeries associated with TB include gastrectomy (224), which is reported to increase risk fivefold, and jejunoileal bypass (225,226). Since both of these procedures lead to weight loss, their effect may be mediated through this mechanism. Among gastrectomy patients who were 15% below ideal body weight, risk of TB was 14 times that of those with normal weight for height (224).

J. Host Genetics

The possibility of that specific host genetic polymorphisms modify the risk of TB has long been suspected based on the observations that populations newly exposed to TB often experience much higher disease and death rates than others (227,228) and that monozygotic twins are twice as likely to have co-occurring TB (i.e., be concordant) as dizygotic twins (229). Early studies also suggested links between genetic traits such as hemophilia (230,231) and specific blood groups (232) and the risk of TB. Furthermore, family studies confirmed the association of specific Mendelian disorders involving the IL-12/23-IFNγ pathway with vulnerability to TB and other mycobacterial infections (233–235). Evidence for more common variants comes from candidate gene studies, in which the presence or absence of a polymorphism is compared in cases and controls and from genome wide association studies which identify regions in the genome that are associated with disease susceptibility without a priori assumptions of which genes are involved. Such studies have identified a number of genetic loci that have modest effects on risk of disease although few have controlled for infection with TB. The candidate genes that have been studied to date were selected because they are orthologs of susceptibility genes identified in animal models or on the basis of their putative role in the acquired or innate host immune response to mycobacteria (236). An example of such a gene is *Nramp1* (SLC11A1), first recognized when infection experiments in inbred mice identified a locus that conferred susceptibility to BCG, leishmania donovanii, and salmonella. Positional cloning pinpointed the affected gene, designated *Nramp* for "natural resistance-associated macrophage protein 1," and subsequent studies of variants within or near the human homolog have confirmed the role of this gene in human susceptibility to a number of infectious and inflammatory diseases (237). A meta-analysis of epidemiologic studies have demonstrated that *Nramp* polymorphisms are associated with TB in a number of different populations in Africa and Asia but not in population of European ancestry with estimated odds ratio of 1.7 in Africans and 1.9 in Asians (238).

Another locus identified in animal models is the Ipr1 gene, of which *SP110* is the nearest homolog (239). Studies have yielded conflicting results on the role of *SP110* variants in pulmonary TB in West Africa with one reporting associations in a series of family studies (240) while another large case control study did not confirm this finding (241). Other studies have focused on MHC genes which have been implicated in other infectious diseases (242); associations have been identified with alleles of the HLA class II DR2 serotype and HLA-DQB1 variants in human populations (243,244).

Other studies have focused on candidate genes known to be involved in innate immunity, such as pattern recognition receptors including mannose binding lectin (MBL), toll-like receptors (TLR), and dendritic cell-specific ICAM-3 grabbing nonintegrin (DC-Sign). Several of these analyses suggested a protective effect of heterozygosity for *MBL2* variant alleles (245,246) while others found association between TLR2 polymorphisms and the risk of pulmonary TB (247,248) and TB meningitis (249). Two promoter variants in the gene encoding *DC-SIGN*, a *M. tuberculosis* receptor on human dendritic cells (250), were linked with TB risk in South Africa (251) while the chemokine monocyte chemoattractant protein-1 was found to be associated with TB in a Mexican and in a South Korean population (252), but not in a Brazilian cohort (253). Heterogeneity in the effects of genetic variants have led some researchers to conclude that the patterns of genetic associations with susceptibility to TB detected are "consistent with the conclusion that unique environmental and natural selective factors have resulted in the development

Table 1   Genes Putatively Associated with TB Susceptibility

Locus	Description
HLA-DRB1	HLA class II molecule
SLC11A1 (Nramp1)	Divalent cation transporter
INF-γ	Interferon-γ cytokine
VDR	Vitamin D receptor
SP110	Transcription factor
IL8	Interleukin-8 cytokine
MAL/TIRAP	TLR signaling pathway adaptor
IL10	Interleukin-10 cytokine
DC-SIGN	C-type lectin receptor on dendritic cells
SP-A	Surfactant protein
CR1	Complement receptor
CCL2	Monocyte chemoattractant protein-1 chemokine
IL12RB1	Interleukin-12 cytokine receptor chain
TLR2	Toll-like recetor-2
MBL2	Mannose-binding lectin
NOD2	Nucleotide-binding domain-2

of ethnic-specific host genetic factors associated with TB susceptibility and resistance worldwide" (254). Table 1 lists current candidate genes under study.

K.   Strain Lineages

Relatively little evidence exists on the contribution of specific *M. tuberculosis* species or strains to the progression of TB disease. Although a number of researchers have assessed the association between specific lineages and clustering of cases in molecular epidemiologic studies of Beijing (255–257), these studies do not distinguish between strain effects on infection and disease. Furthermore, if specific strains circulate within subpopulations which are at higher risk than other communities, such as among immigrants from high burden countries or the homeless, then clustering of these strains may reflect these heterogeneous opportunities for transmission rather than any biological differences between strains. One recent study followed household contacts exposed to *M. africanum* as well as a number of different *M. tuberculosis stricto sensu* lineages including the Beijing strains (98). While there was no difference in the proportion of exposed household members infected, rates of active disease within two years of exposure to different strains differed dramatically. Least likely to lead to disease was exposure to *M. africanum* strains (Table 2), which led to secondary disease in 1% of household contacts. All of the *M. tuberculosis* lineages led to higher rate of disease in those exposed while exposure to Beijing resulted in disease in 5.6% of contacts. This study not only suggests that strain-specific factors may alter the outcome of TB infection but also provide evidence that the bacterial determinants of infection and transmission may differ from those that predispose to disease progression (98).

Other strain genetic differences that have been proposed to lead to differences in disease progression are the mutations associated with drug resistance. Early laboratory data suggested that strains selected for resistance to the anti-TB drug, isoniazid, were less

Table 2 Incidence of TB Within Three Months of Enrollment Among Exposed Household Contacts by Infecting Lineage of Index Case

Lineage	Hazard ratio	95% confidence interval
M. africanum	1	
Beijing	16	2.8–89
DosR	10	2.2–45
RD0182	4.2	0.77–23
RD219	4.2	0.42–43

Source: From Ref. 98.

virulent in animal models than sensitive strains (104,258). Subsequent studies compared the virulence of resistant clinical strains isolated from patients with active TB; these strains exhibited a range of phenotypes including diminished growth, similar growth, and even more increased growth in comparison to sensitive strains (105,259). Epidemiologic studies on the epidemic behavior of multidrug resistant (MDR) and extensively drug resistant (XDR) strains have yielded conflicting results, but like the studies of lineage cited above, most have measured the association between resistance profile and clustering while relatively few have compared rates of progression in those exposed to resistant and sensitive strains and those that have done so have been too small to yield definitive conclusions (260–269). Despite the lack of systematic studies on the risk of progression after exposure to drug resistant TB, recent reports of outbreaks of MDR and XDR TB and the occurrence of resistance in newly diagnosed patients who have not received anti-TB drugs provide evidence that even highly resistant *M. tuberculosis* strains can be transmitted and lead to virulent disease and death (270,271).

L. Reactivation TB

Most of the studies reviewed above have not distinguished between disease that occurs within the first few years after TB infection and disease that occurs later, that is, reactivation disease. There are several reasons why these studies have not addressed risk factors for reactivation disease as distinct from "primary" disease, that is, disease variably defined as that which occurs within the first two or five years after infection. First, in studies that recruit patients who are skin test positive and follow them for outcomes, it is not usually possible to know when a person was infected with the TB bacilli that led to his or her disease episode. Secondly, few studies of converters have followed patients over the many decades during which reactivation might occur. Finally, recent data suggests that reinfection may be responsible for some new episodes of TB disease occurring in people who had previously been infected, so the occurrence of cases many years after skin test conversion does not necessarily imply reactivation disease (270,272–274). Much recent work has focused on identifying risk factors for "recently transmitted" disease in contrast to risk factors for disease that has not spread. These studies use the tools of molecular fingerprinting to identify clusters of cases that share a molecular genotype; in contrast, those cases caused by an *M. tuberculosis* strain that is not shared by other strains from a specific geographic area are considered to be "unique," and are assumed to have arisen through reactivation of a remote infection (275,276). Since some reactivation cases will no doubt go on to spread to others and be clustered with the secondary cases they have given rise to, clustered cases are almost certainly a mixture of reactivation and primary cases while unique cases may represent a purer sample of reactivation cases alone. Comparison among risk factors for clustered and unclustered cases should therefore yield some information on host or pathogen characteristics associated with primary and reactivation TB, at least in so far as risk factors for primary and reactivation disease differ. Of the few host characteristics that distinguish recently transmitted from unique TB across different studies in different geographical and social settings, age > 60 has emerged as the most consistent (277). In low burden settings, foreign birth has also been a determinant of disease caused by an unclustered or unique strain (263,278). Since both older age and birth in a high incidence region are likely to be risk factors for previous infection, these results are not surprising but add little to our understanding of the mechanisms that lead to TB reactivation many years after an initial infection.

M. Reinfection

Evidence for reinfection comes from two different lines of study. Styblo (279) cited the experience of Greenland in the 1950s as evidence that reinfection contributed to the dynamics of TB transmission. He noted that a vigorous intervention program in that country led to a decline in clinical TB, not only among the young people in whom a first infection was averted, but also among the elderly who had almost certainly been previously infected. Had most disease in the elderly been due to reactivation of remote TB, he argued, incidence in that population would not have been affected by a reduction in transmission. Many years later, Nardell and colleagues (280) provided further circumstantial evidence for exogenous reinfection. In a TB outbreak in a Boston homeless shelter, 7 of 25 cases linked both by identical drug resistance pattern and phage type had documentation of previous infection or disease. With the availability of molecular fingerprinting, the debate about the existence of exogenous reinfection has been put to rest. Several groups have shown that reinfection with a second distinct strain can occur in both immunocompromised and immunocompetent individuals (281,282). More recently, researchers have used molecular epidemiologic techniques to quantify the frequency with which exogenous reinfection occurs and to identify the context in which it may contribute substantially to TB dynamics. For example, van Rie et al. (283) enrolled consecutive TB cases over a six-year period from a high incidence South African community. Of the 698 cases identified, 16 had recurrent disease after completing curative therapy and 12 of these 16 were infected with a strain that was different from that isolated during their first episode of disease. Similar studies have been conducted in lower prevalence areas; these have shown that in low risk areas reinfection accounts for fewer of the second episodes of disease (284) than it does in high risk settings and thus in these settings, recurrent disease is more likely to be due to relapse that a new infection.

While these studies suggest that reinfection occurs more commonly than previously believed, they do not provide information on the relative contribution of reinfection to the disease burden of TB. Most cases of reinfection would be expected to occur in people who have been infected in the past but in whom clinical TB did not result from that initial infection. These people will not have *M. tuberculosis* isolates from two distinct episodes of disease and therefore cannot be classified as reinfected cases by typing the strains responsible for recurrent TB. The inability to classify cases of reinfection TB makes it difficult to assess determinants of reinfection. Those studies that have followed people after their initial disease episode for occurrence of a second episode caused by a new strain have accumulated too few endpoints to assess risk factors (283). Nonetheless, one study which assessed the incidence of TB due to reinfection found that rates in persons who had a first episode of TB were higher than in the general population (274). These findings raised the question of whether some form of temporary immunosuppression induced by an initial TB episode had contributed to increasing the risk of infection and disease progression on those afflicted. Future research will no doubt focus on whether there is differential protection against subsequent infection and disease afforded by infection with specific lineages.

N. Relapse

Rates of relapse after TB disease fell markedly with the introduction of increasingly effective chemotherapeutic agents over time (285,286). The risk of relapse after appropriate treatment and cure of pulmonary TB is difficult to assess since relapse after cure cannot be distinguished from disease due to reinfection in the absence of molecular genotyping. Panjabi and colleagues reviewed 32 studies documenting rates of relapse after cure including 18 controlled clinical trials and 14 observational studies (287). Of these, 10 provided data on specific risk factors for relapse (288–297). Rates of relapse were found to be highest in high burden countries with an average of 10,310 cases per 100,000 within the first six months compared to 2380 in low burden countries. This differential might be explained by increased rates of nonadherence to standardized regimens in high burden settings, but could also be due to the increased probability of reinfection in areas where the prevalence of infectious source cases is high. Not surprisingly, rates were also significantly higher in observational studies compared to controlled clinical trials of TB treatment (Fig. 5). All of the studies which examined the effect of HIV infection on

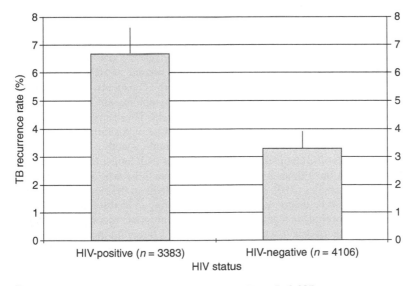

Figure 5 Rate of relapse by HIV status. *Source*: From Ref. 287.

relapse found it played a significant role; coinfected patients had nearly twice the risk of recurrence as HIV-negative TB patients. Two studies used molecular typing to distinguish between relapse and reinfection; both found that HIV infection was a strong risk factor for reinfection with a different strain. In one, HIV also was associated with disease due to the same strain (291) while the other did not confirm this association (288). Among HIV-infected TB patients, the extent of immunosuppression as measured by reduction in CD4 count was also a predictor of recurrence. Two more recent studies have also documented a mitigating effect of HAART on the risk of recurrence of TB in coinfected patients (298,299). In addition to HIV infection, other risk factors associated with relapse include smoking (290), poor treatment adherence (291), drug resistance at initiation of treatment (300–303), residual cavitary disease on completion of treatment (288,290), positive sputum cultures after two months of therapy (292,304), low BMI (304), host HLA-DRB1 polymorphisms (305), and strain type, specifically infection with the Beijing lineage (306).

O. Death

In the prechemotherapeutic era, the risk of death from TB varied with site of disease; TB of the peripheral lymph nodes (307) led to few deaths while TB meningitis was nearly uniformly fatal (308,309). The death rate from pulmonary TB varied by smear status; about two-thirds of those with smear-positive disease died within five years of diagnosis while only 10% to 15% of those who were smear negative died (5). With the advent of effective chemotherapy, TB mortality has plummeted and current risk factors for death often include predictors either of late diagnosis and/or treatment initiation, coexisting morbidities or failure to receive adequate therapy.

Numerous studies have found that TB treatment delays are associated with death (310–316). For example, Pablo-Mendez and colleagues analyzed survival in 229 cases of TB newly diagnosed in one month in New York City in 1991 (313). Of these, 50% were HIV infected and 7% had multi-drug-resistant (MDR) TB. Cumulative all-cause mortality at six months was 40%; risk factors for death included HIV, MDR, and lack of treatment. Among 13 HIV-positive patients who experienced a one-month delay in treatment initiation, 11 died (313). Such findings are not specific to HIV-infected populations in the United States. In a study of newly detected TB patients in The Gambia conducted in 1997, median time from reported onset of symptoms until treatment was 8.6 weeks and 17% experienced a delay of more than 16 weeks. Those reporting a delay of more than eight weeks were five times as likely to die as those with shorter delays (312). Proximal causes of delay vary in different settings. For example, a study of delay in South Africa found that patients who attended a traditional healer took longer to begin anti-TB therapy and were almost three times more likely to die than those who went directly to the government health services (310). In contrast, TB patients in developed low burden countries are often slow to be diagnosed even after presenting to health facilities. In one study of 17 acute care hospitals in Canada, initiation of appropriate therapy was delayed in 30% of patients and these delays were associated with a threefold increase in risk of death (311). A recent systematic review on delays in the diagnosis and treatment of TB identified several broad categories of risk factors: socioeconomic status including low access to health care, rural residence, low education, and poverty; sociopsychological factors including initially seeking care from traditional healers, low level government health facilities, or private practitioners; and demographic factors such as older age and female gender (316).

As TB chemotherapy has improved, deaths among TB patients are increasingly confined to those with comorbid conditions that either complicate TB care or result in death from other causes during the course of TB treatment. HIV infection has been a consistently strong risk factor for death among TB patients in multiple studies (317–320). Duarte conducted a case-control study nested in a cohort of 313,500 patients who were diagnosed with tuberculosis between 2000 and 2004 in Brazil. Of these, 6.6% died during follow-up. The strongest risk factor for death was HIV positivity with an adjusted odds ratio of 11 compared to those who were HIV-negative (317). The introduction of HAART has also had an impact in reducing this HIV effect on TB mortality (321–325). In a recent report from the Netherlands, TB mortality in HIV-positive patients fell between the periods 1993–1995 to 1999–2001 from 22.9 to 11.8%, presumably due to the increased availability of HAART (321). Other comorbidities associated with mortality in TB patients include renal failure (326–328), non-HIV associated immunosuppression (329), malignancies (330), congestive heart failure (331), malnutrition (326,327), and alcoholism (332,333).

Failure to complete an appropriate course of effective therapy is also a major predictor of TB death. Such failure may be due to default from treatment, that is, dropping out of treatment or nonadherence, that is, failure to take all prescribed medications during therapy (334–338). For example, a recent study of 3405 patients treated under the DOTS strategy in India estimated that the adjusted hazard ratio for death among those with incomplete treatment was 6.4 (335). Patients with drug resistant tuberculosis also are at risk for death, either because they are treated with drugs to which their isolates are resistant or because the second line drugs to which their isolates are susceptible are less effective than first line drugs (339). Analysis of risk factors for death among 39,566 TB patients notified in 15 European Union countries found that multi-drug resistance was the strongest predictor of death, with secondary MDR patients, that is, those with a previous history of TB, three times more likely to die than those with drug sensitive disease and those with primary MDR 1.6 times more likely to die (340). Numerous studies conducted throughout the world have demonstrated similar results with the hazard of death among those with MDR highest in regions without access to second line drug regimens (341–343). Not surprisingly, risk of death is even higher in those with XDR tuberculosis, with some areas reporting case fatality of 100% among HIV-TB coinfected patients while other studies report lower rates in non–HIV-infected patients (344–346).

VI. Conclusion

In summary, risk factors for TB death and disease can be understood as determinants of specific steps on the pathogenesis of the disease. Those risk factors that increase the number of infectious cases in the community or the intensity of contact with individual TB patients will increase the risk of TB infection. Risk factors for disease progression often reflect individual's immune status and include overt states of immunosuppression like HIV and malnutrition as well as more subtle indicators such as age at infection, gender, smoking, diabetes, and host genetic polymorphisms that impact the innate or acquired immune response. Factors associated with relapse reflect either failure to complete treatment or immune suppression while those that lead to death are indicators of treatment delay, comorbidities, and failure to complete an adequate course of therapy. Understanding such risk factors is vital to design interventions to reduce transmission, forestall progression and prevent relapse and death among those with disease.

References

1. Fusegawa H, Wang BH, Sakurai K, et al. Outbreak of tuberculosis in a 2000-year-old Chinese population. Kansenshogaku Zasshi 2003; 77:146–149.
2. Zink AR, Sola C, Reischl U, et al. Characterization of Mycobacterium tuberculosis complex DNAs from Egyptian mummies by spoligotyping. J Clin Microbiol 2003; 41:359–367.
3. Konomi N, Lebwohl E, Mowbray K, et al. Detection of mycobacterial DNA in Andean mummies. J Clin Microbiol 2002; 40:4738–4740.
4. Nerlich AG, Haas CJ, Zink A, et al. Molecular evidence for tuberculosis in an ancient Egyptian mummy. Lancet 1997; 350:1404.
5. Rieder HL. Epidemiologic Basis of Tuberculosis Control. Paris, France: International Union Against TB and Lung Disease, 2003.
6. Rieder HL. Opportunity for exposure and risk of infection: The fuel for the tuberculosis pandemic. Infection 1995; 23:1–3.
7. Roese NJ. Counterfactual thinking. Psychol Bull 1997; 121:133–148.
8. Egwaga SM, Cobelens FG, Muwinge H, et al. The impact of the HIV epidemic on tuberculosis transmission in Tanzania. AIDS 2006; 20:915–921.
9. Odhiambo JA, Borgdorff MW, Kiambih FM, et al. Tuberculosis and the HIV epidemic: Increasing annual risk of tuberculous infection in Kenya, 1986–1996. Am J Public Health 1999; 89:1078–1082.
10. Glynn JR, Murray J, Bester A, et al. Effects of duration of HIV infection and secondary tuberculosis transmission on tuberculosis incidence in the South African gold mines. AIDS 2008; 22:1859–1867.
11. Halloran ME, Struchiner CJ. Causal inference in infectious diseases. Epidemiology 1995; 6:142–151.
12. de la Rua-Domenech R. Human Mycobacterium bovis infection in the United Kingdom: Incidence, risks, control measures and review of the zoonotic aspects of bovine tuberculosis. Tuberculosis (Edinb) 2006; 86:77–109.
13. Evans JT, Smith EG, Banerjee A, et al. Cluster of human tuberculosis caused by Mycobacterium bovis: Evidence for person-to-person transmission in the UK. Lancet 2007; 369:1270–1276.
14. Ojo O, Sheehan S, Corcoran GD, et al. Mycobacterium bovis strains causing smear-positive human tuberculosis, Southwest Ireland. Emerg Infect Dis 2008; 14:1931–1934.
15. van der Werf MJ, Borgdorff MW. How to measure the prevalence of tuberculosis in a population. Trop Med Int Health 2007; 12:475–484.
16. Dye C, Bassili A, Bierrenbach AL, et al. Measuring tuberculosis burden, trends, and the impact of control programmes. Lancet Infect Dis 2008; 8:233–243.
17. Dye C, Scheele S, Dolin P, et al. Consensus statement. Global burden of tuberculosis: Estimated incidence, prevalence, and mortality by country. WHO Global Surveillance and Monitoring Project. JAMA 1999; 282:677–686.
18. Hong YP, Kim SJ, Lew WJ, et al. The seventh nationwide tuberculosis prevalence survey in Korea, 1995. Int J Tuberc Lung Dis 1998; 2:27–36.
19. China Tuberculosis Control Collaboration. The effect of tuberculosis control in China. Lancet 2004; 364:417–422.
20. Soemantri S, Senewe FP, Tjandrarini DH, et al. Three-fold reduction in the prevalence of tuberculosis over 25 years in Indonesia. Int J Tuberc Lung Dis 2007; 11:398–404.

21. Tupasi TE, Radhakrishna S, Rivera AB, et al. The 1997 nationwide tuberculosis prevalence survey in the Philippines. Int J Tuberc Lung Dis 1999; 3:471–477.

22. National Center for Tuberculosis and Leprosy Control. National tuberculosis prevalence survey, 2002, Cambodia. Phnom Penh, Cambodia: Royal Government of Cambodia, Ministry of Health, 2005.

23. Sebhatu M, Kiflom B, Seyoum M, et al. Determining the tuberculosis burden in Eritrea: A new approach. Bull World Health Organ 2007; 85:593–599.

24. Dye C. Global epidemiology of tuberculosis. Lancet 2006; 367:938–940.

25. Menzies D. Interpretation of repeated tuberculin tests. Boosting, conversion, and reversion. Am J Respir Crit Care Med 1999; 159(1):15–21.

26. Pai M, Zwerling A, Menzies D. Systematic review: T-cell-based assays for the diagnosis of latent tuberculosis infection: An update. Ann Intern Med 2008; 149:177–184.

27. Lowell AM, Edwards LB, Palmer CE. Tuberculosis. Cambridge, MA: Harvard University Press, 1969:129–166.

28. Roelsgaard E, Iversen E, Blocher C. Tuberculosis in tropical Africa. An Epidemiologic Study. Bull World Health Organ 1964; 30:459–518.

29. Ministry of Health and Welfare, Korean Institute of Tuberculosis. Korean National Tuberculosis Association. Report on the First Tuberculosis Prevalence Survey in Korea – 1965, 1st ed. Soeul: The Korea institute of Tuberculosis, 1966.

30. Shashidhara AN, Chadha VK, Jagannatha PS, et al. The annual risk of tuberculous infection in Orissa State, India. Int J Tuberc Lung Dis 2004; 8:545–51.

31. Chadha VK, Kumar P, Jagannatha PS, et al. Average annual risk of tuberculous infection in India. Int J Tuberc Lung Dis 2005; 9:116–118.

32. Hanifa Y, Grant AD, Lewis J, et al. Prevalence of latent tuberculosis infection among gold miners in South Africa. Int J Tuberc Lung Dis 2009; 13:39–46.

33. Stead WW. Tuberculosis among elderly persons: An outbreak in a nursing home. Ann Intern Med 1981; 94:606–610.

34. Blondet M, Rodríguez W. The prevalence of latent tuberculous infection at nursing homes in the San Juan metropolitan area. P R Health Sci J 2003; 22:343–344.

35. Centers for Disease Control and Prevention (CDC). Tuberculosis transmission in a homeless shelter population–New York, 2000–2003. MMWR Morb Mortal Wkly Rep 2005; 54:149–152.

36. Falchook G, Gaffga C, Eve S, et al. Tuberculosis screening, referral, and treatment in an inner city homeless shelter in Orleans parish. J La State Med Soc 2000; 152(8):398–404.

37. Saunders DL, Olive DM, Wallace SB, et al. Tuberculosis screening in the federal prison system: An opportunity to treat and prevent tuberculosis in foreign-born populations. Public Health Rep 2001; 116:210–218.

38. Chee CB, Teleman MD, Boudville IC, et al. Contact screening and latent TB infection treatment in Singapore correctional facilities. Int J Tuberc Lung Dis 2005; 9(11): 1248–1252.

39. Steenland K, Levine AJ, Sieber K, et al. Incidence of tuberculosis infection among New York State prison employees. Am J Public Health 1997; 87:2012–2014.

40. Stead WW, Lofgren JP, Warren E, et al. Tuberculosis as an endemic and nosocomial infection among the elderly in nursing homes. N Engl J Med 1985; 312:1483–1487.

41. MacIntyre CR, Kendig N, Kummer L, et al. Impact of tuberculosis control measures and crowding on the incidence of tuberculous infection in Maryland prisons. Clin Infect Dis 1997;24:1060–1067.

42. Stead WW. Undetected tuberculosis in prison. Source of infection for community at large. JAMA 1978; 240:2544–2547.

43. Nardell EA. Tuberculosis in homeless, residential care facilities, prisons, nursing homes and other close communities. Semin Respir Infect 1989; 4:206–215.

44. Hill PC, Brookes RH, Fox A, et al. Longitudinal assessment of an ELISPOT test for Mycobacterium tuberculosis infection. PLoS Med 2007; 4:e192.
45. Lienhardt C, Sillah J, Fielding K, et al. Risk factors for tuberculosis infection in children in contact with infectious tuberculosis cases in the Gambia, West Africa. Pediatrics 2003; 111:608–614.
46. Lutong L, Bei Z. Association of prevalence of tuberculin reactions with closeness of contact among household contacts of new smear-positive pulmonary tuberculosis patients. Int J Tuberc Lung Dis 2000; 4:275–277.
47. Bener A, Uduman S, Bin-Othman SA. Factors associated with tuberculin reactivity among children in United Arab Emirates. Respir Med 1996; 90:89–94.
48. Lienhardt C, Fielding K, Sillah J, et al. Risk factors for tuberculosis infection in sub-Saharan Africa: A contact study in The Gambia. Am J Respir Crit Care Med 2003; 168: 448–455.
49. Tornee S, Kaewkungwal J, Fungladda W, et al. Risk factors for tuberculosis infection among household contacts in Bangkok, Thailand. Southeast Asian J Trop Med Public Health 2004; 35:375–383.
50. Sinfield R, Nyirenda M, Haves S, et al. Risk factors for TB infection and disease in young childhood contacts in Malawi. Ann Trop Paediatr 2006; 26:205–213.
51. Rathi SK, Akhtar S, Rahbar MH, et al. Prevalence and risk factors associated with tuberculin skin test positivity among household contacts of smear-positive pulmonary tuberculosis cases in Umerkot, Pakistan. Int J Tuberc Lung Dis 2002; 6:851–857.
52. Marks SM, Taylor Z, Qualls NL, et al. Outcomes of contact investigations of infectious tuberculosis patients. Am J Respir Crit Care Med 2000; 162:2033–2038.
53. Rodrigo T, Caylà JA, García de Olalla P, et al. Characteristics of tuberculosis patients who generate secondary cases. Int J Tuberc Lung Dis 1997; 1:352–357.
54. McPhedran FM, Opie EL. The spread of tuberculosis in families. Am J Hyg 1935; 22:565–643.
55. Hertzberg G. The infectiousness of human tuberculosis. Acta Tuberc Scand 1957; 38(S-1):1–146.
56. Loudon RG, Williamson J, Johnson JM. An analysis of 3485 tuberculosis contacts in the city of Edinburgh during 1954–1955. Am Rev Tuberc 1958; 77:623–643.
57. Grzybowski S, Barnett GD, Styblo K. Contacts of cases of active pulmonary tuberculosis. Bull Int Union Tuberc 1975; 50:90–106.
58. van Geuns HA, Meijer J, Styblo K. Results of contact examination in Rotterdam, 1967–1969. Bull Int Union Tuberc 1975; 50:107–121.
59. Plunkett RE, Weber GW, Siegal W, et al. Development of tuberculosis in a controlled environment. Am J Public Health 1940; 30:229–236.
60. Beeuwkes H, Hahn RG, Putnam P. A survey of persons exposed to tuberculosis in the household: The necessity for prolonged observation of contacts. Am Rev Tuberc 1942; 45:165–193.
61. Twinam CW, Pope AS. Pulmonary tuberculosis resulting from extra-familial contacts. Am J Public Health 1942; 32:1215–1218.
62. Puffer RR, Stewart HC, Gass RS. Tuberculosis in household associates: The influence of age and relationship. Am Rev Tuberc 1945; 52:89–103.
63. Blahd M, Leslie EI, Rosenthal SR. Infectiousness of the "closed case" in tuberculosis. Am J Public Health 1946; 36:723–726.
64. Bluhm I. Is there any risk of infection from gastric lavage positives? Acta Tuberc Scand 1947; 21:70–86.
65. Ross JD, Willison JC. The relationship between tuberculin reactions and the later development of tuberculosis: An investigation among Edinburgh school children in 1960–1970. Tubercle 1971; 52:258–265.

66. Riley RL, Moodie AS. Infectivity of patients with pulmonary tuberculosis in inner city homes. Am Rev Respir Dis 1974; 110:810–812.
67. Liippo KK, Kulmala K, Tala EO. Focusing tuberculosis contact tracing by smear grading of index cases. Am Rev Respir Dis 1993; 148(1):235–236.
68. Tornee S, Kaewkungwal J, Fungladda W, et al. The association between environmental factors and tuberculosis infection among household contacts. Southeast Asian J Trop Med Public Health 2005; 36(suppl 4):221–224.
69. Lin X, Chongsuvivatwong V, Lin L, et al. Dose-response relationship between treatment delay of smear-positive tuberculosis patients and intra-household transmission: A cross-sectional study. Trans R Soc Trop Med Hyg 2008; 102:797–804.
70. Madhi F, Fuhrman C, Monnet I, et al. Transmission of tuberculosis from adults to children in a Paris suburb. Pediatr Pulmonol 2002; 34:159–163.
71. Ramakrishnan CV, Andrews RH, Devadatta S, et al. Influence of segregation of tuberculous patients for one year on the attack rate of tuberculosis in a 2-year period in close family contacts in South India. Bull World Health Organ 1961; 24:129–148.
72. Kamat SR, Dawson JJY, Devadatta S, et al. A controlled study of the influence of segregation of tuberculous patients for one year on the attack rate of tuberculosis in a 5-year period in close family contacts in South India. Bull World Health Organ 1966; 34:517–532.
73. Gunnels JJ, Bates JH, Swindoll H. Infectivity of sputum-positive tuberculous patients on chemotherapy. Am Rev Respir Dis 1974; 109:323–330.
74. Brooks SM, Lassiter NL, Young EC. A pilot study concerning the infection risk of sputum positive tuberculosis patients on chemotherapy. Am Rev Respir Dis 1973; 108:799–804.
75. Aziz A, Ishaq M, Akhwand R. Infection risk of sputum positive tuberculosis patients to their family contacts with and without chemotherapy. J Pak Med Assoc 1985; 35:249–252.
76. Loudon RG, Spohn SK. Cough frequency and infectivity in patients with pulmonary tuberculosis. Am Rev Respir Dis 1969; 99:109–111.
77. Bates JH. Potts WE, Lewis M. Epidemiology of primary tuberculosis in an industrial school. N Engl J Med 1965; 272:714–717.
78. Cruciani M, Malena M, Bosco O, et al. The impact of human immunodeficiency virus type 1 on infectiousness of tuberculosis: A meta-analysis. Clin Infect Dis 2001; 33:1922–1930.
79. Nunn P, Mungai M, Nyamwaya J, et al. The effect of human immunodeficiency virus type 1 on the infectiousness of tuberculosis. Tuber Lung Dis. 1994; 75:25–32.
80. Topley JM, Maher D, Nyong'onya M. Transmission of tuberculosis to contacts of sputum positive adults in Malawi. Arch Dis Child 1996; 74:140–143.
81. Espinal MA, Perez EN, Baez J, et al. Infectiousness of Mycobacterium tuberculosis in HIV-1 infected patients with tuberculosis: A prospective study. Lancet 2000; 355:275–280.
82. Manoff S, Cauthen GM, Stoneburnet RL, et al. TB patients with AIDS: Are they more likely to spread TB? In: Program and abstracts: IV International Conference on AIDS (Stockholm). Washington, DC. 1988.
83. Beck-Sagué C, Dooley S, Hutton MD, et al. Hospital outbreak of multidrug-resistant Mycobacterium tuberculosis infections. Factors in transmission to staff and HIV-infected patients. JAMA 1992; 268:1280–1286.
84. Dooley SW, Villarino M, Lawrence M, et al. Nosocomial transmission of tuberculosis in a hospital unit for HIV-infected patients. JAMA 1992; 267:2632–2655.
85. Di Perri G, Cadeo GP, Castelli F, et al. Transmission of HIV-associated tuberculosis to healthcare workers. Infect Control Hosp Epidemiol 1993; 14:67–72.
86. Ikeda RM, Birkhead GS, DiFerdinando GT, et al. Nosocomial tuberculosis: An outbreak of a strain resistant to seven drugs. Infect Control Hosp Epidemiol 1995; 16:152–159.
87. Wenger P, Otten J, Breeden A, et al. Control of nosocomial transmission of multidrug-resistant Mycobacterium tuberculosis among healthcare workers and HIV-infected patients. Lancet 1995; 345:235–240.

88. Standaert B, Niragira F, Kadende P, et al. The association of tuberculosis and HIV infection in Burundi. AIDS Res Hum Retroviruses 1989; 5:247–251.

89. Elliott AM, Hayes RJ, Halwiindi B, et al. The impact of HIV on infectiousness of pulmonary tuberculosis: A community study in Zambia. AIDS 1993; 7:981–987.

90. Klausner JD, Ryder RW, Baende E, et al. Mycobacterium tuberculosis in household contacts of human immunodeficiency virus type 1–seropositive patients with active pulmonary tuberculosis in Kinshasa, Zaire. J Infect Dis 1993; 168:106–111.

91. Cauthen GM, Dooley SW, Onorato IM, et al. Transmission of Mycobacterium tuberculosis from tuberculosis patients with HIV infection and AIDS. Am J Epidemiol 1996; 14: 69–77.

92. Cayla JA, Garcia de Olalla P, Galdos-Tanguis H, et al. The influence of intravenous drug use and HIV infection in the transmission of tuberculosis. AIDS 1996; 10:95–100.

93. Guwatudde D, Nakeeto MK, Musoke P, et al. The impact of HIV-1 on transmission of tuberculosis in Ugandan households [abstract 13258]. In: Conference record of the 12th World AIDS Conference (Geneva). Geneva: Marathon Multimedia, 1998:137.

94. Zahnow K, Matts JP, Hillman D, et al. Rates of tuberculosis infection in healthcare workers providing service to HIV infected populations. Infect Control Hosp Epidemiol 1998; 19:829–835.

95. Garcia Ordonez MA, Colmenero Castillo JD, Sanchez Simonet MV, et al. Rentabilidad del estudio de los contactos familiares de enfermos con tuberculosis coinfectados por el virus de la immunodeficiencia humana. Rev Clin Esp 1999; 199:275–279.

96. O'Reilly LM, Daborn CJ. The epidemiology of Mycobacterium bovis infections in animals and man: A review. Tubercle Lung Dis 1995; 76(suppl 1):1–46.

97. Collins CH, Yates MD, Grange JM. A study of bovine strains of Mycobacterium tuberculosis isolated from humans in south-east England, 1977–1979. Tubercle 1981; 62:113–116.

98. de Jong BC, Hill PC, Aiken A, et al. Progression to active tuberculosis, but not transmission, varies by Mycobacterium tuberculosis lineage in The Gambia. J Infect Dis 2008; 198:1037–1043.

99. Lillebaek T, Andersen AB, Dirksen A, et al. Mycobacterium tuberculosis Beijing genotype. Emerg Infect Dis 2003; 9:1553–1557.

100. Glynn JR, Whiteley J, Bifani PJ, et al. Worldwide occurrence of Beijing/W strains of Mycobacterium tuberculosis: A systematic review. Emerg Infect Dis 2002; 8:843–849.

101. Sinsimer D, Huet G, Manca C, et al. The phenolic glycolipid of Mycobacterium tuberculosis differentially modulates the early host cytokine response but does not in itself confer hypervirulence. Infect Immun 2008; 76:3027–3036.

102. Caws M, Thwaites G, Dunstan S, et al. The influence of host and bacterial genotype on the development of disseminated disease with Mycobacterium tuberculosis. PLoS Pathog 2008; 4:e1000034.

103. Hanekom M, van der Spuy GD, Streicher E, et al. A recently evolved sublineage of the Mycobacterium tuberculosis Beijing strain family is associated with an increased ability to spread and cause disease. J Clin Microbiol 2007; 45:1483–1490.

104. Middlebrook G, Cohn ML. Some observations on the pathogenicity of isoniazid-resistant variants of tubercle bacilli. Science 1953; 118:297–299.

105. Ordway DJ, Sonnenberg MG, Donahue SA, et al. Drug-resistant strains of Mycobacterium tuberculosis exhibit a range of virulence for mice. Infect Immun 1995; 63:741–743.

106. Billington OJ, McHugh TD, Gillespie SH. Physiological cost of rifampin resistance induced in vitro in Mycobacterium tuberculosis. Antimicrob Agents Chemother 1999; 43: 1866–1869.

107. Pym AS, Saint-Joanis B, Cole ST. Effect of katG mutations on the virulence of Mycobacterium tuberculosis and the implication for transmission in humans. Infect Immun 2002; 70:4955–4960.

108. Snider DE Jr, Kelly GD, Cauthen GM, et al. Infection and disease among contacts of tuberculosis cases with drug-resistant and drug-susceptible bacilli. Am Rev Respir Dis 1985; 132:125–132.

109. Teixeira L, Perkins MD, Johnson JL, et al. Infection and disease among household contacts of patients with multidrug-resistant tuberculosis. Int J Tuberc Lung Dis 2001; 5:321–328.

110. Sutherland I, Fayers PM. The association of the risk of tuberculous infection with age. Bull Int Union Tuberc 1975; 50:70–81.

111. Mossong J, Hens N, Jit M, et al. Social contacts and mixing patterns relevant to the spread of infectious diseases. PLoS Med 2008; 5:e74.

112. Borgdorff MW, Nagelkerke NJ, van Soolingen D, et al. Transmission of tuberculosis between people of different ages in The Netherlands: An analysis using DNA fingerprinting. Int J Tuberc Lung Dis 1999; 3:202–206.

113. Holmes CB, Hausler H, Nunn P. A review of sex differences in the epidemiology of tuberculosis. Int J Tuberc Lung Dis 1998; 2:96–104.

114. Woeltje KF, Kilo CM, Johnson K, et al. Tuberculin skin testing of hospitalized patients. Infect Control Hosp Epidemiol 1997; 18:561–565.

115. Stead WW, Senner JW, Reddick WT, et al. Racial differences in susceptibility to infection by Mycobacterium tuberculosis. N Engl J Med 1990; 322:422–427.

116. Hoge CW, Fisher L, Donnell HD Jr, et al. Risk factors for transmission of Mycobacterium tuberculosis in a primary school outbreak: Lack of racial difference in susceptibility to infection. Am J Epidemiol 1994; 139:520–530.

117. Leung CC, Yew WW, Law WS, et al. Smoking and tuberculosis among silicotic patients. Eur Respir J 2007; 29:745–750.

118. Weis SE, Pogoda JM, Yang Z, et al. Transmission dynamics of tuberculosis in Tarrant county, Texas. Am J Respir Crit Care Med 2002; 166(1):36–42.

119. Klovdahl AS, Graviss EA, Yaganehdoost A, et al. Networks and tuberculosis: An undetected community outbreak involving public places. Soc Sci Med 2001; 52(5):681–694.

120. García-García M, Palacios-Martínez M, Ponce-de-León A, et al. The role of core groups in transmitting Mycobacterium tuberculosis in a high prevalence community in Southern Mexico. Int J Tuberc Lung Dis 2000; 4(1):12–17.

121. Yaganehdoost A, Graviss EA, Ross MW, et al. Complex transmission dynamics of clonally related virulent Mycobacterium tuberculosis associated with barhopping by predominantly human immunodeficiency virus-positive gay men. J Infect Dis 1999; 180(4): 1245–1251.

122. Diel R, Schneider S, Meywald-Walter K, et al. Epidemiology of tuberculosis in Hamburg, Germany: Long-term population-based analysis applying classical and molecular epidemiological techniques. J Clin Microbiol 2002; 40:532–539.

123. Classen CN, Warren R, Richardson M, et al. Impact of social interactions in the community on the transmission of tuberculosis in a high incidence area. Thorax 1999; 54:136–140.

124. Zolnir-Dovc M, Poljak M, Erzen D, et al. Molecular epidemiology of tuberculosis in Slovenia: Results of a one-year (2001) nation-wide study. Scand J Infect Dis 2003; 35:863–868.

125. Lönnroth K, Williams BG, Stadlin S, et al. Alcohol use as a risk factor for tuberculosis – a systematic review. BMC Public Health 2008; 8:289.

126. Wallgren A. The time-table of tuberculosis. Tubercle 1948; 29:245–251.

127. Ferebee SH. Controlled chemoprophylaxis trials in tuberculosis. A general review. Bibl Tuberc 1970; 26:28–106.

128. D'Arcy Hart P, Sutherland I. BCG and vole bacillus vaccines in the prevention of tuberculosis in adolescence and early adult life. Final Report to the Medical Research Council. Br Med J 1977; 2:293–295.

129. Comstock GW, Livesay VT, Woolpert SF. The prognosis of a positive tuberculin reaction in childhood and adolescence. Am J Epidemiol 1974; 99:131–138.

130. Dubos RJ, Dubos J. The White Plague: Tuberculosis, Man and Society. Camden, NJ: Rutgers University Press, 1952.
131. Nagelkerke NJ, de Vlas SJ, MacDonald KS, et al. Tuberculosis and sexually transmitted infections. Emerg Infect Dis 2004; 10(11):2055–2056.
132. National Tuberculosis Institute. Tuberculosis in a rural population of South India: A five-year epidemiological study. Bull World Health Organ 1974; 51:473–488.
133. Comstock GW, Ferebee SH, Hammes LM. A controlled trial of community-wide isoniazid prophylaxis in Alaska. Am Rev Respir Dis 1967; 95:935–943.
134. Gryzbowski S, Allen EA. The challenge of tuberculosis in decline. A study based on the epidemiology of tuberculosis in Ontario, Canada. Am Rev Respir Dis 1964; 90:707–720.
135. Gedde-Dahl T. Tuberculous infection in the light of tuberculin matriculati. Am J Hyg 1952; 56:139–214.
136. Groth-Petersen E, Knudsen J, Wilbek E. Epidemiological basis of tuberculosis eradication in an advanced country. Bull World Health Organ 1959; 21:5–49.
137. Comstock GW, Edwards PQ. The competing risks of tuberculosis and hepatitis for adult tuberculin reactors. Am Rev Respir Dis 1975; 111:573–577.
138. Snider D. Pregnancy and tuberculosis. Chest 1984; 86(3 suppl):10S–13S.
139. Hamadeh MA, Glassroth J. Tuberculosis and pregnancy. Chest 1992; 101:1114–1120.
140. Schwabe KH, Dobstadt HP. Beitr Klin Erforsch Tuberk Lungenkr. 1966;134(2):75–96.
141. Hedvall E. Pregnancy and tuberculosis. Acta Med Scand Suppl 1953; 286:1–101.
142. Crombie JB. Pregnancy and pulmonary tuberculosis. Br J Tuberc Dis Chest 1954; 48(2):97–101.
143. Edge JR. Pulmonary tuberculosis and pregnancy. Br Med J 1952; 1:845–847.
144. Cohen JD, Patton EA, Badger TL. The tuberculous mother; a five- to twenty-year follow-up of 149 women with 401 full-term pregnancies. Am Rev Tuberc 1952; 65:1–23.
145. Palmer CE, Jablon S, Edwards PQ. Tuberculosis morbidity of young men in relation to tuberculin sensitivity and body build. Am Rev Tuberc Pulm Dis 1957; 76:517–539.
146. Edwards LB, Livesay VT, Acquaviva FA, et al. Height, weight, tuberculous infection, and tuberculous disease. Arch Environ Health 1971; 22:106–112.
147. Tverdal A. Height, weight and incidence of tuberculosis. Bull Int Union Tuberc Lung Dis 1988; 63:16–18.
148. Shetty N, Shemko M, Vaz M, et al. An epidemiological evaluation of risk factors for tuberculosis in South India: A matched case control study. Int J Tuberc Lung Dis 2006; 10:80–86.
149. Allen S, Batungwanayo J, Kerlikowske K, et al. Two-year incidence of tuberculosis in cohorts of HIV-infected and uninfected urban Rwandan women. Am Rev Respir Dis 1992; 146:1439–1444.
150. Jick SS, Lieberman ES, Rahman MU, et al. Glucocorticoid use, other associated factors, and the risk of tuberculosis. Arthritis Rheum 2006; 55:19–26.
151. Cegielski JP, McMurray DN. The relationship between malnutrition and tuberculosis: Evidence from studies in humans and experimental animals. Int J Tuberc Lung Dis 2004; 8:286–298.
152. Leung CC, Lam TH, Chan WM, et al. Lower risk of tuberculosis in obesity. Arch Intern Med 2007; 167:1297–1304.
153. Rondinone CM. Adipocyte-derived hormones, cytokines, and mediators. Endocrine 2006; 29:81–90.
154. Antonucci G, Girardi E, Raviglione M, et al. Guidelines of tuberculosis preventive therapy for HIV-infected persons: A prospective, multicentre study. GISTA (Gruppo Italiano di Studio Tubercolosi e AIDS). Eur Respir J 2001; 18:369–375.
155. Selwyn PA, Hartel D, Lewis VA, et al. A prospective study of the risk of tuberculosis among intravenous drug users with human immunodeficiency virus infection. N Engl J Med 1989; 320:545–545.

156. Antonucci G, Girardi E, Raviglione MC, et al. Risk factors for tuberculosis in HIV-infected persons. A prospective cohort study. The Gruppo Italiano di Studio Tubercolosis e AIDS (GISTA). JAMA 1995; 274:143–148.

157. Salami AK, Katibi IA. Human immunodeficiency virus-associated tuberculosis: Pattern and trend in the University of Ilorin Teaching Hospital. Afr J Med Med Sci 2006; 35: 457–460.

158. Whalen CC, Johnson JL, Okwera A, et al. Trial of three regimens to prevent tuberculosis in Ugandan adults infected with the human immunodeficiency virus. Uganda-Case Western Reserve University Research Collaboration. N Engl J Med 1997; 337:801–808.

159. Moreno S, Jarrin I, Iribarren JA, et al; CoRIS-MD. Incidence and risk factors for tuberculosis in HIV-positive subjects by HAART status. Int J Tuberc Lung Dis 2008; 12:1393–1400.

160. Girardi E, Sabin CA, d'Arminio Monforte A, et al.; Antiretroviral Therapy Cohort Collaboration. Incidence of tuberculosis among HIV-infected patients receiving highly active antiretroviral therapy in Europe and North America. Clin Infect Dis 2005; 41:1772–1782.

161. Gupta BN, Mathur N, Mahendra PN, et al. A study of household environmental risk factors pertaining to respiratory diseases. Energy Environment Monitor 1997; 13:61–67.

162. Yu GP, Hsieh CC, Peng J. Risk factors associated with the prevalence of pulmonary tuberculosis among sanitary workers in Shanghai. Tubercle 1988; 69:105–112.

163. Adelstein AM, Rimington J. Smoking and pulmonary tuberculosis: An analysis based on a study of volunteers for mass miniature radiography. Tubercle 1967; 48:219–226.

164. Shah JR, Warawadekar MS, Deshmukh PA, et al. Institutional survey of pulmonary tuberculosis with special reference to smoking habits. Indian J Med Sci 1959; 13:381–392.

165. Lienhardt C, Fielding K, Sillah JS, et al. Investigation of the risk factors for tuberculosis: A case-control study in three countries in West Africa. Int J Epidemiol 1995; 34:914–923.

166. Leung CC, Yew WW, Chan CK, et al. Smoking and tuberculosis in Hong Kong. Int J Tuberc Lung Dis 2003; 7:980–986.

167. Buskin SE, Gale JL, Weiss NS, et al. Tuberculosis risk factors in adults in King County, Washington, 1988 through 1990. Am J Public Health 1994; 84:1750–1756.

168. Lewis JG, Chamberlain DA. Alcohol consumption and smoking habits in male patients with pulmonary tuberculosis. Br J Prev Soc Med 1963; 17:149–152.

169. Brown KE, Campbell AH. Tobacco, alcohol and tuberculosis. Br J Dis Chest 1961; 55:150–158.

170. Wang GJ, Sleigh A, Zhou G, et al. Nonbiologic risk factors of pulmonary tuberculosis among adults in Henan: A case-control study. Zhonghua Liu Xing Bing Xue Za Zhi 2005; 26:92–96.

171. Crampin AC, Glynn JR, Floyd S, et al. Tuberculosis and gender: Exploring the patterns in a case control study in Malawi. Int J Tuberc Lung Dis 2004; 8:194–203.

172. Kolappan C, Gopi PG. Tobacco smoking and pulmonary tuberculosis. Thorax 2002; 57:964–966.

173. Tekkel M, Rahu M, Loit HM, et al. Risk factors for pulmonary tuberculosis in Estonia. Int J Tuberc Lung Dis 2002; 6:887–894.

174. Tocque K, Bellis MA, Beeching NJ, et al. A case-control study of lifestyle risk factors associated with tuberculosis in Liverpool, North-West England. Eur Respir J 2001; 18:959–964.

175. Gupta D, Aggarwal AN, Kumar S, et al. Smoking increases risk of pulmonary tuberculosis. J Environ Med 2001; 3:65–70.

176. Dong B, Ge N, Zhou Y. Smoking and alchohol as risk factor of pulmonary tuberculosis in Chengdu: A matched case-control study. Hua Xi Yi Ke Da Xue Xue Bao 2001; 32:104–106.

177. Alcaide J, Altet MN, Plans P, et al. Cigarette smoking as a risk factor for tuberculosis in young adults: A case-control study. Tuber Lung Dis 1996; 77:112–116.

178. Ariyothai N, Podhipak A, Akarasewi P, et al. Cigarette smoking and its relation to pulmonary tuberculosis in adults. Southeast Asian J Trop Med Public Health 2004; 35:219–227.

179. Lowe CR, An association between smoking and respiratory tuberculosis. Br Med J 1956; 12:1081–1086.
180. Leung CC, Li T, Lam TH, et al. Smoking and tuberculosis among the elderly in Hong Kong. Am J Respir Crit Care Med 2004; 170:1027–1033.
181. Tipayamongkholgul M, Podhipak A, Chearskul S, et al. Factors associated with the development of tuberculosis in BCG immunized children. Southeast Asian J Trop Med Public Health 2005; 36:145–150.
182. Altet MN, Alcaide J, Plans P, et al. Passive smoking and risk of pulmonary tuberculosis in children immediately following infection. A case-control study. Tuber Lung Dis 1966; 77:537–544.
183. Lin HH, Ezzati M, Murray M. Tobacco smoke, indoor air pollution and tuberculosis: A systematic review and meta-analysis. PLoS Med 2007; 4:e20.
184. Mishra VK, Retherford RD, Smith KR. Biomass cooking fuels and prevalence of tuberculosis in India. Int J Infect Dis 1999; 3:119–129.
185. Perez-Padilla R, Perez-Guzman C, Baez-Saldana R, et al. Cooking with biomass stoves and tuberculosis: A case control study. Int J Tuberc Lung Dis 2001; 5:441–447.
186. Paul R. Silicosis in northern Rhodesia copper miners. Arch Environ Health 1961; 2:96–109.
187. Westerholm P, Ahlmark A, Maasing R, et al. Silicosis and risk of lung cancer or lung tuberculosis: A cohort study. Environ Res 1986; 41:339–350.
188. teWaternaude JM, Ehrlich RI, Churchyard GJ, et al. Tuberculosis and silica exposure in South African gold miners. Occup Environ Med 2006; 63:187–192.
189. Cowie RL. The epidemiology of tuberculosis in gold miners with silicosis. Am J Respir Crit Care Med 1994; 150:1460–1462.
190. Kleinschmidt I, Churchyard G. Variation in incidences of tuberculosis in subgroups of South African gold miners. Occup Environ Med 1997; 54:636–641.
191. Hnizdo E, Murray J. Risk of pulmonary tuberculosis relative to silicosis and exposure to silica dust in South African gold miners. Occup Environ Med 1998; 55:496–502. [Erratum in: Occup Environ Med 1999; 56(3):215–216.]
192. Corbett EL, Churchyard GJ, Clayton TC, et al. HIV infection and silicosis: The impact of two potent risk factors on the incidence of mycobacterial disease in South African miners. AIDS 2000; 14:2759–2768.
193. Jeon CY, Murray MB. Diabetes mellitus increases the risk of active tuberculosis: A systematic review of 13 observational studies. PLoS Med 2008; 5(7):e152.
194. Stevenson CR, Critchley JA, Forouhi NG, et al. Diabetes and the risk of tuberculosis: A neglected threat to public health? Chronic Illn 2007; 3:228–245.
195. Kim SJ, Hong YP, Lew WJ, et al. Incidence of pulmonary tuberculosis among diabetics. Tuber Lung Dis 1995; 76:529–533.
196. Chen CH, Lian JD, Cheng CH, et al. Mycobacterium tuberculosis infection following renal transplantation in Taiwan. Transpl Infect Dis 2006; 8:148–156.
197. Pablos-Mendez A, Blustein J, Knirsch CA. The role of diabetes mellitus in the higher prevalence of tuberculosis among Hispanics. Am J Public Health 1997; 87:574–579.
198. Perez A, Brown HS III, Restrepo BI. Association between tuberculosis and diabetes in the Mexican border and non-border regions of Texas. Am J Trop Med Hyg 2006; 74:604–611.
199. Brassard P, Kezouh A, Suissa S. Antirheumatic drugs and the risk of tuberculosis. Clin Infect Dis 2006; 43:717–722.
200. John GT, Shankar V, Abraham AM, et al. Risk factors for post-transplant tuberculosis. Kidney Int 2001; 60:1148–1153.
201. Mori MA, Leonardson G, Welty TK. The benefits of isoniazid chemoprophylaxis and risk factors for tuberculosis among Oglala Sioux Indians. Arch Intern Med 1992; 152:547–550.
202. Rosenman KD, Hall N. Occupational risk factors for developing tuberculosis. Am J Ind Med 1996; 30:148–154.

203. Coker R, McKee M, Atun R, et al. Risk factors for pulmonary tuberculosis in Russia: Case-control study. BMJ 2006; 332:85–87.
204. Ponce-De-Leon A, Garcia-Garcia Md Mde L, Garcia-Sancho MC, et al. Tuberculosis and diabetes in southern Mexico. Diabetes Care 2004; 27:1584–1590.
205. Dyck RF, Klomp H, Marciniuk DD, et al. The relationship between diabetes and tuberculosis in Saskatchewan. Can J Public Health 2007; 98:55–59.
206. Lee MS, Leung CC, Kam KM, et al. Early and late tuberculosis risks among close contacts in Hong Kong. Int J Tuberc Lung Dis 2008; 13:281–287.
207. Personal Communication. Christie Jeon.
208. Espelt A, Borrell C, Roskam AJ, et al. Socioeconomic inequalities in diabetes mellitus across Europe at the beginning of the 21st century. Diabetologia 2008; 51:1971–1979.
209. Kaplan MH, Armstrong D, Rosen P. Tuberculosis complicating neoplastic disease. Cancer 1974; 33:850–858.
210. Feld R, Bodey GP, Gröschel D. Mycobacteriosis in patients with malignant disease. Arch Intern Med 1976; 136:67–70.
211. Kim HR, Hwang SS, Ro YK, et al. Solid-organ malignancy as a risk factor for tuberculosis. Respirology 2008; 13(3):413–419.
212. Kamboj M, Sepkowitz KA. The risk of tuberculosis in patients with cancer. Clin Infect Dis 2006; 42(11):1592–1595.
213. Andrew OT, Schoenfeld PY, Hopewell PC, et al. Tuberculosis in patients with end-stage renal disease. Am J Med 1980; 68:59–65.
214. Belcon MC, Smith EKM, Kahana LM, et al. Tuberculosis in dialysis patients. Clin Nephrol 1982; 17:14–18.
215. Lundin AP, Adler AJ, Berlyne GM, et al. Tuberculosis in patients undergoing maintenance hemodialysis. Am J Med 1979; 67:597–602.
216. Pradhna RP, Katz LA, Nidus BD, et al. Tuberculosis in dialyzed patients. J Am Med Assoc 1974; 229:798–800.
217. Rutsky EA, Rostand SG. Mycobacteriosis in patients with chronic renal failure. Arch Intern Med 1980; 140:57–61.
218. Sasaki S, Akiba T, Suenaga M, et al. Ten years' survey of dialysis-associated tuberculosis. Nephron 1979; 24:141–145.
219. Gardam MA, Keystone EC, Menzies R, et al. Anti-tumour necrosis factor agents and tuberculosis risk: Mechanisms of action and clinical management. Lancet Infect Dis 2003; 3(3):148–155.
220. Horne NW. A critical evaluation of corticosteroids in tuberculosis. Adv Tuberc Res 1966; 15:1–54.
221. Haanaes OC, Bergmann A. Tuberculosis emerging in patients treated with corticosteroids. Eur J Respir Dis 1983; 64:294–297.
222. Schatz M, Patterson R, Kloner R, et al. The prevalence of tuberculosis and positive tuberculinskin tests in a steroid-treated asthmatic population. Ann Intern Med 1976; 84:261–265.
223. Smyllie HC, Connolly CK. Incidence of serious complications of corticosteroid therapy in respiratory disease. A retrospective survey of patients at Brompton Hospital. Thorax 1968; 23:571–581.
224. Thorn PA, Brookes VS, Waterhouse JAH. Peptic ulcer, partial gastrectomy, and pulmonary tuberculosis. Br Med J 1956; 1:603–608.
225. Pickleman JR, Evans LS, Kane JM, et al. Tuberculosis after jejunoileal bypass. J Am Med Assoc 1975; 234:744.
226. Bruce RM, Wise L. Tuberculosis after jejunoileal bypass for obesity. Ann Intern Med 1977; 87:574–576.
227. Cummins SL. Tuberculosis in primitive tribes and its bearing on the tuberculosis of civilized communities. Int J Publ Health 1920; 1:137–171.

228. Sousa AO, Salem JI, Lee FK, et al. An epidemic of tuberculosis with a high rate of tuberculin anergy among a population previously unexposed to tuberculosis, the Yanomami Indians of the Brazilian Amazon. Proc Natl Acad Sci U S A 1997; 94:13227–13232.

229. Comstock GW. Tuberculosis in twins: A re-analysis of the Prophit survey. Am Rev Respir Dis 1978; 117:621–624.

230. Beddall AC, Hill FGH, George RH. Haemophilia and tuberculosis. Lancet 1983; 1:1226.

231. Beddall AC, Hill FGH, George RH, et al. Unusually high incidence of tuberculosis among boys with haemophilia during an outbreak of the disease in hospital. J Clin Pathol 1985; 38:1163–1165.

232. Overfield T, Klauber R. Prevalence of tuberculosis in Eskimos having blood group B gene. Human Biology 1980; 52:87–92.

233. Alcais A, Fieschi C, Abel L, et al. Tuberculosis in children and adults: Two distinct genetic diseases. J Exp Med 2005; 202;1617–1621.

234. Fieschi C. Mendelian susceptibility to mycobacterial disease: Defects in the IL-12/IFNgamma pathway. Presse Med 2006; 35:879–886.

235. Bustamante J, Picard C, Fieschi C, et al. A novel X-linked recessive form of Mendelian susceptibility to mycobacterial disease. J Med Genet 2007; 44:e65.

236. Fortin A, Abel L, Casanova JL, et al. Host genetics of mycobacterial diseases in mice and men: Forward genetic studies of BCG-osis and tuberculosis. Annu Rev Genomics Hum Genet 2007; 8:163–192.

237. Poon A, Schurr E. The NRAMP genes and human susceptibility to common diseases. In: Cellier M, Gros P, eds. The NRAMP Family. New York: Kluwer Acad./Plenum, 2004:29–43.

238. Li HT, Zhang TT, Zhou YQ, et al. SLC11A1 (formerly NRAMP1) gene polymorphisms and tuberculosis susceptibility: A meta-analysis. Int J Tuberc Lung Dis 2006; 10:3–12.

239. Pan H, Yan BS, Rojas M, et al. Ipr1 gene mediates innate immunity to tuberculosis. Nature 2005; 434:767–772.

240. Tosh K, Campbell SJ, Fielding K, et al. Variants in the SP110 gene are associated with genetic susceptibility to tuberculosis in West Africa. Proc Natl Acad Sci U S A 2006; 103:10364–10368.

241. Thye T, Browne EN, Chinbuah MA, et al. No associations of human pulmonary tuberculosis with Sp110 variants. J Med Genet 2006; 43:e32.

242. Casanova JL, Abel L. Genetic dissection of immunity to mycobacteria: The human model. Annu Rev Immunol 2002; 20:581–620.

243. Delgado JC, Baena A, Thim S, et al. Aspartic acid homozygosity at codon 57 of HLA-DQ beta is associated with susceptibility to pulmonary tuberculosis in Cambodia. J Immunol 2006; 176:1090–1097.

244. Goldfeld AE, Delgado JC, Thim S, et al. Association of an HLA-DQ allele with clinical tuberculosis. JAMA 1998; 279:226–228.

245. Garred P, Richter C, Andersen AB, et al. Mannan-binding lectin in the sub-Saharan HIV and tuberculosis epidemics. Scand J Immunol 1997; 46:204–208.

246. Hoal-Van Helden EG, Epstein J, Victor TC, et al. Mannose-binding protein B allele confers protection against tuberculous meningitis. Pediatr Res 1999; 45:459–464.

247. Yim JJ, Lee HW, Lee HS, et al. The association between microsatellite polymorphisms in intron II of the human Toll-like receptor 2 gene and tuberculosis among Koreans. Genes Immun 2006; 7(2):150–155.

248. Ben-Ali M, Barbouche MR, Bousnina S, et al. Toll-like receptor 2 Arg677Trp polymorphism is associated with susceptibility to tuberculosis in Tunisian patients. Clin Diagn Lab Immunol 2004; 11(3):625–626.

249. Thuong NT, Hawn TR, Thwaites GE, et al. A polymorphism in human TLR2 is associated with increased susceptibility to tuberculous meningitis. Genes Immun 2007; 8:422–428.

250. Tailleux L, Schwartz O, Herrmann JL, et al. DC-SIGN is the major Mycobacterium tuberculosis receptor on human dendritic cells. J Exp Med 2003; 197(1):1–5.

251. Barreiro LB, Neyrolles O, Babb CL, et al. Promoter variation in the DC-SIGN-encoding gene CD209 is associated with tuberculosis. PLoS Med 2006; 3:e20.

252. Flores-Villanueva PO, Ruiz-Morales JA, Song CH, et al. A functional promoter polymorphism in monocyte chemoattractant protein-1 is associated with increased susceptibility to pulmonary tuberculosis. J Exp Med 2005; 202:1649–1658.

253. Jamieson SE, Miller EN, Black GF, et al. Evidence for a cluster of genes on chromosome 17q11-q21 controlling susceptibility to tuberculosis and leprosy in Brazilians. Genes Immun 2005; 5:46–57.

254. Delgado JC, Baena A, Thim S, et al. Ethnic-specific genetic associations with pulmonary tuberculosis. J Infect Dis 2002; 186:1463–1468.

255. Johnson R, Warren R, Strauss OJ, et al. An outbreak of drug-resistant tuberculosis caused by a Beijing strain in the western Cape, South Africa. Int J Tuberc Lung Dis 2006; 10:1412–1414.

256. Toungoussova OS, Mariandyshev A, Bjune G, et al. Molecular epidemiology and drug resistance of Mycobacterium tuberculosis isolates in the Archangel prison in Russia: Predominance of the W-Beijing clone family. Clin Infect Dis 2003; 37:665–672.

257. Gagneux S, Burgos MV, DeRiemer K, et al. Impact of bacterial genetics on the transmission of isoniazid-resistant Mycobacterium tuberculosis. PLoS Pathog 2006; 2:e61.

258. Cohn ML, Kovitz C, Oda U, et al. Studies on isoniazid and tubercle bacilli. II. The growth requirements, catalase activities, and pathogenic properties of isoniazid-resistant mutants. Am Rev Tuberc 1954; 70:641–664.

259. Gagneux S, Long CD, Small PM, et al. The competitive cost of antibiotic resistance in Mycobacterium tuberculosis. Science 2006; 312:1944–1946.

260. van Soolingen D, Borgdorff MW, de Haas PE, et al. Molecular epidemiology of tuberculosis in the Netherlands: A nationwide study from 1993 through 1997. J Infect Dis 1999; 180:726–736.

261. Diaz R, Kremer K, de Haas PE, et al. Molecular epidemiology of tuberculosis in Cuba outside of Havana, July 1994-June 1995: Utility of spoligotyping versus IS6110 restriction fragment length polymorphism. Int J Tuberc Lung Dis 1998; 2:743–750.

262. Samper S, Iglesias MJ, Rabanaque MJ, et al. The molecular epidemiology of tuberculosis in Zaragoza, Spain: A retrospective epidemiological study in 1993. Int J Tuberc Lung Dis 1998; 2:281–287.

263. Alland D, Kalkut GE, Moss AR, et al. Transmission of tuberculosis in New York City. An analysis by DNA fingerprinting and conventional epidemiologic methods. N Engl J Med 1994; 330:1710–1716.

264. Small PM, Hopewell PC, Singh SP, et al. The epidemiology of tuberculosis in San Francisco. A population-based study using conventional and molecular methods. N Engl J Med 1994; 330:1703–1709.

265. Marttila HJ, Soini H, Eerola E, et al. A Ser315Thr substitution in KatG is predominant in genetically heterogeneous multidrug-resistant Mycobacterium tuberculosis isolates originating from the St. Petersburg area in Russia. Antimicrob Agents Chemother 1998; 42:2443–2445.

266. Fang Z, Doig C, Rayner A, et al. Molecular evidence for heterogeneity of the multiple-drug-resistant Mycobacterium tuberculosis population in Scotland (1990 to 1997). J Clin Microbiol 1999; 37:998–1003.

267. Niemann S, Rusch-Gerdes S, Richter E. IS6110 fingerprinting of drug-resistant Mycobacterium tuberculosis strains isolated in Germany during 1995. J Clin Microbiol 1997; 35:3015–3020.

268. van Rie A, Warren R, Richardson M, et al. Classification of drug-resistant tuberculosis in an epidemic area. Lancet 2000; 356:22–25.

269. Kruuner A, Pehme L, Ghebremichael S, et al. Use of molecular techniques to distinguish between treatment failure and exogenous reinfection with Mycobacterium tuberculosis. Clin Infect Dis 2002; 35:146–155.

270. Andrews JR, Gandhi NR, Moodley P, et al.; Tugela Ferry Care and Research Collaboration. Exogenous reinfection as a cause of multidrug-resistant and extensively drug-resistant tuberculosis in rural South Africa. J Infect Dis 2008; 198:1582–1589.

271. Gandhi NR, Moll A, Sturm AW, et al. Extensively drug-resistant tuberculosis as a cause of death in patients co-infected with tuberculosis and HIV in a rural area of South Africa. Lancet 2006; 368:1575–1580.

272. Shen G, Xue Z, Shen X, et al. The study recurrent tuberculosis and exogenous reinfection, Shanghai, China. Emerg Infect Dis 2006; 12:1776–1778.

273. Chiang CY, Riley LW. Exogenous reinfection in tuberculosis. Lancet Infect Dis 2005; 5:629–636.

274. Verver S, Warren RM, Beyers N, et al. Rate of reinfection tuberculosis after successful treatment is higher than rate of new tuberculosis. Am J Respir Crit Care Med 2005; 171:1430–1435.

275. Murray M, Nardell E. Molecular epidemiology of tuberculosis: Achievements and challenges to current knowledge. Bull World Health Organ 2002; 80:477–482.

276. Murray M, Alland D. Methodological problems in the molecular epidemiology of tuberculosis. Am J Epidemiol 2002; 155:565–571.

277. Fok A, Numata Y, Schulzer M, et al. Risk factors for clustering of tuberculosis cases: A systematic review of population-based molecular epidemiology studies. Int J Tuberc Lung Dis 2008; 12:480–492.

278. Small PM, Hopewell PC, Singh SP, et al. The epidemiology of tuberculosis in San Francisco. A population-based study using conventional and molecular methods. N Engl J Med 1994; 330(24):1750–1751.

279. Styblo K. Epidemiology of Tuberculosis. 1984. VER Gustav Fischer Verlag Jena. Republished in Selected Papers, Royal Netherlands Tuberculosis Association (KNCV), Vol. 24, The Hague, 1991.

280. Nardell E, McInnis B, Thomas B, et al. Exogenous reinfection with tuberculosis in a shelter for the homeless. N Engl J Med 1986; 315:1570–1574.

281. Small PM, Shafer RW, Hopewell PC, et al. Exogenous reinfection with multidrug-resistant Mycobacterium tuberculosis in patients with advanced HIV infection. N Engl J Med 1993; 328:1137–1144.

282. de Boer AS, van Soolingen D. Recurrent tuberculosis due to exogenous reinfection. N Engl J Med. 2000; 342:1050–1051.

283. van Rie A, Warren R, Richardson M, et al. Exogenous reinfection as a cause of recurrent tuberculosis after curative treatment. N Engl J Med 1999; 341:1174–1179.

284. Jasmer RM, Bozeman L, Schwartzman K, et al.; Tuberculosis Trials Consortium. Recurrent tuberculosis in the United States and Canada: Relapse or reinfection? Am J Respir Crit Care Med 2004; 170:1360–1366.

285. Snider DE, Graczyk J, Bek E, et al. Supervised six months treatment of newly diagnosed pulmonary tuberculosis using isoniazid, rifampin, and pyrazinamide with and without streptomycin. Am Rev Respir Dis 1984; 130:1091–1094.

286. British Thoracic Association. A controlled trial of six months chemotherapy in pulmonary tuberculosis. Second report: Results during the 24 months after the end of chemotherapy. Am Rev Respir Dis 1982; 126:460–462.

287. Panjabi R, Comstock GW, Golub JE. Recurrent tuberculosis and its risk factors: Adequately treated patients are still at high risk. Int J Tuberc Lung Dis 2007; 11:828–837.

288. Sonnenberg P, Murray J, Glynn JR, et al. HIV-1 and recurrence, relapse, and reinfection of tuberculosis after cure: A cohort study in South African mine workers. Lancet 2001; 358:1687–1693.

289. Thomas A, Gopi PG, Santha T, et al. Predictors of relapse among pulmonary tuberculosis patients treated in a DOTS programme in South India. Int J Tuberc Lung Dis 2005; 9:556–561.

290. Mallory KF, Churchyard GJ, Kleinschmidt I, et al. The impact of HIV infection on recurrence of tuberculosis in South African gold miners. Int J Tuberc Lung Dis 2000; 4:455–462.

291. Driver CR, Munsiff SS, Li J, et al. Relapse in persons treated for drug-susceptible tuberculosis in a population with high coinfection with human immunodeficiency virus in New York City. Clin Infect Dis 2001; 33:1762–1769.

292. Aber VR, Nunn AJ. Factors affecting relapse following shortcourse chemotherapy. Bull Int Union 1978; 53(4):260–264.

293. Tam CM, Chan SL, Kam KM, et al. Rifapentine and isoniazid in the continuation phase of a 6-month regimen. Final report at 5 years: Prognostic value of various measures. Int J Tuberc Lung Dis 2002; 6:3–10.

294. Combs DL, O'Brien RJ, Geiter LJ. USPHS tuberculosis short course chemotherapy trial 21: Effectiveness, toxicity, and acceptability. Ann Intern Med 1990; 112:397–406.

295. Pulido F, Pena J-M, Rubio R, et al. Relapse of tuberculosis after treatment in human immunodeficiency virus-infected patients. Arch Intern Med 1997; 157:227–232.

296. Malkin JE, Prazuck T, Simonnet F, et al. Tuberculosis and human immunodeficiency virus infection in west Burkina Faso: Clinical presentation and clinical evolution. Int J Tuberc Lung Dis 1997; 1:68–74.

297. Johnson JL, Okwera A, Vjecha MJ, et al. Risk factors for relapse in human immunodeficiency virus type 1 infected adults with pulmonary tuberculosis. Int J Tuberc Lung Dis 1997; 1:446–453.

298. Picon PD, Bassanesi SL, Caramori ML, et al. Risk factors for recurrence of tuberculosis. J Bras Pneumol 2007; 33(5):572–578.

299. Golub JE, Durovni B, King BS, et al. Recurrent tuberculosis in HIV-infected patients in Rio de Janeiro, Brazil. AIDS 2008; 22(18):2527–2533.

300. Lew W, Pai M, Oxlade O, et al. Initial drug resistance and tuberculosis treatment outcomes: Systematic review and meta-analysis. Ann Intern Med 2008; 149:123–134.

301. Seung KJ, Gelmanova IE, Peremitin GG, et al. The effect of initial drug resistance on treatment response and acquired drug resistance during standardized short-course chemotherapy for tuberculosis. Clin Infect Dis 2004; 39(9):1321–1328.

302. Li J, Munsiff SS, Driver CR, et al. Relapse and acquired rifampin resistance in HIV-infected patients with tuberculosis treated with rifampin- or rifabutin-based regimens in New York City, 1997–2000. Clin Infect Dis 2005; 41:83–91.

303. Quy HT, Cobelens FG, Lan NT, et al. Treatment outcomes by drug resistance and HIV status among tuberculosis patients in Ho Chi Minh City, Vietnam. Int J Tuberc Lung Dis 2006; 10:45–51.

304. Benator D, Bhattacharya M, Bozeman L, et al.; Tuberculosis Trials Consortium. Rifapentine and isoniazid once a week versus rifampicin and isoniazid twice a week for treatment of drug-susceptible pulmonary tuberculosis in HIV-negative patients: A randomised clinical trial. Lancet 2002; 360:528–534.

305. Kim HS, Park MH, Song EY, et al. Association of HLA-DR and HLA-DQ genes with susceptibility to pulmonary tuberculosis in Koreans: Preliminary evidence of associations with drug resistance, disease severity, and disease recurrence. Hum Immunol 2005; 66:1074–1081.

306. Lan NT, Lien HT, Tung le B, et al. Mycobacterium tuberculosis Beijing genotype and risk for treatment failure and relapse, Vietnam. Emerg Infect Dis 2003; 9:1633–1635.

307. Thompson BC. The pathogenesis of tuberculosis of peripheral lymph nodes. A clinical study of 324 cases. Tubercle 1940; 21:217–235.

308. Lincoln EM. Tuberculous meningitis in children. With special reference to serous meningitis. Part I. Tuberculous meningitis. Am Rev Tuberc 1947; 56:75–94.

309. Lincoln EM. Tuberculous meningitis in children. With special reference to serous meningitis. Part II. Serous tuberculous meningitis. Am Rev Tuberc 1947; 56:95–109.

310. Barker RD, Millard FJ, Malatsi J, et al. Traditional healers, treatment delay, performance status and death from TB in rural South Africa. Int J Tuberc Lung Dis 2006; 10(6):670–675.

311. Greenaway C, Menzies D, Fanning A, et al.; Canadian Collaborative Group in nosocomial Transmission of Tuberculosis. Delay in diagnosis among hospitalized patients with active tuberculosis–predictors and outcomes. Am J Respir Crit Care Med 2002; 165:927–933.

312. Lienhardt C, Rowley J, Manneh K, et al. Factors affecting time delay to treatment in a tuberculosis control programme in a sub-Saharan African country: The experience of The Gambia. Int J Tuberc Lung Dis 2001; 5:233.

313. Pablos-Méndez A, Sterling TR, Frieden TR. The relationship between delayed or incomplete treatment and all-cause mortality in patients with tuberculosis. JAMA 1996; 276: 1223–1228.

314. Zafran N, Heldal E, Pavlovic S, et al. Why do our patients die of active tuberculosis in the era of effective therapy? Tuber Lung Dis 1994; 75:329–333.

315. de Meer G, van Geuns HA. Rising case fatality of bacteriologically proven pulmonary tuberculosis in The Netherlands. Tuber Lung Dis 1992; 73:83–86.

316. Storla DG, Yimer S, Bjune GA. A systematic review of delay in the diagnosis and treatment of tuberculosis. BMC Public Health 2008; 8:15.

317. Duarte EC, Bierrenbach AL, Barbosa da Silva Junior J Jr, et al. Associated factors with deaths among pulmonary tuberculosis patients: A case-control study with secondary data. J Epidemiol Community Health 2009; 63(3):233–238.

318. Domingos MP, Caiaffa WT, Colosimo EA. Mortality, TB/HIV co-infection, and treatment dropout: Predictors of tuberculosis prognosis in Recife, Pernambuco State, Brazil. Cad Saude Publica 2008; 24:887–896.

319. Ciglenecki I, Glynn JR, Mwinga A, et al. Population differences in death rates in HIV-positive patients with tuberculosis. Int J Tuberc Lung Dis 2007; 11:1121–1128.

320. Harries AD, Nyangulu DS, Kang'ombe C, et al. Treatment outcome of an unselected cohort of tuberculosis patients in relation to human immunodeficiency virus serostatus in Zomba Hospital, Malawi. Trans R Soc Trop Med Hyg 1998; 92:343–347.

321. Lawn SD, Acheampong JW. Pulmonary tuberculosis in adults: Factors associated with mortality at a Ghanaian teaching hospital. West Afr J Med 1999; 18:270–274.

322. Haar CH, Cobelens FG, Kalisvaart NA, et al. HIV-related mortality among tuberculosis patients in The Netherlands, 1993–2001. Int J Tuberc Lung Dis 2007; 11:1038–1041.

323. Churchyard G J, Kleinschmidt I, Corbett EL, et al. Factors associated with an increased case-fatality rate in HIV-infected and non-infected South African gold miners with pulmonary tuberculosis. Int J Tuberc Lung Dis 2000; 4:705–712.

324. Badri M, Wilson D, Wood R. Effect of highly active antiretroviral therapy on incidence of tuberculosis in South Africa: A cohort study. Lancet 2002; 359:2059–2064.

325. Dheda K, Lampe FC, Johnson MA, et al. Outcome of HIV-associated tuberculosis in the era of highly active antiretroviral therapy. J Infect Dis 2004; 190:1670–1676.

326. Walpola HC, Siskind V, Patel AM, et al. Tuberculosis-related deaths in Queensland, Australia, 1989–1998: Characteristics and risk factors. Int J Tuberc Lung Dis 2003; 7:742–750.

327. Fielder JF, Chaulk CP, Dalvi M, et al. A high tuberculosis case-fatality rate in a setting of effective tuberculosis control: Implications for acceptable treatment success rates. Int J Tuberc Lung Dis 2002; 6:1114–1117.

328. Rao VK, Iademarco EP, Fraser VJ, et al. The impact of comorbidity on mortality following in-hospital diagnosis of tuberculosis. Chest 1998; 114:1244–1252.

329. Vasankari T, Holmström P, Ollgren J, et al. Risk factors for poor tuberculosis treatment outcome in Finland: A cohort study. BMC Public Health 2007; 7:291.

330. Sterling TR, Zhao Z, Khan A, et al.; Tuberculosis Trials Consortium. Mortality in a large tuberculosis treatment trial: Modifiable and non-modifiable risk factors. Int J Tuberc Lung Dis 2006; 10:542–549.

331. Dewan PK, Arguin PM, Kiryanova H, et al. Risk factors for death during tuberculosis treatment in Orel, Russia. Int J Tuberc Lung Dis 2004; 8:598–602.
332. Mathew TA, Ovsyanikova TN, Shin SS, et al. Causes of death during tuberculosis treatment in Tomsk Oblast, Russia. Int J Tuberc Lung Dis 2006; 10:857–863.
333. Franke MF, Appleton SC, Bayona J, et al. Risk factors and mortality associated with default from multidrug-resistant tuberculosis treatment. Clin Infect Dis 2008; 46:1844–1851.
334. Nájera-Ortiz JC, Sánchez-Pérez HJ, Ochoa-Díaz H, et al. Demographic, health services and socio-economic factors associated with pulmonary tuberculosis mortality in Los Altos Region of Chiapas, Mexico. Int J Epidemiol 2008; 37:786–795.
335. Kolappan C, Subramani R, Kumaraswami V, et al. Excess mortality and risk factors for mortality among a cohort of TB patients from rural south India. Int J Tuberc Lung Dis 2008; 12:81–86.
336. Vree M, Huong NT, Duong BD, et al. Mortality and failure among tuberculosis patients who did not complete treatment in Vietnam: A cohort study. BMC Public Health 2007; 7:134.
337. García-García Mde L, Ponce-De-León A, García-Sancho MC, et al. Tuberculosis-related deaths within a well-functioning DOTS control program. Emerg Infect Dis 2002; 8:1327–1333.
338. Mukherjee JS, Rich ML, Socci AR, et al. Programmes and principles in treatment of multidrug-resistant tuberculosis. Lancet 2004; 363:474–481.
339. Lefebvre N, Falzon D. Risk factors for death among tuberculosis cases: Analysis of European surveillance data. Eur Respir J 2008; 31:1256–1260.
340. Kawai V, Soto G, Gilman RH, et al. Tuberculosis mortality, drug resistance, and infectiousness in patients with and without HIV infection in Peru. Am J Trop Med Hyg 2006; 75:1027–1033.
341. Thwaites GE, Lan NT, Dung NH, et al. Effect of antituberculosis drug resistance on response to treatment and outcome in adults with tuberculous meningitis. J Infect Dis 2005; 192:79–88.
342. Lockman S, Kruuner A, Binkin N, et al. Clinical outcomes of Estonian patients with primary multidrug-resistant versus drug-susceptible tuberculosis. Clin Infect Dis 2001; 32:373–380.
343. Kliiman K, Altraja A. Predictors of poor treatment outcome in highly drug-resistant pulmonary tuberculosis. Eur Respir J 2009; 33(5):1085–1094.
344. Silva JM, Fuchs SC, Barcellos NT, et al. Treatment of extensively drug-resistant tuberculosis. Lancet 2009; 373(9657):27.
345. Shah NS, Pratt R, Armstrong L, et al. Extensively drug-resistant tuberculosis in the United States, 1993–2007. JAMA 2008; 300:2153–2160.
346. Keshavjee S, Gelmanova IY, Farmer PE, et al. Treatment of extensively drug-resistant tuberculosis in Tomsk, Russia: A retrospective cohort study. Lancet 2008; 372(9647):1403–1409.
347. Lowe CR. Recent trends in survival of patients with respiratory tuberculosis. Br J Prev Soc Med 1954; 8:91–98.
348. Thompson BC. Survival rates in pulmonary tuberculosis. Br Med J 1943; 2:721.

3

Pathogenesis of Tuberculosis: New Insights

NICHOLAS A. BE and WILLIAM R. BISHAI
Center for Tuberculosis Research, Division of Infectious Diseases, Department of Medicine, Johns Hopkins University School of Medicine, Baltimore, Maryland, U.S.A.

SANJAY K. JAIN
Center for Tuberculosis Research, Division of Infectious Diseases, Department of Medicine, Johns Hopkins University School of Medicine; Department of Pediatrics, Division of Pediatric Infectious Diseases, Johns Hopkins University School of Medicine, Baltimore, Maryland, U.S.A.

I. Introduction

Mycobacterium tuberculosis, the cause of human tuberculosis (TB), has been a scourge of humanity throughout recorded history. Even today, this bacillus claims about two million lives per year, remains one of the leading causes of death among the infectious diseases (1,2) and is the leading killer of people with AIDS (3). Human tuberculosis is a multistage disease. Any rational approach to TB control must be based upon the pathogenic processes at work during these stages.

The pathogenic process begins with inhalation of infectious aerosols. Bacilli lodged in the alveoli are engulfed by the alveolar macrophages. If the bacteria are able to survive this initial encounter with the innate immune system, a period of logarithmic growth ensues, with bacterial doubling every 24 hours. Bacteria released from macrophages are engulfed by new macrophages attracted to the site, thereby continuing this cycle. The bacilli may spread from the initial lesion via the lymphatic and/or circulatory systems to other parts of the body.

After approximately four to six weeks, the host develops specific immunity to the bacilli. The resulting *M. tuberculosis*-specific lymphocytes migrate to the site of infection, surrounding and activating the macrophages there. As the cellular infiltration continues, the center of the cell mass, or granuloma, becomes caseous and necrotic (Fig. 1).

In the majority of cases, the immunocompetent human is able to arrest growth of the bacilli within the primary lesion with little or no signs of illness. The initial lesion, which eventually resolves or calcifies, may still harbor viable bacilli, in which case the host is said to harbor latent TB infection (LTBI; see below). However, in about 10% of infected individuals (4–8) the disease progresses during the initial weeks or months after infection, and the patient develops the typical symptoms of active (or progressive) primary TB: cough, fever, lethargy, and weight loss. In some cases, the granuloma becomes quite large and the caseous material liquefies, a phenomenon referred to as cavitary TB (see below and Fig. 2). This phenomenon is more commonly seen in cases of reactivation of latent TB. If the wall of the cavity erodes into an airway, the patient may become highly infectious as the liquefied contents of the cavity are expelled by coughing. Both

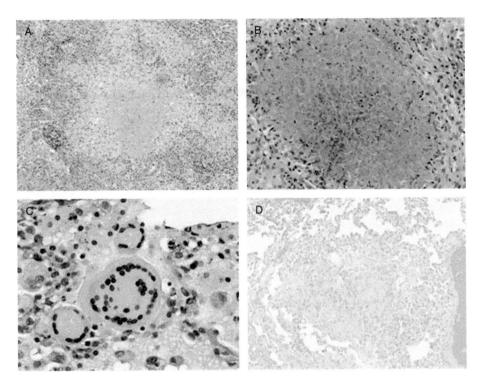

Figure 1 Histopathology of organs following infection of peripherally sensitized rabbits with *M. bovis*. (**A, B**) Necrotic, caseous granuloma (hematoxylin and eosin staining) demonstrating disintegrated epithelioid macrophages at the center and a rim of lymophocytic infiltrate at the periphery. (**C**) Multinucleated (Langhans) giant cell in rabbit lung tissue at five weeks (hematoxylin and eosin staining). (**D**) Rabbit lung tissue demonstrating inflammation and cellular infiltrate. *Source*: Courtesy of G. Nedeltchev, Johns Hopkins University.

caseous granulomas and cavities are devoid of blood supply, impairing both the immune system's ability to fight the infection as well as the clinician's attempts to treat the disease chemotherapeutically.

The progression of TB from infection to either containment of disease or demise of the host has been well characterized anatomically. While the molecular mechanisms responsible for many aspects of TB pathogenesis are unknown, progress has been made in recent years on a number of fronts. This chapter will follow the typical course of the disease through its various stages and describe what is known regarding the molecular processes involved.

II. Infection

Although *M. tuberculosis* can infect by atypical routes and manifest in a number of anatomic sites, this pathogen is acquired in the overwhelming majority of cases by aerosol inhalation. The classic experiments of Wells and Riley (9–12) investigating the

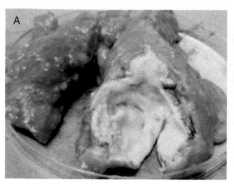
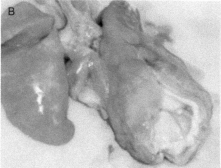

Figure 2 Gross pathology of whole lungs from sensitized New Zealand White rabbits following intratracheal infection with mycobacteria via bronchoscope. Incision reveals a cavitary lesion with extensive caseous necrosis containing thick, liquefied caseous material. (**A**) Rabbit lung infected with *M. bovis*. (**B**) Rabbit lung infected with *M. tuberculosis* CDC1551 *Source*: Courtesy of G. Nedeltchev, Johns Hopkins University.

mechanics of airborne TB transmission have been revisited after more than 40 years in a recent study by Fennelly et al. (13) demonstrating that a large proportion of viable tubercle bacilli expelled by coughing are contained in droplets less than 5 μm in size, consistent with the predictions made by the earlier investigators. Such infectious droplets, being small enough to reach the alveolus, allow the bacillus to avoid the mucociliary clearance mechanisms of the airways.

Once in the alveolus, the bacillus is engulfed by the alveolar macrophage (AM). AMs are continually ingesting inhaled particulates and as a result are usually in a partially activated state, depending on the nature of the particulates and the mechanism by which the material is ingested (e.g., with or without opsonization, specific receptors involved, etc.) (14,15). Phagocytosis by an insufficiently activated AM allows the bacillus to avoid being killed and to begin a phase of exponential replication. That the AM actually contributes to productive *M. tuberculosis* infection is suggested by the observation that selective depletion of AMs from mice using liposome-encapsulated dichloromethylene diphosphonate, which induces apoptosis of AMs, prior to and shortly after infection with *M. tuberculosis* resulted in 100% survival of the mice at 150 days following infection, compared to 60% survival with liposome treatment alone (16). Thus, ironically, the unactivated macrophage is used by the pathogen as a site for intracellular multiplication, and apoptosis of infected macrophages may be an antibacterial host defense mechanism. Additionally, the ultimate mechanism of macrophage cell death has been demonstrated to differ between virulent and avirulent mycobacteria. Following infection with the avirulent strain H37Ra, macrophages develop an apoptotic envelope wherein the bacteria are effectively contained, destroyed, and/or utilized for T-cell priming. Infection with the virulent H37Rv, however, prevents formation of the apoptotic envelope via inhibition of annexin-1 cross-linking (17). This results in reduced membrane integrity (similar to the processes of necrosis) and promotes the spread of viable bacilli.

A few in vitro studies have suggested that *M. tuberculosis* might be capable of invading respiratory epithelial cells (18–21). Sato et al. reported that approximately 10%

of the bacilli observed by electron microscopy in lung sections (from mice intravenously infected with 5×10^7 organisms) were located inside type II alveolar cells at two days postinfection, with the remaining 90% contained within macrophages or neutrophils (22). At 14 days postinfection, few if any mycobacteria were observed within type II alveolar cells. As most natural infections result from the successful aerosol implantation of one or a few bacilli, the relevance of bacillary uptake by respiratory epithelial cells remains to be substantiated.

Additional studies have demonstrated the ability of *M. tuberculosis* to interact with and invade endothelial cells. Menozzi and colleagues have shown that the *M. tuberculosis* encoded protein, heparin-binding hemagglutinin adhesion (HBHA) induces a rearrangement of cytoskeletal networks in bovine capillary endothelial cells via actin remodeling, potentially inducing receptor-mediated endocytosis. In addition, when HBHA is coupled to colloidal gold particles, these particles are observed binding to HEp-2 and A549 epithelial cells as well as within cytoplasmic vacuoles (23). Such results suggest a role for HBHA in extrapulmonary dissemination of bacilli.

M. tuberculosis have also been observed in the invasion of and transcytosis across an in vitro blood–brain barrier composed of human brain microvascular endothelial cells (HBMEC) (24). Similar to the studies in capillary endothelial cells, remodeling of the actin cytoskeleton has been implicated in the mechanisms of bacillary invasion. Further studies in the in vitro model, as well as a murine CNS invasion model have implied that such invasion is likely to be dependent on microbial gene products and their corresponding host–pathogen interactions (24,25).

A. Macrophage Receptors

A great deal of effort has gone into investigating the molecular interactions leading to phagocytosis of *M. tuberculosis* by the macrophage. A number of macrophage cell surface molecules have been shown to bind to and promote internalization of *M. tuberculosis*, including multiple complement receptors (CR1, CR3, and CR4), mannose receptor, CD14, IgG Fcγ receptor and scavenger receptors (26–31). The mechanism by which phagocytosis occurs may influence subsequent cytoplasmic events, thus *M. tuberculosis* may have evolved mechanisms to promote its uptake via specific pathways to avoid intracellular killing. Selectively blocking individual phagocytic pathways with antibody or competitive ligands does not seem to have an appreciable effect on *M. tuberculosis* survival or growth in macrophages (31). However, opsonization of *M. tuberculosis* with specific antibody results in antibody receptor-mediated phagocytosis and subsequent killing of the bacillus after phagosome–lysosome fusion (26), whereas the bacillus is able to prevent phagosome–lysosome fusion otherwise (32). For example, one study found that coating the bacillus with monoclonal antibody to arabinomannan prior to infection had a host protective effect in mice (33).

III. Survival Within the Macrophage

Perhaps more articles have been published on mycobacterial survival within the macrophage than on any other aspect of TB pathogenesis. Ever since the observation that macrophage phagosomes containing *M. tuberculosis* fail to fuse with lysosomes (the normal fate of ingested bacteria) (32), investigators have attempted to unravel the underlying mechanisms of *M. tuberculosis* intracellular survival. The host–pathogen interactions and local environment of the mycobacterial phagosome has been reviewed in depth by Deretic as well as Rohde et al. (34,35).

Whereas the interior of the phagosome ordinarily becomes more acidic as it progresses down the endosomal/lysosomal pathway, phagosomes containing *M. tuberculosis* and other pathogenic mycobacteria do not completely acidify (36,37). This reduced acidification has been attributed to failure of the *M. tuberculosis* phagosome to accumulate vesicular proton-ATPase (36). Consistent with the observation that *M. tuberculosis*-containing phagosomes do not fuse with lysosomes (32), such phagosomes are also lacking in mature lysosomal hydrolases and other lysosomal markers (38–42).

One of the newer mechanisms to be demonstrated as playing a part in immunity against intracellular pathogens is the cellular process of autophagy. Under normal circumstances, autophagy serves as a cellular mechanism for the disposal of damaged or superfluous organelles. Studies by Gutierrez et al. have shown that induction of autophagy in macrophages inhibits intracellular survival of *M. tuberculosis* and promotes phagosome acidification and maturation (43). Autophagy therefore appears to be capable of overcoming the mycobacteria-mediated phagosome block. Induction of this process has been shown to be achieved through the Th1 cytokine interferon-γ as well as the introduction of ATP, resulting in much more rapid killing of intracellular mycobacteria (44,45).

A. Calcium Signaling and Phagosome Maturation

The mechanism responsible for phagosome maturation arrest has been the subject of intense investigation in recent years. Deretic and colleagues have performed extensive characterization of the molecules involved in vesicle trafficking and whether or not these molecules localize normally in *M. tuberculosis*-infected cells (46–51). Chief among their findings were the aberrant accumulation of Rab5 and failure to acquire Rab7 on the mycobacterial phagosome (50,52). Rab5 and Rab7 are small GTP-binding proteins involved in vesicular trafficking, being markers of early and late endosomes, respectively. GTP-binding proteins bind to guanosine triphosphate, thereby becoming activated for interaction with and/or regulation of other specific proteins. The GTP-binding protein also hydrolyzes the GTP to GDP (guanosine diphosphate), thus reverting to an inactive form until the GDP is exchanged for GTP once again. In this way, GTP hydrolysis acts as a molecular timer for protein activation.

Following up on the observed block at the Rab5/Rab7 stage, Fratti et al. discovered that EEA1 (early endosomal autoantigen 1), a Rab5-regulated protein involved in endosome docking and fusion (53), failed to localize to *M. tuberculosis* phagosomes (48). EEA1 also interacts with phosphatidylinositol-3-phosphate (PI3P) (54), generated from membrane phosphatidylinositol (PI) by another protein, hVPS34, a PI kinase (55). This interaction helps to localize EEA1 to the phagosome membrane (54). Vergne et al. showed that hVPS34 interacts with the Ca^{2+}-binding protein calmodulin in a Ca^{2+}-dependent manner (56). These findings intersect with another line of study by Malik et al. demonstrating that *M. tuberculosis* blocks the intracellular rise in Ca^{2+} associated with phagocytosis and that the Ca^{2+}/calmodulin pathway contributes to phagosome–lysosome fusion (57,58). These observations have collectively led to a model (Fig. 3) in which *M. tuberculosis* prevents phagosome maturation by blocking the increase of intracellular Ca^{2+}. Lower intracellular Ca^{2+}, in turn, prevents the Ca^{2+}/calmodulin-dependent activation

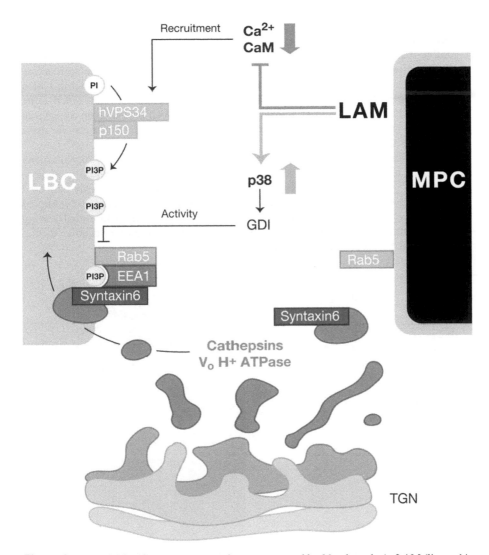

Figure 3   A model for phagosome maturation arrest caused by *M. tuberculosis*. LAM (lipoarabi-nomannan) from the mycobacterial cell wall prevents the normal rise in intracellular Ca^{2+} associated with phagocytosis. This in turn prevents the calcium/calmodulin (CaM) activation of hVPS34 and its subsequent generation of PI3P (phosphatidylinositol-3-phosphate). PI3P synthesized from phago-some membrane phosphatidylinositol (PI) ordinarily serves to recruit both Rab5 and EEA1, which interact with syntaxin-6 on the membrane of vesicles from the trans-Golgi network (TGN) carrying molecules such as cathepsins and the vesicular proton-ATPase. *Abbreviations*: LBC, phagosome containing latex bead; MPC, phagosome containing *M. tuberculosis*. *Source*: From Ref. 59.

of the PI kinase hVPS34, and thus no PI3P is generated on the phagosome membrane to recruit and retain EEA1 (59). Recent studies have produced some contradictory data regarding the role of calcium in phagosome arrest. In work performed by Jayachandran et al., infection of macrophages with pathogenic mycobacteria resulted in an increase in intracellular calcium (60). Jayachandran and colleagues proposed a model in which infection triggers an increase in calcium via the actin-binding protein coronin-1, activating the calcium-dependent protein phosphatase calcineurin, which promotes mycobacterial survival through phagosomal arrest. Additional studies are required to reconcile these findings with previous models.

The failure to synthesize PI3P on the phagosomal membrane would explain many observations regarding the mycobacterial phagosome, including its failure to acquire the vesicular proton-ATPase and lysosomal hydrolases (cathepsins) normally delivered to the phagosome by vesicles of the trans-Golgi network (Fig. 4) (38,41,59). Altered signaling mechanisms may also interfere with recruitment of the endosomal sorting complex required for transport (ESCRT), a host complex required for vacuolar sorting and which has been shown to limit mycobacterial growth (61).

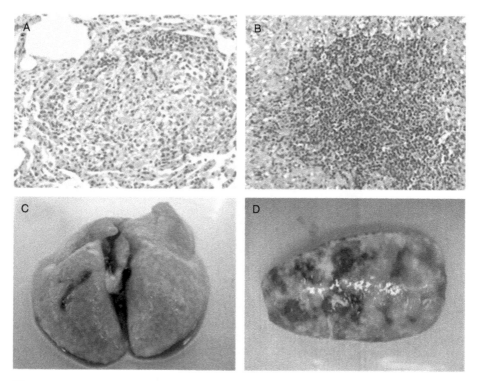

Figure 4 Guinea pig organs following intravenous infection with *M. tuberculosis* CDC1551. Histopathology of (**A**) lung and (**B**) spleen tissue showing cellular infiltrate and granuloma formation (hematoxylin and eosin staining). (**C**) Gross pathology of whole guinea pig lungs showing small, diffuse lesions extending over the full surface of the tissue. (**D**) Gross pathology of whole guinea spleen demonstrating extensive necrosis due to high-dose, disseminated disease.

It has been shown that the *M. tuberculosis* cell wall glycolipid lipoarabinomannan (LAM) inhibits intracellular increases in Ca^{2+} (56). It appears that the *M. tuberculosis*-dependent block of Ca^{2+} elevation occurs via inhibition of host cell sphingosine kinase (62), which has been shown to link a number of cell surface receptors to a rise in cytosolic Ca^{2+} (63,64). One observation that is not explained by this model is the inability of heat- or radiation-killed *M. tuberculosis* to inhibit the Ca^{2+} spike (57). This result seems to be at odds with the aforementioned ability of purified LAM to inhibit Ca^{2+} increase in the macrophage (56), as dead *M. tuberculosis* would still contain LAM. Recent studies have shown that the incorporation of LAM into membrane rafts of the host macrophage cell membrane is required for the blocking of phagosome maturation (65). This mechanism was found to be dependent on insertion of the LAM glycosylphosphatidylinositol (GPI) anchor into the membrane. It is possible that this process, along with potentially active secretion or release of LAM from the cell wall of *M. tuberculosis*, may require bacterial viability. Shabaana et al. demonstrated that the incorporation of LAM into T-cell membrane rafts resulted in an alteration of host cell signaling transduction via raft protein kinases (66). Similar interactions in macrophages may contribute to the mechanism of phagosomal arrest.

Gutierrez et al. have demonstrated another pathogen-mediated mechanism for phagosomal arrest by studying the metabolic state of the bacterium. Using an inducible GFP expression system to monitor bacterial activity, it was observed that metabolically active mycobacteria were primarily found within nonacidified phagosomes, while the less metabolically active mycobacteria were present in acidified phagosomes undergoing phagolysosomal fusion (67). These data suggest that metabolic activity is necessary for preventing phagolysosomal fusion, although definitive causality was not demonstrated.

B. Intersection with Host Phosphorylation

Another proposed mechanism for the prevention of PI3P accumulation on endosomal membranes involves eukaryotic-like phosphatases encoded by mycobacteria. One such lipid phosphatase, SapM, has been demonstrated to hydrolyze host PI3P, thereby inhibiting late endosome–phagosome fusion (68). The protein phosphatase PtpA has also been shown to interfere with host signaling processes. The substrate of PtpA was demonstrated to be the host protein vacuolar protein sorting 33B (VPS33B), essential for proper vesicle trafficking. Bach et al. proposed that dephosphorylation of VPS33B by PtpA results in improper localization of endosomes and hinders phagosome–lysosome fusion, although the precise mechanism by which this occurs has not been demonstrated (69).

Upon sequencing of the *M. tuberculosis* genome, a novel set of encoded proteins were annotated as "eukaryotic-like" serine-threonine protein kinases. Eleven such proteins were identified in *M. tuberculosis*, and it was proposed that they could play a role in the modulation of host responses (70). One of these kinases, PknG, was shown to be required for macrophage survival, as inhibition of the *PknG* gene resulted in lysosomal localization and bacterial cell death. During infection, PknG may be released into the phagosome and may ultimately enter the host cytosol where it may phosphorylate an as-of-yet unidentified host factor, thereby inhibiting this factor from playing a role in phagosome–lysosome fusion (71). New revelations regarding the role of these eukaryotic-like kinases have inspired the consideration of mycobacterial kinases as potential drug targets. Inhibition of a bacterial factor, which promotes lysosomal escape, would allow the host immune system to follow its natural course, resulting in bacterial killing by the macrophage (70).

C.   ESAT-6/CFP-10

The ability of mycobacteria to cause disease is tightly associated with their capacity to survive within the host macrophage. Two of the microbial factors believed to be involved in this process are early secretory antigenic 6 kDa (ESAT-6) protein and culture filtrate protein 10 (CFP-10). Both of these proteins are found in the RD1 region of the mycobacterial genome, present in all virulent strains of the *M. tuberculosis* complex, but absent in the attenuated bacille Calmette-Guérin (BCG) strain (72). Secretion of these proteins is mediated by a specialized system, also encoded by genes within RD1, termed ESX-1 (ESAT-6 secretion-1) (73). This secretion system has been shown to prevent phagosome–lysosome fusion in macrophages following infection with *Mycobacterium marinum*. Furthermore, a unique, novel protein has been found to be cosecreted with ESAT-6 and CFP-10 by the ESX-1 complex (Mh3881c). Secretion of these proteins is codependent and is required for mycobacterial intracellular growth and prevention of phagosome maturation in bone marrow-derived macrophages (74). Such processes are essential to the maintenance of virulence exhibited by members of the *M. tuberculosis* complex, which cause human disease.

In addition to their role in facilitating survival within the macrophage, ESAT-6 and CFP-10 are highly potent T-cell antigens, as measured by interferon-γ production and lymphocyte proliferation (75). Because of the robust host response to these proteins during infection, there is great interest in the potential of these antigens for vaccine applications. Animal studies with ESAT-6 subunit vaccines have demonstrated a protective effect similar to that of BCG (76,77). Also of great interest is the use of this protein complex as a diagnostic test capable of distinguishing *M. tuberculosis* infected patients from individuals who have received the BCG vaccine, due to the fact that the RD1 region is not present in the attenuated strain (78). Such diagnostics tests have been developed and take advantage of the antigenicity of ESAT-6 in development of assays for interferon-γ (79).

D.   Escape from the Macrophage

Aside from preventing phagosome–lysosome fusion, it has been proposed that pathogenic mycobacteria may escape the endosomal compartment completely, spreading into the cytosol of the host. McDonough et al. proposed that *M. tuberculosis* could, under certain conditions, escape into the macrophage cytosol. This concept generated a great deal of skepticism, as it runs counter to the prevailing school of thought, which states that *M. tuberculosis* remain exclusively within endosomal enclosures (80). This notion was revisited more recently in studies which demonstrated that both *M. tuberculosis* and *Mycobacterium leprae* translocate from the phagolysosome to the cytosol. This process was not observed during infection with BCG or heat-killed bacteria and was observed to be contingent upon the secretion of ESAT-6 and CFP-10 (81). The authors propose this phenomenon as a potential explanation for the relatively poor ability of BCG to elicit a $CD8^+$ T-cell response. Further study of this observation is necessary in order to examine the implications of cytosolic translocation, especially during in vivo infection.

IV. Host Response

A. The Inflammasome

The innate immune response to invading bacteria is largely mediated by the host inflammasome, a network of multiple proteins within the host cell cytoplasm responsible for innate recognition of intracellular pathogens. Such systems are largely controlled by intracellular nucleotide-binding oligomerization domain (NOD)-like receptor (NLR) proteins (82). This complex has been implicated in the activation of multiple pathways, including the activation of inflammatory caspases (caspase-1, 4, and 5), which lead to processing and activation of the proinflammatory cytokine IL-1β (83).

Master et al. have recently shown that the *M. tuberculosis* gene *zmp1* plays a significant role in inhibition of the host inflammasome, thereby impeding the processing of IL-1β and arresting phagolysosomal fusion (84). *M. tuberculosis* harboring a mutation in the *zmp1* gene displayed reduced virulence and were present in host phagosomes, which underwent maturation into phagolysosomes. The authors further demonstrated that this phenotype could be reversed through inhibition of host caspase-1, and that phagosomal maturation associated with the *zmp1* mutant did not occur in caspase-1 knockout mice. Such an adaptation by *M. tuberculosis* demonstrates not only a mechanism for phagosome maturation arrest, but also has broad implications for how the pathogen interacts with the host response in general, through inhibition of IL-1β and its associated inflammatory mediators.

In addition to cytokines and chemokines, the host has also been shown to utilize reactive nitrogen species in response to mycobacterial infection, a useful defense due to the multiplicity of bacterial targets. These reactive nitrogen intermediates (RNI) are produced by murine macrophages (85), and mice unable to produce nitric oxide (NO) have demonstrated heightened susceptibility to *M. tuberculosis* infection (86). Recently, Singh et al. have shown that the bicyclic nitroimidazole PA-824 may further promote RNI-mediated bacterial killing via release of intracellular NO (87). PA-824 has been shown to be active against replicating and nonreplicating bacteria (88). It is proposed that reduction of PA-824 by deazaflavin (F_{420})-dependent nitroreductase (Ddn) results in the release of RNI, which correlates with anaerobic killing of mycobacteria. Such findings raise hopes for the potential use of nitroimidazoles as a class of compounds effective in achieving mycobacterial killing under hypoxic conditions.

B. The Dendritic Cell

If successful in preventing phagosome–lysosome fusion, the bacillus replicates within the macrophage, filling the cell with its progeny until the macrophage ruptures to release its microbial cache. These bacilli are in turn engulfed by the more immature monocyte-derived macrophages recruited to the area by chemoattractants such as complement components, bacterial products, and cytokines released by the infected host cell (89). Some of these secondarily infected host cells are dendritic cells (DCs) that migrate to the draining lymph nodes to initiate the onset of the adaptive immune response (90,91). DCs are derived from the monocyte/macrophage lineage and function as effective scavengers that phagocytose, process, and present antigens to T lymphocytes, a necessary event in the development of cell-mediated as well as humoral immunity.

A growing body of literature suggests that *M. tuberculosis* interferes with DC function. Infection of blood monocytes with *M. tuberculosis* prevents their subsequent

IFN-α-induced differentiation into DCs (92). It has also been discovered that the DC-specific intercellular adhesion molecule-grabbing nonintegrin (DC-SIGN) binds to LAM, a prominent glycolipid on the surface of *M. tuberculosis* (93). DC-SIGN has been found to bind to surface molecules of a number of bacterial, parasitic, and viral pathogens, notably human immunodeficiency viruses 1 and 2 (HIV-1 and -2), Ebola virus, and dengue virus (94). The binding of LAM to DC-SIGN has been shown to inhibit both LPS-induced secretion of IL-12 and *Mycobacterium bovis* BCG-mediated DC maturation (93). LAM-DC-SIGN interaction also stimulates secretion of the anti-inflammatory cytokine IL-10 (93). Whether or not the effects of *M. tuberculosis* on DC function play a role in TB pathogenesis, the fact remains that TB patients do develop specific cell-mediated immunity (CMI) and delayed-type hypersensitivity (DTH). It therefore stands to reason that either impairment of DC function by *M. tuberculosis* does not occur in vivo (or at least not to the extent of preventing an adaptive immune response), or that other antigen-presenting cells (e.g., macrophages) must play a role in T-cell activation and proliferation, or both.

C. Granuloma Formation

The rabbit model of tuberculosis, pioneered by Lurie and Dannenberg, has provided a wealth of information regarding the histopathologic changes that occur following aerosol infection with *M. tuberculosis*. Following ingestion of *M. tuberculosis* by the alveolar macrophage and the initial replication within this cell, the resulting bacilli are taken up by the newly arriving macrophages derived from blood monocytes. By two weeks postinfection, infected macrophages at the center of the lesion have acquired an epithelioid morphology. As these cells die, they provide the raw material for the process of caseation necrosis. The periphery of the lesion consists largely of activated macrophages and neutrophils. At four weeks postinfection, the number of mature macrophages seen at the periphery of the caseous lesion has increased. Multinucleated giant cells (Langhans cells; Fig. 1) are often seen by this time, formed by the fusion of activated macrophages. In addition, *M. tuberculosis*-specific lymphocytes have appeared and surrounded the lesion, along with plasma cells and fibroblasts (Fig. 4). The onslaught of the immune response has, by this time, destroyed a large proportion of the bacilli, and by six weeks the rare remaining bacilli are typically found at the edge of the caseous center of the lesion, surrounded by a zone of activated macrophages. Eight weeks following infection, the lesion consists of a caseous necrotic core, surrounded by lymphocytes and a few remaining macrophages. Few if any viable bacilli may be present at this time (95,96).

D. Cell-Mediated Immunity Versus Delayed-Type Hypersensitivity

Dannenberg has made a distinction between mechanisms of macrophage-activating CMI and tissue-damaging DTH (97). In this dual mechanism model, CMI is described as an immunologic mechanism in which macrophages are activated by antigen-specific T cells, thereby acquiring an enhanced ability to destroy bacilli they have ingested. DTH, on the other hand, is viewed as a separate phenomenon whereby bacilli-laden macrophages are themselves destroyed, along with some surrounding tissue, resulting in caseous necrosis. Both CMI and DTH occur within the environment of the granuloma after the onset of adaptive immunity. If the host produces effective CMI, the macrophages attracted to the site of infection become highly activated and surround the existing lesion, engulfing and destroying any bacilli that have been released from dying cells or from the periphery of the caseous center of the granuloma. In this way, the infection is contained and the spread of caseous necrosis is prevented. However, in hosts that fail to mount effective CMI, the incoming macrophages are insufficiently activated and become parasitized by the bacilli, serving as reservoirs for further bacterial replication until they are destroyed by the tissue-damaging DTH response. In this way, more lung tissue is destroyed as the caseous lesion grows larger. While the operational distinction between CMI and DTH is useful in terms of understanding the pathology of the disease, it should be noted that experimental evidence for immunologically distinct mechanisms of CMI and DTH has yet to be conclusively demonstrated. Perhaps a more fundamental way of viewing CMI and DTH as defined above is that these processes represent opposing blades of a double-edged sword; the more effective the immune response at killing or halting replication of the bacilli, the less collateral tissue damage occurs and vice versa.

V. Cavitary TB

In some cases, the caseous lesion becomes quite large and transforms into a liquid-filled cavity. Unfortunately, little is known regarding the process of liquefaction at the molecular level. As more tissue surrounding the cavity is destroyed by caseous necrosis, the cavity expands. The bacilli multiply to high numbers within the liquefied cavity, and if the cavity erodes into the wall of an adjacent blood vessel, the patient may become seeded throughout the body with tubercle bacilli. On the other hand, if the cavity ruptures into an airway, the fluid is expelled as an infectious aerosol as the patient coughs. Thus cavitary TB is one of the most important manifestations of the disease from the perspective of transmission. As with the process of granuloma formation, the rabbit has provided an excellent model for studying the development of cavitary tuberculosis. Whereas the rabbit is usually able to contain and even clear infection with *M. tuberculosis*, infection with *M. bovis* leads to progressive disease. Cavitation in the rabbit is often seen 8 to 12 weeks following infection or reinfection with *M. bovis* (98–100).

Yamamura et al. developed a rabbit model of cavitary TB following direct injection of bacilli or bacterial extracts into the lung through the chest wall (101,102). These investigators found that previous exposure of the rabbit to heat-killed *M. bovis* by subcutaneous injection greatly increased the frequency of cavity formation upon subsequent infection. In fact, Yamamura observed that transthoracic injection of even heat-killed bacilli led to cavitation in 40% to 85% of sensitized rabbits but failed to do so in naïve animals. Therefore, the process of cavitation seems to be purely a host response phenomenon. Immunosuppressive agents (6-mecaptopurine and azathioprine) were found to reduce the occurrence of cavity formation in sensitized rabbits (103). This finding is consistent with the more current observation that TB patients with advanced HIV infection are less likely to develop cavitary disease (104).

VI. Latent TB

Of those who become infected with *M. tuberculosis*, about 10% will progress to active primary disease. The roughly 90% of individuals (4–8) who contain the infection within the initial lesion may still harbor viable bacilli, a condition referred to as LTBI (6). They are at risk for developing secondary (or reactivation) TB, which may manifest as pulmonary or extrapulmonary disease. In the immunocompetent host, the lifetime risk of developing reactivation disease is usually estimated at 5% to 10%. There is good evidence that the use of various immunosuppressive drugs increase the risk of reactivation substantially. TNF-α (tumor necrosis factor-α) inhibitors such as infliximab, etanercept, and adalimumab are associated with an increased incidence of TB, usually within the first months of administration (105–108). Advanced HIV infection has been calculated to increase the relative risk of reactivation TB 10-fold compared to non–HIV-infected patients with LTBI (109).

Given that *M. tuberculosis* can persist for years in the human host before recrudescence of active disease, it follows that either the replication of the bacillus must drastically slow or even cease, or that host bactericidal mechanisms must keep pace with the growth of the bacillus. In fact, this is typically observed in the murine model of TB: after a period of around three weeks of exponential growth of *M. tuberculosis* following inoculation of the mouse, the bacillary burden, as measured by counting bacterial colony-forming units, plateaus. This change in the rate of bacterial growth coincides with the onset of specific immunity. While one might at first conclude this represents "latency," there are important differences between the condition of the mice and that of humans with LTBI. First, the mice continue to harbor high titers of bacilli in their lungs. Second, the mice eventually succumb to the disease, specifically to the loss of airspace in the lungs as a result of progressive inflammatory infiltration. Recent studies by Sherman et al., challenge the notion of reduced bacillary replication in the chronic phase of mouse infection (110). They found that *M. tuberculosis* maintain a state of active replication throughout the chronic stage of infection, and that bacillary load (including live, dead, and isolated organisms) is much higher than would be inferred from direct counting of colony-forming units.

Unfortunately, there are still no truly adequate animal models for LTBI, although the rabbit model shows great promise. Rabbits infected with *M. tuberculosis* form the caseous lesions typical of human TB pathology and, like most humans, are often able to contain the disease such that no cultivable bacilli are recovered from lung homogenates of these animals. If these animals harbor latent bacilli, it may be possible to precipitate reactivation TB through the use of immunosuppressive agents.

A. Hypoxia

Active tuberculosis infection most often occurs in highly oxygenated portions of the lung, with higher bacillary loads being observed in pulmonary cavities with unobstructed access to open airways. In fact, reactivation of latent disease most often occurs in the upper lobes of the lung, which are more extensively oxygenated (111). In vitro models in which *M. tuberculosis* halt replication yet remain viable have been developed to better study the bacterial physiology in LTBI. One of these models, developed by Wayne, is based on the gradual depletion of oxygen from exponentially growing cultures (112). Given the avascular nature of the caseous lesion, and the fact that hypoxia results in a nonreplicating yet viable state, the Wayne model seems to represent a logical hypothesis to explain the change in bacillary metabolism in LTBI. Wayne and colleagues found specific enzyme activities that were induced upon transition to the hypoxic state. Specifically, glycine dehydrogenase activity, catalyzing the reductive amination of glyoxylate to glycine, was significantly increased (113). The production of glycine in this reaction is coupled to the oxidation of NADH to NAD$^+$, and it has been postulated that this regeneration of NAD$^+$ allows the bacillus to complete the current cycle of DNA replication and achieve an orderly metabolic shutdown (113).

The Wayne model results in two distinct models of nonreplicating persistence (NRP). The first, termed NRP1, is a microaerophilic stage characterized by reduced levels of dissolved oxygen, although steady levels of ATP are maintained within the culture. The second, termed NRP2, is an anaerobic state in which bacilli remain viable, but optical density no longer increases and glycine dehydrogenase concentration is reduced (112). The capacity of *M. tuberculosis* to survive the anaerobic conditions of NRP2 is dependent on a gradual reduction in dissolved oxygen and having spent a period of transition in NRP1.

Boon et al. subsequently used the Wayne model to study protein changes in *M. bovis* BCG and found that four proteins were significantly induced (114). Two of these are proteins of unknown function. The third protein, HspX (Acr), belongs to a family of proteins known as chaperones. Chaperones assist in the proper folding (or refolding) of other proteins either during synthesis or after they have become misfolded due to heat shock or chemical stress. The fourth protein, DosR, is a transcriptional regulator that activates the expression of many genes, including *hspX*, in response to hypoxic conditions (115). More recently, whole-genome expression profiling of *M. tuberculosis* identified a host of genes induced in response to hypoxic conditions, including *dosR*, *hspX*, and several genes involved in diverse metabolic pathways, many of which were subsequently found to be regulated by DosR (115). Several genes found to be induced by hypoxia were also found to be induced by low levels of NO, a potent antibacterial molecule implicated in the defense against *M. tuberculosis* (116). Among these genes were *dosR*, *hspX*, *nrdZ* (ribonucleotide reductase class II), *narX* (fused nitrate reductase), *narK2* (nitrite extrusion protein), *ctpF* (cation transport ATPase), and *fdxA* (ferredoxin).

Muttucumaru and colleagues further examined global gene expression profiles in samples taken from both NRP1 and NRP2 cultures grown in the Wayne model of NRP. A number of genes were observed to be upregulated in comparison to aerobically grown cultures, including glycine dehydrogenase, nitrate reductase, the fatty acid metabolism genes *fadD26* and *mas*, and genes under control of the DosR regulator (117). Klinkenberg et al. also employed the Wayne model in order to examine the survival of *M. tuberculosis* mutants with transposon disruptions in genes known to be induced under hypoxic conditions. Out of the 107 mutants tested in this model, 74 were observed to be attenuated relative to the wild-type, with disruptions in genes Rv3134c, Rv1894c, and Rv0020c resulting in greater than 10-fold attenuation (118). Many additional genes potentially involved in dormancy and establishment of LTBI were identified in a comprehensive bioinformatics study by Murphy and Brown (119). In this meta-analysis, gene expression profiles from multiple proposed dormancy models were compiled and analyzed, including nutrient starvation, hypoxia, hollow fiber granulomas, macrophage infections, and in vivo murine models. The most highly induced genes across multiple models were identified as potential drug targets for latent disease. Among these were the dosR regulon and the isopentenyl-pyrophosphate biosynthetic pathway (possibly to promote the maintenance of bacterial membrane integrity). Significantly downregulated were genes associated with ATP and ribosomal synthesis.

A novel *in vivo* granuloma model of tuberculosis infection demonstrating regions of hypoxia was developed by Karakousis et al. using mouse hollow fibers. Organisms within this model display a dormant phenotype analogous to what is observed in human LTBI. In this model, liquid cultures of *M. tuberculosis* are sealed in hollow PVDF fibers and implanted subcutaneously in immunocompetent SKH1 hairless mice. In this microenvironment bacilli exhibit reduced metabolic rates, stationary state growth, and persistence in the presence of antimicrobial treatment (120). Granulomatous lesions develop surrounding the implanted fibers in which microaerophilic conditions were detected using pimonidazole, a maker for hypoxia. Pimonidazole is a 2-nitroimidazole which binds to cellular proteins at low levels of oxygen, forming adducts which may be detected by immunohistochemistry. Degree of hypoxia was observed to be dose dependent, as pimonidazole staining intensity increased with higher bacillary load (118). Transposon disruption mutants for hypoxia-induced genes were then examined in this model, with 67 of these observed to be attenuated for survival in the hollow fiber. Identification of such microbial factors involved in hypoxia will hopefully lead to a more extensive understanding of the driving force behind the shift of the bacilli into a dormant state.

Additional in vivo studies have also been successful in demonstrating reduced oxygen conditions in the guinea pig. Following infection with *M. tuberculosis*, guinea pigs exhibit lung lesions characterized by necrosis, hypoxia, and mineralization, similar to clinical manifestation in humans (Fig. 4). Recent studies have demonstrated hypoxia in guinea pig primary granulomas one month postinfection through pimonidazole staining (121). It was found that, following antimicrobial treatment, persistent bacilli remained in the hypoxic regions of primary lesion necrosis. Such studies support the notion of a hypoxia-induced shift in the state of the bacilli during latent infection.

B. Nutrient Starvation

Another in vitro model that maintains bacterial viability in a state of nonreplication is nutrient starvation. Using whole-genome expression profiling, Betts et al. identified several hundred genes that were induced during nutrient limitation. Among these were *hspX*, discussed above, and four genes (*sigB*, *sigE*, *sigF*, and *sigD*) belonging to the sigma factor family (122). Sigma factors are components of the bacterial RNA polymerase that confer gene target specificity to the polymerase, that is, it is the sigma factor that determines which genes a given molecule of RNA polymerase will recognize and express. Although these genomic studies have identified many genes and metabolic pathways involved in response to starvation or hypoxia, the actual molecular mechanisms by which tubercle bacilli enter a latent state have yet to be elucidated. In fact, it is still not known whether these in vitro conditions truly represent the bacterial physiology at work in LTBI.

Depletion of phosphate from the microenvironment of the bacilli during infection may also play a role in the maintenance of a nonreplicative state (123). Recent studies have demonstrated that phosphate limitation impedes bacterial growth and induces tolerance to treatment with isoniazid. Phosphate deficiency within macrophage phagosomes may, therefore, play a role in nonreplicative persistence during infection of the host.

VII. Conclusion

What, then, does biomedical science have to offer to the fight against TB? One might argue that an effective vaccine would be a beneficial tool. However, roughly 90% of individuals infected with TB are able to contain the infection, and in spite of this successful immune response, many of these individuals are unable to completely eradicate the organism from the body. In addition to protecting newborns from infection, effective vaccination schemes, hence, will also need to protect adults with latent TB infection from reactivation disease. Since reactivation of LTBI most often occurs in the context of a weakened immune system, these goals remain daunting challenges.

New drugs active against the tubercle bacillus are perhaps the most desperately needed weapons in the war on TB. Our current arsenal of drugs contains both bactericidal and sterilizing antibiotics, which work both against active tuberculosis and as secondary prevention in patients with LTBI. It is likely that new anti-TB drugs may also have dual applicability for these two therapeutic needs. Safe, short course, effective therapy against latent infection is certainly a high priority for successful TB control. In fact, bacilli with latent-state physiology may comprise a significant percentage of the bacillary population even during active disease, and may be one reason why such long treatment regimens are required. As more information is gathered on the survival mechanisms of *M. tuberculosis* within the macrophage and during latent infection, new targets for drug intervention may be realized. Clearly it will take a concerted effort on the part of scientists, physicians, and other health care workers, as well as political leaders, to continue making progress against one of the most successful bacterial killers the world has ever known.

References

1. WHO Report 2008: Global Tuberculosis Control-Surveillance, Planning, Financing. Geneva, Switzerland: World Health Organization 2008, 2008:1–294.
2. Dye C, Scheele S, Dolin P, et al. Consensus statement. Global burden of tuberculosis: Estimated incidence, prevalence, and mortality by country. WHO global surveillance and monitoring project. J Am Med Assoc 1999; 282:677–686.
3. Hopewell P, Chaisson R. Tuberculosis and human immunodeficiency virus infection. In: Reichman L, Hershfield E, eds. Tuberculosis: A Comprehensive International Approach, 2nd ed. New York: Marcel Dekker, Inc., 2000:525–552.
4. Ferebee S. Controlled chemoprophylaxis trials in tuberculosis: A general review. Adv Tuberc Res 1969; 17:28–106.
5. Grzybowski S, Barnett G, Styblo K. Contacts of cases of active pulmonary tuberculosis. Bull Int Union Tuberc 1975; 50:90–106.
6. Nuermberger E, Bishai W, Grosset J. Latent Tuberculosis infection. Semin Respir Crit Care Med 2004; 25:317–336.
7. Sutherland I. Recent studies in the epidemiology of tuberculosis, based on the risk of being infected with tubercle bacilli. Adv Tuberc Res 1976; 19:1–63.
8. Sutherland I. The ten-year incidence of clinical tuberculosis following "conversion" in 2550 individuals aged 14 to 19 years. TSTRU Progress Report. The Hague: KNCV, 1968.
9. Riley R, Mills C, Nyka W, et al. Aerial dissemination of pulmonary tuberculosis: A two year study of contagion in a tuberculosis ward. Am J Hyg 1959; 70:185–196.
10. Wells W. On air-borne infection. II: Droplets and droplet nuclei. Am J Hyg 1934; 20:611–618.
11. Wells W, Lurie M. Experimental airborne disease: Quantitative natural respiratory contagion of tuberculosis. Am J Hyg 1941; 34:21–40.
12. Wells W, Ratcliffe H, Crumb C. On the mechanics of droplet nuclei infection. II: Quantitative experimental air-borne tuberculosis in rabbits. Am J Hyg 1948; 47:11–28.
13. Fennelly K, Martyny J, Fulton K, et al. Cough-generated aerosols of *Mycobacterium tuberculosis*. Am J Respir Crit Care Med 2004; 169:604–609.
14. Brown D, Donaldson K, Borm P, et al. Calcium and ROS-mediated activation of transcription factors and TNF-α cytokine gene expression in macrophages exposed to ultrafine particles. Am J Physiol Lung Cell Mol Physiol 2004; 286:L344–L353.
15. Kobzik L, Huang S, Paulauskis J, et al. Particle opsonization and lung macrophage cytokine response. J Immunol 1993; 151:2753–2759.
16. Leemans J, Juffermans N, Florquin S, et al. Depletion of alveolar macrophages exerts protective effects in pulmonary tuberculosis in mice. J Immunol 2001; 166:4604–4611.
17. Gan H, Lee J, Ren F,et al. *Mycobacterium tuberculosis* blocks crosslinking of annexin-1 and apoptotic envelope formation on infected macrophages to maintain virulence. Nat Immunol 2008; 9:1189–1197.

18. Reddy V, Hayworth D. Interaction of *Mycobacterium tuberculosis* with human respiratory epithelial cells (HEp-2). Tuberculosis 2002; 82:31–36.

19. Mehta P, King C, White E, et al. Comparison of in vitro models for the study of *Mycobacterium tuberculosis* invasion and intracellular replication. Infect Immun 1996; 64:2673–2679.

20. Bermudez L, Goodman J. *Mycobacterium tuberculosis* invades and replicates within type II alveolar cells. Infect Immun 1996; 64:1400–1406.

21. Bermudez L, Sangari F, Kolonoski P, et al. The efficiency of the translocation of *Mycobacterium tuberculosis* across a bilayer of epithelial and endothelial cells as a model of the alveolar wall is a consequence of transport within mononuclear phagocytes and invasion of alveolar epithelial cells. Infect Immun 2002; 70:140–146.

22. Sato K, Tomioka H, Shimizu T, et al. Type II alveolar cells play roles in macrophage-mediated host innate resistance to pulmonary mycobacterial infections by producing proinflammatory cytokines. J Infect Dis 2002; 185:1139–1147.

23. Menozzi F, Reddy V, Cayet D, et al. *Mycobacterium tuberculosis* heparin-binding haemagglutinin adhesin (HBHA) triggers receptor-mediated transcytosis without altering the integrity of tight junctions. Microbes Infect 2006; 8:1–9.

24. Jain S, Paul-Satyaseela M, Lamichhane G, et al. *Mycobacterium tuberculosis* invasion and traversal across an in vitro human blood-brain barrier as a pathogenic mechanism for central nervous system tuberculosis. J Infect Dis 2006; 193:1287–1295.

25. Be N, Lamichhane G, Grosset J, et al. Murine model to study the invasion and survival of *Mycobacterium tuberculosis* in the central nervous system. J Infect Dis 2008; 198:1520–1528.

26. Armstrong J, Hart P. Phagosome-lysozome interactions in cultured macrophages infected with virulent tubercle bacilli. Reversal of the usual nonfusion pattern and observations on bacterial survival. J Exp Med 1975; 142:1–16.

27. Ernst J. Macrophage receptors for *Mycobacterium tuberculosis*. Infect Immun 1998; 66: 1277–1281.

28. Peterson P, Gekker G, Hu S, et al. CD14 receptor-mediated uptake of nonopsonized *Mycobacterium tuberculosis* by human microglia. Infect Immun 1995; 63:1598–1602.

29. Schlesinger L. Macrophage phagocytosis of virulent but not attenuated strains of *Mycobacterium tuberculosis* is mediated by mannose receptors in addition to complement receptors. J Immunol 1993; 150:2920–2930.

30. Schlesinger L, Bellinger-Kawahara C, Payne N, et al. Phagocytosis of *Mycobacterium tuberculosis* is mediated by human monocyte complement receptors and complement component C3. J Immunol 1990; 144:2771–2780.

31. Zimmerli S, Edwards S, Ernst J. Selective receptor blockade during phagocytosis does not alter the survival and growth of *Mycobacterium tuberculosis* in human macrophages. Am J Respir Cell Mol Biol 1996; 15:760–770.

32. Armstrong J, Hart P. Response of cultured macrophages to *Mycobacterium tuberculosis*, with observations on fusion of lysosomes with phagosomes. J Exp Med 1971; 134:713–740.

33. Teitelbaum R, Glatman-Freedman A, Chen B, et al. A mAb recognizing a surface antigen of *Mycobacterium tuberculosis* enhances host survival. Proc Natl Acad Sci U S A 1998; 95:15688–15693.

34. Deretic V. Autophagy, an immunologic magic bullet: *Mycobacterium tuberculosis* phagosome maturation block and how to bypass it. Future Microbiol 2008; 3:517–524.

35. Rohde K, Yates R, Purdy G, et al. *Mycobacterium tuberculosis* and the environment within the phagosome. Immunol Rev 2007; 219:37–54.

36. Sturgill-Koszycki S, Schlesinger P, Chakraborty P, et al. Lack of acidification in mycobacterium phagosomes produced by exclusion of the vesicular proton-ATPase. Science 1994; 263:678–681.

37. Crowle A, Dahl R, Ross E, et al. Evidence that vessicles containing living virulent *M. tuberculosis* or *M. avium* in cultured human macrophages are not acidic. Infect Immun 1991; 59:1823–1831.

38. Sturgill-Koszycki S, Schaible U, Russell D. Mycobacterium-containing phagosomes are accessible to early endosomes and reflect a transitional state in normal phagosome biogenesis. EMBO J 1996; 15:6960–6968.
39. Barker L, George K, Falkow S, et al. Differential trafficking of live and dead *Mycobacterium marinum* organisms in macrophages. Infect Immun 1997; 65:1497–1504.
40. Clemens D, Horwitz M. Characterization of the *Mycobacterium tuberculosis* phagosome and evidence that phagosomal maturation is inhibited. J Exp Med 1995; 181:257–270.
41. Fratti R, Chua J, Vergne I, et al. *Mycobacterium tuberculosis* glycosylated phosphatidylinositol causes phagosome maturation arrest. Proc Natl Acad Sci U S A 2003; 100:5437–5442.
42. Xu S, Cooper A, Sturgill-Koszycki S, et al. Intracellular trafficking in *Mycobacterium tuberculosis* and *Mycobacterium avium*-infected macrophages. J Immunol 1994; 153:2568–2578.
43. Gutierrez M, Master S, Singh S, et al. Autophagy is a defense mechanism inhibiting BCG and *Mycobacterium tuberculosis* survival in infected macrophages. Cell 2004; 119:753–766.
44. Harris J, Master S, De Haro S, et al. Th1–Th2 polarisation and autophagy in the control of intracellular mycobacteria by macrophages. Vet Immunol Immunopathol 2008; 128:37–43.
45. Biswas D, Qureshi O, Lee W, et al. ATP-induced autophagy is associated with rapid killing of intracellular mycobacteria within human monocytes/macrophages. BMC Immunol 2008; 9:35.
46. Fratti RA, Chua J, Deretic V. Induction of p38 mitogen-activated protein kinase reduces early endosome autoantigen 1 (EEA1) recruitment to phagosomal membranes. J Biol Chem 2003; 278:46961–46967.
47. Fratti RA, Chua J, Deretic V. Cellubrevin alterations and *Mycobacterium tuberculosis* phagosome maturation arrest. J Biol Chem 2002; 277:17320–17326.
48. Fratti RA, Backer JM, Gruenberg J, et al. Role of phosphatidylinositol 3-kinase and Rab5 effectors in phagosomal biogenesis and mycobacterial phagosome maturation arrest. J Cell Biol 2001; 154:631–644.
49. Fratti RA, Vergne I, Chua J, et al. Regulators of membrane trafficking and *Mycobacterium tuberculosis* phagosome maturation block. Electrophoresis 2000; 21:3378–3385.
50. Via LE, Deretic D, Ulmer RJ, et al. Arrest of mycobacterial phagosome maturation is caused by a block in vesicle fusion between stages controlled by rab5 and rab7. J Biol Chem 1997; 272:13326–13331.
51. Deretic V, Via LE, Fratti RA, et al. Mycobacterial phagosome maturation, rab proteins, and intracellular trafficking. Electrophoresis 1997; 18:2542–2547.
52. Sun J, Deghmane A, Soualhine H, et al. *Mycobacterium bovis* BCG disrupts the interaction of Rab7 with RILP contributing to inhibition of phagosome maturation. J Leukoc Biol 2007; 82:1437–1445.
53. Christoforidis S, McBride HM, Burgoyne RD, et al. The Rab5 effector EEA1 is a core component of endosome docking. Nature 1999; 397:621–625.
54. Simonsen A, Lippe R, Christoforidis S, et al. EEA1 links PI(3)K function to Rab5 regulation of endosome fusion. Nature 1998; 394:494–498.
55. Christoforidis S, Miaczynska M, Ashman K, et al. Phosphatidylinositol-3-OH kinases are Rab5 effectors. Nat Cell Biol 1999; 1:249–252.
56. Vergne I, Chua J, Deretic V. Tuberculosis toxin blocking phagosome maturation inhibits a novel Ca^{2+}/Calmodulin-PI3 K hVPS34 cascade. J Exp Med 2003; 198:653–659.
57. Malik ZA, Denning GM, Kusner DJ. Inhibition of Ca(2+) signaling by *Mycobacterium tuberculosis* is associated with reduced phagosome-lysosome fusion and increased survival within human macrophages. J Exp Med 2000; 191:287–302.
58. Malik ZA, Iyer SS, Kusner DJ. *Mycobacterium tuberculosis* phagosomes exhibit altered calmodulin-dependent signal transduction: Contribution to inhibition of phagosome-lysosome fusion and intracellular survival in human macrophages. J Immunol 2001; 166:3392–3401.

59. Vergne I, Chua J, Singh S, et al. Cell biology of *Mycobacterium tuberculosis* phagosome. Annu Rev Cell Dev Biol 2004; 20:367–394.

60. Jayachandran R, Sundaramurthy V, Combaluzier B, et al. Survival of mycobacteria in macrophages is mediated by coronin 1-dependent activation of calcineurin. Cell 2007; 130:37–50.

61. Philips J, Porto M, Wang H, et al. ESCRT factors restrict mycobacterial growth. Proc Natl Acad Sci U S A 2008; 105:3070–3075.

62. Malik ZA, Thompson CR, Hashimi S, et al. Cutting edge: *Mycobacterium tuberculosis* blocks Ca2+ signaling and phagosome maturation in human macrophages via specific inhibition of sphingosine kinase. J Immunol 2003; 170:2811–2815.

63. Spiegel S, Milstien S. Sphingosine 1-phosphate, a key cell signalling molecule. J Biol Chem 2002; 277:25851–25854.

64. Melendez A, Floto R, Gilooly D, et al. FcγRI coupling to phospholipase D initiates sphingosine kinase-mediated calcium mobilization and vesicular trafficking. J Biol Chem 1998; 273:9393–9402.

65. Welin A, Winberg M, Abdalla H, et al. Incorporation of *Mycobacterium tuberculosis* lipoarabinomannan into macrophage membrane rafts is a prerequisite for the phagosomal maturation block. Infect Immun 2008; 76:2882–2887.

66. Shabaana A, Kulangara K, Semac I, et al. Mycobacterial lipoarabinomannans modulate cytokine production in human T helper cells by interfering with raft/microdomain signalling. Cell Mol Life Sci 2005; 62:179–187.

67. Lee B, Clemens D, Horwitz M. The metabolic activity of *Mycobacterium tuberculosis*, assessed by use of a novel inducible GFP expression system, correlates with its capacity to inhibit phagosomal maturation and acidification in human macrophages. Mol Microbiol 2008; 68:1047–1060.

68. Vergne I, Chua J, Lee H, et al. Mechanism of phagolysosome biogenesis block by viable *Mycobacterium tuberculosis*. Proc Natl Acad Sci U S A 2005; 102:4033–4038.

69. Bach H, Papavinasasundaram K, Wong D, et al. *Mycobacterium tuberculosis* virulence is mediated by PtpA dephosphorylation of human vacuolar protein sorting 33B. Cell Host Microbe 2008; 3:316–322.

70. Pieters J. *Mycobacterium tuberculosis* and the macrophage: Maintaining a balance. Cell Host Microbe 2008; 3:399–407.

71. Walburger A, Koul A, Ferrari G, et al. Protein kinase G from pathogenic mycobacteria promotes survival within macrophages. Science 2004; 304:1800–1804.

72. Stanley S, Raghavan S, Hwang W, et al. Acute infection and macrophage subversion by *Mycobacterium tuberculosis* require a specialized secretion system. Proc Natl Acad Sci U S A 2003; 100:13001–13006.

73. Brodin P, Rosenkrands I, Andersen P, et al. ESAT-6 proteins: Protective antigens and virulence factors? Trends Microbiol 2004; 12:500–508.

74. Xu J, Laine O, Masciocchi M, et al. A unique Mycobacterium ESX-1 protein co-secretes with CFP-10/ESAT-6 and is necessary for inhibiting phagosome maturation. Mol Microbiol 2007; 66:787–800.

75. Berthet F, Rasmussen P, Rosenkrands I, et al. A *Mycobacterium tuberculosis* operon encoding ESAT-6 and a novel low-molecular-mass culture filtrate protein (CFP-10). Microbiology 1998; 144:3195–3203.

76. Brandt L, Elhay M, Rosenkrands I, et al. ESAT-6 subunit vaccination against *Mycobacterium tuberculosis*. Infect Immun 2000; 68:791–795.

77. Olsen A, Hansen P, Holm A, et al. Efficient protection against *Mycobacterium tuberculosis* by vaccination with a single subdominant epitope from the ESAT-6 antigen. Eur J Immunol 2000; 30:1724–1732.

78. Andersen P, Munk M, Pollock J, et al. Specific immune-based diagnosis of tuberculosis. Lancet 2000; 356:1099–1104.

79. Lalvani A. Diagnosing tuberculosis infection in the 21st century: new tools to tackle an old enemy. Chest 2007; 131(6):1898–1906.
80. McDonough K, Kress Y, Bloom B. The interaction of *Mycobacterium tuberculosis* with macrophages: A study of phagolysosome fusion. Infect Agents Dis 1993; 2:232–235.
81. van der Wel N, Hava D, Houben D, et al. *M. tuberculosis* and *M. leprae* translocate from the phagolysosome to the cytosol in myeloid cells. Cell 2007; 129:1287–1298.
82. Sutterwala F, Ogura Y, Flavell R. The inflammasome in pathogen recognition and inflammation. J Leukoc Biol 2007; 82:259–264.
83. Martinon F, Burns K, Tschopp J. The inflammasome: A molecular platform triggering activation of inflammatory caspases and processing of proIL-1B. Mol Cell 2002; 10:417–426.
84. Master S, Rampini S, Davis A, et al. *Mycobacterium tuberculosis* prevents inflammasome activation. Cell Host Microbe 2008; 3:224–232.
85. Chan J, Xing Y, Magliozzo R, et al. Killing of virulent *Mycobacterium tuberculosis* by reactive nitrogen intermediates produced by activated murine macrophages. J Exp Med 1992; 175:1111–1122.
86. MacMicking J, North R, LaCourse R, et al. Identification of nitric oxide synthase as a protective locus against tuberculosis. Proc Natl Acad Sci U S A 1997; 94:5243–5248.
87. Singh R, Manjunatha U, Boshoff H, et al. PA-824 Kills Nonreplicating *Mycobacterium tuberculosis* by intracellular NO release. Science 2008; 322:1392–1395.
88. Barry Cr, Boshoff H, Dowd C. Prospects for clinical introduction of nitroimidazole antibiotics for the treatment of tuberculosis. Curr Pharm Des 2004; 10:3239–3262.
89. Sadek M, Sada E, Toossi Z, et al. Chemokines induced by infection of mononuclear phagocytes with mycobacteria and present in lung alveoli during active pulmonary tuberculosis. Am J Respir Cell Mol Biol 1998; 19:513–521.
90. Jiao X, Lo-Man R, Guermonprez P, et al. Dendritic cells are host cells for mycobacteria in vivo that trigger innate and acquired immunity. J Immunol 2002; 168:1294–1301.
91. Marino S, Pawar S, Fuller C, et al. Dendritic cell trafficking and antigen presentation in the human immune response to *Mycobacterium tuberculosis*. J Immunol 2004; 173: 494–506.
92. Mariotti S, Teloni R, Iona E, et al. *Mycobacterium tuberculosis* diverts alpha interferon-induced monocyte differentiation from dendritic cells into immunoprivileged macrophage-like host cells. Infect Immun 2004; 72:4385–4392.
93. Geijtenbeek T, van Vliet S, Koppel E, et al. Mycobacteria target DC-SIGN to suppress dendritic cell function. J Exp Med 2003; 197:7–17.
94. van Kyook Y, Geijtenbeek T. DC-SIGN: Escape mechanism for pathogens. Nat Rev Immunol 2003; 3:697–709.
95. Lurie M. Resistance to Tuberculosis. Cambridge, MA: Harvard University Press, 1964.
96. Lurie M. The correlation between the histological changes and the fate of living tubercle bacilli in the organs of tuberculous rabbits. J Exp Med 1932; 55:31–54.
97. Dannenberg AM Jr. Roles of cytotoxic delayed-type hypersensitivity and macrophage-activating cell-mediated immunity in the pathogenesis of tuberculosis. Immunobiology 1994; 191:461–73.
98. Dannenberg AM Jr. Pathogenesis of pulmonary *Mycobacterium bovis* infection: Basic principles established by the rabbit model. Tuberculosis 2001; 81:87–96.
99. Lurie M. The fate of tubercle bacilli in the organs of reinfected rabbits. J Exp Med 1929; 50:747.
100. Lurie M. A correlation between the histological changes and the fate of living tubercle bacilli in the organs of reinfected rabbits. J Exp Med 1933; 57:181.
101. Yamamura Y. The pathogenesis of tuberculous cavities. Adv Tuberc Res 1958; 9:13–37.
102. Yamamura Y, Yasaka S, Yamaguchi M, et al. Studies of the experimental tuberculosis cavity: The experimental formulation of the tuberculous cavity in the rabbit lung. Med J Osaka Univ 1954; 5:187–197.

103. Yamamura Y, Ogawa Y, Yamagata H, et al. Prevention of tuberculous cavity formation by immunosuppressive drugs. Am Rev Respir Dis 1968; 98:720.

104. Lucas S, Nelson A. Pathogenesis of tuberculosis in human immunodeficiency virus-infected people. In: Bloom B, ed. Tuberculosis: Pathogenesis, Protection and Control. Washington, DC: American Society for Microbiology, 1994:503–513.

105. Keane J, Gershon S, Wise RP, et al. Tuberculosis associated with infliximab, a tumor necrosis factor alpha-neutralizing agent. N Engl J Med 2001; 345:1098–104.

106. Centers for Disease Control and Prevention. Tuberculosis associated with blocking agents against tumor necrosis factor-alpha–California, 2002–2003. MMWR Morb Mortal Wkly Rep 2004; 53:683–686.

107. Wallis RS, Broder MS, Wong JY, et al. Granulomatous infectious diseases associated with tumor necrosis factor antagonists. Clin Infect Dis 2004; 38:1261–1265.

108. Wallis R, Broder M, Wong J, et al. Granulomatous infections due to tumor necrosis factor blockade: Correction. Clin Infect Dis 2004; 39:1254–1255.

109. Horsburgh CR Jr. Priorities for the treatment of latent tuberculosis infection in the United States. N Engl J Med 2004; 350:2060–2067.

110. Gill WP, Harik NS, Whiddon, MR, et al. A replication clock for Mycobacterium tuberculosis. Nat Med 2009; 15(2):211–214.

111. Adler J, Rose D. Transmission and pathogenesis of tuberculosis. In: Rom W, Garay S, eds. Tuberculosis, 1st ed. Boston: Little, Brown & Company, 1996:1002.

112. Wayne L, Sohaskey C. Nonreplicating persistence of *Mycobacterium tuberculosis*. Annu Rev Microbiol 2001; 55:139–163.

113. Wayne L, Lin K. Glyoxylate metabolism and adaptation of *Mycobacterium tuberculosis* to survival under anaerobic conditions. Infect Immun 1982; 37:1042–1049.

114. Boon C, Li R, Qi R, et al. Proteins of *Mycobacterium bovis* BCG induced in the Wayne dormancy model. J Bacteriol 2001; 183:2672–2676.

115. Park H, Guinn K, Harrell M, et al. Rv3133 c/dosR is a transcription factor that mediates the hypoxic response of *Mycobacterium tuberculosis*. Mol Microbiol 2003; 48:833–843.

116. Voskuil M, Schnappinger D, Visconti K, et al. Inhibition of respiration by nitric oxide induces a *Mycobacterium tuberculosis* dormancy program. J Exp Med 2003; 198:705–713.

117. Muttucumaru D, Roberts G, Hinds J, et al. Gene expression profile of *Mycobacterium tuberculosis* in a non-replicating state. Tuberculosis 2004; 84:239–246.

118. Klinkenberg L, Sutherland L, Bishai W, et al. Metronidazole lacks activity against *Mycobacterium tuberculosis* in an in vivo hypoxic granuloma model of latency. J Infect Dis 2008; 198:275–283.

119. Murphy D, Brown J. Identification of gene targets against dormant phase *Mycobacterium tuberculosis* infections. BMC Infect Dis 2007; 7:84.

120. Karakousis P, Yoshimatsu T, Lamichhane G, et al. Dormancy phenotype displayed by extracellular *Mycobacterium tuberculosis* within artificial granulomas in mice. J Exp Med 2004; 200:647–657.

121. Lenaerts A, Hoff D, Aly S, et al. Location of persisting mycobacteria in a guinea pig model of tuberculosis revealed by R207910. Antimicrob Agents Chemother 2007; 51:3338–3345.

122. Betts J, Lukey P, Robb L, et al. Evaluation of a nutrient starvation model of *Mycobacterium tuberculosis* persistence by gene and protein expression profiling. Mol Microbiol 2002; 43:717–731.

123. Rifat D, Bishai WR, Karakousis PC. Phosphate Depletion: A Novel Trigger for Mycobacterium tuberculosis Persistence. J Infect Dis 2009; 200(7):1126–1135.

4
Diagnosis of Pulmonary and Extrapulmonary Tuberculosis

PHUNG K. LAM and ANTONINO CATANZARO
University of California, San Diego, School of Medicine, San Diego, California, U.S.A.

SHARON PERRY
Stanford University School of Medicine, Division of Geographic Medicine and Infectious Diseases, Stanford, California, U.S.A.

I. Introduction

The diagnosis of active tuberculosis (TB) is, and will always be, a clinical exercise. No single diagnostic test for TB exists at present that can be performed rapidly, simply, inexpensively, and accurately as a stand-alone test for active TB.

Since the landmark discovery over a century ago that TB is caused by *Mycobacterium tuberculosis*, the specific diagnosis of TB had depended one way or another on the demonstration that *M. tuberculosis* or a fragment of the organism is present in a clinical specimen. Many resource-limited settings have developed a heavy dependence on the acid-fast bacillus (AFB) smear microscopy. Unfortunately several technical limitations of this test have lead to the underdiagnosis of active cases of TB when it is the only confirmatory test. In many settings, the limited sensitivity of the AFB smear is augmented by a variety of conventional but less specific methods of diagnosis, such as clinical evaluation, chest radiographs, and chest computed tomography (CT) scans. This practice often leads to overdiagnosis of active TB (1).

Laboratory developers and clinical scientists have developed a number of new methods to aid in the diagnosis of TB infection and TB disease. These new methods include interferon-γ release assays (IGRA), new culture media, microscopic-observation drug-susceptibility (MODS) assay, nucleic acid amplification (NAA), the line-probe assay, tests to identify molecules produced by *M. tuberculosis*, or tests to detect an immune response to antigens of *M. tuberculosis* in biological fluids. These efforts have had mixed results. Rapid and accurate tests tend to be impeded by cost (e.g., culture, NAAs) or technical challenges (e.g., NAAs, MODS) that currently limit their widespread use. Assays that can be performed rapidly, simply, and inexpensively (e.g., serologic or urine tests) have the limitation of low diagnostic accuracy. The lack of specificity between TB infection and active disease can also limit the usefulness of some tests (e.g., IGRAs) in high-burden communities.

Because of the limitations of laboratory-based diagnostic methods, assessment of clinical suspicion of TB (CSTB) remains as the cornerstone of TB diagnosis. Suspicion of TB drives the initiation, the intensity, and the scope of diagnostic inquiries; the suspicion of active TB drives the decision to treat. The influence of clinical suspicion varies in degree from great impact when reliability of a test is low to minimal impact when reliability is high, but it always plays some role in the diagnostic process.

In this chapter, each of the diagnostic modalities is discussed. At the end of the chapter, we describe how to integrate the multiple diagnostic modalities to form an assessment of the CSTB and how to apply that assessment to the rapid diagnosis of TB.

II. Medical History and Physical Examination

TB is generally insidious in onset; symptoms may be minimal or absent until the disease is advanced. With pulmonary TB, the cardinal symptoms are cough, fever, sweats or chills, anorexia, weight loss, and malaise (2,3). Persistent cough, which may be dry or productive, is the most common symptom (4,5). Hemoptysis is usually seen with advanced illness (6). Dyspnea is more likely to occur with pleural involvement (effusion), but with extensive parenchymal or miliary disease frank respiratory failure may ensue (7). Chest pain often results from involvement of the pleura or adjacent parenchyma (6). Individual symptoms and combinations of symptoms lack both sensitivity and specificity for diagnosis. Cough, the most sensitive symptomatic indicator of active disease, is described in 40% to 80% of patients with pulmonary TB, while fever and weight loss generally occur in less than half, and hemoptysis is found in less than one-quarter (2,3,8). In one study, having three of the following four symptoms, cough for greater than 21 days, chest pain for greater than 15 days, absence of expectoration, and absence of dyspnea, was reported to have a sensitivity of 86%, but a specificity of only 49% (5). Similarly, findings of physical examination are both insensitive and nonspecific for diagnosing pulmonary TB (4).

In most settings, even in high-burden communities these symptoms are more likely to be caused by far more common pulmonary conditions like COPD, asthma, bronchiectasis, fungal infections, or lung cancer. This is the reason that the World Health Organization (WHO) and others have insisted on having a positive AFB smear to diagnose TB. Routine laboratory tests may very well be abnormal however are usually not very helpful except perhaps in patients with advanced disease (3). The most common hematologic abnormalities are mild anemia and leukocytosis (2,9). Hyponatremia and hypercalcemia have also been observed (10,11).

III. Microbiological Examination of Respiratory Specimen

A. Acid-Fast Bacillus Smear

If pulmonary TB is suspected based on clinical (or, where promptly available, radiographic evaluation), the next step should be examination of the sputum for mycobacteria. For patients with a productive cough, collection of an early morning, freshly expectorated specimen is recommended (4,12). For patients unable to produce sputum, induction of sputum production via inhalation of nebulized hypertonic saline should be considered (13). For many years it has been standard practice to obtain at least three sputum specimens, collected 24 hours apart (14). Recently several studies have pointed out that the third sputum collection increase case detection by only small percentage points. This has prompted the WHO to recently recommend that "at least two sputum samples" should be collected. Furthermore, the U.S. Centers for Disease Control and Prevention (CDC) has changed its recommendation based on expert opinion to state that it is acceptable to collect sputum for examination as often as every eight hours (15). If it is not possible to collect a sputum sample, even with induction, lavage of gastric secretions to collect aspirated TB organisms should be considered, although this technique has been used primarily in children. Alternatively, bronchoscopy with lavage, brushings or even a transbronchial biopsy, or needle aspiration may be considered. Bronchoscopic sampling can enhance both the speed and likelihood of making a diagnosis for an individual patient (16,17). Recent systematic studies have not found bronchoscopy to provide an aggregate diagnostic yield superior to aerosol-induced sputum sampling, however (18).

Direct microscopic examination of sputum for AFB is inexpensive, rapid, and relatively easy to perform. Compared to mycobacterial culture, the sensitivity of a single sputum AFB smear is 30% to 40%, but increases to 65% to 80% with multiple specimens or concentration of sputum (19,20). The smear is more likely to be positive if disease is extensive, involving multiple lobes or includes cavitary changes (21). Because direct microscopy cannot distinguish between *M. tuberculosis* and nontuberculous mycobacteria (NTM), specificity is a concern. The prevalence of NTM in the environment and disease due to NTM varies widely according to geographic location and patient population. Because of the prevalence of TB in the population tested, many published studies have shown that the AFB smear to continues to have a high specificity (>90%) and positive predictive value (PPV) (70–90%), even in HIV-infected populations where the incidence of NTM may be high (8,22–24). The sensitivity of AFB smear is such that it requires 6000 to 10,000 organism per mL of sample to register as positive. While this limits the sensitivity of microscopy, it also serves to identify patients who are highly infectious and therefore the highest priority for immediate anti-TB treatment.

Methods to improve the sensitivity of AFB smear include fluorescence microscopy, which uses an acid-fast fluorochrome dye with an intense light source. A systematic review showed that fluorescence microscopy has higher sensitivity and comparable specificity to conventional AFB smear (25). Fluorochrome staining is simpler than Ziehl-Neelsen methods, and fluorescence microscopy requires less time and effort from microscopists. In addition, the adaptation of fluorescence microscopes with light-emitting diodes makes fluorescence microscopy more reliable in resource-limited laboratories (26). While fluorescence microscopy was used in predominantly higher-income countries, studies have shown that it may be cost-effective for lower-income countries with high burden of AFB smear examinations (27,28).

B. Mycobacterial Culture

Mycobacterial culture is considerably more sensitive and specific than microscopy for the diagnosis of TB. The classic egg-based solid medium has been used around the world. Clear agar media such as Middlebrook 7H10 have allowed the detection of growth earlier and liquid media are more sensitive and growth is even faster. Liquid medium cultures, coupled with detections systems that detect the release of C 14 from nutrients or color change indicating the consumption of oxygen, are a bit more costly but faster than conventional liquid cultures and allow automation. Even so, the major limitation of culture is the delay in obtaining results. Even using newer liquid-based systems (BACTEC-460 or BACTEC MGIT-960, Becton Dickinson, Sparks, Maryland, U.S.A.), detection and identification of *M. tuberculosis* requires an average of two weeks (29). Using final clinical diagnosis of pulmonary TB as the standard, the sensitivity of sputum culture is greater than 80% (21,22). Mainly because of laboratory contamination of the specimen at the bedside or in the laboratory, false positives also occur with culture. Nevertheless, the specificity of culture has been reported to be as high as 98% (22).

C. Drug Susceptibility Testing

Once *M. tuberculosis* has been isolated from any clinical specimen it can be inoculated into medium that has one or more antibiotics. A tube without antibiotic is used as a control. Any of the media discussed above can be used to perform drug susceptibility testing (DST). The concentration of antibiotics is generally chosen by microbiologists to separate populations that are resistant to an antibiotic from those that are sensitive. Drug susceptibility results are an excellent guide in identifying strains that are likely to be clinically resistant to a particular drug. Drug susceptibility studies generally take much less time to grow out than it took for the original culture.

D. The Microscopic-Observation Drug-Susceptibility Assay

The MODS assay is a microscope-based assay that exploits the fact that *M. tuberculosis* grows more rapidly in liquid broth than solid medium and results in specific "cord" formations that can be seen through the microscope long before colonies on solid medium are visible to the naked eye. The MODS method uses a 24-well culture plate format. Patient sputum samples are processed and placed in wells with culture broth and in wells with broth and drugs. The plates are sealed in plastic bags that are impervious to *M. tuberculosis*. If *M. tuberculosis* grows, a diagnosis of active TB can be made. If *M. tuberculosis* grows in broth alone, but not in drug-containing wells, the isolate is drug sensitive. If *M. tuberculosis* also grows in drug-containing wells, resistant *M. tuberculosis* are present. In addition to the rapid molecular assays described below, the MODS assay is a well-described microbiological technique that has been shown to be reliable, cheap, and easy to implement in low-volume, low-resource settings for susceptibility testing. The assay is flexible in that multiple drugs, even at different concentrations, can be tested at once; the drug panel can be customized to fit specific treatment regimens. When used directly to detect *M. tuberculosis* in sputum, results are available as early as seven days instead of two to three weeks following positive culture (30). Although validated to detect resistance to first-line drugs, reliable methodology for detection of resistance to second-line drugs has not yet been established.

Since initial proof-of-principle development in the late 1990s, the MODS assay has undergone several rounds of evaluation and refinement, culminating in a large-scale validation involving nearly 2000 patients with suspected TB presenting to clinics or hospitals in Lima (30). For smear-positive (1+ and higher) as well as smear-negative sputum specimens, the test has proven to have at least equivalent sensitivity and specificity as standard culture and DST methods used in low TB prevalence settings and superior sensitivity when used in developing countries with high TB prevalence. The sensitivity and specificity values for MODS, respectively, were 97.8% and 99.6% in evaluating for active TB and 88.6% and 100% in evaluating for multidrug-resistant TB (MDR-TB). With direct testing on sputum using MODS, results are available in 7 to 10 days, rivaling gold standard methods for TB identification and far surpassing gold standard DST turnaround times for substantially lower cost. Studies by university-based groups in Ethiopia, Honduras, and Brazil showed essentially the same level of accuracy in detecting active and MDR-TB. While the MODS assay is a freely adaptable technique, a standardized and technically improved MODS kit is currently in the process of development for more widespread use.

IV. Microbiological Examination of Nonrespiratory Specimen

A. Acid-Fast Bacillus Smear and Culture

Extrapulmonary TB is seen in only about 15% of cases in immunocompetent individuals, but is found in up to 70% of patients with advanced HIV (31–33). The most common sites of extrapulmonary TB are peripheral lymph nodes, the pleura, the bones and joints, the genitourinary system, peritoneum, gastrointestinal tract, and the central nervous system (32,33). When disease is isolated to an extrapulmonary site, collection of excretions (urine or stool), aspiration of fluid (e.g., pleural fluid, ascites, cerebral spinal fluid), or tissue biopsy for AFB smear, culture, and histology may be necessary for diagnosis (32,34,35). In addition, for suspected pleural disease, high levels of adenosine deaminase and interferon-γ (IFN-γ) free in the pleural fluid have been associated with pleural TB in numerous studies (36,37). These tests should be considered if available; however, their sensitivity and specificity has not been fully evaluated particularly in low-incidence populations.

V. Chest Radiography

The classic radiographic abnormalities of TB are dramatically different in primary than in reactivation TB. In addition, radiographic abnormalities are altered by comorbidities such as HIV. Primary TB refers to the initial pulmonary infection resulting from inhalation of *M. tuberculosis*-containing droplets. The chest radiograph in primary TB is often completely normal. Alternatively, it may show a small area of nonspecific pneumonitis (usually indistinguishable from bacterial pneumonia) or hilar or paratracheal lymphadenopathy (4,38,39). Enlargement of hilar or mediastinal lymph nodes occurs in up to 43% of adults and 96% of children with primary TB (38,40). Healed parenchymal lesions appear on chest radiograph as nodules, which may eventually calcify (tuberculomas) and are often associated with calcified hilar lymph nodes. In a small percentage of individuals, the initial infection progresses and can manifest as (a) a pleural effusion (less than 10% of patients); (b) extensive pneumonia; or (c) enlargement of tuberculous lymph nodes causing bronchial obstruction (collapse–consolidation lesion, most common in children younger than two years) (38,39). Most of these findings resolve without treatment making the diagnosis elusive. Miliary or disseminated TB, which makes up 1% to 7% of all forms of TB, may also occur as a manifestation of primary TB (38,41).

Reactivation pulmonary TB characteristically presents as an infiltrate in the apical or posterior segments of the upper lobes (38,39). Isolated infiltrates in the anterior segment of the upper lobe or basilar segments of the lower lobe are unusual and are more likely to be seen in combination with disease in the other commonly involved areas listed above (42). The infiltrate may appear as an ill-defined alveolar-filling process (exudative lesion) or may be fibronodular in appearance, although it usually (in about 80% of patients) presents as a combination of both (38). Cavity formation is seen in about 50% of patients, and fibrosis with volume loss occurs in about 30% (38,41). Bronchial stenosis and bronchiectasis are two other relatively common manifestations of reactivation TB. These findings are often easier to see on chest CT scanning than plain films (38). Rapid progression of pulmonary disease with severe ventilation–perfusion disturbances presenting as the adult respiratory distress syndrome is also seen in rare instances (43).

The radiographic appearance of pulmonary TB in HIV-infected patients is often "atypical." Often TB in the setting of HIV may in fact be primary disease, that is, hilar and/or mediastinal adenopathy, there may be infiltrates often without cavitation and the infiltrate is more likely to involve the lower lobes (44,45). Miliary disease has been reported to occur in up to 19% of HIV-infected patients, and pleural effusions are seen in approximately 10% (44,45). Chest radiographs may be normal in 12% to 14% of HIV-infected patients with pulmonary TB confirmed by a positive sputum AFB smear or culture (44,45).

Where there is significant clinical suspicion and plain film findings are ambiguous, CT may provide useful additional diagnostic information. CT has been shown to be more sensitive than plain films for detecting cavities, intrathoracic lymphadenopathy, miliary disease, bronchiectasis, bronchial stenosis, and pleural disease (38,46). At present, magnetic resonance imaging of the chest does not appear to have a role in the diagnosis of TB (46). In some resource-limited settings, the chest X-ray may be performed after the examination of sputum for AFB or not at all.

VI. Molecular Methods for Detection of *M. tuberculosis* and Drug Resistance

A. Nucleic Acid Amplification Assays

With advances in molecular biology, polymerase chain reaction (PCR)-based tests for diagnosis of TB first became available in the 1990s (47,48). These tests are based on amplification of target genomic sequence DNA or RNA that can then be detected with a nucleic acid probe. The method enables detection of as few as 1 to 10 bacilli in clinical specimen such as sputum and other fluids. Relative to smear, which requires a relatively large bacilli load (10^4/mL) and also identifies other acid-fast bacteria, the approach has promised to significantly enhance the sensitivity and specificity of laboratory diagnosis (49). In addition, the tests can be performed within a few hours, making them attractive against culture for rapid diagnosis (50). Because amplification detects dead as well as live organism sequences, the technology is most useful for initial diagnosis and not for treatment follow-up (19).

The basic technical requirements of these tests are now available to most clinical research laboratories in the industrialized world. In addition, a number of commercial kits have been developed, principal among them are the Gen-Probe Amplified *M. tuberculosis* Direct Test (MTD) (51–59), the Roche Amplicor COBAS PCR test (60–64), the Becton-Dickinson ProbeTec ET strand displacement system (65–67), and the Eiken Chemical (Tokyo, Japan) loop-mediated isothermal amplification (LAMP) system (68). The former two have been approved by the U.S. Food and Drug Administration (FDA) for use in the diagnosis of pulmonary disease (69); the Gen-Probe format is currently the only one approved for use in diagnosis of AFB smear-negative as well as AFB smear-positive patients (49,69). Although none of these products are approved in the United States for use in other clinical specimen, including in diagnosis of extrapulmonary disease, there is much interest in their potential for these applications, and the literature offers a number of studies about performance in these specimen (70–77), including reviews of applications in evaluation of lymphadenitis (78), pleuritis (79), and meningitis (80).

In laboratory trials of the FDA-approved NAAs, sensitivity in respiratory specimen has ranged from 50% to 95%, and specificity has ranged from 95% to 100% (19). A recent meta-analysis combining all formats ($n = 125$ studies) estimated overall sensitivity of 85% and specificity of 97% (81). Specificity is consistently very high. Sensitivity is consistently highest in AFB smear-positive specimens, and lowest in specimens from smear-negative (82,83) and/or HIV-positive patients (31,84,85). Nonetheless, the increased sensitivity of the MTD can be useful in detecting additional smear-negative TB cases. Similarly, sensitivity is lower in other specimen, such as gastric fluid (86,87), blood (88–93), CSF (80,94–96), urine (97,98), and most particularly pleural fluid (80,99–101), although specificity again remains high in all settings. Compared to smear and culture, results in some studies have been encouraging for assistance with diagnosis in children (86,102), TB meningitis (80,94,103), or paucibacillary disease (104). Variability in the sensitivity of the NAAs has decreased in more recent trials. In addition to technical improvements, such as refinement of genomic targeting technology, use of inhibition assays and improvements in specimen preparation or volume requirements (105,106), refinements in calibration of output (51,55,107,108) have also improved discrimination.

However, perhaps the most important reason for reduced variability has been the recognition of study design requirements for technology assessment (8,109). This has resulted in better attention to patient selection for study, in particular the selection of patients on the basis of clinical judgment, rather than laboratory specimen availability (110–113). Because laboratory studies do not provide the predictive values, including pretest probabilities, that TB clinicians work with in deciding diagnostic strategies (112,114), performance characteristics in AFB smear-positive and smear-negative groups can be insufficient, in as much as clinicians tend not to rely on any single criteria in their diagnostic assessments (104,115). In an important study (8), PPV of the NAA was 100% in patients classified by physicians as intermediate or high suspicion prior to any laboratory testing, versus 30% (intermediate) and 94% (high) by AFB smear. Conversely, negative predictive values were 99% and 91% in patients considered by physicians to be of low or intermediate suspicion, versus 96% and 71% by smear. In this study, the intermediate suspicion group was highly heterogeneous, containing many HIV-positive and other atypical patients, thus emphasizing the importance of individualized clinical risk assessments in evaluation of laboratory tests.

Head-to-head comparisons of commercial products have not revealed great differences in accuracy or turnaround times (105,116–121), although laboratories may have workflow preferences. As with all PCR-based technologies, cross-contamination within the laboratory can result in amplification of contaminated product and false-positive results (122–124). However, the basic technology has improved considerably in the past decade, and most commercial applications are designed to detect and minimize these errors. The CDC is currently conducting an NAA evaluation program to monitor laboratory protocols for operating PCR-based amplification systems in diagnosis of TB (125). Compared to smear and culture, the commercial tests are relatively expensive; however, the specificity and value of accurate rapid results is difficult to estimate. Laboratories operating in low-incidence areas may find the kits, which require an accumulation of test specimens, difficult to use cost-effectively because of a small number of positives per unit time (126–128). Conversely, in spite of greater usage potential, laboratories operating in low-income countries may find the costs of commercial products prohibitive (129,130).

At the present time, the CDC and American Thoracic Society (ATS) have adopted a cautiously optimistic attitude toward the NAAs, recommending their use as a confirmatory test when clinical suspicion of pulmonary disease has been elevated based on other evaluations including physical, smear, radiographic, and epidemiologic assessments (19,69). Clinicians need to keep in mind the fact that the NAAs have greater sensitivity than the AFB smear, and the MTD can be used in AFB negative cases. Outstanding questions remain regarding the cost-effectiveness of the tests, and their clinical utility, including their clinical utility for diagnosis in immunocompromised patients as well as extrapulmonary disease. However, the introduction of clinical suspicion standards has dramatically shifted the focus of NAA evaluation trials, with the promise of yielding more strategic information about clinical utility and cost-effectiveness in different settings and patient populations. Interpretation of NAA results in the context of clinical suspicion will be further described below.

B.   Line-Probe Assay

Two membrane-bound probe (strip/line) assays are commercially available, the GenoType®MTBDR*plus* assay (Hain Lifesciences, Nehren, Germany,) and the INNO-LiPA Rif.TB (Innogenetics, Ghent, Belgium). Compared to INNO-LiPA Rif.TB, the GenoType®MTBDR*plus* has the major advantage of being able to detect resistance to both INH and RIF simultaneously. Both are highly sensitive and specific when used indirectly on *M. tuberculosis* isolates (131,132), which takes several weeks to grow in culture.

The GenoType®MTBDR*plus* strip has been studied more extensively to rapidly detect *M. tuberculosis* and drug resistance directly in sputum specimens. This assay is based on the principle of amplification of DNA isolated directly from decontaminated patient specimens followed by hybridization with specific membrane-bound probes using a primer-nucleotide mix. The strip has 21 probe sequences. It has been used for the detection of *M. tuberculosis* directly in acid-fast smear-positive clinical specimens (133). A large study using GenoType®MTBDR*plus* on smear-positive sputum specimens from 536 patients with high risk for MDR-TB found sensitivity and specificity of 98.9% and 99.4%, respectively, for detection of rifampin resistance; sensitivity improved to 94.2% with specificity of 99.7% for detection of isoniazid resistance. Results were interpretable for 97% of the specimens within one to two days (134). With this demonstration, it is likely that the GenoType®MTBDR*plus* strip will become available in many more settings. The WHO recommends the use of line-probe assays for rapid detection of MDR-TB, although not as a complete replacement for conventional culture and DST; mycobacteriologic culture remains necessary for smear-negative specimens while conventional DST remains necessary to confirm extensively drug-resistant TB (135).

VII.   Antibody-Detection Tests

A.   Serodiagnosis by Immunoassays

Serodiagnostic tests using various antigens to measure antibodies to *M. tuberculosis* in serum offer several advantages. A variety of assay techniques (e.g., immunochromatographic tests, ELISA) exist, many of which are readily adaptable to regions with high prevalence of TB and limited resources. Serodiagnosis is potentially useful for early diagnosis of both pulmonary and extrapulmonary TB (136), even before clinical manifestation of disease (137). It does not require collection of specimens from the site of disease and is, therefore, especially feasible for TB diagnosis in patients with extrapulmonary disease and in young children who are usually incapable of providing sputum for AFB smear and culture examination (138,139).

There are also several substantial challenges to serodiagnosis of TB. The most favorable tests use purified proteins of limited species distribution, but host antibody response tends to be directed toward shared mycobacterial antigens (136). Variations in test accuracy appear to be population dependent, influenced by factors such as age, geographic origin, exposure to NTM, stage of disease, and past episodes of TB (139–142); in addition, immunosuppressed TB patients such as HIV-positive individuals may test negatively because of their inability to mount an appropriate immune response (140,143).

Laboratory scientists have identified many *M. tuberculosis*-specific antigens with diagnostic potential, several of which have been studied frequently in the clinical context. The first antigen identified was MPT-64, although it remains controversial in TB diagnosis particularly because it has been shown to be present in some bacille Calmette-Guérin (BCG) strains (138). The 38 kDa protein antigen was used in early commercial assays (144) and is considered the "diagnostic antigen of choice" (136). This antigen performed extremely well in Argentina and China, yielding 80% to 90% sensitivity, 84% to 100% specificity, and high predictive values (145,146); however, other studies found low sensitivity, especially in patients who were AFB smear-negative or coinfected with HIV (144). In addition, patients with lepromatous leprosy also produce large amounts of antibodies to the 38 kDa antigen (147). Antigen 60 (A60), obtained from purified protein derivatives, is widely used but has produced discrepant results in various populations (140). A60 contains large amounts of lipoarabinomannan (LAM) polysaccharide antigen, and this constituent may be responsible for variability in A60 tests. In some populations, ELISA with LAM produced favorable results (148), but this has not been the general experience. Use of another antigen, TB glycolipid (TBGL), resulted in increased sensitivity in Japan but different specificity values among patient groups (141). Another potentially useful antigen is 30 kDa, a major protein of mycobacteria. It is a fibronectin-binding protein that may be a major antigen for host recognition of TB. Although widely distributed among mycobacteria, it appears to have species-restricted epitopes and has performed well in serodiagnosis by ELISA (149,150). Recently, two closely-related low-molecular-mass proteins—ESAT-6 and CFP-10—were identified (138,151). They are readily recognized by host immune cells and are absent from BCG strains as well as most environmental mycobacterial species (138). They can detect early active TB and subclinical infection (152,153).

The performance of serodiagnostic tests varies among studies depending on (a) cutoff values selected to discriminate positive from negative test results, (b) target population (e.g., infection with HIV or NTM, or BCG vaccination), and (c) control groups (e.g., healthy controls or patients with other pulmonary disease). Some antigens are of greater value in AFB smear-positive disease (e.g., 38 kDa antigen), while others fare better in smear-negative and culture-positive disease (e.g., 19 kDa antigen) (154). Many studies have compared serodiagnostic tests in known cases of TB against healthy controls. Their use has been disappointing in clinical practice where true TB cases must be distinguished from patients suspected of having TB but who in fact have other conditions.

A number of commercial kits for the detection of antibodies in sera are currently marketed in developing countries. The kits differ in features including test format (i.e., modifications of ELISA or immunochromatographic tests), antigen composition (e.g., secreted and heat shock proteins, lipopolysaccharides, or peptides), and class of detected immunoglobulins (e.g., IgA, IgG, IgM). (155,156) Overall, the range of sensitivity and specificity values for each test varied widely and inconsistently among studies. All studies revealed shortcomings in either sensitivity or specificity, or both. Sensitivity is higher in smear-positive than smear-negative samples. Specificity is higher in healthy volunteers than in patients suspected of having TB. Most of the commercial tests lack adequate studies in smear-negative patients, children, and HIV-infected individuals; these groups are populations that may benefit most from serodiagnostic tests. Currently, no single commercial test can replace the AFB smear.

With increasing numbers of TB antigens identified, combining multiple antigens in polyproteins and mixtures or integrating results from multiple tests has helped to increase diagnostic accuracy in studies of HIV-negative and HIV-positive patients and pulmonary and extrapulmonary TB. For pulmonary TB, single-antigen tests with low sensitivity of 47% to 71% can be increased to 76% to 92% (141,144,150) by combining two to five antigens, and single-antigen tests with low specificity of 18% to 59% can be increased to 78% by combining four test results (157). In addition, combinations of ESAT-6 and CFP-10 yielded sensitivity of 73% to 93% (153,158), compared to 60% for each antigen individually (158), and specificity of 77% to 93% (not reported for antigens individually) (153,158). Furthermore, one study found that a combination of ESAT-6 and CFP-10 is equally accurate in diagnosis of pulmonary and extrapulmonary TB in HIV-negative patients, with sensitivity of 77% and specificity of 94% (151).

A couple of studies used a combination of a number of commercial tests. In a study of HIV-negative subjects, seven test kits individually yielded sensitivity values of 16% to 57% and specificity values of 80% to 97%; all tests performed equally in comparisons between pulmonary and extrapulmonary TB cases and between AFB smear-positive and smear-negative cases (159). In a study of HIV-positive subjects, eight test kits individually yielded sensitivity values of 0% to 63% and specificity values of 39% to 99% (143).

Integrating results from serodiagnostic and other laboratory tests further increases diagnostic accuracy. Combining results of multiantigen tests and AFB smear significantly increased sensitivity from 66% to 76% to 93% (144,157), while the specificity did not change significantly (from 7–76%) (157). A study on a commercial multiantigen test kit also showed that the sensitivity (55%) can be increased to 72% by combining results from the test kit and AFB smear (160); specificity was not reported. In addition, one study found that combining results of the TBGL test and the Amplicor NAA test improved the sensitivity of the individual tests from 57% and 52%, respectively, to 78% (161); specificity values were not reported. Another study also found that combining results of a serodiagnostic kit and the Amplicor test improved the sensitivity of the individual tests from 38% and 57%, respectively, to 75%; specificity values of 87% and 100%, respectively, changed to 90% (104).

Therefore, even with less than optimal diagnostic characteristics as stand-alone tests, serodiagnosis may contribute to rapid, low-cost diagnosis of TB, especially when combined with multiple antigens or used in conjunction with other laboratory tests. Strategies to help integrate serodiagnosis with clinical suspicion are currently being developed. With advances in genomic and microarray technologies, substantial effort is currently placed on discovery of new antigens to improve serodiagnostic tests.

VIII. Antigen-Detection Tests

A. Urine Tests for Detection of LAM

Relatively few studies have examined the detection of circulating or secreted *M. tuberculosis* antigens for the diagnosis of TB. Currently, no commercial test is available for detection of mycobacterial antigens in serum or sputum. Recent studies have focused on ELISA for rapid detection of LAM in urine. Urine offers the advantage of being more easily collected from patients, with lower-risk of collection and handling for health care and laboratory workers.

In a small study by Hamasur et al. (162) with processed urine from 15 TB patients and 26 healthy nursing workers, a LAM ELISA had 93% sensitivity and 96% specificity; using urine from seven of the TB patients and six of the controls, a "dipstick" method yielded 100% sensitivity and specificity. The ELISA and dipstick required two days and four hours, respectively, to complete.

In a larger study by Tessema et al. (163) with 200 TB patients and 800 non-TB patients recruited consecutively from an Ethiopian health center based AFB smear and clinical follow-up, a LAM-ELISA produced 74% sensitivity and 87% specificity. Sensitivity was higher in smear-positive samples (81%) than in smear-negative samples (57%); specificity was higher in healthy control groups (95–100%).

In another large study conducted in Tanzania by Boehme et al. (164), 231 patients with suspected pulmonary TB (69% HIV-positive) and 103 healthy volunteers were screened with standard TB tests and with a new urine LAM-ELISA (Chemogen, Inc., So. Portland, Maine, U.S.A.). Of 132 patients with culture-positive active TB, 106 were positive using the LAM-ELISA (sensitivity 80.3%). Of 17 patients with active TB but negative cultures and negative smears, 13 had positive LAM-ELISA results (sensitivity 76.5%). Of the 82 culture-negative patients without radiographic signs of TB, 74 had negative LAM-ELISA (specificity 90.2%). All but one healthy volunteer had negative results (specificity 99%).

In addition to detecting some smear-negative TB, the urine LAM-ELISA appears to be more sensitive in HIV-infected patients. In contrast, serodiagnostic tests for detection of antibodies to mycobacteria tend to be less sensitive in HIV-infected individuals. Therefore, urine LAM-ELISA may hold promise as supplemental tools to the AFB smear and other tests to improve TB case finding.

IX. Tests of Cellular Immune Reactivity

The tuberculin skin test (TST) was introduced over 100 years ago. The IGRA, QuantiFERON-TB Gold and T-Spot.TB, are introduced more recently and are designed to detect a cellular immune response to *M. tuberculosis*. TB infection or disease are much more likely to be present in a population or individual who has such a response. These tests cannot be used to exclude a TB infection; however, when one is positive, TB infection or disease is much more likely to be the cause of the patient's illness.

A. The Tuberculin Skin Test

The tuberculin skin test (TST) is the time-honored test for TB infection. Over the years, a great deal of information has been amassed on its use in various situations. In order to maximize sensitivity for the diagnosis of active TB, 5 mm induration is taken as positive. The conventional thresholds for TST positivity depend on risk groups, ranging from 5 mm (for high-risk TB suspects such as individuals with HIV infection, household contact, or abnormal chest radiographs), to the standard 10 mm (for moderate-risk suspects such as individuals who reside or work in congregate settings including health care settings, recently emigrated from a TB-endemic country, have certain clinical or immunocompromising conditions, or are children), to 15 mm (for individuals with no known risk factors for TB). Overall, 75% to 90% of patients with active TB react to tuberculin injection (165). The lower sensitivities are typically associated with patients who are more severely ill, have underlying diseases that are immunosuppressive, or are being treated with drugs that are immunosuppressive. Certain groups, such as those with HIV infection, may have rates of false-negative TST results exceeding 50% (165,166). False-positive results also occur commonly, resulting in specificity as low as 50% in many situations. Causes include errors in administering and interpreting the TST, prior vaccination with BCG, and prior infection with NTM (165).

B.   Interferon-γ Release Assays

Immune response to TB infection is known to be associated with a strong Th1 inflammatory response, a hallmark of which is release of the cytokine IFN-γ by CD4 cells. Two techniques have been developed to measure IFN-γ in blood cells in response to *M. tuberculosis-specific* antigens. QuantiFERON®-T Gold (In Tube, and the earlier liquid antigen version; Cellestis Ltd., Melbourne, Australia) uses ELISA (enzyme-linked immunosorbent assay) measure the amount of IFN-γ released in response to in vitro stimulation of whole blood with *M. tuberculosis*-specific antigens. T-Spot (Oxford Immunotec, Oxford, U.K.) uses separated mononuclear cells from peripheral blood and ELISPOT (enzyme-linked immunospot) to count the number of IFN-γ producing cells. Both techniques have the advantage that they measure responses to peptides representing the *M. tuberculosis*-specific antigens, culture filtrate protein 10 (CFP-10) and early secreted antigenic target 6 (ESAT-6), which are encoded from the RD1 region of the *M. tuberculosis* genome. The newer QuantiFERON-TB Gold In Tube format employs an additional peptide from a third highly specific antigen TB 7.7 (Rv2654). Because the genomic regions encoding these antigens are absent from all strains of BCG and the most common environmental mycobacteria such as *Mycobacterium avium intracellulare*, specificity is highly increased compared to the TST (138,167–170).

The first IGRA approved by the FDA was QuantiFERON-TB (Cellestis, Ltd., Melbourne, Australia), which measured IFN-γ release in whole blood stimulated with purified protein derivative. This was followed by FDA approval in December 2005 of QuantiFERON®-TB Gold, which measures responses to the RD1-derived proteins, ESAT-6 and CFP-10, and in October 2007 by the latest In-Tube version of QuantiFERON-TB Gold, which includes an additional antigen: TB 7.7. The "In-Tube" collection system (QFT-IT) enables whole blood to be drawn directly into precoated collection tubes, simplifying the testing procedure. The T-Spot test was approved by the FDA for use in the United States in August 2008. T-Spot involves the purification of monocytes from blood and incubating these with peptides from ESAT-6 and CFP-10 in an IFN-γ ELISPOT assay. The readout for this test is the number of cells producing IFN-γ in response to the peptide antigens.

While both QFT-IT and T-Spot were primarily designed as aids for the diagnosis of latent TB infection, both tests are also highly sensitive for the detection of people with active TB. Sensitivity of QFT-IT for active TB is higher for studies performed in developed countries as distinct from resource-poor settings, where the stage of TB disease may be more advanced and thus more likely for the patients to be anergic. In studies from developed countries, sensitivity of QFT-IT for culture-confirmed active TB ranges from 79% to 93%. Studies of the sensitivity of T-Spot for active TB have been conducted in developed country settings and found a generally higher sensitivity, ranging from 80% to 100% (171,172). As with the TST, both QFT-IT and T-Spot are helpful but insufficient for diagnosing *M. tuberculosis* complex infection or disease in sick patients: a positive result can support the diagnosis of TB disease; however, infections by other mycobacteria (e.g., *Mycobacterium kansasii*) could also cause positive results (173). Other medical and diagnostic evaluations are necessary to confirm or exclude TB disease. What is becoming increasingly clear is that both IGRAs are somewhat more sensitive than the TST for active TB diagnosis.

T-Spot has been widely studied in Europe and in general has similar performance characteristics to QFT-IT. However, the recent FDA evaluation of T-Spot for approval for use in the United States resulted in the approval of a set of cutoffs that are at variance with the cutoffs used with most of the published data. All papers in the literature define a positive T-Spot result as 6 or more spots. The FDA defined a positive T-Spot as 8 spots or more, with 5 to 7 spots returning an equivocal result. This revised definition of a positive T-Spot result causes uncertainty regarding the published literature. "Head-to-head" studies have suggested that sensitivity of the T-Spot is slightly better than QFT-IT, while specificity is lower (174,175); however, these differences must be reevaluated in view of the new U.S. cutoff.

Some studies have suggested the IGRAs may be relatively more sensitive for recent, as opposed to old/cured infection (168,169,176–178). The CDC has recommended that the QFT may be used in "all circumstances" where the TST would be used (179), while in the United Kingdom, interim NICE guidelines recommend a 2-step algorithm, with use of QFT-IT or T-Spot to confirm positive TSTs (180). While this approach does maximize specificity, it is at the cost of reduced sensitivity and should not be used in vulnerable populations such as household contacts or immunosuppressed individuals.

Considerations for use of IGRAs (and even more the case for the TST) as aids for the diagnosis of active TB are their specificities and the fact that they do not differentiate between active and latent TB infection. In a population with a low prevalence of latent TB infection (LTBI), the overall specificity of the test is important, with QFT-IT being more specific than T-Spot, which is more specific than the TST (especially in BCG vaccinated populations). However, both IGRAs should perform well in this situation. However, in a population where the rate of LTBI in the population is high, the diagnostic assistance provided by a positive IGRA or TST for active TB may be low.

Practical advantages of both QFT-IT and T-Spot compared to the TST are that they require a single visit, eliminate observer variability, and do not influence results of future tests. The whole-blood culture assay, QFT-IT, requires less blood and is technically much less demanding than the T-Spot. The cost of IGRA testing is a controversial matter. Published cost-effectiveness studies generally show IGRAs cost less than using the TST alone, but a number of publications show that confirming a positive TST with an IGRA is the least expensive strategy. However, results are variable and depend on the assumptions built into the analysis (181,182). The application of these tests in clinical practice and surveillance is evolving as additional studies are in progress. Insights provided by these new tools are likely to further our understanding of the natural history of infection and improve TB control.

Table 1   Calculations for Sensitivity, Specificity, and Positive and Negative Predictive Values

	TB	No TB	Total
Test +	TP	FP	Tot Test +
Test −	FN	TN	Tot Test −
Total	Tot TB	Tot No TB	Grand Tot

$$PPV = \frac{TP}{Tot\ Test\ +}$$

$$NPV = \frac{TN}{Tot\ Test\ -}$$

Sensitivity =

$$\frac{TP}{Tot\ TB}$$

Specificity =

$$\frac{TN}{Tot\ No\ TB}$$

Abbreviations: TP, True Positive; FN, False Negative; FP, False Positive; TN, True Negative; Tot, Total.

X. Clinical Use of Diagnostic Tests

A. Comparing Sensitivity and Specificity to Positive and Negative Predictive Values

Diagnostic accuracy is conveyed through four basic measures, as calculated in Table 1. The quality of a diagnostic test is evaluated by comparison to a gold standard, which is used to designate "true" TB status, preferably, by both culture examination and response to anti-TB therapy. Sensitivity and specificity values describe the operating characteristics of a diagnostic test by measuring the ability of the test to correctly identify known TB and non-TB cases, respectively. However for individual patients in the clinical setting, PPV and negative predictive value (NPV) are more useful. Given a positive test, the PPV indicates the likelihood that a patient actually has TB; given a negative test, the NPV indicates the likelihood that a patient actually does not have TB.

PPV and NPV depend on disease prevalence in the patient population of interest. Figure 1 shows a hypothetical scenario where the same diagnostic test (i.e., with the same sensitivity and specificity) is used to diagnose TB in patient groups with low, intermediate, and high levels of clinical suspicion. In groups with higher clinical suspicion, higher prevalence of TB leads to higher PPVs but lower NPVs. Therefore, given a test result for an individual patient, clinicians must have a sense of the patient's risk level based on characteristics of the patient pool and the individual before they can assess the likelihood that the patient has or does not have active TB.

XI. Clinical Suspicion of TB

A. CSTB Workup

The diagnosis of TB is a complex clinical exercise that requires integration of all available information, particularly bedside epidemiology. At the University of California San Diego (UCSD) we developed a simple yet powerful tool called the clinical suspicion of TB (CSTB) instrument, which helps clinicians organize diverse information (Table 2). The

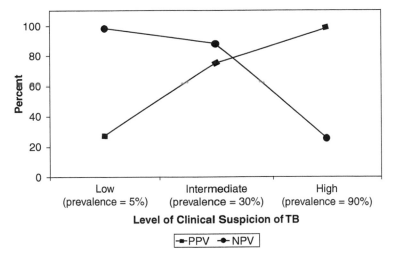

Figure 1   Positive and negative predictive values at varying TB prevalence, using a diagnostic test with sensitivity 70% and specificity 90%.

CSTB instrument asks the clinician to consider clinical data in five domains: (*i*) risk factor analysis, (*ii*) clinical findings, (*iii*) comorbidities, (*iv*) radiology, and (*v*) microbiology. As data is being collected, the clinician answers the question "In your opinion what is the likelihood that, when all the data has been collected, this patient will have active TB?" The answer is given in numerical terms between 1% and 99%. With training and experience in TB diagnosis, both physicians and nonphysicians (e.g., nurses) can use this approach successfully (183).

Risk Factor Analysis or Bedside Epidemiology

The objective of risk factor analysis is to determine the likelihood that the patient has been infected with *M. tuberculosis*. It is fundamental that one cannot have active TB without being infected with *M. tuberculosis*. Bedside epidemiology is the process of conducting risk factor analysis. It is critical to assess these surrogates or risk factors because the clinical features of TB can be mimicked by many disease processes. Given the same set of symptoms, individuals with *M. tuberculosis* infection have considerably higher likelihood of active TB than individuals without the infection. We have biologic tests for TB infection and a set of epidemiologic risk factors that identify populations of persons who are likely to be infected with *M. tuberculosis*.

In low-burden communities, the TST or IGRA should be performed on all patients with suspected TB, while in high-burden settings the role of TST and IGRA is of little value for diagnosis of TB disease. A positive result provides epidemiologic data in support of the diagnosis of TB when other evidence is suggestive. A negative result similarly provides epidemiologic data to suggest that the clinical illness is less likely to be due to TB. The problem with using the TST as a test for active TB is its low specificity, as many persons with a reactive TST have LTBI or are infected with NTM such as BCG or environmental strains (e.g., *M. avium* complex). The vast majority of reactive TSTs are false positive for active TB, either because it indicates a cross-reaction to NTM or the patient has LTBI and another illness that is causing clinical symptoms or findings. The IGRA offers a

Table 2 Key Factors Affecting Clinical Suspicion and Diagnosis of Active Pulmonary
Tuberculosis

Epidemiologic factors	Clinical findings

Demographics
  • Country of birth
  • Recent immigration from country with
    high TB incidence
  • Ethnicity and race
Social history
  • Homelessness or homeless shelter
  • Prison/jail in the past 2 yr
Lifestyle factors
  • Excessive alcohol use
  • Tobacco use
  • Poor nutrition
  • Recreational drug use or participation
    in a drug rehabilitation program
  • Men having sex with men
  • Having multiple partners
History of TB and other mycobacteria
  • Exposure to TB in family, at work, or
    with acquaintances
  • Previous treatment for active TB, with
    or without directly observed therapy
  • History of TST and treatment for latent
    infection
  • History of BCG vaccination
  • History of nontuberculous
    mycobacterial infection
	Symptoms for more than 3 wk
	  • Cough
	  • Hemoptysis
	  • Fever
	  • Night sweats
	  • Weight loss
	  • Enlarged lymph nodes
	Comorbidity
	  • HIV status, viral load, CD4 cell count
	  • Diabetes mellitus
	  • Organ transplant
	  • Silicosis
	  • Immunosuppressive disease (e.g.,
	    malignancy of any type, chronic renal
	    failure) or medications (e.g., steroids,
	    anti-TNF preparations, or other
	    immunosuppressive agents)
	Abnormal physical
	  • Rales, wheezes, pleural changes
	  • Lymphadenopathy or splenomegaly
	Abnormal chest X-ray
	  • Cavity
	  • Fibronodular changes
	  • Adenopathy
	  • Infiltration
	  • Fibrosis
	  • Bronchiectasis

Bacteriologic	**Other findings**

AFB smear results
NAA test results
Culture results
	Diagnosis other than TB
	  • Pneumonia
	  • Bronchitis
	  • Cancer
	  • Histoplasmosis
	  • Coccidioidomycosis
	Response to treatment
	  • Symptoms cleared or improved
	  • Weight gain
	  • Chest X-ray cleared or improved
	  • Microbiology conversion

great improvement over the TST because they use antigens that are highly specific for *M. tuberculosis*. While the utility of the IGRAs is not completely determined, particularly in contrast to each other, it is clear that these tests are much more specific than the TST because they do not react with BCG or most environmental mycobacteria, particularly *M. avium*. However these tests are reactive in patients with latent LTBI as well as those with active TB; therefore, clinical factors must be used to differentiate active TB from LTBI.

Epidemiology offers another approach to assess the likelihood of infection with *M. tuberculosis*. The CDC has identified a set of epidemiologic risk factors and packaged them as recommendations for the Targeted Testing program. The program is designed to identify populations that are at high risk of having LTBI. Those patients may have a TB infection even if the TST or IGRA is nonreactive. These epidemiologic risk factors require an understanding of the epidemiology of TB as a whole and types of TB.

The epidemiology of TB has been well studied over many years in order to develop effective public health policies. The same information can be applied to the diagnostic process. We call it bedside epidemiology. The application of bedside epidemiology to the diagnostic process is the critical component of determining the likelihood of TB infection and progression to active disease.

One of the highest risk factors for TB infection is being in close contact with an active case of TB. There is no single definition regarding how close the contact needs to be. The classic definition has been living in the same abode. Studies have consistently demonstrated that about 25% of household contacts of an active case have been infected at the time the index case is diagnosed. Recently, attention has focused on nonhousehold contact such as working face-to-face or near a patient with active TB. The definitions of four hours per week of direct faced-to-face contact or working within 15 feet of an active case have been used. In addition, some occupations put one at risk of unknowing exposure to an undiagnosed patient with infectious TB such as working in a health care facility, a correctional facility, or a social service facility.

Social circumstances may act as markers of more likely exposure and therefore infection with TB. Factors that increase the likelihood of having TB infection include ethnicity or having been born and lived in a country with a high TB burden, recent immigration, social contacts with drinking friends or association with street drug users, or homelessness.

Demographics can be used to identify groups of individuals that are likely to be infected with *M. tuberculosis*. Every community has a characteristic set of patients who are at increased risk of being infected. In the United States, most patients with active TB are foreign born. Half of the foreign-born patients of TB were born in Mexico, the Philippines, Vietnam, or India. One can use the fact that someone has been immunized with BCG as a marker of increased likelihood of being infected with *M. tuberculosis*. BCG itself does not increase the likelihood of infection with *M. tuberculosis*; however, it is an indication that the individual was in a population that was thought by the local public health officials of being at high risk of TB. In many cases these individuals are infected by *M. tuberculosis*. TST cannot differentiate TB infection from BCG infection; the IGRAs have their greatest utility in this setting.

The past medical history can be very helpful in identifying patients who are infected with *M. tuberculosis* and at risk of having active TB. Specifically, persons who have had active TB disease in the past have clearly been infected. In certain cases, active disease may have been controlled by substandard therapies. Active disease may have been curtailed, but the patient may have persistent *M. tuberculosis* organisms. These may lead to reactivation when the patient's immune status is weakened. This is particularly the case if the treatment was self-administered or did not include rifampin.

Clinical Presentation

Clinical symptoms are one of the main features that distinguish patients with active TB from those with LTBI. Unfortunately symptoms may vary over a very broad spectrum. The cardinal symptoms of TB are generally considered to be chronic cough—three weeks or more particularly when accompanied by sputum production, fever, night sweats, and weight loss. The finding of these symptoms generally will alert the clinician to consider active TB since they are present in the majority of patients with active TB. While one may suspect TB based on clinical symptoms, these symptoms are not specific; however, whenever cough is present for more than three weeks, TB should be considered in the differential diagnosis. While these symptoms are impressive, they are also very common in a variety of other even more common conditions. In any case the clinician must diagnose the cause of these symptoms and treat them. It is appropriate in most cases with these symptoms to start by "ruling out TB."

Some patients may have few respiratory symptoms or mild symptoms (e.g., low-grade fever or fatigue) and still have active TB. This is particularly the case in patients who have comorbid conditions that alter the host immune response to infection. The lack of specificity of these symptoms is particularly problematic in immunosuppressed patients who may be more susceptible to a variety of more common infections. In HIV-positive individuals, the rates of these symptoms are comparable between those with and without TB. However about one-third of patients with active TB have little or no symptoms, even on close questioning. Furthermore, even in high-burden countries, most people are not infected with TB during childhood; when they become infected as adults, they are at risk of developing primary TB. Patients who become infected as adults will have subtle clinical illness and may be misdiagnosed as community-acquired pneumonia or another similar process. Vigilance and application of risk factor analysis is key in interpreting clinical findings.

Not all cases of TB are pulmonary. Classically, 15% of TB cases are extrapulmonary. These cases will manifest symptoms depending on the tissue involved. The most common extrapulmonary site of involvement with TB is cervical adenopathy or scrofula. Tuberculous adenopathy classically causes swelling of the lymph nodes with attachment to underlying tissue, typically with little or no pain or redness. The next most common site is pleural; patients with pleural TB may have pleuritic pain but more commonly may have no symptoms at all. Literally, any organ can be involved with active TB, and the symptoms will depend on the site of infection. When the patient is immunosuppressed due to comorbidity or medications, the frequency of extrapulmonary TB disease will increase dramatically. One-third of patients with extrapulmonary TB may also have pulmonary changes. Unfortunately, as many as one-third of the patients with active TB will have little or no symptoms. This may be true even with extensive, highly contagious forms of TB. The lack of symptoms is no assurance that the patient does not have active TB. On the contrary, if a patient has a manifestation of disease that suggests active infection and there are little or no symptoms, the suspicion of active TB is raised considerably because other pathologies that cause such manifestations usually make the patient very symptomatic.

Comorbidity

Comorbid conditions are common in patients with active TB. These conditions may be a concurrent disease process that impairs the patient's ability to keep the low-grade infection in check or it may be a medication that impairs the patient's defenses. Sometimes the comorbid condition that leads to reactivation may be subtle, such as malnutrition or aging. Immunosuppressive diseases and medications may influence both the frequency and manifestation of TB disease in several ways. They all have one thing in common—reduction in the host immune response to *M. tuberculosis*. HIV, malignancies, diabetes mellitus, and chronic renal failure are the best examples. However, more problematic is immunosuppression induced by medications such as corticosteroids, antineoplasia chemotherapy, and immunosuppressants or immune modifiers used to control transplant rejection or autoimmune disease. Reduction in the host immune response to *M. tuberculosis* results in the reduction of the intensity of chronic low grade symptoms to the point that the patient may be unaware of the slowly progressive infection. When symptoms become evident, the clinical picture may appear to be a short-lived, mild infectious process. If the host has untreated LTBI, the combination of long-standing TB infection and immunosuppression will increase the likelihood of reactivation or postprimary TB due to breakdown of granulomas that may have held live *M. tuberculosis* organisms in check for decades. If the person has a primary infection and a comorbidity, the situation is even more problematic. Symptoms of primary TB tend to be more acute and therefore missing the chronic feature one associates with TB. In this setting, immunosuppression results in poor granuloma formation and progressive infection that may develop into active disease. Frequently, the presentation is more likely to be devoid of the characteristics that are often associated with granulomatous infection—chronic symptoms or fibronodular or cavitary changes on chest radiographs. Many times the disease will be extrapulmonary and involve more than one site, particularly visceral sites.

Chest Radiology

Although neither specific nor conclusive, the chest radiograph is one of the most fundamental tools in diagnosing pulmonary diseases and is used to modulate the suspicion of TB. Radiology of the lungs has been studied extensively. Fibronodular infiltrates, particularly of the posterior segments of the upper lungs with or without cavitation are often present. The classic changes associated with TB are those of reactivation TB. These changes often raise the suspicion of TB when the concern was not raised by consideration of symptoms alone. Unfortunately the changes of primary TB are much more difficult to differentiate from other pulmonary diseases. In many communities, 50% of the new cases are recently acquired or primary TB. In these cases, lower lobe disease predominates; infiltrates may be nondescript alveolar infiltrates lacking the hallmark fibronodular appearance or cavitation. Many have hilar or mediastinal adenopathy.

The diagnosis of pulmonary TB is rarely straightforward. Studies in the 1950s and 1960s investigating the value of a chest X-ray demonstrated a surprisingly poor sensitivity and specificity (2). While chest radiographs increase the diagnostic sensitivity, it often does not allow for the differentiation of active from inactive TB. For this reason, in resource-limited setting the chest radiograph may not be performed in all cases. It is common in those settings to go directly to sputum microscopy. If the sputum is negative for AFB, the patient may have a chest X-ray; if the AFB smear is positive, a chest X-ray may not be performed.

Microbiological Studies

Microbiology is the bedrock of the specific diagnosis of TB. AFB smear, culture, and NAAs are described in detail above.

The Ziehl-Neelsen stain is the time-honored approach to identifying *M. tuberculosis* rapidly in clinical specimen. Any specimen can be stained for AFB. AFB smear is very useful as a rapid screening test for mycobacteria. It is not specific in that it does not differentiate *M. tuberculosis* from NTM such as *M. avium* complex. The process of looking for acid-fast organisms is relatively insensitive. Approximately 6000 to 10,000 organisms per mL of sputum are required for 3 organisms to be seen on examination of a microscope slide. For this reason, smear-positive patients are considered highly infectious. The clinician must be very careful not to be misled into thinking that a series of three negative AFB sputum smears rules out TB. It does not. Nearly half of TB cases in California, for example, are AFB smear-negative. Sensitivity and specificity of the AFB smear are highly dependent on care laboratory staff put into staining and examining a slide and the characteristics of the patient population studied.

There are many culture media available and many ways of identifying mycobacterial growth. The method used in the laboratory greatly influences the outcome. In general, a liquid medium improves sensitivity and, to a lesser extent, the growth rate. The detection of growth by consumption of oxygen or generation of carbon dioxide is more sensitive, therefore more rapid, than visualization of colony growth.

In developed countries, two FDA-approved NAA tests are available as aids in TB diagnosis. Both recognize nucleic acid sequences that are specific for *M. tuberculosis*. The MTD targets RNA with the rationale that each *M. tuberculosis* organism has 1000 copies of RNA, whereas the Amplicor targets DNA. The MTD uses isothermal amplification using transcription-mediated amplification and Amplicor uses classic PCR. The MTD test is approved for use on both AFB smear-negative and smear-positive specimens, whereas Amplicor has been approved only for use in smear-positive samples.

CSTB Assessment

These five domains form the basis for a systematic collection and analysis of clinical information. The systematic framework of the CSTB instrument helps to track clinical suspicion during the extended diagnostic workup. This is done by answering the question, "What do you think is the likelihood that, when all the information is available, this patient will have been proven to have active TB?" A series of CSTB estimates (1–99%) should be documented using information on risk factors and patient history, chest radiograph, and AFB smears and NAA. Once culture data are available, the CSTB estimate should be reassessed, taking into account all available information to make a final diagnosis.

In a multicenter trial of TB diagnosis, we found that the CSTB estimate using the above five domains without using culture at the beginning of the workup closely approximated TB status determined after culture results are available. The prevalence of TB was 4% the patient group with low CSTB, 28% in the intermediate CSTB group, and 85% in the high CSTB group (8).

B.   Applications of CSTB Assessment to the Evaluation of TB Suspects

The application of CSTB assessment will vary according to the prevalence of TB and the clinical needs. For example, the CSTB level can be used to determine additional tests that are needed to make a diagnosis. It can be used to identify false-positive or false-negative test results. The first step is to collect the information discussed above and estimate the CSTB. CSTB estimates <25%, 25% to 75%, and >75% may be considered to have low, intermediate, and high likelihood of active TB, respectively. In all groups of TB suspects (high, low, and intermediate), ask for the collection of three consecutive first morning sputum examinations, with induction using an ultrasonic nebulizer if necessary. A true or false-positive smear result involves consideration of the CSTB as defined below.

CSTB less than 25%

If the CSTB is low, the first sputum should be examined by AFB smear. If the first smear is positive, the sputum should be tested with an MTD or Amplicor to determine if nucleotides specific to *M. tuberculosis* can be identified. If the NAA test is positive, it is likely that the patient has highly infectious TB. If the NAA test is negative, the sputum should be examined for inhibitors of NAA. In a few patients categorized as having a low CSTB (e.g., recent immigrants or household contacts whose presentations are not suggestive of TB), it may be appropriate to use an MTD regardless of the AFB smear results. In this setting, the higher sensitivity of the MTD may identify an occasional case of TB. Patients with low CSTB and negative smear are unlikely to have TB (<2%) and even if they do, do not need to be isolated. If the patient has TB, it is of a low order of infectiousness, and the diagnosis will be made when the cultures is completed.

CSTB Between 25% and 75%

These cases are difficult since the burden of proof is shifted from the bedside to the laboratory. These cases often require AFB testing of all three sputum samples. Any sputum with a positive smear should also be tested with an NAA. If the first two sputum samples are AFB negative or if one is AFB positive, the third sample should be tested by both an AFB smear and an MTD either to confirm that the AFB is *M. tuberculosis* or to take advantage of the greater sensitivity of the MTD.

CSTB over 75%

These patients are very likely to have pulmonary disease. Usually this disease will be active TB but, occasionally, the patient may have NTM disease, fungal disease, or inactive TB or a pulmonary malignancy with a superimposed bacterial infection. These patients need both an AFB smear and MTD. These are best performed on the first specimen. If both the AFB smear and MTD are positive, the diagnosis is established. If the AFB smear is positive and the MTD is negative, the MTD may be a false-negative result due to inhibitors or NTM infection may be present. Laboratory studies for inhibitors can be ordered and a repeat MTD is also a good idea. If three AFB smears and two MTDs are negative the patient probably does not have active TB and needs further diagnostic studies to determine specific abnormalities.

The Application of CSTB in a Low-Incidence Settings

Most patients suspected of having TB will have low CSTB. The TB workup of these patients is focused on excluding TB. This can be accomplished fairly quickly and effectively with a single AFB smear. In patients with low CSTB (e.g., 4% with TB), negative AFB smears further reduce the likelihood of TB by 50% (e.g., 2% with TB). In some cases, one MTD may also need to be performed. If the MTD is positive, it is necessary to confirm with a second positive MTD, particularly if the AFB smear is negative. One must keep in mind that 1% to 2% of these patients may have paucibacillary TB. These patients are not a public health risk, and TB treatment can be started when the culture is found to be positive. Patients with an intermediate or high CSTB (e.g., 28% with TB) and those who are HIV positive are smaller groups in low-incidence settings; in these groups, three negative smears reduce likelihood of TB (e.g., 14% with TB) and negative MTD further reduce the likelihood of TB (e.g., 2–3% with TB). Because of their increased complexity, the greater sensitivity and specificity of the NAA will ultimately be needed; testing the first sample with MTD will save time. The AFB smear is needed in MTD positive patients to determine level of infectiousness. In many cases, one negative MTD is sufficient to exclude *M. tuberculosis*; however, it may be prudent in some cases to have two negative MTD results. Approximately 2% to 3% of TB cases may be missed by this process and can be treated for TB when the culture is found to be positive.

The Application of CSTB in a High-Incidence Population

In developed countries, clinicians depend on routine cultures to diagnose and rule out TB. In resource-limited, high-incidence countries, AFB smears are routinely used for diagnosis; culture can be performed only in reference laboratories, but NAAs are generally not available due to the high cost and lack of skilled personnel and appropriate facilities. In resource limited settings, CSTB estimation may help to determine a small subgroup for further culture examinations to increase diagnostic accuracy over smear alone.

Based on clinical experience, a decision tree was developed (Fig. 2) (184). In this analysis, estimates of diagnostic accuracy of the AFB smear, culture, and decision tree were compared to the final diagnosis. Among all subjects studied, the sensitivity and specificity were 58.1% and 98.9% for smear and 89.9% and 99.6% for culture. When the decision tree (i.e., with CSTB, smear, and a subset of culture results) was used, the sensitivity and specificity were 88.4% and 99.2%, 30% more sensitive and slightly more specific than smear. Essentially, the decision tree was as accurate as culture for all subjects but required cultures for only 37.2% of subjects who most benefited from culture evaluations.

Application of CSTB in the Interpretation of Novel Laboratory Tests

TB control is limited by the lack of rapid and accurate diagnostic tests. However, novel rapid tests tend to be greatly limited as stand-alone tests; CSTB assessment can help to integrate multiple tests, particularly those using different approaches of detection, to improve case detection. In prior work from our laboratory (185), sera of TB suspects were screened by immunoassay (ELISA) for secreted TB antigens [*M. tuberculosis* $H_{37}Rv$

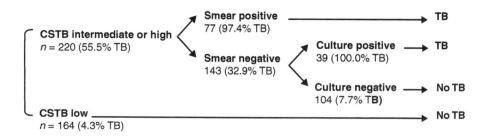

Figure 2   Decision tree using clinical suspicion of tuberculosis (CSTB), smear, and culture findings to determine active TB status, $n = 384$ patients with complete data.

culture filtrate proteins (CFP) as the antigen and serum against Erdman CFP as the primary antibody] and for antibodies to TB by the Rapid Lateral Flow (RLF)-Test (Chembio, Inc., Medford, NY). The sensitivity and specificity for individual tests were 40% and 92% for TB antigen ELISA, 34% and 90% for RLF TB antibody test, 64% and 99% for AFB smear and 83% and 88% for CSTB scores greater than 75%. An algorithm was developed to augment the outcome based on AFB smear alone using the CSTB score, ELISA, and RLF test. When smear-negative patients with high CSTB (>75%) and a positive result with the ELISA or RLF test are considered TB-positive, the overall sensitivity significantly increased to 73% ($p = 0.001$) without a statistically significant decrease in specificity to 97% ($p = 0.50$) compared to smear alone. Integrating different diagnostic modalities that include clinical suspicion and laboratory tests that detect AFB, antigen or antibody levels, yields a strategy that performs better than each of the tests alone.

References

1. Schluger NW. The diagnosis of tuberculosis: what's old, what's new. Semin Respir Infect 2003; 18(4):241–248.
2. Arango L, Brewin AW, Murray JF. The spectrum of tuberculosis as currently seen in a metropolitan hospital. Am Rev Respir Dis 1973; 108(4):805–812.
3. MacGregor RR. A year's experience with tuberculosis in a private urban teaching hospital in the postsanatorium era. Am J Med 1975; 58(2):221–228.
4. Friedman LN, Selwyn PA. Pulmonary tuberculosis: primary, reactivation, HIV related, and non-HIV related. In: Friedman LN, ed. Tuberculosis: Current Concepts and Treatment. Boca Raton, FL: CRC Press, 1994.
5. Samb B, Henzel D, Daley CL, et al. Methods for diagnosing tuberculosis among in-patients in eastern Africa whose sputum smears are negative. Int J Tuberc Lung Dis 1997; 1(1):25–30.
6. Hopewell PC. A clinical view of tuberculosis. Radiol Clin North Am 1995; 33(4):641–653.
7. Murray HW, Tuazon CU, Kirmani N, et al. The adult respiratory distress syndrome associated with miliary tuberculosis. Chest 1978; 73(1):37–43.
8. Catanzaro A, Perry S, Clarridge JE, et al. The role of clinical suspicion in evaluating a new diagnostic test for active tuberculosis: results of a multicenter prospective trial. JAMA 2000; 283(5):639–645.
9. Cameron SJ. Tuberculosis and the blood—a special relationship? Tubercle 1974; 55(1): 55–72.
10. Abbasi AA, Chemplavil JK, Farah S, et al. Hypercalcemia in active pulmonary tuberculosis. Ann Intern Med 1979; 90(3):324–328.
11. Chung DK, Hubbard WW. Hyponatremia in untreated active pulmonary tuberculosis. Am Rev Respir Dis 1969; 99(4):595–597.
12. Christie JD, Callihan DR. The laboratory diagnosis of mycobacterial diseases. Challenges and common sense. Clin Lab Med 1995; 15(2):279–306.
13. Fishman JA, Roth RS, Zanzot E, et al. Use of induced sputum specimens for microbiologic diagnosis of infections due to organisms other than *Pneumocystis carinii*. J Clin Microbiol 1994; 32(1):131–134.
14. Jensen PA, Lambert LA, Iademarco MF, et al. CDC.Guidelines for Preventing the Transmission of *Mycobacterium tuberculosis* in Health-Care Settings, 2005. MMWR Recomm Rep 2005; 54(RR-17); 1–141.
15. Blumberg HM, Burman WJ, Chaisson RE, et al. American Thoracic Society/Centers for Disease Control and Prevention/Infectious Diseases Society of America. Treatment of tuberculosis. Am J Respir Crit Care Med 2003; 167(4):603–662.
16. Baughman RP, Dohn MN, Loudon RG, et al. Bronchoscopy with bronchoalveolar lavage in tuberculosis and fungal infections. Chest 1991; 99(1):92–97.

17. Wallace JM, Deutsch AL, Harrell JH, et al. Bronchoscopy and transbronchial biopsy in evaluation of patients with suspected active tuberculosis. Am J Med 1981; 70(6):1189–1194.

18. Conde MB, Soares SL, Mello FC, et al. Comparison of sputum induction with fiberoptic bronchoscopy in the diagnosis of tuberculosis: Experience at an acquired immune deficiency syndrome reference center in Rio de Janeiro, Brazil. Am J Respir Crit Care Med 2000; 162(6):2238–2240.

19. Diagnostic Standards and Classification of Tuberculosis in Adults and Children. This official statement of the American Thoracic Society and the Centers for Disease Control and Prevention was adopted by the ATS Board of Directors, July 1999. This statement was endorsed by the Council of the Infectious Disease Society of America, September 1999. Am J Respir Crit Care Med 2000; 161(4 Pt 1):1376–1395.

20. Daniel TM. Rapid diagnosis of tuberculosis: Laboratory techniques applicable in developing countries. Rev Infect Dis 1989; 11(suppl 2):S471–S478.

21. Greenbaum M, Beyt BE Jr, Murray PR. The accuracy of diagnosing pulmonary tuberculosis at a teaching hospital. Am Rev Respir Dis 1980; 121(3):477–481.

22. Levy H, Feldman C, Sacho H, et al. A reevaluation of sputum microscopy and culture in the diagnosis of pulmonary tuberculosis. Chest 1989; 95(6):1193–1197.

23. Long R, Scalcini M, Manfreda J, et al. The impact of HIV on the usefulness of sputum smears for the diagnosis of tuberculosis. Am J Public Health 1991; 81(10):1326–1328.

24. Yajko DM, Nassos PS, Sanders CA, et al. High predictive value of the acid-fast smear for *Mycobacterium tuberculosis* despite the high prevalence of *Mycobacterium avium* complex in respiratory specimens. Clin Infect Dis 1994; 19(2):334–336.

25. Steingart KR, Henry M, Ng V, et al. Fluorescence versus conventional sputum smear microscopy for tuberculosis: a systematic review. Lancet Infect Dis 2006; 6(9):570–581.

26. Hung NV, Sy DN, Anthony RM, et al. Fluorescence microscopy for tuberculosis diagnosis. Lancet Infect Dis 2007; 7(4):238–239.

27. Sohn H, Sinthuwattanawibool C, Rienthong S, et al. Fluorescence microscopy is less expensive than Ziehl-Neelsen microscopy in Thailand. Int J Tuberc Lung Dis 2009; 13(2):266–268.

28. Kivihya-Ndugga LE, van Cleeff MR, Githui WA, et al. A comprehensive comparison of Ziehl-Neelsen and fluorescence microscopy for the diagnosis of tuberculosis in a resource-poor urban setting. Int J Tuberc Lung Dis 2003; 7(12):1163–1171.

29. Cruciani M, Scarparo C, Malena M, et al. Meta-analysis of BACTEC MGIT 960 and BACTEC 460 TB, with or without solid media, for detection of mycobacteria. J Clin Microbiol 2004; 42(5):2321–2325.

30. Moore DAJ, Evans CAW, Gilman RH, et al. Microscopic-observation drug-susceptibility assay for the diagnosis of TB. N Engl J Med 2006; 355(15):1539–1550.

31. Havlir DV, Barnes PF. Tuberculosis in patients with human immunodeficiency virus infection. N Engl J Med 1999; 340(5):367–373.

32. Talavera W, Lessnau KK, Handwerger S. Extrapulmonary tuberculosis. In: Friedman LN, ed. Tuberculosis: Current Concepts and Treatment. Boca Raton, FL: CRC Press, 1994:113–151.

33. Thornton GF. Extrapulmonary tuberculosis, excluding the central nervous system. In: Rossman MD, MacGregor RR, eds. Tuberculosis: Clinical Management and New Challenges. New York: McGraw Hill, 1995:173–184.

34. Christensen WI. Genitourinary tuberculosis: Review of 102 cases. Medicine (Baltimore) 1974; 53(5):377–390.

35. Marshall JB. Tuberculosis of the gastrointestinal tract and peritoneum. Am J Gastroenterol 1993; 88(7):989–999.

36. Ribera E, Ocana I, Martinez-Vazquez JM, et al. High level of interferon gamma in tuberculous pleural effusion. Chest 1988; 93(2):308–311.

37. Valdes L, San Jose E, Alvarez D, et al. Diagnosis of tuberculous pleurisy using the biologic parameters adenosine deaminase, lysozyme, and interferon gamma. Chest 1993; 103(2):458–465.

38. McAdams HP, Erasmus J, Winter JA. Radiologic manifestations of pulmonary tuberculosis. Radiol Clin North Am 1995; 33(4):655–678.
39. Palmer PE. Pulmonary tuberculosis—usual and unusual radiographic presentations. Semin Roentgenol 1979; 14(3):204–243.
40. Leung AN, Muller NL, Pineda PR, et al. Primary tuberculosis in childhood: radiographic manifestations. Radiology 1992; 182(1):87–91.
41. Miller WT, Miller WT Jr. Tuberculosis in the normal host: Radiological findings. Semin Roentgenol 1993; 28(2):109–118.
42. Woodring JH, Vandiviere HM, Fried AM, et al. Update: the radiographic features of pulmonary tuberculosis. AJR Am J Roentgenol 1986; 146(3):497–506.
43. Lintin SN, Isaac PA. Miliary tuberculosis presenting as adult respiratory distress syndrome. Intensive Care Med 1988; 14(6):672–674.
44. Greenberg SD, Frager D, Suster B, et al. Active pulmonary tuberculosis in patients with AIDS: Spectrum of radiographic findings (including a normal appearance). Radiology 1994; 193(1):115–119.
45. Pitchenik AE, Rubinson HA. The radiographic appearance of tuberculosis in patients with the acquired immune deficiency syndrome (AIDS) and pre-AIDS. Am Rev Respir Dis 1985; 131(3):393–396.
46. Miller WT. Expanding options for the radiographic evaluation of tuberculosis. In: Rossman MD, MacGregor RR, eds. Tuberculosis: Clinical Management and New Challenges. New York: McGraw Hill, 1995:275–289.
47. Clarridge JE III, Shawar RM, Shinnick TM, et al. Large-scale use of polymerase chain reaction for detection of *Mycobacterium tuberculosis* in a routine mycobacteriology laboratory. J Clin Microbiol 1993; 31(8):2049–2056.
48. Eisenach KD, Sifford MD, Cave MD, et al. Detection of *Mycobacterium tuberculosis* in sputum samples using a polymerase chain reaction. Am Rev Respir Dis 1991; 144(5):1160–1163.
49. Woods GL. The mycobacteriology laboratory and new diagnostic techniques. Infect Dis Clin North Am 2002; 16(1):127–144.
50. Mathur P, Sacks L, Auten G, et al. Delayed diagnosis of pulmonary tuberculosis in city hospitals. Arch Intern Med 1994; 154(3):306–310.
51. Alcala L, Ruiz-Serrano MJ, Hernangomez S, et al. Evaluation of the upgraded amplified *Mycobacterium tuberculosis* direct test (gen-probe) for direct detection of *Mycobacterium tuberculosis* in respiratory and non-respiratory specimens. Diagn Microbiol Infect Dis 2001; 41(1–2):51–56.
52. Bergmann JS, Woods GL. Enhanced Amplified *Mycobacterium Tuberculosis* Direct Test for detection of *Mycobacterium tuberculosis* complex in positive BACTEC 12B broth cultures of respiratory specimens. J Clin Microbiol 1999; 37(6):2099–2101.
53. Bodmer T, Mockl E, Muhlemann K, et al. Improved performance of Gen-Probe Amplified *Mycobacterium Tuberculosis* Direct Test when 500 instead of 50 microliters of decontaminated sediment is used. J Clin Microbiol 1996; 34(1):222–223.
54. Chedore P, Jamieson FB. Routine use of the Gen-Probe MTD2 amplification test for detection of *Mycobacterium tuberculosis* in clinical specimens in a large public health mycobacteriology laboratory. Diagn Microbiol Infect Dis 1999; 35(3):185–191.
55. Coll P, Garrigo M, Moreno C, et al. Routine use of Gen-Probe Amplified *Mycobacterium Tuberculosis* Direct (MTD) test for detection of *Mycobacterium tuberculosis* with smear-positive and smear-negative specimens. Int J Tuberc Lung Dis 2003; 7(9):886–891.
56. Gamboa F, Fernandez G, Padilla E, et al. Comparative evaluation of initial and new versions of the Gen-Probe Amplified *Mycobacterium Tuberculosis* Direct Test for direct detection of *Mycobacterium tuberculosis* in respiratory and nonrespiratory specimens. J Clin Microbiol 1998; 36(3):684–689.

57. Jonas V, Alden MJ, Curry JI, et al. Detection and identification of *Mycobacterium tuberculosis* directly from sputum sediments by amplification of rRNA. J Clin Microbiol 1993; 31(9):2410–2416.

58. O'Sullivan CE, Miller DR, Schneider PS, et al. Evaluation of Gen-Probe amplified *mycobacterium tuberculosis* direct test by using respiratory and nonrespiratory specimens in a tertiary care center laboratory. J Clin Microbiol 2002; 40(5):1723–1727.

59. Smith MB, Bergmann JS, Onoroto M, et al. Evaluation of the enhanced amplified *Mycobacterium tuberculosis* direct test for direct detection of *Mycobacterium tuberculosis* complex in respiratory specimens. Arch Pathol Lab Med 1999; 123(11):1101–1103.

60. Carpentier E, Drouillard B, Dailloux M, et al. Diagnosis of tuberculosis by Amplicor *Mycobacterium tuberculosis* test: A multicenter study. J Clin Microbiol 1995; 33(12): 3106–3110.

61. Cartuyvels R, De Ridder C, Jonckheere S, et al. Prospective clinical evaluation of Amplicor *Mycobacterium tuberculosis* PCR test as a screening method in a low-prevalence population. J Clin Microbiol 1996; 34(8):2001–2003.

62. Rajalahti I, Vuorinen P, Nieminen MM, et al. Detection of *Mycobacterium tuberculosis* complex in sputum specimens by the automated Roche Cobas Amplicor *Mycobacterium Tuberculosis* Test. J Clin Microbiol 1998; 36(4):975–978.

63. Reischl U, Lehn N, Wolf H, et al. Clinical evaluation of the automated COBAS AMPLICOR MTB assay for testing respiratory and nonrespiratory specimens. J Clin Microbiol 1998; 36(10):2853–2860.

64. Shah JS, Liu J, Buxton D, et al. Detection of *Mycobacterium tuberculosis* directly from spiked human sputum by Q-beta replicase-amplified assay. J Clin Microbiol 1995; 33(2): 322–328.

65. Bergmann JS, Keating WE, Woods GL. Clinical evaluation of the BDProbeTec ET system for rapid detection of *Mycobacterium tuberculosis*. J Clin Microbiol 2000; 38(2):863–865.

66. Little MC, Andrews J, Moore R, et al. Strand displacement amplification and homogeneous real-time detection incorporated in a second-generation DNA probe system, BDProbeTecET. Clin Chem 1999; 45(6 Pt 1):777–784.

67. Mazzarelli G, Rindi L, Piccoli P, et al. Evaluation of the BDProbeTec ET system for direct detection of *Mycobacterium tuberculosis* in pulmonary and extrapulmonary samples: a multicenter study. J Clin Microbiol 2003; 41(4):1779–1782.

68. Boehme CC, Nabeta P, Henostroza G, et al. Operational feasibility of using loop-mediated isothermal amplification for diagnosis of pulmonary tuberculosis in microscopy centers of developing countries. J Clin Microbiol 2007; 45(6):1936–1940.

69. Centers for Disease Control and Prevention (CDC). Update: Nucleic acid amplification tests for tuberculosis. MMWR Morb Mortal Wkly Rep 2000; 49(26):593–594.

70. Cloud JL, Shutt C, Aldous W, et al. Evaluation of a Modified Gen-Probe Amplified Direct Test for Detection of *Mycobacterium tuberculosis* complex organisms in cerebrospinal fluid. J Clin Microbiol 2004; 42(11):5341–5344.

71. D'Amato RF, Hochstein LH, Colaninno PM, et al. Application of the Roche Amplicor *Mycobacterium tuberculosis* (PCR) test to specimens other than respiratory secretions. Diagn Microbiol Infect Dis 1996; 24(1):15–17.

72. Ehlers S, Ignatius R, Regnath T, et al. Diagnosis of extrapulmonary tuberculosis by Gen-Probe amplified *Mycobacterium tuberculosis* direct test. J Clin Microbiol 1996; 34(9):2275–2279.

73. Gamboa F, Dominguez J, Padilla E, et al. Rapid diagnosis of extrapulmonary tuberculosis by ligase chain reaction amplification. J Clin Microbiol 1998; 36(5):1324–1329.

74. Portillo-Gomez L, Morris SL, Panduro A. Rapid and efficient detection of extra-pulmonary *Mycobacterium tuberculosis* by PCR analysis. Int J Tuberc Lung Dis 2000; 4(4):361–370.

75. Rajo MC, Perez Del Molina ML, Lado Lado FL, et al. Rapid diagnosis of tuberculous meningitis by ligase chain reaction amplification. Scand J Infect Dis 2002; 34(1):14–16.

76. Rantakokko-Jalava K, Marjamaki M, Marttila H, et al. LCx *Mycobacterium tuberculosis* assay is valuable with respiratory specimens, but provides little help in the diagnosis of extrapulmonary tuberculosis. Ann Med 2001; 33(1):55–62.

77. Woods GL, Bergmann JS, Williams-Bouyer N. Clinical Evaluation of the Gen-Probe amplified *Mycobacterium tuberculosis* direct test for rapid detection of *Mycobacterium tuberculosis* in select nonrespiratory specimens. J Clin Microbiol 2001; 39(2):747–749.

78. Daley P, Thomas S, Pai M. Nucleic acid amplification tests for the diagnosis of tuberculous lymphadenitis: A systematic review. Int J Tuberc Lung Dis 2007; 11(11):1166–1176.

79. Pai M, Flores LL, Hubbard A, et al. Nucleic acid amplification tests in the diagnosis of tuberculous pleuritis: A systematic review and meta-analysis. BMC Infect Dis 2004; 4:6.

80. Pai M, Flores LL, Pai N, et al. Diagnostic accuracy of nucleic acid amplification tests for tuberculous meningitis: a systematic review and meta-analysis. Lancet Infect Dis 2003; 3(10):633–643.

81. Ling DI, Flores LL, Riley LW, et al. Commercial nucleic-acid amplification tests for diagnosis of pulmonary tuberculosis in respiratory specimens: Meta-analysis and meta-regression. PLoS One 2008; 3(2):e1536.

82. Lebrun L, Mathieu D, Saulnier C, et al. Limits of commercial molecular tests for diagnosis of pulmonary tuberculosis. Eur Respir J 1997; 10(8):1874–1876.

83. Sarmiento OL, Weigle KA, Alexander J, et al. Assessment by meta-analysis of PCR for diagnosis of smear-negative pulmonary tuberculosis. J Clin Microbiol 2003; 41(7):3233–3240.

84. Barnes PF, Lakey DL, Burman WJ. Tuberculosis in patients with HIV infection. Infect Dis Clin North Am 2002; 16(1):107–126.

85. Perry S, Catanzaro A. Use of clinical risk assessments in evaluation of nucleic acid amplification tests for HIV/tuberculosis. Int J Tuberc Lung Dis 2000; 4(2)(suppl 1):S34–S40.

86. Delacourt C, Poveda JD, Chureau C, et al. Use of polymerase chain reaction for improved diagnosis of tuberculosis in children. J Pediatr 1995; 126(5 Pt 1):703–709.

87. Pierre C, Olivier C, Lecossier D, et al. Diagnosis of primary tuberculosis in children by amplification and detection of mycobacterial DNA. Am Rev Respir Dis 1993; 147(2):420–424.

88. Condos R, McClune A, Rom WN, et al. Peripheral-blood-based PCR assay to identify patients with active pulmonary tuberculosis. Lancet 1996; 347(9008):1082–1085.

89. Folgueira L, Delgado R, Palenque E, et al. Rapid diagnosis of *Mycobacterium tuberculosis* bacteremia by PCR. J Clin Microbiol 1996; 34(3):512–515.

90. Richter C, Kox LF, Van Leeuwen JV, et al. PCR detection of mycobacteraemia in Tanzanian patients with extrapulmonary tuberculosis. Eur J Clin Microbiol Infect Dis 1996; 15(10):813–817.

91. Ritis K, Tzoanopoulos D, Speletas M, et al. Amplification of IS6110 sequence for detection of *Mycobacterium tuberculosis* complex in HIV-negative patients with fever of unknown origin (FUO) and evidence of extrapulmonary disease. J Intern Med 2000; 248(5):415–424.

92. Rolfs A, Beige J, Finckh U, et al. Amplification of *Mycobacterium tuberculosis* from peripheral blood. J Clin Microbiol 1995; 33(12):3312–3314.

93. Schluger NW, Condos R, Lewis S, et al. Amplification of DNA of *Mycobacterium tuberculosis* from peripheral blood of patients with pulmonary tuberculosis. Lancet 1994; 344(8917):232–233.

94. Hadgu A, Sternberg M. Nucleic acid amplification tests for diagnosis of tuberculous meningitis. Lancet Infect Dis 2004; 4(1):9–10.

95. Kox LF, Kuijper S, Kolk AH. Early diagnosis of tuberculous meningitis by polymerase chain reaction. Neurology 1995; 45(12):2228–2232.

96. Pfyffer GE, Kissling P, Jahn EM, et al. Diagnostic performance of amplified *Mycobacterium tuberculosis* direct test with cerebrospinal fluid, other nonrespiratory, and respiratory specimens. J Clin Microbiol 1996; 34(4):834–841.

97. Fontana D, Pozzi E, Porpiglia F, et al. Rapid identification of *Mycobacterium tuberculosis* complex on urine samples by Gen-Probe amplification test. Urol Res 1997; 25(6): 391–394.
98. Sechi LA, Pinna MP, Sanna A, et al. Detection of *Mycobacterium tuberculosis* by PCR analysis of urine and other clinical samples from AIDS and non-HIV-infected patients. Mol Cell Probes 1997; 11(4):281–285.
99. Mitarai S, Shishido H, Kurashima A, et al. Comparative study of amplicor Mycobacterium PCR and conventional methods for the diagnosis of pleuritis caused by mycobacterial infection. Int J Tuberc Lung Dis 2000; 4(9):871–876.
100. Nagesh BS, Sehgal S, Jindal SK, et al. Evaluation of polymerase chain reaction for detection of *Mycobacterium tuberculosis* in pleural fluid. Chest 2001; 119(6):1737–1741.
101. Villena V, Rebollo MJ, Aguado JM, et al. Polymerase chain reaction for the diagnosis of pleural tuberculosis in immunocompromised and immunocompetent patients. Clin Infect Dis 1998; 26(1):212–214.
102. Smith KC, Starke JR, Eisenach K, et al. Detection of *Mycobacterium tuberculosis* in clinical specimens from children using a polymerase chain reaction. Pediatrics 1996; 97(2): 155–160.
103. Johansen IS, Lundgren B, Tabak F, et al. Improved sensitivity of nucleic acid amplification for rapid diagnosis of tuberculous meningitis. J Clin Microbiol 2004; 42(7):3036–3040.
104. Al Zahrani K, Al Jahdali H, Poirier L, et al. Accuracy and utility of commercially available amplification and serologic tests for the diagnosis of minimal pulmonary tuberculosis. Am J Respir Crit Care Med 2000; 162(4 Pt 1):1323–1329.
105. Piersimoni C, Scarparo C, Piccoli P, et al. Performance assessment of two commercial amplification assays for direct detection of *Mycobacterium tuberculosis* complex from respiratory and extrapulmonary specimens. J Clin Microbiol 2002; 40(11):4138–4142.
106. Sloutsky A, Han LL, Werner BG. Practical strategies for performance optimization of the enhanced gen-probe amplified *Mycobacterium tuberculosis* direct test. J Clin Microbiol 2004; 42(4):1547–1551.
107. Kerleguer A, Koeck JL, Fabre M, et al. Use of equivocal zone in interpretation of results of the amplified *Mycobacterium tuberculosis* direct test for diagnosis of tuberculosis. J Clin Microbiol 2003; 41(4):1783–1784.
108. Middleton AM, Cullinan P, Wilson R, et al. Interpreting the results of the amplified *Mycobacterium tuberculosis* direct test for detection of *M. tuberculosis* rRNA. J Clin Microbiol 2003; 41(6):2741–2743.
109. Rapid diagnostic tests for tuberculosis: what is the appropriate use? American Thoracic Society Workshop. Am J Respir Crit Care Med 1997; 155(5):1804–1814.
110. Chin DP, Yajko DM, Hadley WK, et al. Clinical utility of a commercial test based on the polymerase chain reaction for detecting *Mycobacterium tuberculosis* in respiratory specimens. Am J Respir Crit Care Med 1995; 151(6):1872–1877.
111. Cohen RA, Muzaffar S, Schwartz D, et al. Diagnosis of pulmonary tuberculosis using PCR assays on sputum collected within 24 hours of hospital admission. Am J Respir Crit Care Med 1998; 157(1):156–161.
112. Lim TK, Mukhopadhyay A, Gough A, et al. Role of clinical judgment in the application of a nucleic acid amplification test for the rapid diagnosis of pulmonary tuberculosis. Chest 2003; 124(3):902–908.
113. Schluger NW, Rom WN. The polymerase chain reaction in the diagnosis and evaluation of pulmonary infections. Am J Respir Crit Care Med 1995; 152(1):11–16.
114. Lim TK, Gough A, Chin NK, et al. Relationship between estimated pretest probability and accuracy of automated *Mycobacterium tuberculosis* assay in smear-negative pulmonary tuberculosis. Chest 2000; 118(3):641–647.
115. Wisnivesky JP, Kaplan J, Henschke C, et al. Evaluation of clinical parameters to predict *Mycobacterium tuberculosis* in inpatients. Arch Intern Med 2000; 160(16):2471–2476.

116. Della-Latta P, Whittier S. Comprehensive evaluation of performance, laboratory application, and clinical usefulness of two direct amplification technologies for the detection of *Mycobacterium tuberculosis* complex. Am J Clin Pathol 1998; 110(3):301–310.
117. Gamboa F, Manterola JM, Lonca J, et al. Comparative evaluation of two commercial assays for direct detection of *Mycobacterium tuberculosis* in respiratory specimens. Eur J Clin Microbiol Infect Dis 1998; 17(3):151–157.
118. Ichiyama S, Iinuma Y, Tawada Y, et al. Evaluation of Gen-Probe Amplified *Mycobacterium Tuberculosis* Direct Test and Roche PCR-microwell plate hybridization method (AMPLICOR MYCOBACTERIUM) for direct detection of mycobacteria. J Clin Microbiol 1996; 34(1):130–133.
119. Scarparo C, Piccoli P, Rigon A, et al. Comparison of enhanced *Mycobacterium tuberculosis* amplified direct test with COBAS AMPLICOR *Mycobacterium tuberculosis* assay for direct detection of *Mycobacterium tuberculosis* complex in respiratory and extrapulmonary specimens. J Clin Microbiol 2000; 38(4):1559–1562.
120. Visca P, De Mori P, Festa A, et al. Evaluation of the BDProbeTec strand displacement amplification assay in comparison with the AMTD II direct test for rapid diagnosis of tuberculosis. Clin Microbiol Infect 2004; 10(4):332–334.
121. Iinuma Y, Senda K, Fujihara N, et al. Comparison of the BDProbeTec ET system with the Cobas Amplicor PCR for direct detection of *Mycobacterium tuberculosis* in respiratory samples. Eur J Clin Microbiol Infect Dis 2003; 22(6):368–371.
122. Burkardt HJ. Standardization and quality control of PCR analyses. Clin Chem Lab Med 2000; 38(2):87–91.
123. Noordhoek GT, van Embden JD, Kolk AH. Reliability of nucleic acid amplification for detection of *Mycobacterium tuberculosis*: an international collaborative quality control study among 30 laboratories. J Clin Microbiol 1996; 34(10):2522–2525.
124. Noordhoek GT, Mulder S, Wallace P, et al. Multicentre quality control study for detection of *Mycobacterium tuberculosis* in clinical samples by nucleic amplification methods. Clin Microbiol Infect 2004; 10(4):295–301.
125. Ridderhof JC, Williams LO, Legois S, et al. Assessment of laboratory performance of nucleic acid amplification tests for detection of *Mycobacterium tuberculosis*. J Clin Microbiol 2003; 41(11):5258–5261.
126. Doern GV. Diagnostic mycobacteriology: Where are we today? J Clin Microbiol 1996; 34(8):1873–1876.
127. Dowdy DW, Maters A, Parrish N, et al. Cost-effectiveness analysis of the gen-probe amplified *Mycobacterium tuberculosis* direct test as used routinely on smear-positive respiratory specimens. J Clin Microbiol 2003; 41(3):948–953.
128. Lim TK, Cherian J, Poh KL, et al. The rapid diagnosis of smear-negative pulmonary tuberculosis: A cost-effectiveness analysis. Respirology 2000; 5(4):403–409.
129. Kambashi B, Mbulo G, McNerney R, et al. Utility of nucleic acid amplification techniques for the diagnosis of pulmonary tuberculosis in sub-Saharan Africa. Int J Tuberc Lung Dis 2001; 5(4):364–369.
130. Roos BR, van Cleeff MR, Githui WA, et al. Cost-effectiveness of the polymerase chain reaction versus smear examination for the diagnosis of tuberculosis in Kenya: A theoretical model. Int J Tuberc Lung Dis 1998; 2(3):235–241.
131. Ling DI, Zwerling AA, Pai M. GenoType MTBDR assays for the diagnosis of multidrug-resistant tuberculosis: A meta-analysis. Eur Respir J 2008; 32(5):1165–1174.
132. Morgan M, Kalantri S, Flores L, et al. A commercial line probe assay for the rapid detection of rifampicin resistance in *Mycobacterium tuberculosis*: A systematic review and meta-analysis. BMC Infect Dis 2005; 5:62.
133. Hillemann D, Weizenegger M, Kubica T, et al. Use of the genotype MTBDR assay for rapid detection of rifampin and isoniazid resistance in *Mycobacterium tuberculosis* complex isolates. J Clin Microbiol 2005; 43(8):3699–3703.

134. Barnard M, Albert H, Coetzee G, et al. Rapid molecular screening for multidrug-resistant tuberculosis in a high-volume public health laboratory in South Africa. Am J Respir Crit Care Med 2008; 177(7):787–792.

135. World Health Organization Expert Group. Molecular Line Probe Assays for Rapid Screening of Patients at Risk of Multidrug-Resistant Tuberculosis (MDR-TB): Policy Statement. February 3, 2009.

136. Garg SK, Tiwari RP, Tiwari D, et al. Diagnosis of tuberculosis: Available technologies, limitations, and possibilities. J Clin Lab Anal 2003; 17(5):155–163.

137. Laal S, Samanich KM, Sonnenberg MG, et al. Surrogate marker of preclinical tuberculosis in human immunodeficiency virus infection: Antibodies to an 88-kDa secreted antigen of *Mycobacterium tuberculosis*. J Infect Dis 1997; 176(1):133–143.

138. Andersen P, Munk ME, Pollock JM, et al. Specific immune-based diagnosis of tuberculosis. Lancet 2000; 356(9235):1099–1104.

139. Lodha R, Kabra SK. Newer diagnostic modalities for tuberculosis. Indian J Pediatr 2004; 71(3):221–227.

140. Chan ED, Heifets L, Iseman MD. Immunologic diagnosis of tuberculosis: A review. Tuber Lung Dis 2000; 80(3):131–140.

141. Okuda Y, Maekura R, Hirotani A, et al. Rapid serodiagnosis of active pulmonary *Mycobacterium tuberculosis* by analysis of results from multiple antigen-specific tests. J Clin Microbiol 2004; 42(3):1136–1141.

142. Silva VM, Kanaujia G, Gennaro ML, et al. Factors associated with humoral response to ESAT-6, 38 kDa and 14 kDa in patients with a spectrum of tuberculosis. Int J Tuberc Lung Dis 2003; 7(5):478–484.

143. Talbot EA, Hay B, Hone NM, et al. Tuberculosis serodiagnosis in a predominantly HIV-infected population of hospitalized patients with cough, Botswana, 2002. Clin Infect Dis 2004; 39(1):e1–e7.

144. Houghton RL, Lodes MJ, Dillon DC, et al. Use of multiepitope polyproteins in serodiagnosis of active tuberculosis. Clin Diagn Lab Immunol 2002; 9(4):883–891.

145. Balestrino EA, Daniel TM, de Latini MD, et al. Serodiagnosis of pulmonary tuberculosis in Argentina by enzyme-linked immunosorbent assay (ELISA) of IgG antibody to *Mycobacterium tuberculosis* antigen 5 and tuberculin purified protein derivative. Bull World Health Organ 1984; 62(5):755–761.

146. Ma Y, Wang YM, Daniel TM. Enzyme-linked immunosorbent assay using *Mycobacterium tuberculosis* antigen 5 for the diagnosis of pulmonary tuberculosis in China. Am Rev Respir Dis 1986; 134(6):1273–1275.

147. Bothamley G, Beck JS, Britton W, et al. Antibodies to *Mycobacterium tuberculosis*-specific epitopes in lepromatous leprosy. Clin Exp Immunol 1991; 86(3):426–432.

148. Sada E, Brennan PJ, Herrera T, et al. Evaluation of lipoarabinomannan for the serological diagnosis of tuberculosis. J Clin Microbiol 1990; 28(12):2587–2590.

149. Sada E, Ferguson LE, Daniel TM. An ELISA for the serodiagnosis of tuberculosis using a 30,000-Da native antigen of *Mycobacterium tuberculosis*. J Infect Dis 1990; 162(4):928–931.

150. Uma Devi KR, Ramalingam B, Raja A. Antibody response to *Mycobacterium tuberculosis* 30 and 16kDa antigens in pulmonary tuberculosis with human immunodeficiency virus coinfection. Diagn Microbiol Infect Dis 2003; 46(3):205–209.

151. Munk ME, Arend SM, Brock I, et al. Use of ESAT-6 and CFP-10 antigens for diagnosis of extrapulmonary tuberculosis. J Infect Dis 2001; 183(1):175–176.

152. Doherty TM, Demissie A, Olobo J, et al. Immune responses to the *Mycobacterium tuberculosis*-specific antigen ESAT-6 signal subclinical infection among contacts of tuberculosis patients. J Clin Microbiol 2002; 40(2):704–706.

153. Scarpellini P, Tasca S, Galli L, et al. Selected pool of peptides from ESAT-6 and CFP-10 proteins for detection of *Mycobacterium tuberculosis* infection. J Clin Microbiol 2004; 42(8):3469–3474.

154. Bothamley GH, Rudd R, Festenstein F, et al. Clinical value of the measurement of *Mycobacterium tuberculosis* specific antibody in pulmonary tuberculosis. Thorax 1992; 47(4): 270–275.

155. Steingart KR, Dendukuri N, Henry M, et al. Performance of purified antigens for serodiagnosis of pulmonary tuberculosis: A meta-analysis. Clin Vaccine Immunol 2009; 16(2):260–276.

156. Steingart KR, Henry M, Laal S, et al. A systematic review of commercial serological antibody detection tests for the diagnosis of extrapulmonary tuberculosis. Postgrad Med J 2007; 83(985):705–712.

157. Kanaujia GV, Lam P, Perry S, et al. Integration of microscopy and serodiagnostic tests to screen for active tuberculosis. Int J Tuberc Lung Dis 2005; 9(10):1120–1126.

158. van Pinxteren LA, Ravn P, Agger EM, et al. Diagnosis of tuberculosis based on the two specific antigens ESAT-6 and CFP10. Clin Diagn Lab Immunol 2000; 7(2):155–160.

159. Pottumarthy S, Wells VC, Morris AJ. A comparison of seven tests for serological diagnosis of tuberculosis. J Clin Microbiol 2000; 38(6):2227–2231.

160. Perkins MD, Conde MB, Martins M, et al. Serologic diagnosis of tuberculosis using a simple commercial multiantigen assay. Chest 2003; 123(1):107–112.

161. Maekura R, Kohno H, Hirotani A, et al. Prospective clinical evaluation of the serologic tuberculous glycolipid test in combination with the nucleic acid amplification test. J Clin Microbiol 2003; 41(3):1322–1325.

162. Hamasur B, Bruchfeld J, Haile M, et al. Rapid diagnosis of tuberculosis by detection of mycobacterial lipoarabinomannan in urine. J Microbiol Methods 2001; 45(1):41–52.

163. Tessema TA, Bjune G, Assefa G, et al. Clinical and radiological features in relation to urinary excretion of lipoarabinomannan in Ethiopian tuberculosis patients. Scand J Infect Dis 2002; 34(3):167–171.

164. Boehme C, Molokova E, Minja F, et al. Detection of mycobacterial lipoarabinomannan with an antigen-capture ELISA in unprocessed urine of Tanzanian patients with suspected tuberculosis. Trans R Soc Trop Med Hyg 2005; 99(12):893–900.

165. Huebner RE, Schein MF, Bass JB, Jr. The tuberculin skin test. Clin Infect Dis 1993; 17(6): 968–975.

166. Canessa PA, Fasano L, Lavecchia MA, et al. Tuberculin skin test in asymptomatic HIV seropositive carriers. Chest 1989; 96(5):1215–1216.

167. Lein AD, von Reyn CF, Ravn P, et al. Cellular immune responses to ESAT-6 discriminate between patients with pulmonary disease due to *Mycobacterium avium* complex and those with pulmonary disease due to *Mycobacterium tuberculosis*. Clin Diagn Lab Immunol 1999; 6(4):606–609.

168. Arend SM, Thijsen SF, Leyten EM, et al. Comparison of two interferon-gamma assays and tuberculin skin test for tracing tuberculosis contacts. Am J Respir Crit Care Med 2007; 175(6):618–627.

169. Brock I, Weldingh K, Lillebaek T, et al. Comparison of tuberculin skin test and new specific blood test in tuberculosis contacts. Am J Respir Crit Care Med 2004; 170(1):65–69.

170. Harada N, Higuchi K, Yoshiyama T, et al. Comparison of the sensitivity and specificity of two whole blood interferon-gamma assays for M. *tuberculosis* infection. J Infect 2008; 56(5):348–353.

171. Kim SH, Choi SJ, Kim HB, et al. Diagnostic usefulness of a T-cell based assay for extrapulmonary tuberculosis. Arch Intern Med 2007; 167(20):2255–2259.

172. Soysal A, Torun T, Efe S, et al. Evaluation of cut-off values of interferon-gamma-based assays in the diagnosis of M. *tuberculosis* infection. Int J Tuberc Lung Dis 2008; 12(1): 50–56.

173. Clinicians Guide to QuantiFERON-TB Gold. Melbourne, AUS, Cellestis Ltd. January 13, 2005.

174. Higuchi K, Kawabe Y, Mitarai S, et al. Comparison of performance in two diagnostic methods for tuberculosis infection. Med Microbiol Immunol 2009; 198(1):33–37.

175. Pai M, Zwerling A, Menzies D. Systematic review: T-cell-based assays for the diagnosis of latent tuberculosis infection: An update. Ann Intern Med 2008; 149(3):177–184.

176. Diel R, Loddenkemper R, Meywald-Walter K, et al. Comparative performance of tuberculin skin test, QuantiFERON-TB-Gold In Tube Assay, and T-Spot. TB Test in contact investigations for tuberculosis. Chest 2009; 135(4):1010–1018.

177. Ewer K, Deeks J, Alvarez L, et al. Comparison of T-cell-based assay with tuberculin skin test for diagnosis of *Mycobacterium tuberculosis* infection in a school tuberculosis outbreak. Lancet 2003; 361(9364):1168–1173.

178. Hill PC, Brookes RH, Fox A, et al. Large-scale evaluation of enzyme-linked immunospot assay and skin test for diagnosis of *Mycobacterium tuberculosis* infection against a gradient of exposure in The Gambia. Clin Infect Dis 2004; 38(7):966–973.

179. Mazurek GH, Jereb J, LoBue P, et al. Guidelines for using QuantiFERON-TB Gold test for detecting *Mycobacterium tuberculosis* infection. MMWR Recomm Rep 2005; 54(RR-15):49–55.

180. Health Protection Agency Tuberculosis Programme Board. Health Protection Agency Position Statement on the Use of Interferon Gamma Release Assay (IGRA) Tests for Tuberculosis (TB). February 3, 2009.

181. Diel R, Nienhaus A, Lange C, et al. Cost-optimisation of screening for latent tuberculosis in close contacts. Eur Respir J 2006; 28(1):35–44.

182. Oxlade O, Schwartzman K, Menzies D. Interferon-gamma release assays and TB screening in high-income countries: A cost-effectiveness analysis. Int J Tuberc Lung Dis 2007; 11(1):16–26.

183. Lam PK, Lobue PA, Catanzaro A. Clinical diagnosis of tuberculosis by specialists and non-specialists. Int J Tuberc Lung Dis 2009; 13(5):659–661.

184. Catanzaro A, Lam PK, Bothamley G, et al. Using Clinical Suspicion to Identify Smear-Negative Cases for Culture of *Mycobacterium tuberculosis*. Kagoshima, Japan: 41st Joint Tuberculosis/Leprosy Conference. 2006.

185. Rao SP, Lam PK, Bothamley G, et al. Integrating laboratory tests and clinical suspicion in tuberculosis (TB) diagnosis. Am J Respir Crit Care Med 2007; 175:A419.

5
Treatment of Tuberculosis

PHILIP C. HOPEWELL
Division of Pulmonary and Critical Care Medicine, San Francisco General Hospital, Francis J. Curry National Tuberculosis Center, Department of Medicine, University of California, San Francisco, California, U.S.A.

I. Tuberculosis Treatment as a Public Health Measure

Prompt, accurate diagnosis and effective treatment for tuberculosis are the key elements in the public health response to tuberculosis and are the cornerstones of tuberculosis control (1). Effective treatment not only restores the health of the individual with the disease but, also, quickly renders the patient noninfectious and no longer a threat to the community. Thus, all providers who undertake treatment of patients with tuberculosis must recognize that not only are they treating an individual but they are assuming an important public health function that also entails a high level of responsibility to the community as well as to the individual patient (2). To discharge this responsibility, clinicians must have a sound understanding of the drugs and treatment regimens used and the ability to ensure that treatment is taken as prescribed.

II. History of Antituberculosis Chemotherapy

Effective treatment for tuberculosis is a relatively recent development (3). Streptomycin, the first effective antituberculosis drug, was introduced into experimental clinical use in 1945 (4). Soon thereafter it was observed that although there was striking initial improvement in patients who received streptomycin, their condition subsequently worsened, and the organisms isolated from these patients were found to be resistant to streptomycin (5). The findings of clinical failure caused by drug-resistant organisms identified the major bacteriologic principle on which successful chemotherapy for tuberculosis depends: wild strain populations of *Mycobacterium tuberculosis* are not uniform in their susceptibility to antimycobacterial agents, thus, it is always necessary to treat with more than one drug to which the organisms are susceptible. The effectiveness of multiple-drug chemotherapy was first demonstrated in a British Medical Research Council study in which streptomycin was given in combination with p-aminosalicylic acid (PAS) (3,6).

Antituberculosis chemotherapy that was both effective and well tolerated became a reality in 1952 with the introduction of isoniazid—an effective, well-tolerated, and cheap drug (7). Again, however, it was found that single drug treatment with isoniazid was inadequate and that resistance developed quickly. Thus, the combination of isoniazid and PAS with or without streptomycin came to be the standard therapy for tuberculosis.

Effective therapy using optimum combinations of isoniazid, streptomycin, and PAS produced a revolution in the care of patients with tuberculosis (8). Springett (9) reviewed death rates for cohorts of patients in Birmingham, England, for the years 1947, 1950, 1953, 1956, and 1959. The study found that there was a dramatic decrease in deaths during the 10 years after diagnosis, associated with the increasing use of chemotherapy. Nearly all of the reduction was accounted for by improvements in survival during the first year after diagnosis. In addition, not only were there many more survivors but among the survivors there were many fewer who continued to have persistently positive sputum and, thus, served as ongoing sources of new infections.

In 1967 the effectiveness of ethambutol as a substitute for PAS was documented (10). Ethambutol was found to be much more tolerable and less toxic as a companion drug for isoniazid than PAS. Subsequently, it was demonstrated that the combination of isoniazid and rifampin (introduced in the early 1970s), generally with ethambutol or streptomycin, could shorten the necessary duration of treatment from the standard 18–24 months to 6–9 months (11).

Investigators then began to focus on the differential effects of antituberculosis drugs and especially on the potential role of pyrazinamide (12,13). Dickinson and coworkers (14) demonstrated that streptomycin, rifampin, and isoniazid are quickly bactericidal for rapidly growing *M. tuberculosis* in vitro. The in vitro conditions could be likened to the in vivo conditions under which the extracellular organisms in tuberculous lesions are living. Although both rifampin and isoniazid are rapidly bactericidal, Mitchison and Dickinson (15) demonstrated that rifampin is more effective in killing organisms that grow in spurts rather than continuously. Although both isoniazid and rifampin are effective in killing intracellular organisms, pyrazinamide is especially effective in this regard, suggesting that the addition of pyrazinamide would strengthen the isoniazid–rifampin combination. Two studies have substantiated that the addition of pyrazinamide for two months to a regimen of isoniazid and rifampin improves the effectiveness of a six-month regimen (16,17). Thus, a core regimen of isoniazid and rifampin, supplemented by pyrazinamide and ethambutol for the initial two months, is now recommended as standard treatment for both pulmonary and extrapulmonary tuberculosis (18,19).

III. Antituberculosis Drugs

As shown in Table 1, there are 10 drugs currently approved by the U.S. Food and Drug Administration for treating tuberculosis plus 6 other drugs that are effective but not approved for this indication (18). The table lists the drugs, available preparations, and the doses that are recommended.

A. First-Line Drugs

For a succinct review of the mechanisms of action of current and potential antituberculosis drugs, see Ref. 21.

Isoniazid

Isoniazid is a prodrug that requires conversion to its active form by the catalase-peroxidase enzyme system in *M. tuberculosis* (22,23). Once activated, in susceptible organisms the drug has profound early bactericidal activity, reducing bacillary populations by about 2 logs within 48 hours. Most strains of *M. tuberculosis* are inhibited by concentrations of isoniazid of 0.05 to 0.20 µg/mL. It is readily absorbed from the gastrointestinal tract; peak blood concentrations of approximately 5 µg/mL occur one to two hours after the

Table 1 Antituberculosis Drugs, Preparations, and Doses

Drug/Preparation	Adults/children	Daily	Doses 2/wk	3/wk
First-line drugs				
Isoniazid: Tablets (50 mg, 100 mg, 300 mg); elixir (50 mg/5 mL); aqueous solution (100 mg/mL) for intravenous or intramuscular injection	Adults (max.)	5 mg/kg (300 mg)	15 mg/kg (900 mg)	10 mg/kg (600 mg)
	Children (max.)	10–15 mg/kg (300 mg)	20–30 mg/kg (900 mg)	15–20 mg/kg (600 mg)
Rifampin: Capsule (150 mg, 300 mg); powder may be suspended for oral administration; aqueous solution for intravenous injection	Adults‡(max.)	10 mg/kg (600 mg)	10 mg/kg (600 mg)	10 mg/kg (600 mg)
	Children (max.)	10–20 mg/kg (600 mg)	10–20 mg/kg (600 mg)	10–20 mg/kg (600 mg)
Rifabutin: Capsule (150 mg)	Adults‡(max.)	5 mg/kg (300 mg)	5 mg/kg (300 mg)	5 mg/kg (300 mg)
	Children	Appropriate dosing for children is unknown	Appropriate dosing for children is unknown	Appropriate dosing for children is unknown
Rifapentine: Tablet (150 mg, film-coated)	Adults	Approved for once/wk in continuation phase (600 mg)	—	—
	Children	The drug is not approved for use in children		
Pyrazinamide: Tablet (500 mg, scored)	Adults (max)	20–30 mg/kg (2.0 g)	40–50 mg/kg (4.0 g)	30–40 mg/kg (3.0 g)
	Children (max.)	30–40 mg/kg/day (2.0 g)	50 mg/kg (2.0 g)	40 mg/kg (2.0 g)
Ethambutol: Tablets (100 mg, 400 mg)	Adults (max)	15–20 mg/kg (1.6 g)	35–50 mg/kg (4.0 g)	25–35 mg/kg (2.4 g)
	Children§(max.)	15–25 mg/kg/day (1.0 g)	50 mg/kg (2.5 g)	30 mg/kg (2.0 g)

Table 1 Antituberculosis Drugs, Preparations, and Doses (*Continued*)

Drug/Preparation	Adults/children	Doses		
		Daily	2/wk	3/wk
Second-line drugs				
Cycloserine: Capsule (250 mg)	Adults (max.)	10–15 mg/kg/day (1.0 g in two doses), usually 500–750 mg/day in two doses	There are no data to support intermittent administration	There are no data to support intermittent administration
	Children (max.)	10–15 mg/kg/day (1.0 g/day)	—	—
Ethionamide: Tablet (250 mg)	Adults#(max.)	15–20 mg/kg/day (1.0 g/day), usually 500–750 mg/day in a single daily dose or two divided doses#	There are no data to support intermittent administration	There are no data to support intermittent administration
	Children (max.)	15–20 mg/kg/day (1.0 g/day)	There are no data to support intermittent administration	There are no data to support intermittent administration
Streptomycin: Aqueous solution (1-g vials) for intravenous or intramuscular administration	Adults (max.)	**	**	**
	Children (max.)	20–40 mg/kg/day (1 g)	20 mg/kg (1 g)	20 mg/kg (1 g)
Amikacin: Aqueous solution (500-mg and kanamycin 1-g vials) for intravenous or intramuscular administration	Adults (max.)	**	**	**
	Children (max.)	15–30 mg/kg/day (1 g) intravenous or intramuscular as a single daily dose	15–30 mg/kg (1 g)	15–30 mg/kg (1 g)

			**	**
Capreomycin: Aqueous solution (1-g vials) for intravenous or intramuscular administration	Adults (max.)	15–30 mg/kg/day (1 g) as a single daily dose	15–30 mg/kg (1 g)	15–30 mg/kg (1 g)
	Children (max.)		There are no data to support intermittent administration	There are no data to support intermittent administration
p-Aminosalicylic acid (PAS): Granules (4-g packets) can be mixed with food; tablets (500 mg) are still available in some countries, but not in the United States; a solution for intravenous administration is available in Europe.	Adults	8–12 g/day in two or three to four divided doses (10 g)	There are no data to support intermittent administration	There are no data to support intermittent administration
	Children		There are no data to support intermittent administration	There are no data to support intermittent administration
Levofloxacin: Tablets (250 mg, 500 mg, 750 mg); aqueous solution (500 mg vials) for intravenous injection	Adults	500–1000 mg daily	There are no data to support intermittent administration	There are no data to support intermittent administration
	Children	△	-	-

(Continued)

Table 1 Antituberculosis Drugs, Preparations, and Doses (*Continued*)

| Drug/Preparation | Adults/children | Daily | Doses | | |
			2/wk	3/wk
Moxifloxacin: Tablets (400 mg); aqueous solution (400 mg/250 mL) for intravenous injection	Adults	400 mg daily	There are no data to support intermittent administration	There are no data to support intermittent administration
	Children	△	-	-
Gatifloxacin: Tablets (400 mg); aqueous solution (200 mg/20 mL; 400 mg/40 mL) for intravenous injection	Adults	400 mg daily	There are no data to support intermittent administration	There are no data to support intermittent administration
	Children	△	-	-

§Dose per weight is based on ideal body weight. Children weighing more that 40 kg should be dosed as adults.

#For purposes of this document adult dosing begins at age 15 years.

†Dose may need to be adjusted when there is concomitant use of protease inhibitors or nonnucleoside reverse transcriptase inhibitors.

††The drug can likely be used safely in older children but should be used with caution in children younger than 5 years in whom visual acuity cannot be monitored. In younger children, EMB at the dose of 15 mg/kg/day can be used if there is suspected or proven resistance to INH or RIF.

*It should be noted that, although this is the dose recommended generally, most clinicians with experience using cycloserine indicate that it is unusual for patients to be able to tolerate this amount. Serum concentration measurements are often useful in determining the optimum dose for a given patient.

**The single daily dose can be given at bedtime or with the main meal.

xx15 mg/kg/day (1 g) and 10 mg/kg in persons older than 59 years of age (750 mg). Usual dose 750 to 1000 mg IM or IV typically given as a single dose for five to seven days a week and reduced to two to three times a week after first two to four months or after culture conversion, depending on the efficacy of the other drugs in the regimen.

△ The long-term (>several weeks) use of fluoroquinolones in children and adolescents has not been approved because of concerns about effects on bone and cartilage growth. However, most experts agree that the drug should be considered for children with tuberculosis caused by organisms resistant to both INH and RIF. The optimal dose is not known.

Source: From Ref. 20.

administration of a dose of 3 to 5 mg/kg body weight. The serum half-life varies, depending on whether a person is a rapid or slow acetylator; it is 2 to 4 hours in slow acetylators and 0.5 to 1.5 hours in rapid acetylators (24). The drug penetrates well into all body fluids and cavities, producing concentrations similar to those found in serum. Isoniazid exerts its effect mainly by inhibiting cell wall mycolic acid synthesis (21,25).

In any wild strain population of *M. tuberculosis,* the frequency of isoniazid-resistant mutants is approximately one in 3.5×10^6 organisms (26). However, when isoniazid is used alone, a population of organisms resistant to the drug emerges rapidly. This was demonstrated in an early clinical trial in which 11%, 52%, and 71% of patients to whom isoniazid alone was given developed resistant strains after one, two, and three months of treatment, respectively (27).

Several different mutations result in resistance to isoniazid. The most common of these occur in the gene, *kat g,* coding for catalase-peroxidase production and result in decreased or absent function of the enzyme that converts isoniazid to its active form. Mutations in the *inh, a* promoter, also result in resistance to isoniazid but are less common. Together *kat g* and *inh a* mutations account for a large majority of isoniazid-resistant strains (25).

Hepatitis is the major toxic effect of isoniazid. Asymptomatic aminotransferase elevations up to five times the upper limit of normal occur in 10% to 20% of persons receiving INH alone for treatment of latent tuberculosis infection (28). However, data from a large observational cohort indicate that the incidence of clinical hepatitis is lower than was previously thought. In 11,141 patients managed in an urban tuberculosis control program and who were receiving INH alone as treatment for latent tuberculosis infection, hepatitis occurred in only 0.1% to 0.15% (29). A meta-analysis of six studies estimated the rate of clinical hepatitis in patients given INH to be only 0.6% (30). When isoniazid was given in combination with rifampin, the rate of clinical hepatitis averaged 2.7% in 19 reports. For INH alone, the risk of hepatotoxicity increases with increasing age; it is uncommon among persons younger than 20 years of age but is nearly 2% in persons aged 50 to 64 years (31). The risk also may be increased in persons with underlying liver disease, in those with a history of heavy alcohol consumption, and in the postpartum period, particularly among Hispanic women (31,32). A large survey estimated the rate of fatal hepatitis to be 0.023%, but more recent studies suggest the rate is substantially lower (29,33,34). Death has been associated with continued administration of INH despite onset of symptoms of hepatitis (34). The possible mechanisms for isoniazid-induced hepatotoxicity are reviewed in Ref. 35.

Peripheral neuropathy, the second most frequent serious adverse reaction associated with isoniazid, occurs especially with other disorders that may cause neuropathy (HIV infection, diabetes mellitus, uremia, alcoholism). The neuropathy can nearly always be prevented or reversed by administration of pyridoxine 25 to 50 mg/day.

Rifamycins

Of the rifamycins (rifampin, rifabutin, and rifapentine), rifampin is by far the most widely used. Like isoniazid, rifampin is also rapidly bactericidal for *M. tuberculosis*. It is quickly absorbed from the gastrointestinal tract; serum concentrations of 6 to 7 μg/mL occur 1.5 to 2 hours after ingestion. The half-time in blood is 3 to 3.5 hours, although this may be decreased in persons who have been taking the drug for several weeks (36). The half-time increases with increasing doses of the drug. For sensitive strains of *M. tuberculosis,* the minimum inhibitory concentration is approximately 0.5 µg/mL, although there is variation among strains (37). Approximately 75% of the drug is protein-bound, but it penetrates well into tissues and cells. Penetration through noninflamed meninges is poor; however, therapeutic concentrations are achieved in cerebrospinal fluid when the meninges are inflamed (38).

Among the wild strains of *M. tuberculosis,* the rate of rifampin resistance–conferring mutations is approximately 10×10^{10} per bacterium per generation (26). Rifampin exerts its effect by binding to the β subunit of RNA polymerase (21,39,40). For this reason, it has activity against many bacteria other than *M. tuberculosis.* Approximately 96% of rifampin-resistant strains have mutations in the *rpoB* gene, the product of which is the β subunit of RNA polymerase (21,39). The mechanism for resistance in the remaining 4% is not known. Resistance to rifampin, unaccompanied by resistance to other antituberculosis drugs, has been reported to occur nearly exclusively among patients with HIV infection, particularly among patients being treated with highly (once or twice weekly) intermittent regimens (40–43).

Adverse reactions to rifampin when it is given daily include rashes, hepatitis, gastrointestinal upset, and, rarely, thrombocytopenia. The rate of these reactions has been variable, but in general is quite low (18). Hepatitis occurred in 3.1% of the patients in the U.S. Public Health Service study of six-month isoniazid–rifampin treatment (44). Twice weekly administration of higher doses of rifampin is associated with several immunologically mediated reactions, including thrombocytopenia, an influenza-like syndrome, hemolytic anemia, and acute renal failure (45).

Drug–drug interactions due to induction of hepatic microsomal enzymes by rifampin are relatively common and are of particular concern in patients with HIV infection. The rifamycins interact with the protease inhibitor and non-nucleoside reverse transcriptase inhibitor classes of antiretroviral agents (18). The interaction of these classes of drugs is bidirectional: protease inhibitors decrease clearance of rifamycins, and rifamycins, by inducing hepatic P-450 cytochrome oxidases, accelerate clearance of protease inhibitors (46,47). Of the rifamycin derivatives, rifabutin has the least effect on the concentration of antiretroviral agents. Rifampin induces the metabolism of a number of other drugs, including methadone, warfarin, oral contraceptives, digoxin, macrolide antibiotics, and ketoconazole (18). [A complete list of interactions with the rifamycins is given in Ref. (18)]. Doses of these drugs need to be adjusted when rifampin is given. Ketoconazole and, to a lesser extent, fluconazole interfere with absorption of rifampin, thereby decreasing its serum concentration.

Rifabutin, although not approved by the U.S. Food and Drug Administration for tuberculosis, may be used as a substitute for rifampin in treating tuberculosis (18). Because of its lesser propensity to induce cytochrome P450 enzymes, rifabutin is generally reserved for patients who are taking any medication for which there are unacceptable interactions with rifampin. It may also be used for patients who are intolerant of rifampin. There is nearly complete cross-resistance among the rifamycins. The toxicity profile of rifabutin is similar to that of rifampin, except that in some studies with HIV-infected patients neutropenia has been reported and uveitis has been described when the drug is given with a macrolide antibiotic (clarithromycin, azithromycin) that reduces rifabutin clearance (18).

Rifapentine, which has the longest serum half-life of the rifamycins, has been shown in controlled clinical trials to be effective in combination with isoniazid given once weekly in the continuation phase of treatment for pulmonary tuberculosis (48). It should be emphasized, however, that there are important limitations on the use of this regimen. It is not to be used for patients with HIV infection, for patients who have cavitary lesions on chest film, or who have positive sputum smears at the end of the initial phase of treatment; thus, a once-weekly rifapentine regimen should not be used when radiographic examination and HIV testing are not available (or not performed routinely). The toxicity profile of rifapentine is similar to that of rifampin.

Ethambutol

Ethambutol in usual doses of 15 mg/kg body weight has a static effect on *M. tuberculosis*. It is used mainly to reduce the risk of rifampin resistance in patients with tuberculosis caused by strains that have primary resistance to isoniazid. Peak plasma concentrations occur two to four hours after ingestion. With doses of 15 mg/kg, the peak concentration is approximately 4 μg/mL (49). The concentration increases proportionally with increasing doses. In persons with normal renal function, the half-time in blood is approximately four hours. Minimum inhibitory concentrations of the drug for *M. tuberculosis* range from 1 to 5 μg/mL. Cerebrospinal fluid concentrations of ethambutol, even in the presence of meningeal inflammation, are low (50). Ethambutol appears to exert its effect by interfering with cell wall biosynthesis. Specifically, the target for ethambutol is thought to be an arabinosyl transferase (21). Mutations in the *embB* gene, which, together with *embA* and *embC*, code for arabinosyl transferases, are found in approximately 70% of ethambutol-resistant strains (39). The rate of resistance-conferring mutations is 0.5×10^4 for ethambutol (26).

Retrobulbar neuritis is the main adverse effect of ethambutol. Symptoms include blurred vision, central scotomata, and red–green color blindness. This complication is dose-related, occurring in 15% of patients given 50 mg/kg, 1% to 5% with 25 mg/kg, and less than 1% with 15 mg/kg (18,51). The frequency of ocular effects is increased in patients with renal failure, presumably in relation to increased serum concentrations of the drug.

Pyrazinamide

Pyrazinamide is active against *M. tuberculosis* at an acid pH, which suggests that the drug is activated under these conditions (21,52). The drug is particularly active against dormant or semidormant *M. tuberculosis* in macrophages, or in the acidic environment within areas of caseation, and is rapidly bacteriostatic but only slowly bactericidal. Peak serum concentrations occur approximately two hours after ingestion. Concentrations generally range from 30 to 50 μg/mL with doses of 20 to 25 mg/kg. The serum half-life is 9 to 10 hours. At a pH of 5.5, the minimal inhibitory concentration of pyrazinamide for *M. tuberculosis* is 20 μg/mL. The mechanism of action of pyrazinamide is thought to be the disruption of membrane energy metabolism (21).

The genetic mechanism of mycobacterial resistance to pyrazinamide appears to be any of a large number of mutations in the *pncA* gene, which encodes the enzyme pyrazinamidase (21,39). This enzyme appears to be necessary for the intracellular conversion of pyrazinamide to its active form, pyrazanoic acid. Mutations in the *pncA* gene are found in approximately 70% of pyrazinamide-resistant strains (21,39).

The most important adverse reaction to pyrazinamide is liver injury, which is dose-related. In a large U.S. Public Health Service study in which pyrazinamide was given in a dose of 25 mg/kg daily for six months, hepatotoxicity occurred in 2% to 3% of patients (53). At a dose of 40 mg/kg per day, also given for six months, 6% of patients developed hepatitis. All patients were receiving isoniazid and PAS in addition to pyrazinamide. An increased frequency of hepatotoxicity has been reported in studies of pyrazinamide combined with rifampin in a two-month treatment regimen for latent tuberculosis infection in persons without HIV infection (54).

Hyperuricemia occurs in nearly all patients taking pyrazinamide. Although gout is not common, diffuse arthralgias, apparently unrelated to the hyperuricemia, occur frequently. The drug may also cause nausea and vomiting, and skin rashes, including photosensitive dermatitis.

Streptomycin

Streptomycin was widely used in the past as a first-line drug. However, currently because of increasing resistance and the need for parental administration, its use is limited. The drug is rapidly bactericidal, although its effectiveness is inhibited by an acid pH (18). Peak serum concentrations occur approximately one hour after an intramuscular dose. With a dose of 15 mg/kg, the peak concentration is in the range of 40 μg/mL. The half-time in blood is approximately five hours. Sensitive strains of *M. tuberculosis* are inhibited by streptomycin in a concentration of 8 μg/mL. The drug has good tissue penetration; however, it enters the cerebrospinal fluid only in the presence of meningeal inflammation. Streptomycin and ethambutol have been found to be of approximately equal effect in combination regimens; however, because of a relatively high prevalence of resistance to streptomycin, particularly in developing countries and because it requires injection, its usefulness is limited.

Streptomycin exerts its effect by interfering with ribosomal protein synthesis. This effect is mediated by binding of the drug to 16S rRNA inhibiting initiation of translation (21). Mutations in the genes that code for 16S rRNA (*rrs* and *rpsL*) have been found in 65% to 77% of resistant strains. Mutations in *rpsL* have been associated with high-level streptomycin resistance while low-level resistance has been associated with *rrs* mutations (39). The rate of resistance-conferring mutations is one in 3.8×10^6 generations (26).

Ototoxicity is the most common serious adverse effect of streptomycin (18). This usually results in vertigo, but hearing loss may also occur. The risk of ototoxicity is related both to cumulative dosage and to peak serum concentrations. In general, peak concentrations of greater than 40 to 50 μg/mL should be avoided, and the total dose should not exceed 100 to 120 g (18). Because of its effect on fetal auditory system development, streptomycin is contraindicated in pregnancy. Streptomycin should be used with caution in patients with renal insufficiency because of increased risk of nephrotoxicity and ototoxicity. The dosing frequency should be reduced to two to three times a week (18).

B. Second-Line Drugs

There are four additional agents approved by the U.S. Food and Drug Administration for treating tuberculosis: PAS, ethionamide, cycloserine, and capreomycin. In addition, fluoroquinolones, amikacin, kanamycin, and linezolid have antituberculosis effects and are used in treating patients with tuberculosis caused by drug-resistant organisms or those intolerant of first-line drugs (18,55).

Of the second-line drugs, the fluoroquinolones are perhaps most useful and, therefore, the most widely used (56,57). The fluoroquinolones should not be considered as first-line agents but should be reserved for patients with drug-resistant organisms or those who cannot tolerate first-line drugs (18,58,59). The target of the fluoroquinolones is DNA gyrase—an enzyme that operates to increase coiling of DNA. Inhibition of gyrase in turn inhibits DNA synthesis. Resistance to these agents is mediated by mutations in *gyrA* and *gyrB* genes that encode for DNA gyrase (39). Not many strains have been sequenced, but *gyrA* or *gyrB* mutations have been found in 42% to 85% of resistant isolates.

The quinolones are generally well-tolerated. The most frequent adverse effects include nausea, vomiting, dizziness, anxiety, and other central nervous system effects. Because of the broad spectrum of antimicrobial action, diarrhea may be associated with the quinolones. Photosensitivity and arthropathy may also occur (60). There are few clinical studies regarding the usefulness of quinolones in multiple-drug regimens. Optimal dosages and durations of quinolone administration are not known. Both animal and limited human data suggest that moxifloxacin is the most potent of the existing quinolones and is the most promising of this class of drugs (61–63).

All of the other oral second-line agents are difficult to administer because of adverse effects. It is recommended that an expert be consulted before these drugs are used (18). (Ref. 18 contains a more detailed discussion of the adverse effects of second-line drugs.) Administration of PAS is associated with a high frequency of gastrointestinal upset. Hypersensitivity reactions occur in 5% to 10% of patients taking the drug. In addition, the usual dose of 10 to 12 g/day requires ingestion of 20 to 24 tablets. Administration has been made somewhat easier by use of a granular formulation of the drug. Similarly, ethionamide causes a high frequency of gastrointestinal side effects, often necessitating discontinuation of the drug. Cycloserine causes behavioral disturbances in a large number of patients to whom the drug is administered. These disturbances range from irritability and depression to psychosis. In addition, seizures and peripheral neuropathy occur, especially with high doses and when cycloserine and isoniazid are given together. In addition to the adverse effects, neither PAS, ethionamide, or cycloserine is particularly potent against *M. tuberculosis*. Kanamycin, amikacin, and capreomycin are not absorbed from the gastrointestinal tract and thus require parenteral administration. All three drugs may cause hearing loss related both to peak concentrations and to cumulative doses and, in addition, may impair renal function.

IV. Promoting Adherence to Treatment

For antituberculosis chemotherapy to be effective in both its individual and public health roles, it must be conducted properly. Accomplishing the goals of therapy requires individualization of the means of patient supervision, often with creative innovations, to enable assessment of adherence and to address poor adherence when it is identified. It must be emphasized that, because of the public health considerations related to tuberculosis, successful therapy is the responsibility of those supervising the care of the patient. Health care providers undertaking to treat patients with tuberculosis must provide a means for ensuring that therapy is completed successfully (2).

The reasons for poor adherence to treatment for tuberculosis are complex and numerous, and prediction of who will be adherent and who will not is unreliable (64). It is clear that there is no single approach to management that is effective for all patients, conditions, and settings. Consequently, interventions that target adherence must be tailored or customized to the particular situation of a given patient (18,65). Concordance, defined in this context as an agreement between a patient with tuberculosis and the health care provider, reinforces their mutual contribution and responsibility to achieve successful treatment (66). Components of this approach include setting clinic hours to suit the patient's schedule; providing treatment support in the clinic, the patient's home, or other locations; and offering incentives and enablers, such as transportation reimbursements. Such an approach must be developed in close collaboration with the patient to achieve optimum adherence. This patient-centered, individualized approach to treatment support is a core element of all tuberculosis care and control efforts.

A central element in ensuring completion of therapy is giving the drugs under direct observation [directly observed therapy (DOT)] (18). Ancillary measures, such as pill counting or testing for drug metabolites in urine, may also be useful for assessment of adherence. The use of DOT has been shown to be associated with improved outcomes of therapy in several cohort analyses (67–69). Patient-centered approaches using the full range of accepted measures to ensure medication ingestion are central to the WHO Stop TB Strategy—the first component of which is DOTS—comprising four elements in addition to DOT (70,71). The success of the strategy has been demonstrated most clearly in Peru and China (72,73). However, concerns have been raised that the direct observation of medication ingestion, not the full DOTS strategy, does not lead to better outcomes compared with self-supervised treatment (74).

V. Current Treatment Regimens

The tuberculosis treatment regimens that are recommended currently by the American Thoracic Society, Centers for Disease Control and Prevention, and the Infectious Diseases Society of America (ATS/CDC/IDSA) (18) are given in Table 2. These recommendations are intended to guide treatment in areas where mycobacterial culture, drug-susceptibility testing, chest radiography, and second-line drugs are available routinely. The treatment recommendations of the World health Organization (WHO) (19) (Table 3) are directed toward low- and middle-income countries where the above resources are not available routinely.

The basic treatment regimen recommended by both ATS/CDC/IDSA and WHO for patients who have not been treated previously consists of an initial phase of isoniazid, rifampin, pyrazinamide, and ethambutol for two months, followed by four months of isoniazid and rifampin (18,19). As shown in Table 2, there are several variations in the pattern of administration of the basic regimen. In large part these variations are designed to enable closer supervision of medication ingestion. Previous WHO recommendations included a continuation phase of isoniazid and ethambutol given daily for six months when circumstances did not allow for effective supervision beyond the initial phase. This was intended to minimize the likelihood of rifampin resistance developing. However, in a comparative clinical trial, the isoniazid– ethambutol continuation phase regimen was significantly less effective that the isoniazid– rifampin continuation phase regimen (75). Moreover it has been shown that in patients with HIV infection the outcome is significantly better when the regimen contains rifampin throughout (76).

Where quality-assured laboratory facilities are available, initial isolates should have drug-susceptibility tests performed. If resistance is identified, regimens can be tailored to suit the specific pattern. Drug-susceptibility tests should be repeated if *M. tuberculosis* is isolated after three or more months of treatment.

Table 2 Drug Regimens for Pulmonary Tuberculosis Caused by Drug-Susceptible Organisms

	Initial phase			Continuation phase			Range of total doses (minimum duration)	RATING[a] (Evidence)[b]	
Regimen	Drugs	Regimen	Interval and doses[c] (minimum duration)	Regimen	Drugs	Interval and doses[c,d] (minimum duration)		HIV−	HIV+
1	INH RIF PZA EMB		Seven days per week for 56 doses (8 weeks) *or* five days per week for 40 doses (8 weeks)[e]	1a	INH/RIF	Seven days per week for 126 doses (18 weeks) *or* five days per week for 90 doses (18 weeks)[e]	182–130 (26 weeks)	A (I)	A (II)
				1b	INH/RIF	Twice-weekly for 36 doses (18 weeks)	92–76 (26 weeks)	A (I)	A (II)[g]
				1c[f]	INH/RPT	Once weekly for 18 doses (18 weeks)	74 or 58 (26 weeks)	B (I)	E (I)
2	INH RIF PZA EMB		Seven days per week for 14 doses (2 weeks) *then* twice-weekly for 12 doses (6 weeks) *or* five days per week for 10 doses (2 weeks)[e] *then* twice weekly for 12 doses (6 weeks)	2a	INH/RIF	Twice-weekly for 36 doses (18 weeks)	62–58 (26 weeks)	A(II)	B (II)[g]
		2b[f]		2b[f]	INH/RPT	Once weekly for 18 doses (18 weeks)	44 or 40 (26 weeks)	B(I)	E (I)
3	INH RIF PZA EMB		Thrice-weekly for 24 doses (8 weeks)	3a	INH/RIF	Thrice-weekly for 54 doses (18 weeks)	78 (26 weeks)	B (I)	B (II)

(Continued)

Table 2 Drug Regimens for Pulmonary Tuberculosis Caused by Drug-Susceptible Organisms (*Continued*)

	Initial phase			Continuation phase			RATING[a] (Evidence)[b]	
Regimen	Drugs	Interval and doses[c] (minimum duration)	Regimen	Drugs	Interval and doses[c,d] (minimum duration)	Range of total doses (minimum duration)	HIV−	HIV+
4	INH RIF EMB	Seven days per week for 56 doses (8 weeks) *or* five days per week for 40 doses (8 weeks)[e]	4a	INH/RIF	Seven days per week for 217 doses (31 weeks) *or* five days per weeks for 155 doses (28 weeks)[e]	273–195 (39 weeks)	C (I)	C (II)
			4b	INH/RIF	Twice-weekly for 62 doses (31 weeks)	118–102 (39 weeks)	C (I)	C (II)

[a]Definitions of evidence ratings: A = preferred; B = acceptable alternative; C = offer when A and B cannot be given; E = should never be given.

[b]Definitions of evidence ratings: I = randomized clinical trial; II = data from clinical trials that were not randomized or were conducted in other populations; III = expert opinion.

[c]When DOT is used, drugs may be given 5 days/wk and the necessary number of doses adjusted accordingly. Although there are no studies that compare 5 with 7 daily doses, extensive experience indicates this would be an effective practice.

[d]Patients with cavitation on initial chest radiograph and positive cultures at completion of two months of therapy should receive a seven-month [28 week; either 196 doses (daily) or 56 doses (twice-weekly)] continuation phase.

[e]Five-days-a-week administration is always given by DOT. Rating for five-days-a-week regimens is AIII.

[f]Options 1c and 2b should be used only in HIV-negative patients who have negative sputum smears at the time of completion of two months of therapy and who do not have cavitation on the initial chest radiograph (see text). For patients started on this regimen and found to have a positive culture at two months, treatment should be extended for an extra three months.

[g]Not recommended for HIV-infected patients with CD4 cell counts <100 cells/mL.

Abbreviations: INH, isoniazid; RIF, rifampin; RPT, rifapentine; PZA, pyrazinamide; EMB, ethambutol.

Source: From Ref. 20.

Table 3 Recommended Treatment for Persons Not Treated Previously

Initial phase	Continuation phase
INH, RIF, PZA, EMB[a,b] daily, 2 months	INH, RIF daily, 4 months
INH, RIF, PZA, EMB[a,b] 3×/week, 2 months	INH, RIF 3×/week, 4 months

[a] Streptomycin may be substituted for EMB.
[b] EMB may be omitted in uncomplicated childhood tuberculosis.
Abbreviations: INH, isoniazid; RIF, rifampicin; PZA, pyrazinamide; EMB, ethambutol.
Source: From Ref. 19.

The recommendation of a four-drug initial phase is based, in part, on findings of the British Medical Research Council (BMRC) (77) that strongly suggest that where the prevalence of initial resistance to isoniazid is likely to be high, treatment regimens should include an initial two-month, 4-drug initial phase, and rifampin plus isoniazid should be given for a four-month continuation phase. The results of this regimen in the BMRC were nearly as good in the presence of resistance to isoniazid as for fully susceptible organisms. However, a recent systematic review suggests that even single drug (usually isoniazid) initial resistance is associated with a higher frequency of acquired drug resistance (78). In the review, the pooled estimate of the cumulative incidence of acquired drug resistance with initially pan-sensitive strains was 0.8% (95% CI, 0.5–1.0%) compared with 6% (CI, 4–8%) with initially single drug–resistant strains and 14% (CI, 9–20%) with initially polydrug-resistant strains. Failure and relapse were associated with initial drug resistance. Failure was also associated with shorter duration of rifampin therapy and nonuse of streptomycin, whereas the rate of relapse was higher with a shorter duration of rifampin therapy and nonuse of pyrazinamide. These results reinforce the importance of using an initial phase of four drugs, including pyrazinamide, and maintaining rifampin throughout the full six months of treatment.

Several factors have been found to be predictive of a poor therapeutic outcome (18,48,79). In United States Public Health Service Study 22, the presence of cavitation on the initial chest film and sputum culture positivity at the time of completion of the initial phase of treatment were highly predictive of an adverse outcome—either treatment failure or relapse (48). For this reason for patients with cavitation on the initial chest film and who have positive sputum cultures at the end of the initial phase of treatment, prolongation of the continuation phase to seven months, making a total of nine months of treatment is recommended by the ATS, CDC, IDSA treatment guidelines (18). These recommendations differ from those of WHO. In many parts of the world, radiographic examination and cultures are not available, thus, following these guidelines is not possible. Additional factors that have been associated with poor clinic attendance and, therefore, with a lower chance of favorable response include use of alcohol, younger age (but above 18 years), and unmarried status (18).

After two to three months of chemotherapy, 75% to 90% of patients taking regimens containing isoniazid and rifampin should have negative sputum cultures. Failure of the sputum to become negative may indicate that either the patient is not taking the drugs or, less commonly, the organisms are resistant to the drugs being used. In patients who continue to have *M. tuberculosis* in their sputum after two to three months of treatment, DOT should be re-enforced and drug-susceptibility tests should be performed, if facilities are available. If resistance is found, the regimen should be modified based on the results. If sputum samples are still positive after four to five months of therapy, the regimen should be considered to have failed and a new regimen begun, ideally, based on recent drug-susceptibility test results.

VI. Drug Resistance

The fourth (most recent) Global Drug Surveillance Project conducted by the WHO and The Union, including data from 76 countries, shows that drug resistance, in general, is ubiquitous and that there are areas of the world in which rates of multiple drug–resistant (MDR) tuberculosis (tuberculosis caused by organisms that are resistant to at least isoniazid and rifampin) among persons without previous treatment are truly alarming (80). These include several former Soviet republics, several oblasts in Russia, the Baltic countries, and two provinces in China.

Clinical errors that commonly lead to the emergence of drug resistance include failure to provide effective treatment support and assurance of adherence; failure to recognize and address patient nonadherence; inadequate drug regimens; adding a single new drug to a failing regimen; and failure to recognize existing drug resistance (58). In addition, co-morbid conditions associated with reduced serum levels of anti-tuberculosis drugs (e.g., malabsorption, rapid transit diarrhea, HIV infection, use of antifungal agents) may also lead to the acquisition of drug resistance (58).

Patients with drug-resistant tuberculosis can spread the drug-resistant bacilli to their contacts. Transmission of drug-resistant strains of *M. tuberculosis* has been well described in congregate settings and in susceptible populations, notably HIV-infected persons (81–84). However, MDR tuberculosis (tuberculosis caused by organisms that are resistant to, at least, isoniazid and rifampin) may spread in the population at large as has been evident in China, the Baltic States, and countries of the former Soviet Union (58).

According to the WHO/IUATLD Global Project on Anti-TB Drug Resistance Surveillance, the strongest factor associated with drug resistance in an individual patient is previous anti-tuberculosis treatment (80,85). In previously treated patients, the odds of any resistance are at least 4-fold higher and that of MDR at least 10-fold higher than in new (untreated) patients (58). Patients with chronic tuberculosis (sputum positive after re-treatment) and those who fail treatment (sputum-positive after five months of treatment) are at highest risk of having MDR tuberculosis, especially if rifampicin was used throughout the course of treatment (58). The likelihood of resistance is directly related to the duration of previous treatment (86). Resistance to isoniazid increases approximately 4% per month of treatment for durations of less than one year. Resistance to streptomycin increases at approximately 2.5% per month of prior treatment.

Persons who are in close contact with confirmed MDR tuberculosis patients, especially children and HIV-infected individuals, also are at high risk of being infected with MDR strains. In some closed settings prisoners, persons staying in homeless shelters, and certain categories of immigrants and migrants are at increased risk of MDR-tuberculosis. (58,80,85). These factors are summarized and presented in descending order of level of risk in Table 4.

By the midnineties, most countries participating in the WHO-Union global survey of anti-tuberculosis drug resistance registered cases of MDR tuberculosis. Not surprisingly,

Table 4   Assessing Risk for Drug Resistance

Risk factors for resistance	Comments
Failure of re-treatment regimen	Patients who are still sputum smear positive at the end of a re-treatment regimen have perhaps the highest MDR-TB rates of any group, often exceeding 80%.
Close contact with a known drug-resistant case	Most studies have shown the tuberculosis occurring in close contacts of MDR-TB patients to have high rates of MDR-TB.
Failure of the initial treatment regimen	Patients who fail to become sputum smear negative while on treatment are likely to have drug-resistant organisms. However, the likelihood depends on a number of factors, including whether rifampicin was used in the continuation phase and whether DOT was used throughout treatment. Thus, a detailed history of drugs used is essential. This is especially true for patients treated by private providers, often with non-standard regimens.
Relapse after apparently successful treatment	In clinical trials most patients who relapse have fully susceptible organisms. However under programs conditions, an apparent relapse, especially an early relapse, may, in fact, be an unrecognized treatment failure and thus have a higher likelihood of drug resistance.
Return after default without recent treatment failure	The likelihood of varies substantially in this group, depending in part on the amount of treatment taken and the degree of adherence before default.
Exposure in institutions that have DR-TB outbreaks or a high DR-TB prevalence	Patients who frequently stay in homeless shelters; prisoners in many countries; and health care workers in clinics, laboratories, and hospitals can have high rates of DR-TB.
Residence in areas with high DR-TB prevalence	DR-TB rates in many areas of the world can be high enough to justify routine DST in all new cases.

Source: From Ref. 58.

in 2006, extensively drug-resistant (XDR) tuberculosis, defined as tuberculosis caused by *M. tuberculosis* resistant to at least isoniazid and rifampin of the first-line drugs as well as to any one of the fluoroquinolones and to at least one of three injectable second-line drugs (amikacin, capreomycin, or kanamycin), was identified. Subsequent reports have identified XDR tuberculosis in all regions of the world and, to date, treatment outcomes have been significantly worse than MDR tuberculosis outcomes (87–89). In one cohort from KwaZulu-Natal, 98% of XDR tuberculosis patients co-infected with HIV died, with a median time of death of only 16 days from time of specimen collection (87).

The two strongest risk factors for (or predictors of) XDR tuberculosis are (*i*) failure of a tuberculosis treatment containing second-line drugs, including an injectable agent and a fluoroquinolone, and (*ii*) close contact with an individual with documented XDR tuberculosis or with an individual for whom treatment with a regimen including second-line drugs is failing or has failed.

DST for first-line drugs is currently recommended for all patients with a history of previous anti-tuberculosis treatment: patients who have failed treatment, especially those who have failed a standardized re-treatment regimen, and chronic cases are the highest priority (58). Patients who develop tuberculosis and are known to have been in close contact with persons known to have MDR tuberculosis also should have DST performed on an initial isolate. Although HIV infection has not been conclusively shown to be an independent risk factor for drug resistance, MDR tuberculosis outbreaks in HIV settings and high mortality rates in persons with MDR tuberculosis and HIV infection justify routine DST in all HIV-infected tuberculosis patients, resources permitting (58). All patients suspected of having MDR/XDR tuberculosis should have DST to isoniazid, rifampin, the second-line injectable agents, and a fluoroquinolone. When epidemiological or other factors suggest that there is a risk for MDR/XDR tuberculosis in a person with HIV infection, liquid media or other validated rapid techniques for DST of first- and second-line drugs is recommended.

The basic principle of treatment for patients whose organisms are resistant to one or more of the first-line drugs is the administration of at least two (but generally three to four) agents to which there is demonstrated or presumed sensitivity (18,58). Unfortunately, there are no data to provide evidence-based guidelines as to the relative effectiveness of various regimens and the necessary duration of treatment. Clearly, if the organism is susceptible to isoniazid and rifampin, a usual regimen can be expected to be successful. In the presence of resistance to isoniazid, treatment with rifampin and ethambutol, supplemented by pyrazinamide, also is likely to be successful. There are data that suggest 12 months of treatment with rifampin and ethambutol is sufficient (18); however, in patients with organisms resistant to isoniazid, such decisions should be made on a case-by-case basis.

Tuberculosis caused by MDR and XDR organisms presents particularly difficult management problems (18,19,58,90–96). At least in part, the outcome of treatment depends on the number of agents to which the organisms are susceptible, the promptness and appropriateness of therapy, the number of previous courses of therapy, and the HIV status of the patient. For example, in a group of patients with MDR tuberculosis who had undergone multiple previous courses of chemotherapy, the rate of successful outcome was only slightly better than 50% (90). However, both in New York and in San Francisco non–HIV-infected patients with MDR tuberculosis who had not been extensively treated previously had a much better rate of success (92% and 97%, respectively), albeit with a much shorter follow-up time (91,92). In the report from San Francisco, the prognosis for patients with HIV infection and MDR tuberculosis was very poor, with all 11 patients dying during the period of the study, although this group of patients was treated prior to the availability of HAART (92).

As would be expected, the outcome of treatment of patients with XDR tuberculosis is generally less good than the outcome for patients with MDR disease (93–96). Outcome data for patients with XDR tuberculosis are scarce. Rates of successful completion of treatment among patients without HIV infection range from approximately 30% to 60%. Consultation with an expert is advised in treating patients with MDR/XDR tuberculosis. Often, the regimen chosen represents the last best chance for cure and treatment must be done correctly. The regimen should be based on the results of drug-susceptibility tests when available. In most instances, however, the results are not known until several weeks after therapy is started. In such instances, treatment should be determined on the basis of the patient's history of prior therapy, avoiding reliance on agents taken previously, and on the prevailing resistance patterns in the community or subpopulation of which the patient is a member.

VII. Treatment in Special Situations

A. Infection with Human Immunodeficiency Virus

The recommended treatment regimen for HIV-infected patients with tuberculosis consists of the same six-month regimen as described for non–HIV-infected patients (18,19). However, there are several important areas in which therapy for patients with tuberculosis and HIV infection differs. There is an association between HIV infection and acquired rifampin resistance (40,42,43). The cause of rifampin monoresistance is not clear but both resistance and an increased rate of adverse outcomes have been associated with the use of highly intermittent (twice or once weekly) drug administration in the continuation phase. Rifamycin monoresistance has also been associated with prior use of rifabutin as prophylaxis for *Mycobacterium avium* complex infections (97). Because of the increased risk of adverse outcomes and of rifamycin resistance, the rifapentine once-weekly regimen is contraindicated for any patient with HIV infection and a twice-weekly regimen is not recommended for HIV-infected patients with CD4 cell counts of <100/ mL (18).

An important consideration in treating tuberculosis in patients with HIV infection is the potential for interactions of antituberculosis agents, especially the rifamycins, with other drugs, especially the protease inhibitor class of antiretroviral agents. (Reviewed in detail in Ref. 18.) The most practical means of minimizing the effects of the interactions is to use an antiretroviral regimen that excludes protease inhibitors and consists of two nucleoside reverse transcriptase inhibitors plus efavirenz (because animal studies suggest a possibility of congenital abnormalities with efavirenz, pregnant women should be treated with nevirapine.), and rifabutin, although much more expensive, should be used in place of rifampin. Monitoring serum drug concentrations may be useful in avoiding the adverse consequences of the interactions (98). However, in many parts of the world neither rifabutin nor therapeutic drug concentration measurements are available, and thus, treatment for both diseases must be given under careful clinical monitoring. The optimum time to initiate an antiretroviral regimen in patients being treated for tuberculosis has not been determined. The general recommendation is that an antiretroviral regimen should be started for patients with tuberculosis and HIV infection having <200 CD4 cells/mL (99). With CD4 cell counts of 200 to 350/mL the possible benefits are less clear, but treatment should be considered.

Because of the potential for frequent changes in recommendations for treating tuberculosis in patients with HIV infection, the information on the CDC Web site (http://www.cdc.gov/nchstp/tb/TBHIVDrugs/TOC.htm) and the NIH Web site (http://www.aidsinfo.nih.gov/guidelines) is regularly updated. These sites should be consulted for the most up-to-date recommendations.

Another feature of tuberculosis treatment in patients with HIV infection is the paradoxical worsening (immune reconstitution syndrome), which may occur in patients in whom antiretroviral therapy is initiated (100–103). Presumably these reactions are the result of reconstitution of the immune response to mycobacteria. Typical features include new onset of fever, lymphadenopathy, and worsening appearance of lesions on chest films (100–103). When these features occur, it is important to rule out treatment failure as well as other opportunistic diseases. Treatment is usually symptomatic with nonsteroidal anti-inflammatory agents. In some instances the reactions are sufficiently severe as to warrant the use of corticosteroids, although this approach is not of proven benefit.

Finally, in large part because of high death rates early in the course of treatment of HIV-infected persons with tuberculosis, rates of treatment success are less than in cohorts of non–HIV-infected patients. Apart from these deaths that, often, are due to advanced HIV infection, the rate of treatment success is nearly equal to that of persons without HIV infection. However, as indicated by the increased rates of treatment failure and relapse with highly intermittent therapy, there is less margin of safety for drug administration in patients with HIV-infection. Thus, direct observation of therapy is extremely important to be certain of a high level of adherence. If there are problems with treatment, such as breaks in therapy, delayed conversion, or persistence of symptoms, prolonging therapy beyond six months should be strongly considered (18).

B. Pregnancy and Breast-feeding

Active untreated tuberculosis is more of a hazard to a pregnant woman and her fetus than is treatment for the disease. In a pregnant woman or a mother of a young infant, it is important that the most effective therapy for tuberculosis be given. Thus, treatment should be initiated with isoniazid, rifampin, and ethambutol. Pyrazinamide is included in WHO's recommendations for treating tuberculosis in pregnant women, but it has not been included in the ATS/CDC/IDSA recommendations because of insufficient information about possible harmful effects (18,19). Without pyrazinamide in the regimen, treatment must be given for a total of nine months. Streptomycin, which interferes with development of the ear and may cause congenital deafness, is the only antituberculosis drug documented to have harmful effects on the fetus. This potential is presumably shared by amikacin, kanamycin, and capreomycin; however, there is little or no information about the effects of these drugs as well as of cycloserine and ethionamide on the fetus.

Although several antituberculosis drugs are present in breast milk, their concentrations and the total amounts that could possibly be ingested by a nursing infant are so small that adverse effects would be unlikely. Thus, no modifications of treatment regimens are necessary for nursing mothers.

C. Other Associated Conditions

Tuberculosis occurs in association with many other conditions either because an underlying disorder alters immune responsiveness, thereby predisposing to tuberculosis, or because the accompanying condition may occur frequently in the same social and cultural milieu as does tuberculosis. Examples of the former class of disorders include hematological or reticuloendothelial malignancies, immunosuppressive therapy, HIV infection, chronic renal failure, diabetes mellitus, and malnutrition. Alcoholism and its accompanying disorders and other forms of substance abuse are also very common in patients with tuberculosis. All of these conditions may influence the therapy. The response of the impaired host to treatment may not be as satisfactory as that of a person with normal host responsiveness. For this reason, therapeutic decisions must be made on a much more individualized basis and, when possible, steps taken to correct the immunosuppression.

In patients with impaired renal function, streptomycin, kanamycin, amikacin, and capreomycin should be avoided if at all possible or given two to three times a week in the usual dose. If there is severe impairment of renal function, reduction in the frequency of administration of ethambutol and pyrazinamide to two to three times a week may be necessary (18). The drugs should be administered after hemodialysis.

Liver disease, particularly alcoholic hepatitis and cirrhosis, is common among patients with tuberculosis. For isoniazid, rifampin, and pyrazinamide, there is an increased frequency of hepatotoxicity in the presence of preexisting liver disease (104). Moreover, detecting hepatotoxicity, if it occurs, may be difficult because of the preexisting liver function abnormalities. Additionally, what in a person with normal liver function would be minor hepatotoxicity, in a patient with severe liver disease could have major consequences. Options in treating patients with severe liver disease include treatment without pyrazinamide, using isoniazid, rifampin, and ethambutol for 9 months; treatment with only one potentially hepatotoxic drug, usually retaining rifampin and adding ethambutol and a fluoroquinolone for a total of 12 to 18 months; and treatment with a regimen that contains no hepatotoxic drugs, i.e., streptomycin, ethambutol, a fluoroquinolone, and perhaps another second-line drug such as cycloserine plus capreomycin or and aminoglycoside for 18 to 24 months (18,105). In patients with severe liver disease, routine testing of liver function should be performed at baseline and during treatment. Patients should be questioned regularly to detect symptoms suggestive of hepatotoxicity.

VIII. Adjunctive Treatments for Pulmonary Tuberculosis

A. Corticosteroids

The use of corticosteroids in pulmonary tuberculosis has been and remains controversial. However, corticosteroids may, under certain conditions, be of at least short-term benefit in patients with pulmonary tuberculosis (106). A systematic review of 11 clinical trials of adjunctive corticosteroids in pulmonary tuberculosis concluded that there were significant benefits in patients with advanced disease in terms of weight gain, defervescence, and length of hospital stay. Sputum conversion was not affected. It should be noted, however, that only two of the studies used modern, rifampin-containing treatment regimens. Nevertheless, the data suggest a potential role for corticosteroid treatment is in patients with severe tuberculosis and severe systemic effects. Although not considered in the systematic review, steroids may also be of benefit in patients with marked abnormalities of gas exchange and respiratory failure (107). It should be emphasized, however, that before using corticosteroid treatment in patients with severe pulmonary tuberculosis, one must be confident that adequate antituberculosis chemotherapy is being given.

B. Surgical Interventions

Surgical resection may be indicated in several situations. In patients with tuberculosis caused by MDR organisms that is anatomically limited within the lung, resection may be an effective therapeutic option (108). Before an operation in such patients, it is important to reduce the bacillary population as much as possible with drugs to which the organism is susceptible. Determining the optimum time to perform surgery, however, can be difficult, because the effectiveness of a limited second-line drug regimen cannot always be predicted. Resection may also be necessary because of massive hemoptysis associated with current or old tuberculosis or a mycetoma in a residual cavity, because of residual lung damage with recurrent bacterial infections or because of a bronchopleural fistula with (usually) a tuberculous empyema. In addition to these therapeutic indications for surgery, it is fairly common for tuberculosis to be diagnosed by examination of a resected pulmonary mass or nodule thought to be malignant.

In any situation involving possible lung surgery in patients with or suspected of having tuberculosis, including the resection of a solitary nodule in a patient with a positive tuberculin reaction, it is desirable for the patient to have been receiving adequate antituberculosis chemotherapy before the operation. This will minimize the possibility of spread of tuberculosis within the lung and of bronchial stump infection and empyema. The optimum duration of treatment before operation is not clear. In emergencies, such as massive hemoptysis, at least single doses of the drugs should be given, whereas with elective procedures, it is best to wait at least until the sputum smear is negative.

IX. Extrapulmonary Tuberculosis

A. Disseminated Tuberculosis
Standard antituberculosis chemotherapeutic regimens should be employed for disseminated tuberculosis unless meningitis is present in which case the recommended duration is 9 to 12 months (18). Corticosteroids may be useful, as mentioned previously, for severe pulmonary disease with respiratory failure.

B. Lymphatic Tuberculosis
A six-month regimen is recommended for treatment of tuberculous lymphadenitis (109–111). However, even with effective regimens, the rate of response is much slower than with pulmonary tuberculosis. Lymph nodes may enlarge, new nodes may appear, and fistulas may develop during treatment that ultimately proves effective, but true bacteriologic relapse after completion of therapy is unusual. Corticosteroid treatment has been used to shrink intrathoracic nodes and relieve bronchial obstruction, primarily in children. In a controlled study, Nemir and coworkers (112) demonstrated that corticosteroids increase the rate of resolution of radiographic changes thought to be due to bronchial narrowing by lymph nodes or endobronchial lesions in children with primary tuberculosis. Apart from this indication, there is no clear role for corticosteroids in lymphatic tuberculosis.

Surgical intervention may be necessary to make a diagnosis of tuberculous lymphadenitis, and on occasion surgical incision and drainage are needed to prevent spontaneous drainage and fistula formation. Surgical excision of involved nodes, strictly as an adjunct to chemotherapy, is associated with perhaps a slightly worse outcome than medical treatment with aspiration of the node or medical treatment alone (113).

C. Pleural Tuberculosis
Treatment of the hypersensitivity variety of tuberculous pleural effusion consists of standard antituberculosis drug regimens (18). Drainage via tube thoracostomy is rarely

necessary, although repeat thoracenteses may be required to relieve symptoms. Occasionally, early in the course of eventually successful therapy, the amount of fluid in the thorax increases before decreasing. In general, the amount of residual pleural scarring is small. The use of corticosteroids may increase the rate of resolution and decrease the residual fluid, but such treatment is rarely indicated.

The second variety of tuberculous involvement of the pleura is a true empyema. This is much less common than tuberculous pleurisy with effusion and results from a large number of organisms spilling into the pleural space, usually from rupture of a cavity or an adjacent parenchymal focus via a broncho-pleural fistula. Although standard chemotherapy should be instituted for tuberculous empyema, it is unlikely to clear the pleural space infection, probably because penetration of the antituberculosis agents into the pleural cavity is limited. For this reason, surgical drainage is often necessary and may be required for a prolonged period of time both as treatment for the infection and because of the frequent association with a broncho-pleural fistula. Drainage may be accomplished with a standard thoracostomy tube. In selected patients, creation of an Eloesser flap, in which a small portion of rib overlying the empyema space is resected and the skin is sutured to the pleura, is the procedure of choice.

D. Genitourinary Tuberculosis

There are several treatment considerations for genitourinary tuberculosis apart from standard chemotherapy (114). In patients who have tuberculosis caused by MDR organisms and who can tolerate removal of a kidney, nephrectomy may be indicated. Nephrectomy may also be indicated for patients who have recurrent pyogenic bacterial infections in a kidney destroyed by tuberculosis, for persistent pain and for massive hematuria. Surgical or endoscopic procedures may also be necessary to correct ureteral strictures and to augment the capacity of a contracted bladder.

E. Bone and Joint Tuberculosis

Standard chemotherapy of six to nine months duration is highly successful in skeletal tuberculosis, but surgery is occasionally a necessary adjunct. The longer duration of treatment has been suggested because of the difficulties in assessing response. Several controlled studies have documented that chemotherapy conducted largely on an ambulatory basis is effective in curing spinal tuberculosis without the need for immobilization (115,116). The role of emergency spinal cord decompression in patients with Pott's disease and early neurologic findings is not clear, and if paraplegia is already present, the benefit of surgical intervention is even less clear. Moreover, there is no well-defined surgical procedure of choice. Surgery may be indicated in other forms of articular tuberculosis when there is extensive destruction of the joint or surrounding soft tissues, in which case synovectomy and joint fusions may be necessary.

F. Central Nervous System Tuberculosis

Isoniazid penetrates the blood–brain barrier quite readily, and in the presence of meningeal inflammation, rifampin enters the cerebrospinal fluid in concentrations sufficient to inhibit the growth of the organism. Although data are limited, pyrazinamide seems to penetrate the barrier easily, at least in the presence of inflammation, and streptomycin achieves inhibitory concentrations when there is meningitis. Ethambutol penetrates poorly, and doses of 25 mg/kg body weight produce subinhibitory concentrations. In view of the potential catastrophic consequences of poorly treated tuberculous meningitis, the possibility that no organisms can be isolated, and the length of time required for drug-susceptibility studies to be done, the potential for resistant organisms should be taken into account when the treatment is initiated. If there are no epidemiological indicators of possible resistance a regimen of isoniazid, rifampin, pyrazinamide, and ethambutol should be effective. The recommended length of the continuation phase is 7 months for a total treatment duration of 9 to 12 months, although there are no clinical trials that serve to define the optimum treatment duration (18).

Corticosteroid treatment has a beneficial effect in patients with tuberculous meningitis and cerebral edema (113,117–119). In addition, in the presence of high cerebrospinal fluid protein concentration, corticosteroids reduce the frequency of adhesive arachnoiditis and spinal fluid block. In children with less severe stages of disease, corticosteroid therapy has been shown to decrease the frequency of sequelae (118,119). Given the severity of the process, reasonably good data supporting corticosteroid use in more severe forms of the disease, and a paucity of information in patients with less severe tuberculosis meningitis, corticosteroid treatment, specifically with dexamethasone, is recommended for all patients, especially those with alterations in their level of consciousness. The recommended dose of dexamethasone is 12 mg/day for three weeks then decreased gradually during the next three weeks.

The other major central nervous system form of tuberculosis, the tuberculoma, presents a more subtle clinical picture than does tuberculous meningitis. The response to antituberculosis chemotherapy is good, and corticosteroids are indicated only if there is an increase in intracranial pressure. Tuberculomas seem relatively more common in patients with HIV infection and may worsen with life-threatening consequences with the immune reconstitution syndrome.

G. Abdominal Tuberculosis

Standard chemotherapy is quite effective in abdominal tuberculosis. Corticosteroids have been advocated in tuberculous peritonitis to reduce the risk of adhesions causing intestinal obstructions, but this recommendation is controversial because the low frequency of obstruction is generally low. Surgery is often necessary to establish a diagnosis and, in addition, may be necessary to relieve intestinal obstruction if it should occur.

H. Pericardial Tuberculosis

Because of the potentially life-threatening nature of pericardial tuberculosis, treatment with antituberculosis agents should be instituted promptly once the diagnosis is made or strongly suggested. It appears that the likelihood of pericardial constriction is greater in patients who have had symptoms longer; thus, early therapy may reduce the incidence of this complication. Several studies have suggested that corticosteroids have a beneficial effect in treating both tuberculous pericarditis with effusion and constrictive pericarditis (113,120,121). However, a meta-analysis of studies examining the effects of corticosteroids in tuberculous pericarditis concluded that, although steroids could have an important effect, the studies were too small and heterogeneous to be conclusive

(121,122). Nevertheless, given the potentially serious consequences of tuberculous pericarditis, recommendations in both the United States and the United Kingdom support the administration of corticosteroids to patients receiving adequate antituberculosis therapy and who have no major contraindications (18,113). The optimum regimen is not known, but prednisone, 60 mg/day for four weeks, followed by 30 mg/day for four weeks, 15 mg/day for two weeks, and 5 mg/day for one week is the recommended regimen (18). In general, if hemodynamic compromise occurs, pericardiectomy is necessary. Although pericardiocentesis generally improves the circulatory status, the improvement is usually temporary. Pericardial windows with drainage into the left pleural space also generally provide only temporary relief.

X. New Drugs for Tuberculosis

The goals of new antituberculosis drug development are, first, to develop a drug that will enable shortening of the minimum duration of treatment for bacteriologically proven tuberculosis from the current six months to one to two months; second, to provide new drugs for treating MDR/XDR tuberculosis; and third, to develop more effective treatments for latent tuberculosis infection (123). (See chap. 14 for a detailed discussion on new drugs for tuberculosis.) Currently there are a number of drugs with antituberculosis activity that undergoing clinical testing in humans and others that are in preclinical testing (124). Drugs in human trials include the existing quinolones (moxifloxacin and gatifloxacin), a nitroimidazole (PA-824), a diarylquinoline, and a pyrrole (LL-3858). The quinolones have been discussed previously and have been used fairly extensively, albeit, without a clear definition of the role and maximal benefit for these agents. However, there is preliminary evidence that inclusion of a quinolone, probably moxifloxacin because of its greater potency, may shorten the duration of treatment (56,57).

PA-824 is a prodrug that is thought to act on cell wall lipid biosynthesis (125). It is active against MDR organisms, suggesting that the target enzyme is new, and is as active as isoniazid against susceptible organisms, having an MIC of 0.015 to 0.25 μg/mL. It appears safe in mice, but human data are not yet available.

The diarylquinolines are thought to act by inhibiting the proton pump of ATP synthase, and the lead compound has an MIC of 0.030 to 0.120 μg/mL both for fully susceptible and for resistant strains of *M. tuberculosis* (126,127). The drug appears to be specific for mycobacteria and is active against a wide range pathogenic and saprophytic members of the family. The frequency of resistance mutations ranges from 5×10^{-7} to 5×10^{-8} depending on the drug concentration, a frequency comparable to that of rifampin. The drug has an early bactericidal effect comparable to or greater than that of isoniazid and a delayed effect that exceeds that of rifampin. It also has a long plasma and tissue half-life in mice, facilitating its time-dependant killing properties. Although the drug has undergone only limited human testing, its properties suggest that it may be an exceptionally effective agent in treating tuberculosis.

Although there are a number of promising new drugs for treating tuberculosis, as was pointed out by Dye (128), without effective systems for their delivery, even the best antituberculosis drugs will not have their potential benefit realized. Moreover, to make major advances against the global tuberculosis epidemic, similar advances will be necessary in diagnostics and vaccine development (129,130).

References

1. Hopewell PC, Pai M. Tuberculosis, vulnerability, and access to quality care. JAMA 2005; 293:2790–2793.
2. Hopewell PC, Pai M, Maher D, et al. International standards for tuberculosis care. Lancet Infect Dis 2006; 6:710–725.
3. Mitchison DA. The diagnosis and therapy of tuberculosis during the past 100 years. Am J Respir Crit Care Med 2005; 171:699–706.
4. Hinshaw H, Feldman WH. Streptomycin in the treatment of clinical tuberculosis: A preliminary report. Proc Staff Meet Mayo Clin 1945; 20:313–318.
5. McDermott W, Muschenheim C, Hadley SJ, et al. Streptomycin in the treatment of tuberculosis in humans: I. Meningitis and generalized hematogenous tuberculosis. Ann Intern Med 1947; 27:769–822.
6. Medical Research Council. Treatment of pulmonary tuberculosis with streptomycin and para-aminosalicylic acid. BMJ 1950; 2:1073–1085.
7. Robitzek EH, Selikoff IJ. Hydrazine derivative of isonicotinic acid (Rimifon, Marsalid) in the treatment of acute progressive caseous-pneumonic tuberculosis. A preliminary report. Am Rev Tuberc 1952; 65:402–428.
8. Medical Research Council. Long-term chemotherapy in the treatment of chronic pulmonary tuberculosis with cavitation. Tubercle 1962; 43:201–211.
9. Springett VH. Ten-year results during the introduction of chemotherapy for tuberculosis. Tubercle 1971; 52:73–87.
10. Bobrowitz ID, Robins DE. Ethambutol-isoniazid versus PAS-isoniazid in original treatment of pulmonary tuberculosis. Am Rev Respir Dis 1967; 96:428–438.
11. Fox W, Mitchison DA. Short-course chemotherapy for tuberculosis. Am Rev Respir Dis 1975; 111:325–353.
12. Mackaness GB. The intracellular activation of pyrazinamide and nicotinamide. Am Rev Tuberc 1956; 74:718–728.
13. Fox W, Ellard GA, Mitchison DA. Studies on the treatment of tuberculosis undertaken by the British Medical Research Council tuberculosis units, 1946–1986, with relevant subsequent publications. Internat J Tuberc Lung Dis 1999; 3(10)(suppl 2):S231–S279.
14. Dickinson JM, Aber VR, Mitchison DA. Bactericidal activity of streptomycin, isoniazid, rifampin, ethambutol and pyrazinamide alone and in combination against *Mycobacterium tuberculosis*. Am Rev Respir Dis 1977; 116:627–635.
15. Mitchison DA, Dickinson JM. Bactericidal mechanisms in short-term chemotherapy. Bull Int Union Tuberc 1978; 53:270–275.
16. Snider DE Jr, Graczyk J, Bek E, et al. Supervised six-month treatment of newly diagnosed pulmonary tuberculosis using isoniazid, rifampin and pyrazinamide with and without streptomycin. Am Rev Respir Dis 1984; 130:1091–1094.
17. Coombs DL, O'Brien RJ, Geiter LJ. USPHS tuberculosis short-course therapy trial 21: Effectiveness toxicity and acceptability. The report of the final result. Ann Intern Med 1990; 112:407–415.
18. American Thoracic Society; Centers for Disease Control and Prevention; Infectious Diseases Society of America. Treatment of tuberculosis. Am J Respir Crit Care Med 2003; 167: 604–661.
19. World Health Organization. Treatment of Tuberculosis: Guidelines for National Programmes. WHO/CDS/TB/2003.313. Geneva, Switzerland: World Health Organization, 2003. (Updated on line, 2004.) http://www.who.int/tb/publications/cds_tb_2003_313/en/index.html.
20. Centers for Disease Control and Prevention. Treatment of Tuberculosis, American Thoracic Society, Centers for Disease Control and Prevention, and Infectious Diseases Society of America. MMWR Morb Mortal Wkly Rep 2003; 52(No. RR-11):1–77.
21. Zhang Y. The magic bullets and tuberculosis drug targets. Ann Rev Pharmacol Toxicol 2005; 45:529–564.

22. Zhang Y, Heym B, Allen B, et al. The catalase-peroxidase gene and isoniazid resistance of *Mycobacterium tuberculosis*. Nature 1992; 358:591–593.
23. Heym B, Zhang Y, Poulet S, et al. Characterization of the *Katg* gene encoding a catalase-peroxidase required for the isoniazid susceptibility of *Mycobacterium tuberculosis*. J Bacteriol 1993; 175:4255–4259.
24. Ellard GA. Variations between individuals and populations in the acetylation of isoniazid and its significance for the treatment of pulmonary tuberculosis. Clin Pharmacol Ther 1976; 19:610–625.
25. Vilchèze C, Jacobs WR Jr. The mechanism of isoniazid killing: Clarity through the scope of genetics. Ann Rev Microbiol 2007; 61:35—50.
26. David H L. Probability distribution of drug-resistant mutants in unselected populations of *Mycobacterium tuberculosis*. Appl Microbiol 1970; 20:810–814.
27. Medical Research Council. The treatment of pulmonary tuberculosis with isoniazid. BMJ 1952; 2:735–746.
28. Mitchell JR, Zimmerman HJ, Ishak KG, et al. Isoniazid liver injury: Clinical spectrum, pathology and probably pathogenesis. Ann Intern Med 1976; 84:181–192.
29. Nolan CM, Goldberg SV, Buskin SE. Hepatotoxicity associated with isoniazid preventive therapy. JAMA 1999; 281:1014–1018.
30. Steele MA, Burk RF, DesPrez RM. Toxic Hepatitis with Isoniazid and Rifampin. Chest 1999; 99:465–471.
31. Kopanoff DE, Snider DE Jr, Caras GJ. Isoniazid-related hepatitis. A US Public Health Service cooperative surveillance study. Am Rev Respir Dis 1978; 117:991–1001.
32. Franks AL, Binkin NJ, Snider DE Jr, et al. Isoniazid hepatitis among pregnant and postpartum Hispanic patients. Pub Health Rep 1989; 104:151–155.
33. Snider DE Jr, Caras GJ. Isoniazid-associated hepatitis deaths: A review of available information. Am Rev Respir Dis 1992; 145:494–497.
34. Salpeter S. Fatal isoniazid-induced hepatitis: Its risk during chemoprophylaxis. West J Med 1993; 159:560–564.
35. Tostmann A, Boeree MJ, Aarnoutse RE, et al. Antituberculosis drug-induced hepatotoxicity: Concise up-to-date review. Gastroenterol Hepatol 2008; 23:192–202.
36. Acocella G, Nicolis FB. Kinetic studies on rifampicin. Chemotherapy 1971; 16: 356–370.
37. Lorian V, Finland M. In vitro effect of rifampin on mycobacteria. Appl Microbiol 1969; 17:202–207.
38. D'Oliveira JJG. Cerebrospinal fluid concentrations of rifampin in meningeal tuberculosis. Am Rev Respir Dis 1972; 106:432–437.
39. Ramaswamy S, Musser JM. Molecular genetic basis of antimicrobial agent resistance in Mycobacterium tuberculosis: 1998 update. Tuberc Lung Dis 1998; 79:3–29.
40. Wallis RS, Weyer K, Fourie PB. Acquired rifamycin resistance pharmacology and biology. Expert Rev Anti Infect Ther 2008; 6:223–230.
41. Bradford WZ, Martin JN, Reingold AL, et al. The changing epidemiology of acquired drug-resistant tuberculosis in San Francisco, USA. Lancet 1996; 348:928–931.
42. Vernon, A, Burman W, Benator D, et al. Acquired rifamycin monoresistance in patients with HIV-related tuberculosis treated with once-weekly rifapentine and isoniazid. Lancet 1999; 353:1843–1847.
43. Centers for Disease Control and Prevention. Notice to Readers: Acquired rifamycin resistance in persons with advanced HIV disease being treated for active tuberculosis with intermittent rifamycin-based regimens. MMWR Morb Mortal Wkly Rep 2002; 51:214–215.
44. Snider DE Jr, Long MW, Cross FS, et al. Six-months isoniazid-rifampin therapy for pulmonary tuberculosis: Report of a United States Public Health Service cooperative trial. Am Rev Respir Dis 1984; 129:573–579.
45. Girling DJ, Hitze KL Adverse reactions to rifampicin. Bull WHO 1979; 57:45–49.

46. Burman WJ, Jones BE. Treatment of HIV-related tuberculosis in the era of effective antiretro-viral therapy. Am J Respir Crit Care Med 2001; 164:7–12.

47. McIlleron H, Meintjes G, Burman WJ, et al. Complications of antiretroviral therapy in patients with tuberculosis: Drug interactions, toxicity, and immune reconstitution inflammatory syndrome. J Infect Dis 2007; 196(suppl 1):S63–S75.

48. Benator D, Bhattacharya M, Bozeman L, et al. Rifapentine and isoniazid once a week versus rifampicin and isoniazid twice a week for treatment of drug-susceptible pulmonary tuberculosis in HIV-negative patients: A randomized clinical trial. Lancet 2002; 360: 528–534.

49. Lee CS, Gambertoglio JG, Brater DC, et al. Kinetics of ethambutol in the normal subject. Clin Pharmacol Ther 1977; 22:615–621.

50. Bobrowitz ID. Ethambutol in tuberculous meningitis. Chest 1972; 61:629–632.

51. Chan RY, Kwok AK. Ocular toxicity of ethambutol. Hong Kong Med J 2006; 12:56–60.

52. McDermott W, Tompsett R. Activation of pyrazinamide and nicotinamide in acidic environments. Am Rev Tuberc 1954; 70:748–753.

53. United States Public Health Service Tuberculosis Therapy Trial. Hepatic toxicity of pyrazinamide used with isoniazid in tuberculous patients. Am Rev Respir Dis 1959; 80:371–387.

54. United States Public Health Service. Update. Adverse event data and revised American thoracic Society/CDC recommendations against the use of rifampin and pyrazinamide for treatment of latent tuberculosis infection—United States, 2003. MMWR Morb Mortal Wkly Rep 2003; 52:735.

55. Ntziora F, Falagas ME. Linezolid for the treatment of patients with mycobacterial infections: A systematic review. Int J Tuberc Lung Dis 2007; 11:606–11.

56. Kennedy N, Berger L, Curram, J, et al. Randomized controlled trial of a drug regimen that includes ciprofloxacin for the treatment of pulmonary tuberculosis. Clin Infect Dis 1996; 22:827–833.

57. Gillespie SH, Kennedy N. Fluoroquinolones: A new treatment for tuberculosis? Int J Tuberc Lung Dis 1998; 2:265–271.

58. World Health Organization. Guidelines for the programmatic management of drug-resistant tuberculosis. WHO/HTM/TB/2008.402. Geneva, Switzerland: World Health Organization.

59. Ziganshina LE, Squire SB. Fluoroquinolones for treating tuberculosis. Cochrane Database Syst Rev 2008; (1):CD004795. doi: 10.1002/14651858.CD004795.pub3.

60. Lipsky BA, Baker CA. Fluoroquinolone toxicity profiles: A review focusing on newer agents. Clin Infect Dis 1999; 28:352–364.

61. Sato A, Tomioka K, Sano H, et al Comparative antimicrobial activities of gatifloxacin, sitafloxacin and levofloxacin against *Mycobacterium tuberculosis* replicating within Mono Mac 6 human macrophage and A-549 type II alveolar cell lines. J Antimicrobial Chemotherapy 2003; 52:199–203.

62. Nuernberger EL, Yoshimatsu T, Tyagi S, et al. Moxifloxacin-containing regimens of reduced duration produce a stable cure in murine tuberculosis. Am Rev Respir Dis 2004; 170: 1131–1134.

63. Sulochana S, Rahman F, Paramasivan CN. In vitro activity of fluoroquinolones against *Mycobacterium tuberculosis*. J Chemother 2005; 17:169–173.

64. World Health Organization. Adherence to long-term therapies: Evidence for action. Geneva, Switzerland: World Health Organization; 2003.

65. Munro SA, Lewin SA, Smith HJ, et al. Patient adherence to tuberculosis treatment: A systematic review of qualitative research. PLoS Med 2007; 4: e238.

66. Maher D, Uplekar M, Blanc L, et al. Concordance and tuberculosis treatment (editorial). BMJ 2003; 327:822–823.

67. Chaulk CP, Moore-Rice K, Rizzo R, et al. Eleven years of community-based directly observed therapy for tuberculosis. JAMA 1995; 274:945–951.

68. Weiss, SE, Slocum PC, Blin FX, et al. The effect of directly-observed therapy on the rates of drug resistance and relapse in tuberculosis. N Engl J Med 1994; 330:1179–1184.
69. China Tuberculosis Control Collaboration. Results of directly-observed short-course chemotherapy in 112,842 Chinese patients with smear-positive tuberculosis. Lancet 1996; 347:807–809.
70. World Health Organization, WHO Tuberculosis Programme. Framework for Effective Tuberculosis Control. WHO Report WHO/TB/94.179. Geneva, Switzerland: World Health Organization; 1994.
71. World Health Organization. The Stop TB Strategy: vision, goal, objectives and targets. WHO/HTM/TB 2006.368. Geneva, Switzerland: World Health Organization.
72. Suarez PG, Watt CJ, Alarcon E, et al. The dynamics of tuberculosis in response to 10 years of intensive control effort in Peru. J Infect Dis 2001; 184:473–478.
73. Chen F, Zhao H, Duanmu H,et al. The DOTS strategy in China; results and lessons after 10 years. Bull World Health Organ 2002; 80:430–436.
74. Volmink J, Matchaba P, Garner P. Directly observed therapy and treatment adherence. Lancet 2000; 355:1345–1350.
75. Jindani A, Nunn AJ, Enarson DA. Two 8-month regimens of chemotherapy for treatment of newly diagnosed pulmonary tuberculosis: International multicentre randomised trial. Lancet 2004; 364:1244–1251.
76. Korenromp EL, Scano F, Williams BG, et al. Effects of human immunodeficiency virus infection on recurrence of tuberculosis after rifampin-based treatment: An analytical review. Clin Infect Dis 2003; 37:101–112.
77. Mitchison DA, NunnAJ. Influence of initial drug resistance on the response to short-course chemotherapy of pulmonary tuberculosis. Am Rev Respir Dis 1986; 133:423–430.
78. Lew W, Pai M, Oxlade O, et al. Initial drug resistance and tuberculosis treatment outcomes: Systematic review and meta-analysis. Ann Intern Med 2008; 149:123–134.
79. Darbyshire JH, Aber VR, Nunn AJ. Predicting a successful outcome in short-course chemotherapy. Bull Int Union Tuberc 1984; 59:22–23.
80. World Health Organization. Antituberculosis Drug Resistance in the World: Fourth Global Report. Geneva, Switzerland: World Health Organization, 2008. WHO/HTM/TB/2008.394.
81. Coninx R, Mathieu C, Debacker M, et al. First-line tuberculosis therapy and drug-resistant Mycobacterium tuberculosis in prisons. Lancet. 1999; 353:969–973.
82. Edlin BR, Tokars JI, Grieco MH, et al. An outbreak of multidrug-resistant tuberculosis among hospitalized patients with the acquired immunodeficiency syndrome. N Engl J Med 1992; 326:1514–1521.
83. Fischl MA, Uttamchandani RB, Daikos GL, et al. An outbreak of tuberculosis caused by multiple-drug-resistant tubercle bacilli among patients with HIV infection. Ann Intern Med 1992; 117:177–183.
84. Schaaf HS, Van Rie A, Gie RP, et al. Transmission of multidrug-resistant tuberculosis. Pediatr Infect Dis J 2000; 19:695–699.
85. Aziz MA, Wright A, Laszlo A, et al. Epidemiology of antituberculosis drug resistance (the Global Project on Anti-tuberculosis Drug Resistance Surveillance): An updated analysis. Lancet 2006; 368:2142–2154.
86. Costello HD, Caras GJ, Snider DE Jr. Drug resistance among previously treated tuberculosis patients: A brief report. Am Rev Respir Dis 1980; 121:313–316.
87. Gandhi NR, Moll A, Sturm AW, et al. Extensively drug-resistant tuberculosis as a cause of death in patients co-infected with tuberculosis and HIV in a rural area of South Africa. Lancet 2006; 368:1575–1580.
88. Shah NS, Wright A, Bai GH, et al. Worldwide emergence of extensively drug-resistant tuberculosis. Emerg Infect Dis 2007; 13:380–387.

89. Migliori GB, Ortmann J, Girardi E, et al. Extensively drug-resistant tuberculosis, Italy and Germany. Emerg Infect Dis 2007; 13:780–782.

90. Goble M, Iseman MDR, Madsen LA, et al. Treatment of pulmonary tuberculosis resistant to isoniazid and rifampin: Results in 171 cases. N Engl J Med 1993; 32:527–532.

91. Telzak EE, Sepkowitz K, Alpert P, et al. Multidrug resistant tuberculosis in patients without HIV infection. N Engl J Med 1995; 333:907–911.

92. Burgos M, Gonzalez LC, Paz EA, et al. Treatment of multidrug resistant tuberculosis in San Francisco: an outpatient –based approach. Clin Infect Dis 2005; 40:968–975.

93. Kim HR, Hwang SS, Kim HJ, et al. Impact of extensive drug resistance on treatment outcomes in non-HIV-infected patients with multidrug-resistant tuberculosis. Clin Infect Dis 2007; 45:1290–1295.

94. Kim DH, Kim HJ, Park SK, et al. Treatment outcomes and long-term survival in patients with extensively drug-resistant tuberculosis. Am J Respir Crit Care Med 2008; 178:1075–1082.

95. Mitnick CD, Shin SS, Seung KJ, et al. Comprehensive treatment of extensively drug-resistant tuberculosis. N Engl J Med 2008; 359:563–574.

96. Bonilla CA, Crossa A, Jave HO, Management of extensively drug-resistant tuberculosis in Peru: Cure is possible. PLoS ONE 2008; 3:e2957.

97. Bishai WR, Graham NN, Harrington S, et al. Brief report: Rifampin resistant tuberculosis in a patient receiving rifabutin prophylaxis. N Engl J Med 1996; 334:1573–1575.

98. Burman, W, Gallicano K, Peloquin C. Therapeutic implications of drug interactions in the treatment of HIV-related tuberculosis. Clin Infect Dis 1999; 28:419–430.

99. World Health organization. Scaling Up Antiretroviral Therapy in Resource-limited Settings. Geneva, Switzerland: World Health Organization, 2002.

100. Narita M, Ashkin D, Hollander ES, et al. Paradoxical worsening of tuberculosis following antiretroviral therapy in patients with AIDS. Am J Respir Crit Care Med 1998; 158:157–161.

101. Wendel KA, Alwood KS, Gachuhi R, et al. Paradoxical worsening of tuberculosis in HIV-infected persons. Chest 2001; 120:193–197.

102. Ramos A, Asensio A, Perales I, et al. Prolonged paradoxical reaction of tuberculosis in an HIV infected patient after initiation of highly active antirtetroviral therapy. Eur J Clin Microbiol Infect Dis 2003; 22:374–376.

103. Meintjes G, Lawn SD, Scano F, et al. Tuberculosis-associated immune reconstitution inflammatory syndrome: Case definitions for use in resource-limited settings. Lancet Infect Dis 2008; 8:516–523.

104. Forget EJ, Menzies D. Adverse reactions to first-line antituberculosis drugs. Expert Opin Drug Saf 2006; 5:231–249.

105. Saukkonen JJ, Cohn DL, Jasmer RM, et al. An official ATS statement: Hepatotoxicity of antituberculosis therapy. Am J Respir Crit Care Med 2006; 174:935–952.

106. Smego RA, Ahmed N. A systematic review of the adjunctive use of systemic corticosteroids for pulmonary tuberculosis. Int J Tuberc Lung Dis 2003; 7:208–213.

107. Kim YJ, Pack KM, Jeong E, et al. Pulmonary tuberculosis with acute respiratory failure. Eur Respir J 2008; 32:1625–1630.

108. Chan ED, Laurel V, Strand MJ, et al. Treatment and outcome analysis of 205 patients with multidrug-resistant tuberculosis. Am J Respir Crit Care Med 2004; 169:1103–1109.

109. Campbell IA. The treatment of superficial tuberculous lymphadenitis. Tubercle 1990; 71:1–3.

110. Campbell IA, Dyson AJ. Lymph node tuberculosis: A comparison of various methods of treatment. Tubercle 1977; 58:171–179.

111. British Thoracic Society Research Committee. Short course therapy for tuberculosis of lymph nodes: A controlled trial. BMJ 1985; 290:1106–1108.

112. Nemir RL, Cardona J, Vagiri F, et al. Prednisone as an adjunct in the chemotherapy of lymph node-bronchial tuberculosis in childhood, a double blind study: II. Further term observations. Am Rev Respir Dis 1967; 95:402–410.

113. Evans DJ. The use of adjunctive corticosteroids in the treatment of pericardial, pleural and meningeal tuberculosis: do they improve outcome? Respir Med 2008; 102:793–800.

114. Gow JG. Genitourinary tuberculosis: A study of short course regimens. J Urol 1976; 115: 707–711.

115. Medical Research Council Working Party on Tuberculosis of the Spine. A five-year assessment of controlled trials of in-patient and out-patient treatment and of plaster-of-Paris jackets for tuberculosis of the spine in children on standard chemotherapy. J Bone Joint Surg 1976; 58:399–411.

116. Medical Research Council Working Party on Tuberculosis of the Spine. Five-year assessments of controlled trials of ambulatory treatment, debridement and anterior spinal fusion in the management of tuberculosis of the spine. J Bone Joint Surg 1978; 60:163–177.

117. O'Toole RD, Thornton GF, Mukherjee MK, et al. Dexamethasone in tuberculous meningitis. Ann Intern Med 1969; 70:39–48.

118. Giris NI, Forid Z, Kilpatrick ME, et al. Dexamethasone as an adjunct to treatment of tuberculous meningitis. Pediatr Infect Dis 1991; 10:179–185.

119. Wang JT, Hung CC, Sheng WH, et al. Prognosis of tuberculous meningitis in adults in the era of modern antituberculous chemotherapy. J Microbiol Immunol Infect 2002; 35:215–222.

120. Strang JIG, Kakaza HHS, Gibson DG, et al. Controlled trial of prednisolone as an adjunct in treatment of tuberculous constrictive pericarditis in Transkei. Lancet 1987; 2:1418–1422.

121. Mayosi BM, Ntsekhe M, Volmink JA, et al. Interventions for treating tuberculous pericarditis. Cochrane Database Syst Rev 2002; (4) CD000526.

122. Mayosi BM, Burgess LJ, Doubell AF, Tuberculous pericarditis. Circulation 2005; 112: 3608–3616.

123. O'Brien RJ, Nunn PP. The need for new drugs against tuberculosis. Am J Respir Crit Care Med 2001; 163:1055–1058.

124. Ginsberg AM. Emerging drugs for active tuberculosis. Semin Respir Crit Care Med 2008; 29:552–559. Epub 2008 Sep 22.

125. Stover CK, Warrener P, Vandevantner DR, et al. A small molecule nitroimidazpyran drug candidate for the treatment of tuberculosis. Nature 2000; 405:962–966.

126. Andries K, Verhasselt P, Guillemont J, et al. A diarylquinoline drug active on the ATP synthase of *Mycobacterium tuberculosis*. Science 2005; 307:223–227.

127. Cole ST, Alzari PM. TB—a new target, a new drug. Science 2005; 307:214–215.

128. Dye C. The science of social diseases. Science 2005; 307:181.

129. Stop TB partnership and World Health Organization. The global plan to stop TB: 2006–2015. Geneva, Switzerland: World health Organization, 2006. WHO/HTM/STB/2006.35.

130. Young DB, Perkins MD, Duncan K, et al. Confronting the scientific obstacles to global control of tuberculosis. J Clin Invest 2008; 118:1255–1265.

6

Tuberculosis/HIV Coinfection: Epidemiology, Clinical Aspects, and Programmatic Interventions

ALASDAIR REID
Joint United Nations Programme on HIV/AIDS (UNAIDS), Geneva, Switzerland

HAILEYESUS GETAHUN
Stop TB Department, World Health Organization, Geneva, Switzerland

ENRICO GIRARDI
Clinical Epidemiology Unit, National Institute for Infectious Diseases "L. Spallanzani," Rome, Italy

I. Introduction

The World Health Organization's (WHO) new Stop TB Strategy recognizes that the pandemic of human immunodeficiency virus (HIV) and the spread of drug-resistant TB are the greatest threats to global tuberculosis (TB) control (1). Similarly, TB is the commonest cause of morbidity and mortality in people living with HIV in Africa and a significant cause in the rest of the world, despite being largely preventable and curable. The increasing overlap between the epidemics of HIV and drug-resistant TB is of even greater global concern with potentially disastrous consequences for global TB and HIV control (2,3). Despite these threats, there are opportunities. Greater collaboration between the TB and HIV programs can bring benefits to both programs and the communities they serve. Implementation of the "Three I's for HIV/TB" (intensified TB case finding, isoniazid preventive therapy (IPT), and infection control), as an integral part of HIV care can reduce the burden of TB among people living with HIV (4). Furthermore, well-resourced TB programs can play an important role in scaling up towards universal access to comprehensive HIV prevention, diagnosis, treatment, and care services.

II. History

TB was first associated with the recently described acquired immunodeficiency syndrome (AIDS) in the early 1980s. Researchers recognized that Haitians with AIDS frequently presented with atypical TB early on in the course of HIV disease (5–8). In 1986, the halt in the decline of TB cases in the United States was ascribed to the impact of the HIV epidemic (9). In the same year, Jonathan Mann and colleagues identified high HIV prevalence rates among TB patients in Zaire, heralding the devastating interaction between the epidemics of TB and HIV in sub-Saharan Africa and beyond (10). Despite the early recognition of a strong association between TB and HIV, the national and international public health approach to addressing the diseases has been largely separate. It was not until 2004 that the WHO published their "Interim policy on collaborative TB/HIV activities," which established the policy framework for a more integrated approach toward the interlinked epidemics (11). There has been some progress in implementing collaborative TB/HIV activities globally but this is far too slow to avoid hundreds of thousands of preventable TB deaths in people living with HIV and to achieve the Stop TB Partnership and Millennium Development Goal targets (12,13).

III. Global Epidemiology

The WHO estimates that one-third of the world's population is infected with *Mycobacterium tuberculosis* (12). This suggests that at least 11 million people living with HIV are also infected with the tubercle bacillus and thus are at an increased risk of developing TB disease. There were an estimated 9.3 million new cases of TB in 2007, of which 1.37 million (15%) occurred among people living with HIV and resulted in 456,000 deaths in 2007 (14). Country data on HIV prevalence among newly diagnosed TB cases has greatly improved with direct measurement of the proportion of TB cases that are co-infected with HIV reported from 64 countries in 2008 (compared to 15 countries in 2007) (14). These new measurements suggest that people living with HIV are about 20 times more likely than HIV-negative people to develop TB in countries with a generalized HIV epidemic (14). These revised estimates were applied to countries where direct measurements were not available, resulting in an almost doubling of the global estimates for the burden of HIV related TB compared to 2006. Applying these improved estimates to previous years suggests that the numbers of HIV-positive TB cases and deaths are actually declining and were estimated to have peaked in 2005, at 1.39 million cases (15% of all incident cases) and 480,000 deaths (14).

Global incidence of TB per capita continues to decline following a peak in 2004. This decline follows a similar pattern to the decline in global HIV prevalence (14). The decline in incidence rates in Africa first reported in 2008 appears to continue (12,14). However, this decline in Africa lags behind the declines seen elsewhere in the world as a result of the impact of HIV combined with the weaknesses of the health systems in the region (12). Many countries with a high burden of HIV-related TB have developed national policies in line with WHO recommendations to reduce the burden of TB in people living with HIV, however, implementation of these policies is often lacking (11). Although 39% (84/213) of countries reported having a national policy for delivering IPT to people living with HIV, only 11% (24/213) reported implementation of the policy (15). Only 0.6 million people living with HIV were reportedly screened for TB in all countries in 2007 and less than 30,000 people living with HIV were started on IPT (14). Fifty-five countries reported the outcome of TB treatment by HIV status for the 2006 cohort. An analysis of these data suggests that HIV positive TB patients were six times more likely to die during TB treatment than HIV negative TB patients (14). Recently there have been reports of the close association between HIV and multidrug-resistant (MDR) TB and extensively drug-resistant (XDR) TB (2). Latvia and Donetsk Oblast in Ukraine showed significantly higher rates of MDR TB among people living with HIV compared to HIV-negative TB patients (2). The link between HIV and XDR TB is of even greater concern, and although successful treatment completion has been reported in up to 66% of XDR TB cases, these have come from settings with low HIV prevalence (16,17). A South African outbreak of XDR TB showed it to be almost universally fatal in people living with HIV (3). The complexity of treatment, poor availability of effective second-line drugs, drug interactions with antiretroviral therapy, diagnostic delays, and weakened immune systems suggest that treatment success will be considerably less in XDR TB occurring in people living with HIV in low-income settings (3).

IV. Pathogenesis

The host's ability to mount an effective immune response is a major determinant of the natural history of TB infection and progress to disease. The immune response to *M. tuberculosis* is primarily cell-mediated and T lymphocytes are central to the control of infection. It is therefore not surprising that the progressive and severe impairment of cell-mediated immunity caused by HIV represents one of the most potent risk factors for the development of active TB.

A.   Impact of HIV on the Natural History of TB

Observational studies indicate that the risk of TB in people living with HIV is correlated with direct ($CD4^+$cell count) and indirect (clinical staging or duration of infection) measures of immunosuppression (18–20). The risk of TB increases very early in the course of HIV infection suggesting a specific immune defect that promotes progression to active TB, independent of $CD4^+$ cell counts (20,21). HIV-induced immune suppression increases the risk of rapid progression of a recently acquired infection and the risk of reactivation of latent TB infection compared to HIV-negative people (18,22). Rates of TB disease in people living with HIV, mainly those with symptomatic HIV infection or AIDS, exposed to TB in institutional settings, range from 9% to 39%, with an incubation period of one to six months (23). The risk of reactivation of latent TB infection is increased among tuberculin-positive people living with HIV with an annual incidence of TB ranging from 4.5 to 16 per 100 and higher than that recorded in tuberculin-negative subjects (23). TB disease in people living with HIV may also result from exogenous reinfection (24–26). The proportion of recurrence due to reinfection varies greatly between studies and may differ according to the background patterns of TB transmission (26,27). The increased risk of reinfection in people living with HIV who have been treated for active TB may be due to their impaired ability to develop a protective immune response.

B.   Impact of TB on the Natural History of HIV Disease

Experimental evidence suggests that TB can induce HIV-1 replication and increase rates of HIV infection of macrophages, $CD4^+$ cells, and dendritic cells at sites of active *M. tuberculosis* infection such as in the lung or pleura of patients who are coinfected with HIV and TB (28). The clinical significance of these observations, however, remains unclear (29). A pooled estimate from eight studies suggested that TB may be associated with a slight increase in the risk of death in people living with HIV (30), and a recent prospective study estimated that TB is associated with a more than twofold increase in the hazard of AIDS-related mortality (30). However, the presence of latent TB infection is not associated with more rapid progression of HIV (31), and a systematic review of treatment of latent TB infection with isoniazid in people living with HIV provided no evidence of a reduction in all-cause mortality (32).

V. Clinical Features

HIV infection changes the natural history and clinical presentation of TB (33) as the progression of TB infection is fundamentally regulated by the host's immune system (34). During early HIV infection, patients present with typical sputum smear-positive pulmonary TB, with little to distinguish between it and TB in HIV-negative individuals. Later in HIV infection, there is a higher proportion of sputum smear-negative pulmonary and extrapulmonary TB. Institution-based studies showed that the proportion of smear-negative pulmonary TB among people living with HIV ranged from 26% to 61% whereas extrapulmonary TB ranged from 10% to 40% (35). In one study from the United States, extrapulmonary TB was found in 28% of HIV-positive TB patients with CD4 count >300 cells/mm^3 but rose to 70% in those with $\leq$100 CD4 cells/mm^3 (36). Extrapulmonary TB can affect virtually any part of the body and thus a high index of suspicion for TB should be held for all symptomatic people living with HIV. Clinical manifestations of extrapulmonary TB depend on the site involved, for example, patients with central nervous system involvement may present with indolent meningitis with headache, stiff neck, vomiting and cranial nerve deficits, or with focal signs; or abdominal pain may be the presenting symptom in patients with peritonitis or gastrointestinal involvement. Involvement of more than one site and mycobactaremia (especially with CD4$^+$ cell count $\leq$100/mm^3) (36) may be observed but a pulmonary focus is often present and sputum for smear microscopy and culture should always be part of the diagnostic process (37). Constitutional signs and symptoms may be the only clinical manifestation of extrapulmonary TB, and *M. tuberculosis* may be a common cause of fever of unknown origin in HIV-positive patients (38). Fever and weight loss are more common presenting symptoms and cough and hemoptysis are less common in pulmonary TB patients living with HIV than in those without HIV (39). Moreover, several studies particularly in sub-Saharan Africa have shown that people living with HIV, including those with a higher CD4$^+$ count, can present with culture-positive TB without discernable signs and symptoms, which has been referred to as subclinical disease (40–43).

The radiological findings of pulmonary TB also vary according to levels of immunosuppression. The upper zone infiltrates, typical of classic postprimary TB, are most frequently observed in patients with less advanced HIV disease. In contrast among patients with a CD4$^+$ cell count below 200/mm^3, an atypical pattern is common which includes lower- or midzone infiltrates, adenopathy, interstitial and nodular pattern, or normal radiograph. Pleural effusion is observed over a wide range of immunosuppression (44,45).

Differential diagnosis of pulmonary TB may be particularly challenging given the wide range of other pulmonary conditions with a similar clinical picture, including opportunistic infections and HIV-associated cancers. In addition, the occurrence of neoplastic or infectious pulmonary illnesses that are common to nonimmunosuppressed individuals should also be considered (37). In one U.S. study, Pneumocystis jiroveci pneumonia was the most common opportunistic infection, whereas TB accounted for approximately 1% of recorded episodes (46). In contrast, TB is the most common diagnosis among HIV-positive patients presenting with pulmonary symptoms in sub-Saharan Africa, accounting for 30% to 70% of diagnoses. Bacterial pneumonia, most commonly caused by *Streptococcus pneumoniae*, is the second most frequent HIV-associated pulmonary complication and Pneumocystis jiroveci pneumonia is increasingly observed. Other HIV-associated respiratory illnesses such as nocardiosis, cryptococcosis, Kaposi's sarcoma, and histoplasmosis appear to be infrequent but are probably underdiagnosed (47). $CD4^+$ cell counts can be a useful adjunct to refining the differential diagnosis. Bacterial pneumonias, including TB, can present over a wide range of $CD4^+$ counts, whereas the frequency of other conditions varies by $CD4^+$ cell count (46). Pneumocystis jiroveci and Cryptococcus neoformans pneumonia are most common when the $CD4^+$ cell count falls below $200/mm^3$, and in case of a count below $100 CD4^+$ cells/mm^3, pulmonary Kaposi's sarcoma and Toxoplasma pneumonia may also occur. In those with most severely immunosuppressed cell counts ($CD4^+$ cell count below $50/mm^3$) other pathogens such as, Histoplasma capsulatum, Coccidioides immitis, cytomegalovirus, Mycobacterium avium complex, Aspergillus species, and Candida species need to be considered.

VI. Diagnostic Challenges of HIV-Related TB

The clinical challenges described above highlight the difficulties of diagnosing TB among people living with HIV, especially in the absence of an efficient and rapid diagnostic test. Although, there is now considerable effort to develop the ideal diagnostic tool, its realization is still far from reality; TB diagnosis in most parts of the world depends on microscopy of sputum smears stained with Ziehl-Neelsen stain, which has even lower sensitivity in people living with HIV. There are methods that optimize the utility of smear microscopy such as sputum processing (liquefaction or concentration through sedimentation) and the use of fluorescence microscopy. Although the specific impact of sputum processing among people living with HIV is not well understood, fluorescence microscopy can increase the sensitivity of diagnosis by up to 10%, irrespective of HIV status (35).

Mycobacterial culture is the gold standard for TB diagnosis and is now routinely recommended to assist the diagnosis of TB among people living with HIV (48). Mycobacteria are slow-growing organisms (6–8 weeks) and due to the lower bacillary load among people living with HIV, incubation time may need to be longer (35). Culture can be performed on either egg- or agar-based conventional solid (Lowenstein-Jensen) media or broth-based liquid (Bactec™ or MGIT™) media. Liquid media can reduce the duration of mycobacterial growth by half (49), but there is an increased risk of contamination with liquid media compared to solid media (50). Culture requires more sophisticated facilities and technical expertise, which limits its utility particularly in resource-limited settings.

The Mantoux tuberculin skin test (TST) is used to identify infection with *M. tuberculosis*. TST has low specificity among BCG-vaccinated populations and also in those who are exposed to nontuberculosis Mycobacteria (NTM). Moreover, due to anergy its sensitivity is diminished among people living with HIV (51). T-cell based assays, often referred to as interferon gamma release assays (IGRA) are also used to assist the diagnosis of TB infection and disease. There are two types of IGRA available—the Quantiferon® TB Gold In-Tube Assay (Cellestis Ltd, Carnegie, Victoria, Australia) and the T-SPOT® TB assay (Oxford Immunotec Limited, Abingdon, Oxon, U.K.), which are based on the specific interferon gamma release of activated T-cells that are incubated with antigens specific to *M. tuberculosis* [early secretory antigen target-6 (ESAT-6) and culture filtrate protein 10 (CFP-10)]. Quantiferon is an ELISA test that quantifies interferon gamma in plasma, whereas ELISPOT quantifies the number of interferon gamma secreting cells (52). Although there are data suggesting the 75% to 90% of sensitivity of IGRA in active disease, the tests cannot differentiate between active disease and latent infection (52). IGRAs are widely used in low TB incidence and developed countries, but there is limited information about their use in people living with HIV in high TB prevalence and resource-limited settings. Studies from developed countries among people living with HIV showed that IGRAs are comparable to or more sensitive than TST but with low agreement of positive test (53) and low sensitivity in people living with HIV (54). Moreover, it is suggested that the immunological impairment of people living with HIV may affect the performance of these tests (55).

Nucleic acid amplification tests (NAAT) are a group of tests that detect mycobacteria nucleic acid using a polymerase chain reaction technique. These tests vary in which nucleic acid sequence they detect. They have higher specificity than TST but widely variable sensitivity, particularly for smear-negative and extrapulmonary TB (56). They also require sophisticated infrastructure and technical expertise as they involve three distinct steps of specific processing: nucleic acid extraction, amplification, and then detection of amplified products. Tests with better performance are under development, such as genoType® MTBDRplus assay (Hain Lifescience GmbH, Nehren, Germany), loop-mediated isothermal amplification (LAMP), and Xpert MTB (Cepheid, Sunnyvale, California, U.S.A.). Line probe assays [INNO-LiPA® Rif.TB kit (Innogenetics, Ghent, Belgium) and the GenoType® MTBDRplus assay] use polymerase chain reaction and reverse hybridization techniques that can detect mutations associated with drug-resistant strains. These are recommended by WHO due to their superior performance over conventional drug-susceptibility testing (57). However, the recommendations are only for AFB smear-positive specimens and culture isolates. Moreover, nucleic acid amplification tests have not been extensively validated in people living with HIV.

VII. Treatment Issues

The treatment of TB in people living with HIV is the same as in those who are HIV negative. Isoniazid, rifampicin, ethambutol, and pyrazinamide for two months followed by isoniazid and rifampicin for four months is the treatment of choice for people living with HIV with new pulmonary (both smear-positive and smear-negative) or extrapulmonary TB (58). Studies show no difference in the rates of treatment failure between HIV-positive and HIV-negative TB patients treated with this regimen (59–61). However, there is evidence that the rate of recurrence is higher in people living with HIV, which was inversely correlated with the duration of rifampicin treatment and increased with background TB incidence, probably reflecting the increased risk of reinfection (62). Observational data suggest that the rate of relapse may be lower in people living with HIV treated for more than six months (63) but clinical trial data, demonstrating the advantage of a longer course of treatment, is lacking. Some experts currently recommend a seven-month continuation phase in patients with cavitary disease on chest radiograph and who are still sputum positive two months after initiation of treatment and for those with central nervous system disease (64,65). Mortality rates are also higher in HIV-positive TB patients compared to those who are HIV negative. A systematic review of studies conducted in sub-Saharan Africa has shown that case fatality rates ranged between 16% and 35% among TB patients who are HIV positive compared to 4% to 9% among those who are HIV negative, and the death rate among HIV-positive TB patients was highest in the first three months after starting TB treatment (66). In studies in which the specific cause of death was available, death was attributed to TB itself in only one-third of HIV-positive TB cases, whereas among HIV-negative patients most of the deaths were due to TB (66). It is likely that other HIV-related diseases account for at least part of the increased mortality observed in HIV-positive TB patients. Interestingly, similar death rates were reported from industrialized countries in patients who had TB before combination antiretroviral therapy (ART) became widely available and $CD4^+$ cell count at the time of TB diagnosis was an important predictor of the risk of death (67,68). The use of trimethoprim-sulfamethoxazole (cotrimoxazole) preventive therapy has been shown to reduce death rate by 46% and hospitalization by 43% among HIV-positive TB patients in a randomized clinical trial in Cote d'Ivoire (69). Subsequent studies conducted in African countries confirmed these findings and also demonstrated the feasibility of implementing this intervention in TB treatment programs (70–72). The role of cotrimoxazole treatment in the context of increased access to ART remains to be determined.

People living with HIV are at an increased risk of developing adverse reactions during TB treatment. Clinical hepatitis; biochemical signs of hepatotoxicity; neurological, gastrointestinal, and cutaneous side effects; and fever appear to be increased among people living with HIV (73,74). Thiacetazone is contraindicated in HIV-positive TB patients because of the increased risk of life-threatening mucocutaneous hypersensitivity and toxic epidermal necrolysis (75). The reason for the increased risk of adverse reactions is unclear. Immune mechanisms linked to immunosuppression may be involved (73,76) and other coinfections such as hepatitis C may also play a role (77).

A. Cotreatment of TB and ART

Incidence of adverse reactions and drug–drug interactions is increased, usually during the initial phase of treatment, among people on concomitant treatment with antituberculous and antiretroviral drugs that may lead to treatment discontinuation (74,78). Rifampicin is a potent inducer of a series of enzymes and drug-transporting molecules, including cytochrome P-450, and thus may cause clinically important reductions in the levels of many other drugs, including antiretrovirals (79). The plasma levels of the currently available protease inhibitors (PI) (with the possible exception of ritonavir) are greatly decreased by rifampicin and these drugs should not be administered together. Serum levels of nonnucleoside reverse transcriptase inhibitors (NNRTIs) are also decreased by simultaneous administration of rifampicin, although the magnitude of this effect varies for different drugs in this class. Plasma concentrations of efavirenz are reduced by 20% to 25% but the clinical impact of this effect appears to be limited (80). Presently, efavirenz (600 mg) is considered a first choice drug for antiretroviral treatment in TB patients treated with rifampicin (65,81), although some guidelines recommend increasing the dose to 800 mg in patients weighing more than 60 kg (65). Nevirapine concentration in the plasma may be reduced by 20% to 50% by rifampicin; nonetheless there is some evidence that this does not affect efficacy of nevirapine (79). Thus, nevirapine can be considered a possible alternative to efavirenz, although, because of increased risk of severe hepatic damage, close clinical and laboratory monitoring of liver enzymes is recommended for patients receiving nevirapine plus rifampicin (81). Rifampicin should not be used with delaviridine as it is predicted to interfere with the pharmacokinetics of the second generation NNRTI etravirine (82). There is no evidence of a clinically important effect of rifampicin on the efficacy of nucleoside reverse transcriptase inhibitors (NRTIs), which can thus be used in combination with an NNRTI in TB patients. As for the other novel therapeutic drug classes, there is evidence that rifampicin does not modify as the pharmacokinetics of the fusion inhibitor enfuvirtide (83), though it is likely to affect concentrations of CCR5 coreceptor antagonists such as maraviroc (82). Moreover it appears to decrease plasma concentration of the integrase inhibitor raltegravir, although the clinical significance of this interaction is unclear (82). Other rifamycins, such as rifabutin, are less potent enzyme inducers and have been proposed for use with PI-based antiretroviral treatment in people living with HIV in whom NNRTI cannot be administered (82). However, rifabutin is expensive and not available in many resource-limited countries and its concomitant use with PI's is complicated. Rifapentine is attractive because of its once-a-week administration; however, it has been associated with increased risk of relapse with rifamycin monoresistant strains and thus it is not presently recommended (84).

In the last decade, successful antiretroviral treatment has been shown to improve, in most cases, the quantity and function of $CD4^+$ T-cells and specific *M. tuberculosis* immune responses (85). This immune restoration results in reduced TB incidence, although incidence remains higher than in HIV-negative individuals (86,87). ART-induced immune reconstitution can impact on the presentation and clinical course of TB and may lead to a paradoxical worsening of clinical condition in TB patients. This phenomenon was previously recognized in HIV-negative TB patients, caused by the reversion of *M. tuberculosis*-specific immune anergy after starting effective treatment (88). This paradoxical worsening may present in 8% to 40% of people living with HIV on TB treatment after initiation of ART, usually after an initial improvement in the TB signs and symptoms, and has been coined TB-associated immune reconstitution inflammatory syndrome (TB-IRIS) (89,90). Symptoms may include constitutional symptoms, respiratory symptoms, lymph node enlargement, abscesses, or other focal, localization, and central nervous system involvement. New or worsening radiological features of TB may be also observed. Risk factors for TB-IRIS include low $CD4^+$ cells count at initiation of ART and a short time interval between initiation of TB treatment and initiation of ART. Clinical manifestations are usually mild and self-limiting; however, in some instances they may require hospitalization or result in death (90). Diagnosis of TB-IRIS is made on clinical criteria, and requires careful exclusion of other possible conditions that may cause clinical deterioration such as TB treatment failure, other HIV-associated illnesses, or adverse drug reactions (89). Evidence for treatment of paradoxical TB-IRIS is limited. For mild forms, symptomatic treatment with nonsteroidal anti-inflammatory agents without a change in anti-TB treatment or ART is recommended. For severe reactions the use of prednisone or methylprednisolone used at a dose of approximately 1 mg/kg body weight and gradually reduced after one to two weeks, is suggested (65).

Recent cohort studies of people on ART have shown that the risk of TB is highest in the period just after initiation of ART (91). The explanation for this is not yet clear. The immune recovery related to ART may take months to achieve a significant reduction in the risk of developing TB. It is also possible that increased clinical attention during initiation of ART may lead to case ascertainment bias and identification of previously undiagnosed TB. Finally, some patients may have a clinically unapparent active disease at the time they start ART. In these patients, the restoration of immune response against *M. tuberculosis* antigens may result in disease becoming clinically apparent with prominent acute inflammatory features (91,92). The term "ART-associated tuberculosis" has been proposed for cases of TB occurring during ART and the term "unmasking

TB-associated IRIS" for cases of ART-associated TB, characterized by a heightened intensity of clinical manifestations or by the occurrence of paradoxical reaction once the patient is put on TB treatment (89). Increased clinical vigilance is required during the first month of ART in order to rapidly identify TB-IRIS. Patients with unmasking TB-IRIS may have had constitutional symptoms before staring ART and present with a clinical picture suggestive of an exaggerated inflammatory response including lymphadenitis or TB abscesses, respiratory failure due to adult respiratory distress syndrome, or a marked systemic inflammatory syndrome (89,91,92).

The factors discussed above: toxicity, drug–drug interactions, and paradoxical TB-IRIS, suggest that ART initiation should be delayed, if possible until completion of TB treatment. However, HIV-associated TB has a high mortality, especially during the first months that is at least in part due to HIV disease and could thus be reduced by early initiation of ART. A number of trials designed to assess the best timing of ART initiation in patients on TB treatment are ongoing (93), but preliminary data from one of these trials appears to indicate a favorable impact of early ART on the death rate of HIV-positive TB patients (94). Current WHO guidelines suggest starting ART between two and eight weeks after the start of TB therapy, in patients with a $CD4^+$ cell count below 200 cells/mm^3 or for whom a $CD4^+$ cell count is not available (81). Similar recommendations have been issued by the CDC, NIH, and IDSA (65). In particular it is recommended to start ART after at least two weeks of TB treatment in patients with a $CD4^+$ cell count <100/mm^3 and to consider delaying ART until the end of the two-month intensive phase of TB treatment in persons with a $CD4^+$ cell count between 100 and 200/mm^3. Both guidelines recommend starting ART during the continuation phase of TB treatment in those with a sustained $CD4^+$ cell count above 200/mm^3, and after completion of TB treatment in those with more than 350 $CD4^+$ cells/mm^3. For patients who present with TB during ART, the ART regimen should be modified if it poses an increasing risk of interaction with anti-TB drugs and/or there is evidence of treatment failure based on laboratory data ($CD4^+$ cell count and HIV viremia) when available, or on clinical criteria (such as clinical presentation of TB and occurrence of other HIV-associated illnesses) (81).

VIII. Other Interventions To Reduce the Impact of HIV-Related TB

A. Reducing the Burden of TB in People Living with HIV (Three I's)

Intensified TB Case Finding

People living with HIV should be regularly and routinely screened for symptoms and signs of TB, and based on the outcome of screening, patients should be started on either TB preventive therapy or treatment of active TB disease (11). Intensified TB case-finding and treatment of TB among people living with HIV interrupts disease transmission by infectious cases, delays mortality, and decreases the risk of nosocomial TB transmission (95–98). TB can occur at any level of CD4 cell count of a person living with HIV, and hence screening for TB to identify active cases of TB should be a routine part of HIV care (99). Screening activities include simple questionnaires, which can be administered by health care personnel as a part of the routine clinical exam. If screening is positive, additional investigations for active TB should be pursued (99). Depending on the particular symptoms and signs used in the screening questionnaire, studies have shown sensitivity ranges from 91% to 100% and specificity from 10% to 88% for identifying TB among people living with HIV (41,100,101). TB screening strategies are likely to vary according to the epidemiology of HIV and TB and the availability of resources. High rates of undetected TB among people living with HIV are common in many HIV- and TB-prevalent and resource-constrained settings (42,102). In these settings, TB screening questionnaires are simple and can be mainstreamed into preexisting HIV services with little additional cost (103). Trained counselors and lay health workers using simple TB screening tools can detect previously undiagnosed TB in up to 11% of people living with HIV and attending HIV testing and care services (100,102–104). Expediting the diagnosis of TB in people living with HIV through strengthening household and community systems such as through the screening of household contacts (99) and enhancing the role of community members in identification and referral of people suspected to have TB is crucial (105). Screening of household members of HIV-positive persons with active TB has been shown to be feasible and high yielding in Malawi and Zambia (99). The screening tool should be based on the TB case definition of the national TB control guidelines and should incorporate appropriate respiratory and constitutional symptoms applicable to the specific setting and clinical practice. The screening tool should also include guidance on how to administer TB preventive therapy with isoniazid if people living with HIV are free from TB symptoms and signs.

Isoniazid Preventive Therapy

TB preventive therapy should be given to all people living with HIV who have latent TB infection (LTBI) in order to reduce their risk of developing active TB (11). Several randomized trials have shown, isoniazid preventive therapy is effective in reducing the incidence of TB in people living with HIV, with the greatest reduction observed in positive tuberculin skin test patients [RR 0.8 (95% CI, 0.63–1.02)] (106). In clinical trials, rifampicin- and pyrazinamide-containing regimens are shown to be as effective as isoniazid-containing regimens, but they are more likely to be discontinued due to side effects. Treatment of LTBI with rifampicin and pyrazinamide in HIV-negative individuals resulted in more hepatotoxicity than isoniazid (32,107,108). This risk appears to be limited to HIV-negative individuals, as a rigorous re-analysis of a large trial of rifampicin and pyrazinamide in HIV-positive patients confirmed a lack of serious toxicity (108).

The effectiveness of IPT in patients who also receive ART has been examined in one observational cohort study in Brazil, which showed an additive benefit of combining IPT and ART (109). Secondary preventive therapy (treatment of latent TB in those who have already been treated for active TB) is not currently recommended, but studies suggest possible benefit (110).

Despite proven effectiveness, global uptake of TB preventive therapy has been slow, with less than 30,000 people living with HIV reported to have received IPT in 2007 (14). Concerns about promoting drug resistance, low adherence, risk of reinfection, and questions around optimal frequency and methods for screening are often cited by TB program managers as reasons for reluctance to roll out IPT. A number of studies are under way to try to respond to these concerns and the WHO is currently promoting IPT as part of the Three I's strategy to reduce the burden of TB in people living with HIV (4).

TB Infection Control

The atypical presentation of TB in people living with HIV, limited access to drug sensitivity testing, poor infection control, and inadequate facilities to isolate patients with drug-resistant TB contributed to the outbreak of drug-resistant TB in the 1990s among people living with HIV in the West (111–114). These same factors are now contributing to the spread of drug-resistant TB among people living with HIV in Africa (3,115). The increasing number of people living with HIV who are accessing HIV treatment and care in resource-limited countries in the absence of effective infection control measures, is bringing together those most vulnerable to infection (people living with HIV) with the most infectious (undiagnosed TB cases), with predictable consequences (3). An effective infection control policy for TB should include a hierarchy of interventions: administrative controls, environmental measures, and individual protective measures for exposed workers (116–118). Administrative controls aim to prevent individuals without TB infection from being exposed to infectious droplet nuclei containing *M. tuberculosis* by promoting prompt identification, isolation, and treatment of infectious TB patients. This requires the development and implementation of a TB infection control plan in each health care facility, education of staff and patients, early identification of TB suspects and separation from other patients, and surveillance of TB infection and disease among health care workers (118). Environmental control measures are aimed at reducing the concentration and length of time that infectious droplet nuclei remain in the air in health care and other closed settings. Isolation of all infectious TB cases in single negative pressure ventilated rooms in hospitals is largely unfeasible today in the developing world (116,119). But ventilation systems for hospital wards need not be expensive; hospital rooms can be designed and managed in order to favor natural ventilation, and fans may also assist in removing droplet nuclei from enclosed spaces (118). Ultraviolet lamps may help in decontaminating the air by killing the mycobacteria, but their efficacy may be reduced if humidity exceeds 70% and if the lamps are not maintained properly (120). Personal respiratory protection may add further protection for health care workers in settings where exposure to MDR/XDR TB is likely and while performing high risk cough-inducing procedures, for example, bronchoscopy and sputum induction. Paper surgical masks do not protect the wearer from inhalation of infected airborne particles. Fitted filtering personal respirators that comply with appropriate standards (e.g., N95 respirators in the United States or FFP2 respirators in Europe) should be used to protect health workers (116,119). These respirators are expensive and uncomfortable. They require proper fit testing and staff should be fully trained in their use.

B.   Reducing the Burden of HIV in TB Patients

HIV Testing and Counseling for TB Patients

Providing HIV testing for TB suspects and patients is an important gateway to appropriate HIV prevention, care, and support (48,101,121–125). Provider-initiated HIV testing and counseling is recommended for all adults, adolescents, and children who present with signs and symptoms suggestive of TB (TB suspects) and all confirmed TB patients as a standard of care (48). Uptake is generally high and can be improved by simplifying procedures, such as the use of rapid tests in the same room by the TB clinician (126,127). National scale-up of quality rapid HIV testing requires well-trained health workers at all service delivery points and uninterrupted supplies of rapid HIV tests available in all inpatient and outpatient settings (128). Rapid nationwide expansion of HIV testing for TB patients has been achieved in countries such as Thailand, Rwanda, and Malawi that are testing over 65% of all TB patients (14).

HIV Prevention, Treatment, Care, and Support for TB Patients

TB facilities and health care workers can provide an opportunity to expand access to HIV prevention, information, and methods. All TB suspects and patients who have accepted HIV testing should receive post-test counseling tailored to their HIV serostatus and focused on appropriate HIV prevention advice according to an assessment of individual risks. The provision of HIV prevention, treatment, and care needs to consider local epidemiological and social contexts, appraisal of available resources, and prevailing standards of HIV prevention, treatment, care and support, and judgments about the social and legal protections available to people living with HIV or at risk of exposure to it (129). Providing quality HIV prevention to TB patients in TB clinics or through referral to HIV services is feasible in high HIV and TB settings (103,104). TB control programs should implement comprehensive HIV preventive strategies aimed at reduction of sexual, parenteral, and vertical transmission of HIV (11). Particular emphasis has to be given for injecting drug use where it drives the HIV epidemic namely in Europe and in central and east Asia; TB prevention, diagnosis, and treatment need to be integrated with harm reduction strategies, wherever applicable (130). As HIV is the most important risk factor for TB disease it is in the best interest of TB programs, especially in high HIV prevalence settings, to play a major role in delivering effective HIV prevention information and methods.

HIV-positive TB patients should have access to comprehensive HIV care and support services including effective referral mechanisms (11). Stigma needs special attention as it leads people to either hide their TB diagnosis, delay seeking treatment, or refrain altogether from getting help out of fear (131). Extending effective and appropriate psychological and social support will be crucial to address stigma issues and improve the quality of life of HIV-positive patients. Treatment literacy efforts should also be strengthened to generate demand for services by affected communities and also improve the quality of care and support services.

IX. TB/HIV in Special Situations

A. TB/HIV in Children

Approximately 11% (1 million) of global TB cases occur in children under the age of 15 years (132). The WHO reports the number of notifications of sputum smear–positive TB cases in children annually (48,000 in 2007) (14). This may underestimate the burden of TB in children in general and in children living with HIV in particular, because of the difficulties in collecting sputum from children and the complexities of making a definitive clinical diagnosis (133). Data on the burden of TB in children living with HIV are scarce due to these diagnostic challenges and lack of standardized case definitions (134). There does, however, appear to be a real increased risk of TB disease (up to 20-fold) in HIV-positive children associated with poorer treatment outcome (135–144). The burden of HIV in confirmed and clinical cases of TB in children ranges from 11% to 70% (135,140,145–148). The new Stop TB Strategy aims to overcome the chronic neglect of childhood TB and calls for equitable access to standard TB care for adults and children alike, regardless of HIV status (1).

Children, especially those living with HIV, are more likely to progress to active disease following infection than adults, and children under two years of age are most likely to develop severe forms of TB (135,149,150). The clinical presentation and radiological findings of TB in children are similar in HIV-positive and negative children

(140,148,151–153). Presentation is frequently nonspecific and easily confused with the signs and symptoms of HIV, malnutrition, and other causes of pneumonia in children. Clinical algorithms and score charts have been developed to improve the clinical diagnosis of TB in children (154–156) and a number of methods have been developed to improve the quality of samples for bacteriological diagnosis, such as gastric lavage, induced sputum, and string tests (157–159). The tuberculin skin test is less reactive in children living with HIV (140,148,151–153); however, it can still be a useful adjunct in establishing the diagnosis. Advances in molecular and culture methods may refine the diagnosis of TB in HIV-positive children but the immunological methods are as yet unable to distinguish between active disease and latent TB infection (134,160,161). The urgent need for more research into reliable diagnostics for TB is even more acute for children living with HIV than adults (162). The recommended treatment for TB in HIV-positive children is the same as for HIV-negative children (132), although some have suggested prolonging treatment in HIV-positive children as recurrence has been shown due to relapse (163). Similarly malabsorption of TB drugs related to HIV may require dose adjustment (164). Cotreatment of TB and HIV in children is prone to the same complications of treatment in adults including drug interactions and the risks of immune reconstitution syndrome (165). Children living with HIV who are on TB treatment should be considered for ART as soon as they are stable on TB treatment (166). BCG vaccination is no longer recommended for HIV-positive children because of the high risk of disseminated BCG infection (167,168). Isoniazid preventive therapy is recommended for children living with HIV who live in areas with high TB prevalence or are household contacts of people with TB following exclusion of active TB disease (132,166).

B. TB/HIV in Prisons

Prisons have been associated with disease transmission as far back as 1666 (169). TB rates among prisoners can be more than fifty times higher than the rate in the general population; they are even higher in prisoners living with HIV and they appear to be linked with the length of time in prison; furthermore, prisoners are more likely to die or default from treatment (170–181). Prisons create the "perfect storm" of environmental, individual, and health system factors that enhance the development and spread of TB and drug resistance (182). The overcrowded, unhygienic, and poorly ventilated living conditions with low natural sunlight combine with malnutrition, drug use, and high HIV prevalence, which may be difficult to prevent because of the illicit or underground nature of risk factors, for example, injecting drug use, tattooing, piercing, unprotected sex (178,183–188). Add to this poor access to comprehensive health services and poor continuity between prison and public health services (189–191), and the heavy burden of TB and drug-resistant TB in prisoners is easy to understand (2,192–195). Remand prisoners are often at greater risk (196). TB in prisons also negatively impacts on prison staff and the surrounding community (171,193,197–201), and can persist for many years (202). Prisons can, however, provide an ideal opportunity to deliver integrated TB and HIV prevention, diagnostic, and treatment services to marginalized populations (e.g., drug users) that often have poor access to services in the community (203). Prisons should not, however, be used to substitute for poor public health services or better collaboration between prison and public health, and extending a prison stay solely to complete investigation or treatment of TB would constitute an infringement of human rights (196).

Intensified efforts should be made to identify and isolate TB suspects and ensure rapid effective treatment of cases and other infection control procedures should be put in place to minimize risk of TB transmission inside the prison (118). Screening prisoners for TB on entry to prison identifies previously undiagnosed TB and cases where treatment was interrupted on arrest (204). Methods for screening will depend on available resources but simple symptom screens may miss a significant number of cases (171,205,206). Chest X-ray and sputum culture may pick up additional cases (206–209) and are particularly useful for diagnosing TB in prisoners living with HIV. HIV testing and care should be voluntary and delivered under the same standards of confidentiality as in the general population. Efforts to prevent HIV transmission in prisons will ultimately reduce the risk of TB disease. Care must be taken to avoid the perverse incentives that better conditions (prison hospital, better food, avoidance of work) that prisoners with TB may benefit from (196). Treatment of latent TB infection is also feasible in prisons but adherence may be low (203). Provision of opiate substitution therapy can promote adherence to TB treatment among injecting drug users in prison and can reduce the risk of HIV transmission (210).

C. TB/HIV and Drug Users

Drug users are at increased risk of TB infection and TB disease, even if HIV negative, and this risk is significantly higher if they are HIV positive or have a history of imprisonment (184,211–216). Injection drug use has been associated more with extrapulmonary disease and poorer TB treatment outcomes (217–220). The epidemics of injection drug use, HIV- and multidrug-resistant TB are increasingly overlapping in marginalized populations in Eastern Europe and Asia (2,221). Injection drug use is also rising in eastern and southern Africa, which experienced the greatest increases in opiate use between 2005 and 2006 (222).

Managing HIV, drug-resistant TB, and other comorbidities in drug users who are frequently marginalized and have poor access to services requires special effort. WHO guidelines recommend an integrated approach to the management of TB, HIV, and the harmful effects of drug use, in order to better prevent, diagnose, and treat the common comorbidities associated with drug use (223). Drug users should have universal access to comprehensive TB, HIV, and drug use services at every entry point, which necessitates close collaboration between TB and HIV programs, specialist drug services, and the criminal justice system (223). Adherence to prescribed treatment can be poor in drug users (224–226), but high adherence rates can be achieved cost-effectively with appropriate adherence support mechanisms (227–233). Drug users should not be denied services on the grounds of their drug use or the presence of other common comorbidities, such as viral hepatitis. Infection control is a priority to reduce transmission of blood-borne pathogens and TB in all care and detention settings as well as in the community (118). Particular attention needs to be paid to ensuring continuity of care as drug users move between community, detention centers, and health care facilities.

X. Conclusions

The interaction between the epidemics of TB and HIV has had a negative impact on the global control and care of both diseases, with the greatest impact occurring in some of the poorest regions of the world and the most marginalized members of society. Although our ability to effectively prevent, diagnose, and treat TB among people living with HIV is restricted by the limitations of current technology and weak health systems, significant reductions in morbidity and mortality can be achieved through closer collaboration between the TB and HIV programs to ensure optimal implementation of the proven interventions that are available today.

References

1. World Health Organization. The Stop TB Strategy – Building on and enhancing DOTS to meet the TB-related Millennium Development Goals. Geneva, Switzerland: World Health Organization 2006. WHO/HTM/TB/2006.368.
2. World Health Organization. Anti-tuberculosis drug resistance in the world – Report no. 4 – The WHO/IUATLD global project on anti-tuberculosis drug resistance surveillance. Geneva, Switzerland: World Health Organization 2008. WHO/HTM/TB/2008.394.
3. Gandhi NR, Moll A, Sturm AW, et al. Extensively drug-resistant tuberculosis as a cause of death in patients co-infected with tuberculosis and HIV in a rural area of South Africa. Lancet 2006; 368:1575–1580.
4. World Health Organization. WHO Three 'I's meeting – Intensified Case Finding (ICF), Isoniazid Preventive Therapy (IPT) and TB Infection Control (IC) for people living with HIV. Report of a joint WHO HIV/AIDS and TB Department meeting, 2–4 April, 2008. Geneva, Switzerland: World Health Organization 2008.
5. Pitchenik AE, Fischl MA, Dickinson GM, et al. Opportunistic infections and Kaposi's sarcoma among Haitians: Evidence of a new acquired immunodeficiency state. Ann Intern Med 1983; 98:277–284.
6. Pape JW, Liautaud B, Thomas F, et al. Characteristics of the acquired immunodeficiency syndrome (AIDS) in Haiti. N Engl J Med 1983; 309:945–950.
7. Pitchenik AE, Cole C, Russell BW, et al. Tuberculosis, atypical mycobacteriosis, and the acquired immunodeficiency syndrome among Haitian and non-Haitian patients in south Florida. Ann Intern Med 1984; 101:641–645.
8. Guerin JM, Malebranche R, Elie R, et al. Acquired immune deficiency syndrome: Specific aspects of the disease in Haiti. Ann N Y Acad Sci 1984; 437:254–263.
9. Centers for Disease Control and Prevention (CDC). Tuberculosis–United States, 1985–and the possible impact of human T-lymphotropic virus type III/lymphadenopathy-associated virus infection. MMWR Morb Mortal Wkly Rep 1986; 35:74–76.
10. Mann J, Snider DE Jr, Francis H, et al. Association between HTLV-III/LAV infection and tuberculosis in Zaire [letter]. JAMA 1986; 256:346.
11. World Health Organization. Interim policy on collaborative TB/HIV activities. Geneva, Switzerland: World Health Organization 2004. WHO/HTM/TB/2004.330; WHO/HTM/HIV/2004.1.
12. World Health Organization. Global tuberculosis control: Surveillance, planning, financing. WHO Report 2008. Geneva, Switzerland: World Health Organization 2008. WHO/HTM/TB/2008.393.
13. World Health Organization/Stop TB Partnership. Actions for Life. Towards a world free of tuberculosis. The Global Plan to Stop Tuberculosis 2006–2015. Geneva, Switzerland: World Health Organization 2006. WHO/HTM/STB/2006.35.
14. World Health Organization. Global Tuberculosis Control: epidemiology, strategy, financing – WHO report 2009. Geneva, Switzerland: World Health Organization 2009. WHO/HTM/TB/2009.411
15. Gunneberg C, Hosseini SM, Scheele S, et al. Isoniazid preventative therapy and screening for TB: The need to move from policy to action. In: XVII International AIDS Conference (AIDS 2008) Abstract WEPE0142. Mexico City, DF: International AIDS Society, 2008.

16. Keshavjee S, Gelmanova IY, Farmer PE, et al. Treatment of extensively drug-resistant tuberculosis in Tomsk, Russia: A retrospective cohort study. Lancet 2008; 372:1403–1409.

17. Kwon YS, Kim YH, Suh GY, et al. Treatment outcomes for HIV-uninfected patients with multidrug-resistant and extensively drug-resistant tuberculosis. Clin Infect Dis 2008; 47:496–502.

18. Antonucci G, Girardi E, Raviglione MC, et al. Risk factors for tuberculosis in HIV-infected persons. A prospective cohort study. The Gruppo Italiano di Studio Tubercolosi e AIDS (GISTA). JAMA 1995; 274:143–148.

19. van der Sande MA, Schim van der Loeff MF, Bennett RC, et al. Incidence of tuberculosis and survival after its diagnosis in patients infected with HIV-1 and HIV-2. AIDS 2004; 18:1933–1941.

20. Glynn JR, Murray J, Bester A, et al. Effects of duration of HIV infection and secondary tuberculosis transmission on tuberculosis incidence in the South African gold mines. AIDS 2008; 22:1859–1867.

21. Geldmacher C, Schuetz A, Ngwenyama N, et al. Early Depletion of Mycobacterium tuberculosis-Specific T Helper 1 Cell Responses after HIV-1 Infection. J Infect Dis 2008; 198:1590–1598.

22. Markowitz N, Hansen NI, Hopewell PC, et al. Incidence of tuberculosis in the United States among HIV-infected persons. Ann Intern Med 1997; 126:123–132.

23. Girardi E, Raviglione MC, Antonucci G, et al. Impact of the HIV epidemic on the spread of other diseases: The case of tuberculosis. AIDS 2000; 14(suppl 3):S47–S56.

24. Small PM, Hopewell PC, Singh SP, et al. The epidemiology of tuberculosis in San Francisco. A population-based study using conventional and molecular methods. N Engl J Med 1994; 330:1703–1709.

25. Alland D, Kalkut GE, Moss AR, et al. Transmission of tuberculosis in New York City. An analysis by DNA fingerprinting and conventional epidemiologic methods. N Engl J Med 1994; 330:1710–1716.

26. Lambert ML, Hasker E, Van Deun A, et al. Recurrence in tuberculosis: Relapse or reinfection? Lancet Infect Dis 2003; 3:282–287.

27. Sonnenberg P, Murray J, Glynn JR, et al. HIV-1 and recurrence, relapse, and reinfection of tuberculosis after cure: A cohort study in South African mineworkers. Lancet 2001; 358:1687–1693.

28. Toossi Z. Virological and immunological impact of tuberculosis on human immunodeficiency virus type 1 disease. J Infect Dis 2003; 188:1146–1155.

29. Reid A, Scano F, Getahun H, et al. Towards universal access to HIV prevention, treatment, care, and support: The role of tuberculosis/HIV collaboration. Lancet Infect Dis 2006; 6:483–495.

30. Lopez-Gatell H, Cole SR, Margolick JB, et al. Effect of tuberculosis on the survival of HIV-infected men in a country with low tuberculosis incidence. AIDS 2008; 22:1869–1873.

31. Manoff SB, Farzadegan H, Munoz A, et al. The effect of latent Mycobacterium tuberculosis infection on human immunodeficiency virus (HIV) disease progression and HIV RNA load among injecting drug users. J Infect Dis 1996; 174:299–308.

32. Woldehanna S, Volmink J. Treatment of latent tuberculosis infection in HIV infected persons. Cochrane Database Syst Rev 2004; 1:CD000171.

33. Colebunders R, Bastian I. A review of the diagnosis and treatment of smear-negative pulmonary tuberculosis. Int J Tuberc Lung Dis 2000; 4:97–107.

34. Ducati RG, Ruffino-Netto A, Basso LA, et al. The resumption of consumption–a review on tuberculosis. Mem Inst Oswaldo Cruz 2006; 101:697–714.

35. Getahun H, Harrington M, O'Brien R, et al. Diagnosis of smear-negative pulmonary tuberculosis in people with HIV infection or AIDS in resource-constrained settings: Informing urgent policy changes. Lancet 2007; 369:2042–2049.

36. Jones BE, Young SM, Antoniskis D, et al. Relationship of the manifestations of tuberculosis to CD4 cell counts in patients with human immunodeficiency virus infection. Am Rev Respir Dis 1993; 148:1292–1297.

37. Goozé L, Daley CL. Tuberculosis and HIV. In: Peiperl L, Coffey S, Bacon O, Volberding PA, eds. HIV InSite Knowledge Base. San Francisco: UCSF, 2003. Available at: http://hivinsite.ucsf.edu/InSite?page = kb-05–01-06. Accessed January26, 2009.

38. Bissuel F, Leport C, Perronne C, et al. Fever of unknown origin in HIV-infected patients: A critical analysis of a retrospective series of 57 cases. J Intern Med 1994; 236:529–535.

39. World Health Organization. TB/HIV – A clinical manual. Geneva, Switzerland: World Health Organization, 2004. WHO/HTM/TB/2004.329.

40. Mtei L, Matee M, Herfort O, et al. High rates of clinical and subclinical tuberculosis among HIV-infected ambulatory subjects in Tanzania. Clin Infect Dis 2005; 40:1500–1507.

41. Day JH, Charalambous S, Fielding KL, et al. Screening for tuberculosis prior to isoniazid preventive therapy among HIV-infected gold miners in South Africa. Int J Tuberc Lung Dis 2006; 10:523–529.

42. Wood R, Middelkoop K, Myer L, et al. Undiagnosed tuberculosis in a community with high HIV prevalence: Implications for tuberculosis control. Am J Respir Crit Care Med 2007; 175:87–93.

43. Corbett EL, Bandason T, Cheung YB, et al. Epidemiology of tuberculosis in a high HIV prevalence population provided with enhanced diagnosis of symptomatic disease. PLoS Med 2007; 4:e22.

44. Keiper MD, Beumont M, Elshami A, et al. CD4 T lymphocyte count and the radiographic presentation of pulmonary tuberculosis. A study of the relationship between these factors in patients with human immunodeficiency virus infection. Chest 1995; 107:74–80.

45. Post FA, Wood R, Pillay GP. Pulmonary tuberculosis in HIV infection: Radiographic appearance is related to CD4$^+$ T-lymphocyte count. Tuber Lung Dis 1995; 76:518–521.

46. Wallace JM, Rao AV, Glassroth J, et al. Respiratory illness in persons with human immunodeficiency virus infection. The Pulmonary Complications of HIV Infection Study Group. Am Rev Respir Dis 1993; 148(6)(Pt 1):1523–1529.

47. Murray JF. Pulmonary complications of HIV-1 infection among adults living in Sub-Saharan Africa. Int J Tuberc Lung Dis 2005; 9:826–835.

48. World Health Organization. Improving the diagnosis and treatment of smear-negative pulmonary and extrapulmonary tuberculosis among adults and adolescents – Recommendations for HIV-prevalent and resource-constrained settings. Geneva, Switzerland: World Health Organization, 2007. WHO/HTM/TB/2007.379 & WHO/HIV/2007.1.

49. Tortoli E, Cichero P, Piersimoni C, et al. Use of BACTEC MGIT 960 for recovery of mycobacteria from clinical specimens: Multicenter study. J Clin Microbiol 1999; 37:3578–3582.

50. Diraa O, Fdany K, Boudouma M, et al. Assessment of the Mycobacteria Growth Indicator Tube for the bacteriological diagnosis of tuberculosis. Int J Tuberc Lung Dis 2003; 7:1010–1012.

51. Pai M, Kalantri S, Dheda K. New tools and emerging technologies for the diagnosis of tuberculosis: Part I. Latent tuberculosis. Expert Rev Mol Diagn 2006; 6:413–422.

52. Pai M, O'Brien R. New diagnostics for latent and active tuberculosis: State of the art and future prospects. Semin Respir Crit Care Med 2008; 29:560–568.

53. Luetkemeyer AF, Charlebois ED, Flores LL, et al. Comparison of an interferon-gamma release assay with tuberculin skin testing in HIV-infected individuals. Am J Respir Crit Care Med 2007; 175:737–742.

54. Stephan C, Wolf T, Goetsch U, et al. Comparing QuantiFERON-tuberculosis gold, T-SPOT tuberculosis and tuberculin skin test in HIV-infected individuals from a low prevalence tuberculosis country. AIDS 2008; 22:2471–2479.

55. Brock I, Ruhwald M, Lundgren B, et al. Latent tuberculosis in HIV positive, diagnosed by the M. tuberculosis specific interferon-gamma test. Respir Res 2006; 7:56.
56. Pai M, Ling DI. Rapid diagnosis of extrapulmonary tuberculosis using nucleic acid amplification tests: What is the evidence? Future Microbiol 2008; 3:1–4.
57. World Health Organization. Molecular line probe assays for rapid screening of patients at risk of multidrug resistant tuberculosis (MDR TB): Policy statement. Geneva, Switzerland: World Health Organization, 2008.
58. World Health Organization. Treatment of Tuberculosis: Guidelines for National Programmes, 3rd ed. Geneva, Switzerland: World Health Organization, 2003. WHO/CDS/TB/2003.313.
59. Perriens JH, St Louis ME, Mukadi YB, et al. Pulmonary tuberculosis in HIV-infected patients in Zaire. A controlled trial of treatment for either 6 or 12 months. N Engl J Med 1995; 332:779–784.
60. Kassim S, Sassan-Morokro M, Ackah A, et al. Two-year follow-up of persons with HIV-1- and HIV-2-associated pulmonary tuberculosis treated with short-course chemotherapy in West Africa. AIDS 1995; 9:1185–1191.
61. Chaisson RE, Clermont HC, Holt EA, et al. Six-month supervised intermittent tuberculosis therapy in Haitian patients with and without HIV infection. Am J Respir Crit Care Med 1996; 154:1034–1038.
62. Korenromp EL, Scano F, Williams BG, et al. Effects of human immunodeficiency virus infection on recurrence of tuberculosis after rifampin-based treatment: An analytical review. Clin Infect Dis 2003; 37:101–112.
63. Nahid P, Gonzalez LC, Rudoy I, et al. Treatment outcomes of patients with HIV and tuberculosis. Am J Respir Crit Care Med 2007; 175:1199–1206.
64. Pozniak AL, Miller RF, Lipman MCI, et al. BHIVA treatment guidelines for tuberculosis (TB)/HIV infection 2005. HIV Med 2005; 6(suppl 2):62–83.
65. Panel on Antiretroviral Guidelines for Adults and Adolescents. Guidelines for the use of antiretroviral agents in HIV-1-infected adults and adolescents. Department of Health and Human Services, November 3, 2008: 1–139. Available at: http://www.aidsinfo.nih.gov/ContentFiles/AdultandAdolescentGL.pdf. Accessed January 26, 2009.
66. Mukadi YD, Maher D, Harries A. Tuberculosis case fatality rates in high HIV prevalence populations in sub-Saharan Africa. AIDS 2001; 15:143–152.
67. Whalen C, Horsburgh CR Jr, Hom D, et al. Site of disease and opportunistic infection predict survival in HIV-associated tuberculosis. AIDS 1997; 11:455–460.
68. Girardi E, Palmieri F, Cingolani A, et al. Changing clinical presentation and survival in HIV-associated tuberculosis after highly active antiretroviral therapy. J Acquir Immune Defic Syndr 2001; 26:326–331.
69. Wiktor SZ, Sassan-Morokro M, Grant AD, et al. Efficacy of trimethoprim-sulphamethoxazole prophylaxis to decrease morbidity and mortality in HIV-1-infected patients with tuberculosis in Abidjan, Cote d'Ivoire: A randomised controlled trial [published erratum appears in Lancet 1999 Jun 12; 353(9169):2078] [see comments]. Lancet 1999; 353:1469–1475.
70. Nunn AJ, Mwaba P, Chintu C, et al. Role of co-trimoxazole prophylaxis in reducing mortality in HIV infected adults being treated for tuberculosis: Randomised clinical trial. BMJ 2008; 337:a257.
71. Grimwade K, Swingler. Cotrimoxazole prophylaxis for opportunistic infections in adults with HIV. Cochrane Database Syst Rev 2003; 3:CD003108.
72. Chimzizi RB, Harries AD, Manda E, et al. Counselling, HIV testing and adjunctive cotrimoxazole for TB patients in Malawi: From research to routine implementation. Int J Tuberc Lung Dis 2004; 8:938–944.
73. Yimer G, Aderaye G, Amogne W, et al. Anti-tuberculosis therapy-induced hepatotoxicity among Ethiopian HIV-positive and negative patients. PLoS One 2008; 3:e1809.
74. Breen RA, Miller RF, Gorsuch T, et al. Adverse events and treatment interruption in tuberculosis patients with and without HIV co-infection. Thorax 2006; 61:791–794.

75. Nunn P, Kibuga D, Gathua S, et al. Cutaneous hypersensitivity reactions due to thiacetazone in HIV-1 seropositive patients treated for tuberculosis. Lancet 1991; 337:627–630.
76. Okwera A, Johnson JL, Vjecha MJ, et al. Risk factors for adverse drug reactions during thiacetazone treatment of pulmonary tuberculosis in human immunodeficiency virus infected adults. Int J Tuberc Lung Dis 1997; 1:441–445.
77. Ungo JR, Jones D, Ashkin D, et al. Antituberculosis drug-induced hepatotoxicity: The role of hepatitis C virus and the human immunodeficiency virus. Am J Respir Crit Care Med 1998; 157:1871–1876.
78. Dean GL, Edwards SG, Ives NJ, et al. Treatment of tuberculosis in HIV-infected persons in the era of highly active antiretroviral therapy. AIDS 2002; 16:75–83.
79. McIlleron H, Meintjes G, Burman WJ, et al. Complications of antiretroviral therapy in patients with tuberculosis: Drug interactions, toxicity, and immune reconstitution inflammatory syndrome. J Infect Dis 2007; 196(suppl 1):63S–75S.
80. Manosuthi W, Sungkanuparph S, Thakkinstian A, et al. Efavirenz levels and 24-week efficacy in HIV-infected patients with tuberculosis receiving highly active antiretroviral therapy and rifampicin. AIDS 2005; 19:1481–1486.
81. World Health Organization. Scaling up antiretroviral therapy in resource-limited settings. Updated guidelines for a public health approach. May 2006. Geneva, Switzerland: World Health Organization, 2006.
82. Centers for Disease Control and Prevention. Managing Drug Interactions in the Treatment of HIV-Related Tuberculosis 2007. Available at: http://www.cdc.gov/tb/tb_hiv_Drugs/default.htm. Accessed Jan 26, 2009.
83. Boyd MA, Zhang X, Dorr A, et al. Lack of enzyme-inducing effect of rifampicin on the pharmacokinetics of enfuvirtide. J Clin Pharmacol 2003; 43:1382–1391.
84. Li J, Munsiff SS, Driver CR, et al. Relapse and acquired rifampin resistance in HIV-infected patients with tuberculosis treated with rifampin- or rifabutin-based regimens in New York City, 1997–2000. Clin Infect Dis 2005; 41:83–91.
85. Sutherland R, Yang H, Scriba TJ, et al. Impaired IFN-gamma-secreting capacity in mycobacterial antigen-specific CD4T cells during chronic HIV-1 infection despite long-term HAART. AIDS 2006; 20:821–829.
86. Girardi E, Sabin CA, Monferte AD, et al. Incidence of tuberculosis among HIV-infected patients receiving highly active antiretroviral therapy in Europe and North America. Clin Infect Dis 2005; 41:1772–1782.
87. Lawn SD, Bekker LG, Wood R. How effectively does HAART restore immune responses to Mycobacterium tuberculosis? Implications for tuberculosis control. AIDS 2005; 19:1113–1124.
88. Smith H. Paradoxical responses during the chemotherapy of tuberculosis. J Infect 1987; 15:1–3.
89. Meintjes G, Lawn SD, Scano F, et al. Tuberculosis-associated immune reconstitution inflammatory syndrome: Case definitions for use in resource-limited settings. Lancet Infect Dis 2008; 8:516–523.
90. Lawn SD, Bekker LG, Miller RF. Immune reconstitution disease associated with mycobacterial infections in HIV-infected individuals receiving antiretrovirals. Lancet Infect Dis 2005; 5:361–373.
91. Manabe YC, Breen R, Perti T, et al. Unmasked Tuberculosis and Tuberculosis Immune Reconstitution Inflammatory Disease: A Disease Spectrum after Initiation of Antiretroviral Therapy. J Infect Dis 2009; 199:437–444.
92. Breen RAM, Smith CJ, Cropley I, et al. Does immune reconstitution syndrome promote active tuberculosis in patients receiving highly active antiretroviral therapy? AIDS 2005; 19:1201–1206.
93. Blanc FX, Havlir DV, Onyebujoh PC, et al. Treatment strategies for HIV-infected patients with tuberculosis: Ongoing and planned clinical trials. J Infect Dis 2007; 196(suppl 1):46S–51S.

94. ACC Editors. Concurrent ART/TB treatment finally proven to be beneficial. AIDS Clin Care 2008. Available at: http://aids-clinical-care.jwatch.org/cgi/content/full/2008/929/1. Accessed January 26, 2009.
95. Harries AD, Maher D, Nunn P. Practical and affordable measures for the protection of health care workers from tuberculosis in low-income countries. Bull World Health Organ 1997; 75:477–489.
96. De Cock KM, Chaisson RE. Will DOTS do it? A reappraisal of tuberculosis control in countries with high rates of HIV infection. Int J Tuberc Lung Dis 1999; 3:457–465.
97. Lawn SD, Shattock RJ, Griffin GE. Delays in the diagnosis of tuberculosis: A great new cost. Int J Tuberc Lung Dis 1997; 1:485–486.
98. Nachega J, Coetzee J, Adendorff T, et al. Tuberculosis active case-finding in a mother-to-child HIV transmission prevention programme in Soweto, South Africa. AIDS 2003; 17:1398–1400.
99. Havlir DV, Getahun H, Sanne I, et al. Opportunities and challenges for HIV care in overlapping HIV and TB epidemics. JAMA 2008; 300:423–430.
100. Mohammed A, Ehrlich R, Wood R, et al. Screening for tuberculosis in adults with advanced HIV infection prior to preventive therapy. Int J Tuberc Lung Dis 2004; 8:792–795.
101. Chheng P, Tamhane A, Natpratan C, et al. Pulmonary tuberculosis among patients visiting a voluntary confidential counseling and testing center, Cambodia. Int J Tuberc Lung Dis 2008; 12(3)(suppl 1):54–62.
102. Kimerling ME, Schuchter J, Chanthol E, et al. Prevalence of pulmonary tuberculosis among HIV-infected persons in a home care program in Phnom Penh, Cambodia. Int J Tuberc Lung Dis 2002; 6:988–994.
103. World Health Organization. Report of a "lessons learnt" workshop on the six ProTEST pilot projects in Malawi, South Africa and Zambia. Geneva, Switzerland: World Health Organization, 2004. WHO/HTM/TB2004.336.
104. Burgess AL, Fitzgerald DW, Severe P, et al. Integration of tuberculosis screening at an HIV voluntary counselling and testing centre in Haiti. AIDS 2001; 15:1875–1879.
105. Getahun H, Maher D. Contribution of 'TB clubs' to tuberculosis control in a rural district in Ethiopia. Int J Tuberc Lung Dis 2000; 4(2):174–178.
106. Centers for Disease Control and Prevention (CDC). Preventive therapy against tuberculosis in people living with HIV. Wkly Epidemiol Rec 1999; 74:385–398.
107. Centers for Disease Control and Prevention (CDC); American Thoracic Society. Update: Adverse event data and revised American Thoracic Society/CDC recommendations against the use of rifampin and pyrazinamide for treatment of latent tuberculosis infection–United States, 2003. MMWR Morb Mortal Wkly Rep 2003; 52:735–739.
108. Gordin FM, Cohn DL, Matts JP, et al. Hepatotoxicity of rifampin and pyrazinamide in the treatment of latent tuberculosis infection in HIV-infected persons: Is it different than in HIV-uninfected persons? Clin Infect Dis 2004; 39:561–565.
109. Golub JE, Saraceni V, Cavalcante SC, et al. The impact of antiretroviral therapy and isoniazid preventive therapy on tuberculosis incidence in HIV-infected patients in Rio de Janeiro, Brazil. AIDS 2007; 21:1441–1448.
110. Churchyard GJ, Scano F, Grant AD, et al. Tuberculosis preventive therapy in the era of HIV infection: Overview and research priorities. J Infect Dis 2007; 196(suppl 1):S52–S62.
111. Di Perri G, Cruciani M, Danzi MC, et al. Nosocomial epidemic of active tuberculosis among HIV-infected patients. Lancet 1989; 2:1502–1504.
112. Centers for Disease Control and Prevention (CDC). Nosocomial transmission of multidrug-resistant tuberculosis to health-care workers and HIV-infected patients in an urban hospital–Florida. MMWR Morb Mortal Wkly Rep 1990; 39:718–722.
113. Centers for Disease Control and Prevention (CDC). Nosocomial transmission of multidrug-resistant tuberculosis among HIV-infected persons–Florida and New York, 1988–1991. MMWR Morb Mortal Wkly Rep 1991; 40:585–591.

114. Moro ML, Gori A, Errante I, et al. An outbreak of multidrug-resistant tuberculosis involving HIV-infected patients of two hospitals in Milan, Italy. AIDS 1998; 12:1095–1102.

115. Sacks LV, Pendle S, Orlovic D, et al. A comparison of outbreak- and nonoutbreak-related multidrug-resistant tuberculosis among human immunodeficiency virus-infected patients in a South African hospital. Clin Infect Dis 1999; 29:96–101.

116. Jensen PA, Lambert LA, Iademarco MF, et al. Guidelines for preventing the transmission of Mycobacterium tuberculosis in health-care settings, 2005. MMWR Recomm Rep 2005; 54:1–141.

117. World Health Organization. Guidelines for the prevention of tuberculosis in health care facilities in resource-limited settings. WHO/TB/99.269. Geneva, Switzerland: World Health Organization, 1999.

118. World Health Organization and Centers for Disease Control and Prevention. Tuberculosis infection control in the era of expanding HIV care and treatment (Addendum to WHO Guidelines for the Prevention of Tuberculosis in Health Care Facilities in Resource-Limited Settings, 1999) Atlanta, United States: Centers for Disease Control and Prevention, 2006.

119. National Collaborating Centre for Chronic Conditions, inventor Royal College of Physicians, assignee. Tuberculosis: Clinical diagnosis and management of tuberculosis, and measures for its prevention and control 2006. Available at: http://www.rcplondon.ac.uk/pubs/contents/dfb1d46a-bc32–4538-b631–1d82f4b6c8aa.pdf. Accessed Jan 26, 2009.

120. Bock NN, Jensen PA, Miller B, et al. Tuberculosis infection control in resource-limited settings in the era of expanding HIV care and treatment. J Infect Dis 2007; 196(suppl 1): 108S–113S.

121. World Health Organization, UNAIDS. Guidance on provider-initiated HIV testing and counselling in health facilities. Geneva, Switzerland: World Health Organization, 2007.

122. UNAIDS, World Health Organization. UNAIDS/WHO policy statement on HIV testing. Geneva, Switzerland: UNAIDS/WHO, 2004. Available at: http://www.unaids.org/html/pub/una-docs/hivtestingpolicy_en_pdf.htm. Accessed Jan 26, 2009.

123. Odhiambo J, Kizito W, Njoroge A, et al. Provider-initiated HIV testing and counselling for TB patients and suspects in Nairobi, Kenya. Int J Tuberc Lung Dis 2008; 12(3)(suppl 1): 63–68.

124. Shetty PV, Granich RM, Patil AB, et al. Cross-referral between voluntary HIV counselling and testing centres and TB services, Maharashtra, India, 2003–2004. Int J Tuberc Lung Dis 2008; 12(3)(suppl 1):26–31.

125. Munthali L, Mwaungulu JN, Munthali K, et al. Using tuberculosis suspects to identify patients eligible for antiretroviral treatment. Int J Tuberc Lung Dis 2006; 10:199–202.

126. Zachariah R, Spielmann MPL, Chinji C, et al. Voluntary counselling, HIV testing and adjunctive cotrimoxazole reduces mortality in tuberculosis patients in Thyolo, Malawi. AIDS 2003; 17:1053–1061.

127. Chakaya JM, Mansoer JR, Scano F, et al. National scale-up of HIV testing and provision of HIV care to tuberculosis patients in Kenya. Int J Tuberc Lung Dis 2008; 12:424–429.

128. World Health Organization. Report of the fourth global TB/HIV Working Group meeting. Geneva, Switzerland: World Health Organization, 2005.

129. UNAIDS. Practical Guidelines for Intensifying HIV Prevention – Towards Universal Access. Geneva, Switzerland: UNAIDS, 2007. UNAIDS/07.07E /JC1274E.

130. World Health Organization, UNODC, UNAIDS. Policy guidelines for collaborative TB and HIV services for injecting and other drug users: An integrated approach. Geneva, Switzerland: World Health Organization, 2008.

131. Thomas C. A literature review of the problems of delayed presentation for treatment and non-completion of treatment for tuberculosis in less developed countries and ways of addressing these problems using particular implementations of the DOTS strategy. J Manag Med 2002; 16:371–400.

132. World Health Organization. Guidance for national tuberculosis programmes on the management of tuberculosis in children. Geneva, Switzerland: World Health Organization, 2006. WHO/HTM/TB.2006.371.

133. de Charnace G, Delacourt C. Diagnostic techniques in paediatric tuberculosis. Paediatr Respir Rev 2001; 2:120–126.

134. Newton SM, Brent AJ, Anderson S, et al. Paediatric tuberculosis. Lancet Infect Dis 2008; 8:498–510.

135. Coovadia HM, Jeena P, Wilkinson D. Childhood human immunodeficiency virus and tuberculosis co-infections: Reconciling conflicting data. Int J Tuberc Lung Dis 1998; 2:844–851.

136. Graham SM, Harries AD. Childhood TB/HIV co-infection: Correction, confusion and compliance. Int J Tuberc Lung Dis 1999; 3:1144.

137. Graham SM, Coulter JB, Gilks CF. Pulmonary disease in HIV-infected African children. Int J Tuberc Lung Dis 2001; 5:12–23.

138. Luo C, Chintu C, Bhat G, et al. Human immunodeficiency virus type-1 infection in Zambian children with tuberculosis: Changing seroprevalence and evaluation of a thioacetazone-free regimen. Tuber Lung Dis 1994; 75:110–115.

139. Sassan-Morokro M, De Cock KM, Ackah A, et al. Tuberculosis and HIV infection in children in Abidjan, Cote d'Ivoire. Trans R Soc Trop Med Hyg 1994; 88:178–181.

140. Mukadi YD, Wiktor SZ, Coulibaly IM, et al. Impact of HIV infection on the development, clinical presentation, and outcome of tuberculosis among children in Abidjan, Cote d'Ivoire. AIDS 1997; 11:1151–1158.

141. Madhi SA, Petersen K, Madhi A, et al. Increased disease burden and antibiotic resistance of bacteria causing severe community-acquired lower respiratory tract infections in human immunodeficiency virus type 1-infected children. Clin Infect Dis 2000; 31:170–176.

142. Jeena PM, Pillay P, Pillay T, et al. Impact of HIV-1 co-infection on presentation and hospital-related mortality in children with culture proven pulmonary tuberculosis in Durban, South Africa. Int J Tuberc Lung Dis 2002; 6:672–678.

143. Palme IB, Gudetta B, Bruchfeld J, et al. Impact of human immunodeficiency virus 1 infection on clinical presentation, treatment outcome and survival in a cohort of Ethiopian children with tuberculosis. Pediatr Infect Dis J 2002; 21:1053–1061.

144. Chintu C, Mudenda V, Lucas S, et al. Lung diseases at necropsy in African children dying from respiratory illnesses: A descriptive necropsy study. Lancet 2002; 360:985–990.

145. Nelson LJ, Wells CD. Global epidemiology of childhood tuberculosis. Int J Tuberc Lung Dis 2004; 8:636–647.

146. Madhi SA, Huebner RE, Doedens L, et al. HIV-1 co-infection in children hospitalised with tuberculosis in South Africa. Int J Tuberc Lung Dis 2000; 4:448–454.

147. Schaaf HS, Gie RP, Beyers N, et al. Primary drug-resistant tuberculosis in children. Int J Tuberc Lung Dis 2000; 4:1149–1155.

148. Kiwanuka J, Graham SM, Coulter JB, et al. Diagnosis of pulmonary tuberculosis in children in an HIV-endemic area, Malawi. Ann Trop Paediatr 2001; 21:5–14.

149. Cotton MF, Schaaf HS, Hesseling AC, et al. HIV and childhood tuberculosis: The way forward. Int J Tuberc Lung Dis 2004; 8:675–682.

150. Beyers N, Gie RP, Schaaf HS, et al. A prospective evaluation of children under the age of 5 years living in the same household as adults with recently diagnosed pulmonary tuberculosis. Int J Tuberc Lung Dis 1997; 1:38–43.

151. Espinal MA, Reingold AL, Perez G, et al. Human immunodeficiency virus infection in children with tuberculosis in Santo Domingo, Dominican Republic: Prevalence, clinical findings, and response to antituberculosis treatment. J Acquir Immune Defic Syndr Hum Retrovirol 1996; 13:155–159.

152. Jeena PM, Mitha T, Bamber S, et al. Effects of the human immunodeficiency virus on tuberculosis in children. Tuber Lung Dis 1996; 77:437–443.

153. Schaaf HS, Geldenduys A, Gie RP, et al. Culture-positive tuberculosis in human immunode-ficiency virus type 1-infected children. Pediatr Infect Dis J 1998; 17:599–604.

154. Van Rheenen P. The use of the paediatric tuberculosis score chart in an HIV-endemic area. Trop Med Int Health 2002; 7:435–441.

155. Marais BJ, Gie RP, Hesseling AC, et al. A refined symptom-based approach to diagnose pulmonary tuberculosis in children. Pediatrics 2006; 118:e1350–1359.

156. Starke JR. Diagnosis of tuberculosis in children. Pediatr Infect Dis J 2000; 19:1095–1096.

157. Zar HJ, Hanslo D, Apolles P, et al. Induced sputum versus gastric lavage for microbiological confirmation of pulmonary tuberculosis in infants and young children: A prospective study. Lancet 2005; 365:130–134.

158. Iriso R, Mudido PM, Karamagi C, et al. The diagnosis of childhood tuberculosis in an HIV-endemic setting and the use of induced sputum. Int J Tuberc Lung Dis 2005; 9:716–726.

159. Mwinga A. Challenges and hope for the diagnosis of tuberculosis in infants and young children. Lancet 2005; 365:97–98.

160. Marais BJ, Graham SM, Cotton MF, et al. Diagnostic and management challenges for child-hood tuberculosis in the era of HIV. J Infect Dis 2007; 196(suppl 1):S76–S85.

161. Oberhelman RA, Soto-Castellares G, Caviedes L, et al. Improved recovery of Mycobacterium tuberculosis from children using the microscopic observation drug susceptibility method. Pediatrics 2006; 118:e100–e106.

162. Donald PR, Maher D, Qazi S. A research agenda to promote the management of childhood tuberculosis within national tuberculosis programmes. Int J Tuberc Lung Dis 2007; 11: 370–380.

163. Schaaf HS, Gie RP, van Rie A, et al. Second episode of tuberculosis in an HIV-infected child: Relapse or reinfection? J Infect 2000; 41:100–103.

164. Graham SM, Bell DJ, Nyirongo S, et al. Low levels of pyrazinamide and ethambutol in children with tuberculosis and impact of age, nutritional status, and human immunodeficiency virus infection. Antimicrob Agents Chemother 2006; 50:407–413.

165. Puthanakit T, Oberdorfer P, Akarathum N, et al. Immune reconstitution syndrome after highly active antiretroviral therapy in human immunodeficiency virus-infected Thai children. Pediatr Infect Dis J 2006; 25:53–58.

166. World Health Organization. Antiretroviral therapy of HIV infection in infants and chil-dren: Towards universal access. Recommendations for a public health approach. Geneva, Switzerland: World Health Organization, 2007.

167. Revised BCG vaccination guidelines for infants at risk for HIV infection. Wkly Epidemiol Rec 2007; 82:193–196.

168. Hesseling AC, Marais BJ, Gie RP, et al. The risk of disseminated Bacille Calmette-Guerin (BCG) disease in HIV-infected children. Vaccine 2007; 25:14–18.

169. Stern V. Problems in prisons worldwide, with a particular focus on Russia. Ann N Y Acad Sci 2001; 953:113–119.

170. World Health Organization, International Committe of the Red Cross. Tuberculosis control in prisons: A manual for programme managers. Geneva, Switzerland: World Health Organi-zation, 2000.

171. Centers for Disease Control and Prevention (CDC). Rapid assessment of tuberculosis in a large prison system–Botswana, 2002. MMWR Morb Mortal Wkly Rep 2003; 52:250–252.

172. Nyangulu DS, Harries AD, Kang'ombe C, et al. Tuberculosis in a prison population in Malawi. Lancet 1997; 350:1284–1287.

173. Koffi N, Ngom AK, Aka-Danguy E, et al. Smear positive pulmonary tuberculosis in a prison setting: Experience in the penal camp of Bouake?, Ivory Coast. Int J Tuberc Lung Dis 1997; 1:250–253.

174. Rutta E, Mutasingwa D, Ngallaba S, et al. Tuberculosis in a prison population in Mwanza, Tanzania (1994–1997). Int J Tuberc Lung Dis 2001; 5:703–706.

175. MacNeil JR, Lobato MN, Moore M. An unanswered health disparity: Tuberculosis among correctional inmates, 1993 through 2003. Am J Public Health 2005; 95:1800–1805.
176. Coninx R, Mathieu C, Debacker M, et al. First-line tuberculosis therapy and drug-resistant Mycobacterium tuberculosis in prisons. Lancet 1999; 353:969–973.
177. Sretrirutchai S, Silapapojakul K, Palittapongarnpim P, et al. Tuberculosis in Thai prisons: Magnitude, transmission and drug susceptibility. Int J Tuberc Lung Dis 2002; 6:208–214.
178. MacIntyre CR, Kendig N, Kummer L, et al. Impact of tuberculosis control measures and crowding on the incidence of tuberculous infection in Maryland prisons. Clin Infect Dis 1997; 24:1060–1067.
179. Bellin EY, Fletcher DD, Safyer SM. Association of tuberculosis infection with increased time in or admission to the New York City jail system. JAMA 1993; 269:2228–2231.
180. Ferreira MM, Ferrazoli L, Palaci M, et al. Tuberculosis and HIV infection among female inmates in Sao Paulo, Brazil: A prospective cohort study. J Acquir Immune Defic Syndr Hum Retrovirol 1996; 13:177–183.
181. Martin V, Cayla JA, Bolea A, et al. Evolution of the prevalence of Mycobacterium tuberculosis infection in a penitentiary population on admission to prison from 1991 to 1996. Med Clin (Barc) 1998; 111:11–16.
182. Chaves F, Dronda F, Cave MD, et al. A longitudinal study of transmission of tuberculosis in a large prison population. Am J Respir Crit Care Med 1997; 155:719–725.
183. Niveau G. Prevention of infectious disease transmission in correctional settings: A review. Public Health 2006; 120:33–41.
184. Drobniewski FA, Balabanova YM, Ruddy MC, et al. Tuberculosis, HIV seroprevalence and intravenous drug abuse in prisoners. Eur Respir J 2005; 26:298–304.
185. Braun MM, Truman BI, Maguire B, et al. Increasing incidence of tuberculosis in a prison inmate population. Association with HIV infection. JAMA 1989; 261:393–397.
186. Snider DE Jr, Hutton MD. Tuberculosis in correctional institutions. JAMA 1989; 261(3): 436–437.
187. Martin V, Gonzalez P, Cayla JA, et al. Case-finding of pulmonary tuberculosis on admission to a penitentiary centre. Tuber Lung Dis 1994; 75:49–53.
188. Chaves F, Dronda F, Gonzalez Lopez A, et al. Tuberculosis in a prison population: A study of 138 cases. Med Clin (Barc) 1993; 101:525–529.
189. Lobato MN, Roberts CA, Bazerman LB, et al. Public health and correctional collaboration in tuberculosis control. Am J Prev Med 2004; 27:112–117.
190. Coker R. Detention and mandatory treatment for tuberculosis patients in Russia. Lancet 2001; 358:349–350.
191. Coker RJ, Dimitrova B, Drobniewski F, et al. Tuberculosis control in Samara Oblast, Russia: Institutional and regulatory environment. Int J Tuberc Lung Dis 2003; 7:920–932.
192. Mohle-Boetani JC, Miguelino V, Dewsnup DH, et al. Tuberculosis outbreak in a housing unit for human immunodeficiency virus-infected patients in a correctional facility: Transmission risk factors and effective outbreak control. Clin Infect Dis 2002; 34:668–676.
193. McLaughlin SI, Spradling P, Drociuk D, et al. Extensive transmission of Mycobacterium tuberculosis among congregated, HIV-infected prison inmates in South Carolina, United States. Int J Tuberc Lung Dis 2003; 7:665–672.
194. Lafontaine D, Slavuski A, Vezhnina N, et al. Treatment of multidrug-resistant tuberculosis in Russian prisons. Lancet 2004; 363:246–247.
195. Spradling P, Nemtsova E, Aptekar T, et al. Anti-tuberculosis drug resistance in community and prison patients, Orel Oblast, Russian Federation. Int J Tuberc Lung Dis 2002; 6:757–762.
196. Levy MH, Reyes H, Coninx R. Overwhelming consumption in prisons: Human rights and tuberculosis control. Health Hum Rights 1999; 4:166–191.
197. Jones TF, Craig AS, Valway SE, et al. Transmission of tuberculosis in a jail. Ann Intern Med 1999; 131:557–563.

198. Jones TF, Woodley CL, Fountain FF, et al. Increased incidence of the outbreak strain of Mycobacterium tuberculosis in the surrounding community after an outbreak in a jail. South Med J 2003; 96(2):155–157.

199. Stead WW. Undetected tuberculosis in prison. Source of infection for community at large. JAMA 1978; 240:2544–2547.

200. Pelletier AR, DiFerdinando GT Jr, Greenberg AJ, et al. Tuberculosis in a correctional facility. Arch Intern Med 1993; 153:2692–2695.

201. Seidler A, Nienhaus A, Diel R. Review of epidemiological studies on the occupational risk of tuberculosis in low-incidence areas. Respiration 2005; 72:431–446.

202. Munsiff SS, Nivin B, Sacajiu G, et al. Persistence of a highly resistant strain of tuberculosis in New York City during 1990–1999. J Infect Dis 2003; 188:356–363.

203. Lobato MN, Leary LS, Simone PM. Treatment for latent TB in correctional facilities: A challenge for TB elimination. Am J Prev Med 2003; 24:249–253.

204. White MC, Tulsky JP, Portillo CJ, et al. Tuberculosis prevalence in an urban jail: 1994 and 1998. Int J Tuberc Lung Dis 2001; 5:400–404.

205. Sanchez A, Gerhardt G, Natal S, et al. Prevalence of pulmonary tuberculosis and comparative evaluation of screening strategies in a Brazilian prison. Int J Tuberc Lung Dis 2005; 9: 633–639.

206. Layton MC, Henning KJ, Alexander TA, et al. Universal radiographic screening for tuberculosis among inmates upon admission to jail. Am J Public Health 1997; 87:1335–1337.

207. Puisis M, Feinglass J, Lidow E, et al. Radiographic screening for tuberculosis in a large urban county jail. Public Health Rep 1996; 111:330–334.

208. Jones TF, Schaffner W. Miniature chest radiograph screening for tuberculosis in jails: A cost-effectiveness analysis. Am J Respir Crit Care Med 2001; 164:77–81.

209. Reyes H, Coninx R. Pitfalls of tuberculosis programmes in prisons. BMJ 1997; 315: 1447–1450.

210. Marco A, Cayla JA, Serra M, et al. Predictors of adherence to tuberculosis treatment in a supervised therapy programme for prisoners before and after release. Study Group of Adherence to Tuberculosis Treatment of Prisoners. Eur Respir J 1998; 12:967–971.

211. Reichman LB, Felton CP, Edsall JR. Drug dependence, a possible new risk factor for tuberculosis disease. Arch Intern Med 1979; 139:337–339.

212. Selwyn PA, Hartel D, Lewis VA, et al. A prospective study of the risk of tuberculosis among intravenous drug users with human immunodeficiency virus infection. N Engl J Med 1989; 320:545–550.

213. Martin V, Cayla JA, Bolea A, et al. Mycobacterium tuberculosis and human immunodeficiency virus co-infection in intravenous drug users on admission to prison. Int J Tuberc Lung Dis 2000; 4:41–46.

214. Alvarez Rodriguez M, Godoy Garcia P. Prevalence of tuberculosis and HIV infections among participants in an intravenous drug user risk-control program. Rev Esp Salud Publica 1999; 73:375–381.

215. Robles RR, Marrero CA, Reyes JC, et al. Risk behaviors, HIV seropositivity, and tuberculosis infection in injecting drug users who operate shooting galleries in Puerto Rico. J Acquir Immune Defic Syndr Hum Retrovirol 1998; 17:477–483.

216. Reyes JC, Robles RR, Colon HM, et al. Mycobacterium tuberculosis infection among crack and injection drug users in San Juan, Puerto Rico. P R Health Sci J 1996; 15: 233–236.

217. Jones JL, Burwen DR, Fleming PL, et al. Tuberculosis among AIDS patients in the United States, 1993. J Acquir Immune Defic Syndr Hum Retrovirol 1996; 12:293–297.

218. Tansuphasawadikul S, Amornkul PN, Tanchanpong C, et al. Clinical presentation of hospitalized adult patients with HIV infection and AIDS in Bangkok, Thailand. J Acquir Immune Defic Syndr 1999; 21:326–332.

219. Nissapatorn V, Kuppusamy I, Rohela M, et al. Extrapulmonary tuberculosis in Peninsular Malaysia: Retrospective study of 195 cases. Southeast Asian J Trop Med Public Health 2004; 35(suppl 2):39–45.

220. Kourbatova EV, Borodulin BE, Borodulina EA, et al. Risk factors for mortality among adult patients with newly diagnosed tuberculosis in Samara, Russia. Int J Tuberc Lung Dis 2006; 10:1224–1230.

221. Morozova I, Riekstina V, Sture G, et al. Impact of the growing HIV-1 epidemic on multidrug-resistant tuberculosis control in Latvia. Int J Tuberc Lung Dis 2003; 7:903–906.

222. UNODC. World Drug Report 2007. Vienna, Austria: UNODC, 2007.

223. World Health Organization. Policy guidelines for collaborative TB and HIV services for injecting and other drug users – An integrated approach. Geneva, Switzerland: World Health Organization, 2008.

224. Wobeser W, Yuan L, Naus M. Outcome of pulmonary tuberculosis treatment in the tertiary care setting–Toronto 1992/93. Tuberculosis Treatment Completion Study Group. CMAJ 1999; 160:789–794.

225. Altice FL, Mezger JA, Hodges J, et al. Developing a directly administered antiretroviral therapy intervention for HIV-infected drug users: Implications for program replication. Clin Infect Dis 2004;38(suppl 5):376–387S.

226. Ngamvithayapong J, Uthaivoravit W, Yanai H, et al. Adherence to tuberculosis preventive therapy among HIV-infected persons in Chiang Rai, Thailand. AIDS 1997; 11:107–112.

227. Gourevitch MN, Alcabes P, Wasserman WC, et al. Cost-effectiveness of directly observed chemoprophylaxis of tuberculosis among drug users at high risk for tuberculosis. Int J Tuberc Lung Dis 1998; 2:531–540.

228. Gourevitch MN, Hartel D, Selwyn PA, et al. Effectiveness of isoniazid chemoprophylaxis for HIV-infected drug users at high risk for active tuberculosis. AIDS 1999; 13:2069–2074.

229. Gourevitch MN, Wasserman W, Panero MS, et al. Successful adherence to observed prophylaxis and treatment of tuberculosis among drug users in a methadone program. J Addict Dis 1996; 15:93–104.

230. Jansa JM, Serrano J, Cayla JA, et al. Influence of the human immunodeficiency virus in the incidence of tuberculosis in a cohort of intravenous drug users: Effectiveness of anti-tuberculosis chemoprophylaxis. Int J Tuberc Lung Dis 1998; 2:140–146.

231. Chaisson RE, Barnes GL, Hackman J, et al. A randomized, controlled trial of interventions to improve adherence to isoniazid therapy to prevent tuberculosis in injection drug users. Am J Med 2001; 110:610–615.

232. Scholten JN, Driver CR, Munsiff SS, et al. Effectiveness of isoniazid treatment for latent tuberculosis infection among human immunodeficiency virus (HIV)-infected and HIV-uninfected injection drug users in methadone programs. Clin Infect Dis 2003; 37:1686–1692.

233. Perlman DC, Gourevitch MN, Trinh C, et al. Cost-effectiveness of tuberculosis screening and observed preventive therapy for active drug injectors at a syringe-exchange program. J Urban Health 2001; 78:550–567.

7

Diagnosis and Treatment of Drug-Resistant Tuberculosis

KWONJUNE SEUNG and MICHAEL L. RICH

Partners In Health and Brigham and Women's Hospital, Division of Global Health Equity, Boston, Massachusetts, U.S.A.

I. Introduction

The goal of tuberculosis (TB) control programs is to cure patients with disease due to infection with *Mycobacterium tuberculosis*, in order to avert deaths, prevent the development of new cases, and prevent the emergence of drug resistance. Nevertheless, drug-resistant TB (DR-TB) is bound to appear in even the best-run programs. There is considerable evidence that drug resistance has emerged and is on the upsurge in many parts of the world (1). This chapter focuses on the care of patients with DR-TB and examines the origins, prevention, diagnosis, and impact of drug resistance on TB control.

A. History

Resistance to antituberculous agents was first documented in the 1940s, when patients who initially responded to monotherapy with streptomycin, the only available medication at the time, relapsed with disease that was clearly resistant to the agent (2–4). By 1950, the drug's manufacturer recognized that solo administration of streptomycin caused most cases of TB to become resistant to the drug after two to four months of therapy (5). It was later documented that strains with acquired resistance did not revert to a susceptible phenotype even after the drug in question was no longer administered. Unless new antituberculous drugs were administered and/or localized lesions surgically resected, the disease took its course leading too often to early death. Soon it was determined that *p*-aminosalicylic acid (PAS) given in combination with streptomycin prevented or postponed the development of resistance. This finding eventually led to the principle of treatment with multiple drugs at the same time. Current regimens for multidrug-resistant TB (MDR-TB), defined as resistance to at least isoniazid and rifampicin, often consist of four to six antituberculous agents (6).

B. Definitions and Mechanisms of Resistance

The terms mono-, poly-, and multidrug resistance have been traditionally used in the Western medical literature. Monodrug resistance is defined as resistance to only one antituberculous agent; polydrug resistance is defined as resistance to more than one antituberculous agent but not both isoniazid and rifampicin; and MDR as resistance to at least isoniazid and rifampicin. Since 2006, there has been a further subclassification of MDR-TB designated as extensively drug-resistant TB (XDR-TB). Specifically, XDR-TB is defined as TB resistant in vitro to the effects of isoniazid and rifampicin as well as to any one of the fluoroquinolones and to at least one of three injectable second-line drugs (amikacin, capreomycin, or kanamycin).

Mycobacteria achieve drug resistance through three basic mechanisms: (*i*) the creation of a lipid-rich cell wall that can reduce the permeability of drugs; (*ii*) the production of enzymes that degrade or modify compounds, rendering them useless; and (*iii*) spontaneous chromosomal mutations of key drug targets (7). The third mechanism, the development of drug resistance in *M. tuberculosis* through random genetic mutations, is considered the most significant. In any large population of *M. tuberculosis* bacilli, there are naturally occurring mutants and there is no mobile resistance factor (i.e., no plasmid mechanism) as seen with gram-negative rods. The mutations are unlinked and occur at low but predictable frequencies in the range of one mutation per 10^6 to 10^9 replications.

In clinical practice, acquired resistance occurs when the patient is originally infected with a drug-susceptible strain, and, through inadequate therapy, develops resistance. Inadequate therapy may be due to patient noncompliance, physician error (suboptimal dosing, insufficient number of active agents, noncompliance with established guidelines, or no existing guidelines), lack of access or stockouts of medications, low-quality drugs, poor drug absorption, or the organizational failure of the TB control program. Patient nonadherence is often considered the most common cause of acquired drug resistance (8); however, it has also been argued that the noncompliant patient's contribution to acquired resistance is minimal (9–11). In fact, the organizational failure of TB programs, lack of available drugs, and physician error are likely to be the significant contributors to acquired resistance. Once the patient's bacterial population is resistant to a single drug, any subsequent inadequate treatment (i.e., treatment regimens that may have only one or two effective agents) may select for further acquired resistance. The result is that strains resistant to one or two agents can become sequentially resistant to several agents if the initial resistance is not recognized and addressed.

When drug resistance develops, patients may transmit resistant strains to others who then present with preformed or "primary" drug resistance. If drug-susceptibility testing (DST) is done before the start of the patient's first TB treatment, any resistance documented is primary resistance. If additional resistance is found when DST is later repeated and genetic testing confirms that it is the same strain, only then can one conclude the strain has acquired resistance. If either DST or genetic testing is not available, it is impossible to distinguish acquired resistance from primary resistance. Therefore, in most settings around the world, acquired resistance is not distinguishable from primary resistance.

C. Cross-Resistance

There is well-known cross-resistance between some of the antibiotics used to treat TB. Resistance mutations to one antituberculous drug may confer resistance to some or all members of its drug family and, less commonly, to members of different antibiotic families. There are two classes of drugs that have significant cross-resistance that impacts the choice of therapy and interpretation of DST. There is significant cross-resistance within the aminoglycoside/polypeptide class, which includes such drugs as streptomycin, kanamycin, amikacin (aminoglycosides), and capreomycin (polypeptide). Resistance to the aminoglycoside kanamycin is associated with high cross-resistance to the structurally similar aminoglycoside amikacin (12,13). Likewise, resistance to capreomycin is associated with resistance to viomycin, a structurally similar polypeptide. In contrast, there is less cross-resistance between kanamycin and streptomycin (14,15) and between kanamycin and capreomycin.

There is significant cross-resistance across the fluoroquinolone class of antibiotics (16–22). Strains resistant to early-generation fluoroquinolones such as ciprofloxacin may also be resistant to later-generation fluoroquinolones such as moxifloxacin. Depending on the DST technique and the choice of breakpoints, some isolates may be resistant to early-generation fluoroquinolones but "susceptible" or "intermediate" to later-generation fluoroquinolones. The clinical implications of this, however, are not yet fully understood.

There is partial cross-resistance between isoniazid and thiacetazone (23,24) and between isoniazid and ethionamide (25–29). There is close-to-complete cross-resistance between rifampicin and rifabutin (30–33).

D.   Pathogenicity, Transmissibility, and Drug Resistance

Resistant strains of TB have traditionally been considered less pathogenic, also referred to as less virulent (i.e., less likely to progress to active disease in persons infected with such strains). This assumption was primarily based on the observation by Cohn et al. that virulent strains of *M. tuberculosis,* when selectively bred in the laboratory for high-level resistance to isoniazid, became significantly less capable of producing infection in animal models (34). The technique used to select these particular mutants was associated with the loss of catalase enzyme activity by the bacilli; the catalase was either a direct or a surrogate indicator of attenuated virulence (35).

Some studies have attempted to look at the transmissibility of DR-TB compared to drug-susceptible strains. A small cluster study by Garcia-Garcia et al. examined 25 MDR-TB cases and revealed that drug-resistant strains had decreased propensity to cluster (36). Clustering is associated with recent transmission, and less clustering could be explained by either decreased ability of the MDR-TB strains to infect individuals (decreased transmissibility) or decreased ability of the strains to cause disease once the individual has been infected (decreased pathogenicity). A study by Burgos et al. demonstrated in the context of an effective TB program in San Francisco, CA, that strains that were resistant to isoniazid either alone or in combination with other drugs were less likely to result in secondary cases than were drug-susceptible strains (37).

However, there is substantial evidence that MDR-TB strains are not always less pathogenic or transmissible (38). There are many examples of normal hosts who, once infected with strains resistant to isoniazid, develop serious, even lethal disease. The classic study is the 1996 report on the multiinstitutional spread of the notorious "strain W" in New York City in the early 1990s. This study provides insight into the nature of isoniazid resistance and virulence (39). Contrary to traditional assumptions, the "W" strain is catalase-positive and grows rapidly in both culture medium and animals despite mutations at the katG locus (35).

Furthermore, epidemiological data from the field confirms that resistance is not always accompanied by decreased transmission. Snider et al. performed a retrospective case–control analysis to compare the likelihood of contact infection by patients with drug-susceptible versus drug-resistant strains. They observed that overall tuberculin skin test conversion rates were comparable for young, high-risk persons whether they were contacts of susceptible or resistant cases (33.6% and 39.8%, respectively). Among those who had contact with drug-resistant cases with prior treatment, the risk of conversion was even higher (49%), presumably reflecting extended periods of exposure. In addition, the attack rate of active infection did not differ statistically whether the patient was in contact with a drug-susceptible or a drug-resistant case [6 of 252 (2.38%) vs. 4 of 239 (1.67%), respectively] (40).

Even if MDR-TB is less transmissible or pathogenic, MDR-TB cases can in absolute terms nevertheless generate more secondary cases than pan-sensitive ones because they remain infectious for longer, owing both to the lower cure rates and to the fact that treatment is often unavailable. Blower and Chou (41) have used models to show that, even when MDR-TB strains are less fit (and thus less transmissible and/or less pathogenic) than pan-sensitive strains, hot zones for MDR-TB can emerge. They concluded that MDR-TB levels are driven by case finding rates, cure rates, and amplification probabilities, rather than by just strain fitness. Furthermore, it is highly likely that the relative fitness of MDR-TB strains is heterogeneous, with some strains being less and others more fit. Through mathematical modeling, Cohen and Murray (42) demonstrated that, even when the average fitness of MDR-TB strains is lower, a small subpopulation of a relatively fit strain may eventually out-compete both the drug-sensitive strains and the less-fit MDR-TB strains. Gagneux et al. showed that even though drug-resistant strains can be created with varying degrees of fitness in the laboratory, drug-resistant strains taken from patients tend to have higher fitness, indicating that high-fitness–resistant mutants are the ones that are selected in patients during treatment (43).

Overall, there is a preponderance of evidence indicating that current drug-resistant strains can produce progressive disease in both normal and immunosuppressed contacts. New studies examining transmission patterns in urban settings (44–49) and nosocomial transmissions (50–54) have reported unexpectedly high rates of recently transmitted disease among MDR-TB patients. These studies underscore the point that the transmissibility of MDR-TB should not be dismissed and indicate that treatment of active MDR-TB cases and investigating the contacts of MDR-TB patients should be a high priority.

E. Impact of Drug Resistance on TB Control

Many areas of the world are recording alarmingly high DR-TB rates. The World Health Organization (WHO) estimates that 50 million people are infected with strains resistant to at least one first-line antituberculous agent (55). Estimates on the worldwide incidence of DR-TB are not well characterized. WHO estimated the total number of 2006 incident cases of MDR-TB globally to be approximately 489,000 (56). A 2008 WHO/IUALTD report confirmed that many areas of the world are facing epidemics of DR-TB. MDR-TB was found in 5.3% of all TB cases globally, with exceptionally high rates found in countries of the former Soviet Union and P.R. China (1).

DR-TB is clearly already endemic and is threatening to undermine recent gains in some settings with well-performing national TB control programs (e.g., Peru) as well as in settings where TB programs are recently under expansion (e.g., India). Once MDR-TB strains are well-established in a population, short-course chemotherapy (SCC) will fail to cure a growing proportion of TB patients. The WHO category II re-treatment regimen, when used in MDR-TB cases, has been documented to be successful in a very low percentage of patients—on average, 29% in data from six different countries (57). Close to 30% of MDR-TB cases that are deemed cured with SCC under WHO outcome definitions later relapse (58). Furthermore, there is evidence that challenging drug-resistant strains with SCC actually amplifies already existing resistance to first-line drugs, known as the "amplifier effect of short-course therapy." (59–61) Most MDR-TB cases in the world are resistant to three or four drugs (1); the repeated use of categories I and II treatment regimens in patients with DR-TB most certainly has played a role.

In 14 countries, MDR-TB rates have risen above 6% in new cases, meaning that MDR strains have become so widespread that large numbers of healthy people are becoming exposed and infected. In four countries of the former Soviet Union, MDR-TB rates in new cases were found to be above 15% (1). Blower and Chou (41) determined that MDR-TB prevalence can be three times greater than its incidence; their model indicates that some areas will develop prevalence rates of MDR-TB as high as 40%. These alarming prevalence rates are not just theoretical and have in fact been seen in settings such as Tomsk, Russia, where 530 (40.6%) of the 1302 registered prevalent smear-positive TB cases had MDR strains in 2001 (62).

Some authors have proposed using certain cut-off points (e.g., 1.5% MDR-TB in new cases) where MDR-TB should be considered less of a program priority (63). However, the cut-off point for when universal SCC will lead to treatment failure in a significant proportion of patients and thus compromise DOTS program performance remains unclear. We believe a good TB control programs should not let MDR-TB go unchecked and untreated in any circumstance.

The interaction between MDR-TB and HIV is addressed later in this chapter; however, it is worth mentioning that there have been numerous outbreaks with documented dismal outcomes for co-infected individuals (64). Prompt diagnosis and treatment of MDR-TB in HIV co-infected patients, along antiretroviral therapy (ART), may decrease these outbreaks and improve outcomes. There is reason to believe that HIV will have a similar effect on MDR-TB as it has on fueling the TB epidemic in general.

Because DR-TB is not readily contained by national borders, hospital walls, or prison bars, the full impact of the outbreaks that have been documented worldwide are yet to be fully felt. A universal strategy that includes appropriate treatment of all TB patients may be the best way to prevent resistance from overwhelming TB control efforts. This requires the coordination of many partners and is described in more detail in chapter 10.

F. Extensively Drug-Resistant Tuberculosis

XDR-TB—MDR-TB that is additionally resistant to fluoroquinolones and at least one second-line injectable drug—was first described in 2006, when a report emerged from the KwaZulu-Natal province of South Africa. In this cohort 98% of patients infected with XDR-TB died, with a median time of death of only 16 days from sputum collection (65). In a molecular epidemiology study of 10 years of clinical isolates from KwaZulu-Natal, Pillay and Sturm showed how a common South African strain of tuberculosis progressively developed resistance to more than seven TB drugs (66). They went on to speculate that South African XDR-TB was likely created through re-treatment regimens with an inadequate number of drugs: first the commonly used WHO category II regimen, followed by a standardized MDR-TB treatment regimen of second-line antituberculous drugs. The "new" phenomenon of XDR-TB shows clearly how poor diagnosis and treatment of DR-TB can create increasingly resistant strains that can have devastating public health impact.

A survey was conducted in 2006 to determine the extent of resistance to second-line drugs globally. Surveying the WHO/IUATLD (International Union Against Tuberculosis and Lung Disease) network of supranational reference laboratories (SRLs), over 17,000 isolates from 49 countries were included, all of which had been tested for resistance to at least three classes of second-line drugs. While results are not representative of the general population of patients with TB, the survey found that of the isolates tested against second-line drugs in the 49 contributing countries, 20% were found to be MDR-TB and 2% to be XDR-TB (67). Strains of XDR-TB have been reported in every region of the world, with as many as 19% of MDR strains found to be XDR in some areas (68).

XDR-TB poses a serious threat to global TB control. Even in cohorts of HIV-negative patients, failure and death are often increased (68). Treatment recommendations for XDR-TB are given in section IV.K.

II. Preventing the Evolution and Transmission of Drug Resistance

While there is no known way to completely prevent mutations that give rise to drug resistance, adequate TB treatment can minimize the selection of resistance in both treatment-naive patients and those undergoing re-treatment (69). Assurance of top-notch adherence to appropriate regimens is essential, as is the prevention of exposure to MDR-TB strains through proper infection control measures. The role of the BCG vaccine and of preventive therapy in decreasing the spread of MDR-TB is less clear.

A. Appropriate Regimens

Using multiple drugs for TB treatment is now the accepted standard of care. Appropriate regimens for drug-susceptible TB are described in chapter 5. For DR-TB, a regimen based on reliable DST and a review of treatment history is the gold standard of care. When MDR-TB is not suspected, a regimen that includes only first-line medications is appropriate while awaiting DST. If there is a possibility of primary resistance, a more ample regimen that includes both first- and second-line drugs is indicated. Empirical and definitive regimens are discussed in more detail in the treatment section of this chapter. Inappropriate regimens can lead not only to poor outcomes but also to amplification or acquired drug resistance (70). The use of multiple courses of first-line drugs despite repeated treatment failures has resulted in loss of susceptibility to all first-line drugs. This amplifier effect has been documented by Farmer et al. in Peruvian patients (71), by Seung et al. in Russian patients (61), and by Rigouts and Portaels in Rwandan patients (72).

B. Assurance of Adherence

A treatment regimen is effective only if it is taken correctly. Resistance can emerge if a patient takes only a reduced (ineffective) dose or omits one or more drugs (69). Treatment completion rates for pulmonary TB are most likely to exceed 90% when treatment is based on a patient-centered approach incorporating directly observed therapy (DOT) with multiple enablers and enhancers (73,74). DOT also appears to be cost-effective when compared to self-administered therapy, although cost-effectiveness data are limited (74).

C. Exposure Prevention and Infection Control

Adequate infection control requires a number of complementary interventions and is discussed elsewhere in this book. Special considerations should be included for DR-TB suspects and documented DR-TB patients. Implementing infection control measures is a high priority in preventing the spread of DR-TB.

D. BCG Vaccination

Some experts advocate BCG vaccination for those who have not had the vaccination, are PPD skin test negative, and will have unavoidable contact with DR-TB patients in the future. However, not all experts are in agreement on this approach. The debate is focused around the uncertain efficacy of BCG, the fact that BCG makes the tuberculin test un-interpretable and therefore limits identification of new infections and the option for chemoprophylaxis, and questions of whether persons will accept the ulcer and subsequent scarring that result from the BCG vaccine (75).

E. Prevention with Chemoprophylaxis in MDR-TB Contacts

The pros and cons of secondary prevention for contacts of MDR-TB patients are discussed in chapter 4, which addresses treatment of latent TB.

III. Diagnosis of DR-TB

A. Identification of DR-TB Patients

Assuming adequate resources and technical capacity, in order to ensure identification of DR-TB cases, sputum should be sent for susceptibility testing to at least isoniazid, rifampicin, ethambutol, and streptomycin prior to treatment initiation. If drug resistance is found, testing to second-line drugs and the first-line drug pyrazinamide may be indicated. For patients who initially test pan-susceptible, a repeat DST is indicated if they have persistently positive acid-fast bacilli smear or culture or clinical progression of TB while on therapy.

In some areas, resources to do DST may be limited. In such settings, only patients with suspected MDR-TB should have their sputum sent for culture and DST. Table 1 lists the categories of patients for whom DST is a priority, in descending order of higher to lower risk. Patients in whom treatment is failing or recently failed under DOT and with rifampicin in the continuation phase may have extremely high MDR-TB rates (see sect. V on standardized regimens for a more detailed discussion of the probability of having MDR-TB after failing a first-line drug regimen). In addition, close contacts of MDR-TB patients are very likely to have MDR-TB and DST profiles similar to that of the index case (also see sect. IV.C for a more lengthy discussion on the probability of a contact case having MDR-TB).

DST is strongly recommended for all TB/HIV co-infected patients, since unidentified MDR-TB is especially lethal in this population. It is likely that HIV patients in some settings have an increased risk of developing drug resistance (77,78) but other surveillance data indicate that globally HIV is not an independent risk factor for DR-TB (1). More MDR-TB epidemiological surveillance in HIV-infected patients is needed to fully assess whether drug-resistance rates are growing in co-infected patients.

Table 1 Groups of Patients for Targeted Drug-Susceptibility Testing in Low-Resource Areas

In settings where DST capacity is limited, priority should be given to

- chronic TB cases, patients in whom WHO retreatment SCC regimens failed;
- patients who have had significant exposure to a known MDR-TB case;
- patients in whom WHO category I SCC failed;
- patients in whom private-sector TB treatment failed;
- relapsed and returned after default cases (previous TB treatment with multiple drugs, but no history of recent failure);
- nonadherent patients;
- patients in institutions that have had MDR-TB outbreaks;
- patients from areas with high MDR-TB prevalence;
- patients in whom the use of antituberculous drugs of poor quality is suspected or documented;
- patients who have a history of using medications while on TB treatment that directly compete with antituberculosis drug absorption or alter the metabolism of antituberculous drugs, resulting in reduced serum levels;
- patients treated in programs that operate poorly, including programs with recent and/or frequent drug stockouts;
- patients with comorbid conditions associated with malabsorption or rapid transit diarrhea;
- HIV-positive patients in some settings.

Source: Adapted from Ref. (76).

B. Drug-Susceptibility Testing

A number of different techniques are available for DST. Phenotypic methods involve culturing of *M. tuberculosis* in the presence of anti-TB drugs to detect inhibition of growth. Phenotypic methods allow the detection of drug resistance regardless of mechanism or molecular basis. Genotypic approaches detect the genetic determinants of resistance rather than the resistance phenotype. Genetic testing is often referred to as "rapid molecular testing" since results can be available with less than one day turn around time.

Both phenotypic and genotypic DST methods can be performed as direct or indirect tests. In the direct test, the test is performed with a directly inoculated concentrated specimen. An indirect test involves inoculation with a pure culture grown from the specimen. Some of the newer techniques in TB diagnostics, including whether they can be performed directly or indirectly on specimens, have not yet been field-tested comprehensively in low-resource settings and further standardization studies are needed. More information on DST and rapid DST is presented in chapter 4.

Reliable and valid DST is essential for optimal DR-TB treatment. Many regional laboratories are able to perform susceptibility testing for only four first-line drugs: isoniazid, rifampicin, ethambutol, and streptomycin. Pyrazinamide-susceptibility testing is especially challenging and cannot be done using conventional solid media (79). Typically, second-line drug susceptibility is tested in SRL or in other specialized centers. Regular quality control of results is required for all laboratories.

In general, susceptibility testing for many antituberculous drugs is not as simple as testing for isoniazid and rifampicin, partly because critical drug concentrations defining resistance are much closer to the minimal inhibitory concentrations in the former than in the latter. Nonetheless, reasonably consistent, clinically validated criteria for drug resistance testing were determined almost 50 years ago, for the proportion method on Lowenstein-Jensen medium for kanamycin, capreomycin, viomycin, D-cycloserine, ethionamide, and PAS (80). Guidelines for DST on second-line drugs are also available (81,82).

There has been much debate on the reliability (the ability of the results to be consistently reproducible) of second-line DST (83). It is true that proficiency metrics equivalent to those obtained for first-line drug testing are not available for second-line drug testing. Without such data, little can be said about the reliability of second-line DST. Fortunately a proficiency testing exercise among SRLs to understand the reproducibility of DST is ongoing (83). Even if the reliability for anti-TB DST is determined to be adequate under standardized testing methods, the validity (the correlation between testing resistant and the lack of clinical efficacy of a drug) for many drugs is not well characterized. A validity study of second-line DST is currently underway (84).

In summary, many uncertainties exist in reliability and validity of DST, especially for second-line drugs. Nevertheless, these do not negate the usefulness of in vitro susceptibility testing for antituberculous drugs; many treatment facilities and programs have obtained adequate outcome results with regimens based on first- and second-line DST (6). Any DST results should be interpreted with care, taking into consideration local resistance prevalence, the patient's drug history, and the quality of the testing laboratory. The need persists for improving and better understanding the methodologies presently in use.

C. Rapid Molecular Testing

Screening for resistance with rapid molecular testing is becoming the standard of care in most areas with the resources to do so. These tests are becoming cheaper and easier and have been shown to detect both isoniazid and rifampicin resistance with a high degree of accuracy (85). If done directly on sputum, results can be available within one day. Unfortunately, direct molecular testing generally requires a high bacterial load in the sputum, which essentially excludes smear-negative TB patients from this strategy.

WHO guidelines recommend that patients with a positive rapid molecular test be started on a standardized regimen for MDR-TB (76). At the same time, sputum can be sent for phenotypic culture-based DST to additional first- and second-line drugs. When these more complete results are available, the treatment regimen may be modified accordingly. The use of rapid molecular testing in this way significantly reduces the time to effective treatment for MDR-TB patients, and also decreases nosocomial transmission by quickly identifying highly infectious MDR-TB patients.

D. Prior Anti-TB Treatment History

While DST is an important component of identifying the patient with drug resistance, the use of a good medical history that includes all previous anti-TB treatments, outcomes of treatments, and DST patterns of contacts can also help identify patients with drug resistance. The treatment history and contact history should always be used together with the DST results to help determine whether a drug may be effective against the infecting strain in a patient. This is further discussed in the section.

IV. Treatment of DR-TB

A thorough treatment history, knowledge of local drug resistance patterns, and reliable DST results are key inputs in designing an appropriate MDR-TB treatment regimen. Patients harboring strains resistant to both isoniazid and rifampicin (MDR-TB) are at a high risk for treatment failure and acquired resistance if they are not promptly placed on adequate regimens. Definitive randomized or controlled trials have been performed on patients with various drug resistance patterns. In fact, to date there have been very few randomized trials directly comparing two MDR-TB treatment regimens in a blinded and controlled study setting. Regimen design is thus based on a mixture of nonideal evidence, general principles, extrapolations, and expert opinions (82).

A. Principles of Treatment and Medications

Second-line drugs for the treatment of MDR-TB are more toxic, not as efficacious, and must be administered for longer periods of time than their first-line counterparts. It is recommended that treatment be supervised by a physician specialized in DR-TB, although treatment programs that depend on highly trained nurses and health promoters have also been successful (86,87). The main consideration lies in the choice between a standardized regimen, where all patients in a specific group receive the same regimen and DST is not done for all individuals; or individualized regimens, where treatment is based on each patient's DST profile (an empiric regimen is used while awaiting DST results). The following is a list of general principles for the treatment of MDR-TB patients using either a standardized or individualized approach:

- Early detection and prompt initiation of treatment are critical factors in ensuring successful outcomes.
- Treatment regimens should take into consideration the patient's treatment history. If a patient has taken a drug for an extended period of time (generally defined as longer than one month) with persistently positive smears or cultures, the patient's TB should be considered resistant to that drug even if DST reports indicate susceptibility.
- Care providers should take into consideration local treatment practices and the history of drug availability in the population, including commonly used drugs and first- and second-line drug-resistance patterns.
- Treatment regimens should consist of at least four effective drugs and preferably five. When the susceptibility pattern is unknown, or drug efficacy unclear for whatever reason, as many as six or seven drugs may be used. Recently, a study from Latvia (88) showed the use of five or fewer drugs for three months or more was an independent predictor of poor outcome.
- In the initial phase of treatment, drugs are administered six to seven days a week, usually twice a day (to lessen side effects). In later phases, the drugs are generally given six days a week; however, some programs have given drugs in later phases of treatment five times a week. When possible, pyrazinamide and ethambutol should be given in once-a-day dosing if they are included in the

treatment regimen, since the high peaks attained in once-a-day dosing may be more efficacious. Once-a-day dosing is acceptable for other second-line drugs depending on patient tolerance, but data on the relative efficacy of once-a-day dosing versus twice-a-day dosing with some drugs is unclear.

- Drug dosage should be adjusted to the patient's weight; when a dosage range is suggested, the highest dosage within that range tolerated by the patient is recommended (see Table 2).
- Some drugs (thioamides, cycloserine, PAS) can be introduced at lower doses and increased over 3 to 10 days.
- If available, pharmacokinetic studies (drug serum level testing) can be performed to determine the optimal dosing for maximal serum concentrations in the therapeutic range and to avoid levels above the therapeutic range that may be more likely to cause side effects.
- An injectable agent (an aminoglycoside or capreomycin) should be used for a minimum of 6 months and the treatment with other drugs should last for 24 months (see below for more discussion on length of injectable agent and treatment).
- DOT should be used for all patients for the entire duration of treatment. Strong patient support and aggressive side effects management should be available.
- The use of drugs that have demonstrated in vitro resistance is not recommended (assuming the laboratory testing is accurate), especially when alternative medicines are available. An exception may be in patients whose strain test resistant to low-level isoniazid but is susceptible to high concentrations (greater than 1.0 μg/mL). Isoniazid use was associated with better survival rates in patients with strain W of MDR-TB that was susceptible to higher isoniazid concentrations on susceptibility testing (39,89).
- A full assessment of DST reliability and clinical correlation for some first-line and most second-line antituberculous drugs has not yet been achieved. Nonetheless, regimens should include at least four drugs thought to be efficacious based on DST and/or the patient's treatment history.
- The newer rifamycins have high levels of cross-resistance to rifampicin and should be considered ineffective if DST indicates rifampicin resistance. Amikacin should be considered ineffective if kanamycin tests resistant and vice versa.
- Pyrazinamide can be used for the entire duration of treatment if it is thought to be efficacious. Many MDR-TB patients have chronically inflamed lungs, which theoretically produces the acidic environment in which pyrazinamide is active.
- Analysis of patient cohorts should follow internationally recommended case registration and outcome definitions (90).

B. Drugs Used in DR-TB Treatment

Table 2 is a summary of antituberculous drugs and their mechanism of action, metabolism, recommended dosing, common side effects, and monitoring requirements. Note that rare side effects and drug–drug interactions are available from other sources (96). Drugs not included in Table 2 but applicable in some situations of high resistance include clofazimine, amoxicillin-clavulanate, and clarithromycin (6,82). While some of these

Table 2 Antituberculous Medications and Their Side Effects

Drug name (abbreviation)	Description and adult dose	Side effects	Monitoring requirements and comments
Isoniazid (H)	**Description:** Bactericidal; inhibits mycolic acid synthesis most effectively in dividing cells; hepatically metabolized **Dose:** 300–600 mg/day	**Common:** Hepatitis (10–20% have elevated level of transaminases), peripheral neuropathy (dose-related; increased risk with malnutrition, alcoholism, diabetes, concurrent use of AG or ETO) **Less common:** Gynecomastia, rash, psychosis, seizure	**Monitoring:** Consider baseline and monthly SGOT, especially if age greater than 50 years **Comments:** Give with pyridoxine 50 mg/day if using large dose or if patient is at risk for peripheral neuropathy (diabetes, alcoholism, HIV, etc.)
Rifampicin (R) (Rifampin)	**Description:** Bactericidal; inhibits protein synthesis by blocking mRNA transcription and synthesis; hepatically metabolized **Dose:** 600 mg/day	**Common:** Orange-colored bodily secretions, transient transaminitis, hepatitis, GI distress **Less common:** Cholestatic jaundice	**Monitoring:** Baseline SGOT and bilirubin, repeat if symptoms (jaundice, fatigue, anorexia, weakness, or nausea and vomiting for more than 3 days).
Pyrazinamide (Z)	**Description:** Bactericidal; mechanism unclear; effective in acidic milieu (e.g., cavitary disease, intracellular organisms); hepatically metabolized, renally excreted **Dose:** 30–40 mg/kg/day	**Common:** Arthritis/arthralgias, hepatotoxicity, hyperuricemia, abdominal distress **Less common:** Impaired diabetic control, rash	**Monitoring:** Baseline and monthly SGOT; uric acid can be measured if arthralgias, arthritis, or symptoms of gout are present **Comments:** Usually given once daily, but can split dose initially to improve tolerance
Ethambutol (E)	**Description:** Bacteriostatic at conventional dosing (15 mg/kg); inhibits lipid and cell wall metabolism; renally excreted. **Dose:** 25 mg/kg, consider decreasing to 15 mg/kg once patient is culture-negative	**Common:** Generally well-tolerated **Less common:** Optic neuritis, GI distress, arthritis/arthralgia	**Monitoring:** Baseline and monthly visual acuity and red/green color vision test when dosed at greater than 15 mg/kg/day (more than 10% loss is considered significant) (91); regularly question patient about visual symptoms

(Continued)

Table 2 (*Continued*)

Drug name (abbreviation)	Description and adult dose	Side effects	Monitoring requirements and comments
Aminoglycosides; Amikacin (AMK); Kanamycin (K); Streptomycin (S); Polypeptides; Capreomycin (CM); Viomycin (VM);	**Description:** Bactericidal; aminoglycosides inhibit protein synthesis through disruption of ribosomal function; less effective in acidic, intracellular environments; polypeptides appear to inhibit translocation of the peptidyl-rRNA and the initiation of protein synthesis; renally excreted **Dose:** 15–20 mg/kg/day	**Common:** Pain at injection site, proteinuria, serum electrolyte disturbances **Less common:** Cochlear otoxocity (hearing loss, dose-related to cumulative and peak concentrations, increased risk with renal insufficiency; may be irreversible), nephrotoxicity (dose-related to cumulative and peak concentrations, increased risk with renal insufficiency, often irreversible), peripheral neuropathy, rash, vestibular toxicity (nausea, vomiting, vertigo, ataxia, nystagmus), eosinophilia Otoxocity potentiated by certain diuretics, especially loop diuretics	**Monitoring:** Baseline and then biweekly creatinine, urea, and serum potassium more frequently in high-risk patients; if potassium is low, check magnesium and calcium; baseline audiometry and monthly monitoring in high-risk patients (high-risk patients = elderly, diabetic, or HIV-positive patients, or patients with renal insufficiency) **Comments:** Observe for problems with balance; increase dosing interval or reduce dose and monitor serum drug concentrations as needed to control side effects Electrolyte disturbances are more common in patients receiving CM; (92)
Fluoroquinolones; Ciprofloxacin (CPX); Ofloxacin (OFX); Levofloxacin (LFX); Moxifloxacin (MFX); Gatifloxacin (GFX);	**Description:** Bactericidal; DNA-gyrase inhibitor; renally excreted **Dose:** Ciprofloxacin, 1500 mg/day Ofloxacin, 800 mg/day Levofloxacin, 750 mg/day Moxifloxacin, 400 mg/day Gatifloxacin, 400 mg/day	**Common:** Generally well-tolerated, well-absorbed **Less common:** Diarrhea, dizziness, GI distress, headache, insomnia, photosensitivity, rash, vaginitis, psychosis, seizure (CNS effects seen almost exclusively in elderly)	**Monitoring:** No laboratory monitoring requirements **Comments:** Do not administer with antacids, sucralfate, iron, zinc, calcium, or oral potassium and magnesium replacements; LFX, MFX, GFX have the most activity against *M. tuberculosis*; data on long-term safety and tolerability are limited on MFX and GFX, thus LFX is currently the preferred fluoroquinolone (82).

Drug	Description / Dose	Adverse effects	Monitoring / Comments
Cycloserine (CS)	**Description**: Bacteriostatic; alanine analogue; interferes with cell-wall proteoglycan synthesis; renally excreted **Dose**: 500–1000 mg/day	**Common**: Neurologic and psychiatric disturbances, including headaches, irritability, sleep disturbances, aggression, and tremors **Less common**: Psychosis, peripheral neuropathy, seizures (increased risk of CNS effects with concurrent use of ethanol, H, ETO, or other centrally acting medications), hypersensitivity	**Monitoring**: Consider serum drug monitoring to establish optimal dosing **Comments**: Give 50 mg for every 250 mg of CS (to lessen neurological adverse effects)
Thiamides; Ethionamide (ETO); Prothionamide (PTO);	**Description**: May be bactericidal or bacteriostatic depending on susceptibility and concentrations attained at the infection site; the carbotionamide group, also found on thiacetazone, and the pyridine ring, also found on H, appear essential for activity; (93) hepatically metabolized, renally excreted **Dose**: 500–1000 mg/day	**Common**: GI distress (nausea, vomiting, diarrhea, abdominal pain, loss of appetite), dysgeusia (metallic taste), hypothyroidism (especially when taken with PAS) **Less common**: Arthralgias, dermatitis, gynecomastia, hepatitis, impotence, peripheral neuropathy, photosensitivity	**Monitoring**: Consider baseline and monthly SGOT **Comments**: May split dose or give at bedtime to improve tolerability; ETO and PTO efficacies are considered similar; PTO may cause fewer GI side effects (94)
para-Aminosalicylic acid (PAS)	**Description**: Bacteriostatic; disrupts folic acid metabolism (thought to inhibit the biosynthesis of coenzyme F in the folic acid pathway); hepatic acetylation, renally excreted. **Dose**: 500–1000 mg/day	**Common**: GI distress (nausea, vomiting, diarrhea), hypersensitivity, hypothyroidism (especially when taken with ETO) **Less common**: Hepatitis, electrolyte abnormalities **Drug interactions**: Decreased INH acetylation, decreased R absorption in nongranular preparation, decreased B12 uptake	**Monitoring**: No laboratory monitoring requirements **Comments**: Some formulas of enteric-coated granules need to be administered with an acidic food or beverage (i.e., yogurt or acidic juice)

Source: Adapted from Ref. (95).

agents have been successfully used against nontuberculous mycobacterial infections and may have some proven in vitro activity against *M. tuberculosis*, their clinical efficacy in MDR-TB treatment has not been established. Thioacetazone is not commonly used for MDR-TB because of its modest antituberculous activity, potential for life-threatening toxicity in HIV-infected patients, and cross-resistance to thioamides. Linezolid appears to have antituberculous activity; however, it is anecdotally very toxic when given for extended periods of time (97). Clinical trials are currently underway to determine if alternative dosages will reduce toxicity. Finally, there are a number of additional new compounds that are currently in or entering into phase II clinical trials (98–100). If successful, several new antituberculous drugs could be on the market within the next few years.

C. Empiric Treatment of DR-TB

Patients are started on an empiric regimen when DST results are not available. With a few exceptions, most patients deemed to have a high probability of drug-resistant disease should immediately be placed on an empiric regimen as soon as adequate specimens are obtained for culture and DST in order to prevent clinical deterioration and transmission to contacts. Clinicians are often reluctant to start second-line antituberculous drugs empirically, without laboratory confirmation of resistance to isoniazid and rifampicin. But in situations where DST is not easily accessible, the reliance on laboratory diagnosis can become a bottleneck to life-saving treatment. Early treatment is particularly critical in patients who are immunocompromised from HIV co-infection. Several studies in the 1980s and 1990s of MDR-TB in HIV co-infected patients from Europe and the United States reported mortality rates exceeding 70%, often within four to eight weeks of diagnosis and before laboratory confirmation of MDR-TB (101). In a 2006 report from the KwaZulu-Natal province of South Africa, 52/53 (98%) of patients with XDR-TB died within a median of 16 days from the time of sputum collection for diagnosis (65).

Even in settings where there is ready access to culture and DST, empiric MDR-TB treatment is a strategy that can decrease the time to effective treatment. If rapid DST methods are readily available, consideration may be given to wait for DST results if the patient is clinically very stable. However, most commonly available DST methods use culture on solid or liquid media, which require several weeks or months—ample time for a patient to clinically worsen or die while receiving ineffective first-line drugs. In settings where DST is readily available, there is little to be lost by a starting a well-designed empiric MDR-TB treatment regimen in high-risk patients. If DST subsequently shows the patient to be infected with drug-susceptible TB, the patient can be simply switched back to a first-line regimen.

WHO guidelines for the management of DR-TB provide clear protocols to help clinicians in identifying which patients are at high-risk for MDR-TB and should start empiric treatment (Table 3) (76). Close contacts of MDR-TB patients who develop active disease have MDR-TB in more than two-thirds of cases; they should be started on empiric regimens based on the index patient's DST pattern. A review of literature that searched for any study that examined more than 100 contacts of MDR-TB patients (Table 4) reveals that most of the contacts that developed active disease had drug-resistant forms (49,102–105).

Concordance between the index case and the contact may be lower in case of resistance to drugs other than isoniazid and rifampicin because additional resistance can develop over time in the strain of either the index or the contact patient, and this is often

Table 3 Recommended Empiric Treatment Strategies for Different Programmatic Situations

Patient group	Background-susceptibility data	Recommended strategy
New patient with active TB	Resistance uncommon to moderately common (i.e., a country where a low-to-moderate rate of new cases have MDR-TB) Resistance common (i.e., a country where a high rate of new cases have MDR-TB)	• Start category I treatment • Perform DST of at least H and R in patients not responsive to category I • Rapid DST techniques are preferable • Perform DST of H and R in all patients before treatment starts • Rapid DST techniques are preferable • Start category I treatment while awaiting DST • Adjust regimen to a category IV regimen if DST reveals DR-TB
Patient in whom category I failed	Low percentage of failures of category I have MDR-TB Second-line drug resistance is rare High percentage of failures of category I have MDR-TB Second-line drug resistance is rare High percentage of failures of category I have MDR-TB Second-line drug resistance is common	• Perform DST of H and R at a minimum in all patients before treatment starts • Rapid DST is preferable • Start category II treatment while awaiting DST • Adjust regimen to a category IV regimen if DST reveals DR-TB • Perform DST of isoniazid and rifampicin at a minimum in all patients before treatment starts • Perform DST of isoniazid and rifampicin at a minimum in all patients before treatment starts • Start category IV treatment: IA-FQ- two group 4 agents- +/– Z • Perform DST of H, R, IA, FQ before treatment starts • Start category IV treatment: IA-FQ-three group 4 agents- +/– Z while awaiting DST • Adjust regimen according to DST results if using an individualized approach

(Continued)

Table 3   (*Continued*)

Patient group	Background-susceptibility data	Recommended strategy
Patient in whom category II failed	High percentage of failures of category II have MDR-TB Second-line drug resistance is rare	• Perform DST of H and R at a minimum in all patients before treatment starts • Start category IV treatment: IA-FQ- two group 4 agents- +/– Z while awaiting DST • Adjust regimen according to DST results if using an individualized approach
	High percentage of failures of category II have MDR-TB Second-line drug resistance is common	• Perform DST of H, R, IA, FQ before treatment starts • Start category IV treatment: IA-FQ- three group 4 agents- +/– Z while awaiting DST • Adjust regimen according to DST results if using an individualized approach
Patient with history of relapse or patient returning after default	Low-to-moderate rate of MDR-TB in this group of patients is common	• Perform DST of H and R at a minimum in all patients before treatment starts • Start category II treatment while awaiting DST • Adjust regimen to a category IV regimen if DST returns DR-TB
Contact of MDR-TB patient now with active TB (contact resistance pattern known)	Close contact with high risk of having the same strain	• Perform rapid diagnosis and DST of H and R at a minimum in all patients before treatment starts • Start category IV treatment based on the DST pattern and treatment history of the contact while awaiting DST • Adjust regimen according to DST results
	Casual contact with low risk of having the same strain	• Perform rapid diagnosis and DST of H and R at a minimum in all patients before treatment starts • Start category I treatment while awaiting DST • Adjust regimen according to DST results

(*Continued*)

Table 3 (*Continued*)

Patient group	Background-susceptibility data	Recommended strategy
Patient with documented MDR-TB	Documented, or almost certain, susceptibility	• Start category IV treatment: IA-FQ- two group 4 agents- +/– Z to a FQ and IA
	Documented, or almost certain, susceptibility to FQ	• Start category IV treatment: IA-FQ- three group 4 agents- +/– Z
	Documented, or almost, resistance to an IA	• Use an IA with documented susceptibility • If the strain is resistant to all IAs, use one for which resistance is relatively rare
	Documented, or almost certain, resistance to a FQ	• Start category IV treatment: IA-FQ- three group 4 agents- +/– Z
	Documented, or almost certain, susceptibility to IA	• Use a later-generation FQ
	Documented, or almost certain, resistance to a FQ and IA	• Start category IV treatment for XDR-TB

Injectable agents: streptomycin, amikacin, kanamycin, capreomycin, and viomycin.
Oral second-line agents: ethionamide or prothionamide, cycloserine, *p*-aminosalicylic acid. In cases of very high resistance where four drug regimens cannot be formed, alternative oral agents may include clarithromycin, amoxicillin/clavulanate, linezolid, and/or clofazimine.
Abbreviations: H, isoniazid; R, rifampicin; E, ethambutol; Z, pyrazinamide; S, streptomycin.
Source: Adapted from Ref. (76).

Table 4 Rates of MDR-TB Among Contacts of MDR-TB Patients

Study	Country	Number of contacts	Percentage of patients with MDR-TB (# of TB case/total # with active TB)
Kritski et al. (49)	Brazil	218	62% (8/13)
Schaaf et al. (102)	South Africa	149	83% (5/6)
Texeira et al. (103)	Brazil	133	83% (5/6)
Schaaf et al. (104)	South Africa	119	75% (3/4)
Bayona et al (105)	Peru	945	84% (35/42)

due to inadequate therapy after the time of infection transmission. This may result in decreased confidence in the ability to predict the exact DST pattern of a contact's isolate from the index case's isolate. Therefore, the empiric regimen should be designed based on the treatment histories of both the index and the contact cases (in relation to when the exposure took place) and on the DST of the index case. As with all empiric treatments, the regimen should be adjusted once the DST of the contact case becomes available.

In patients who have previously received antituberculosis treatment, obtaining a detailed clinical history is crucial. Every effort should be made to supplement the patient's recall with objective records from previous health care providers. A detailed treatment history can help suggest which drugs are likely to be ineffective. The probability of acquired drug resistance increases with the amount of time that a drug is administered. While some clinicians use a lower limit of one month as the minimum administration time before drug resistance can develop, in fact there is no lower limit. In the case of inadequate regimen administration, drug resistance can develop within weeks or even days, as has been documented in case reports of patients with drug allergies (106).

Drug resistance surveys are very helpful in identifying groups of patients who are at increased risk for MDR-TB. For example, patients in whom category II treatment fails (chronic cases) in well-run TB control programs almost always have MDR-TB (107,108) and this group, in the vast majority of instances, can start treatment of presumptive MDR-TB without individual confirmation of resistance. However, surveillance DST in this group should still be performed, as it will both confirm that this practice is justified and aid in the design of the specific standardized re-treatment regimen to be used.

Whether failures of WHO category I treatment can routinely enter a standardized MDR-TB treatment regimen is often unclear and depends on a number of factors. The MDR-TB rate in these patients may be related to the drugs used in the continuation phase as well as to the level of DOT. In many TB control programs, category I regimen failures that use isoniazid–rifampicin in the continuation phase have high MDR-TB rates, ranging from 62% to 88% in published studies (109–111). It has been speculated that if isoniazid–rifampicin and strict DOT is used in the continuation phase, the presence of MDR-TB is the main plausible cause of failure. Much lower rates of MDR-TB (22–33%) have been reported if isoniazid–ethambutol or isoniazid–thiacetazone are used or if DOT was not part of the continuation phase (70,109,112).

However, the above observations do not always hold true. A study from Vietnam reported a very high rate of MDR-TB (80%) in failures of category I treatment with unsupervised isoniazid–ethambutol in the continuation phase (113). The high MDR-TB rates among the category I failures in this cohort may have been a result of high rates of primary resistance (both isoniazid resistance and MDR-TB) and past medical practices in the country. Drug resistance survey data are extremely useful to confirm that certain groups of patients that are receiving empiric MDR-TB treatment are likely to have MDR-TB. The surveillance data in these groups will need to be repeated periodically.

The programmatic approach to the identification and treatment of DR-TB is discussed in further detail in chapter 10.

D.   Standardized Regimens

There is a long history of standardized treatment regimens in TB programs. These have been generally beneficial because it can be easy for clinicians to make mistakes in the prescription and administration of the complicated multidrug regimens used in TB treatment. DR-TB requires even more complicated multidrug regimens and so standardized re-treatment regimens can be very helpful to clinicians, particularly in settings where DR-TB is common.

In the past, the WHO and the IIUATLD recommended that all re-treatment cases receive the same regimen, referred to as category II re-treatment regimen (114,115) In many resource-limited settings, the category II regimen continues to be inappropriately used for re-treatment, even in patients with high likelihood for MDR-TB. The WHO currently recommends that several standardized re-treatment regimens be designed by program managers; clinicians may then choose the appropriate regimen based on the characteristics and treatment history of the patient.

Standardized re-treatment regimens may be used for empiric treatment of patients with suspected MDR-TB, but without laboratory confirmation of resistance to isoniazid and rifampicin. They may also be used for patients who are found to have MDR-TB, via rapid molecular testing, and before DST to other drugs are available, as described in the previous section. Standardized re-treatment regimens can be used as the initial phase of treatment and modified after DST results are available. Finally, standardized re-treatment regimens may be used for the entire duration of therapy in settings where DST is not available or in patients who do not have DST results for one reason or another.

The number of drugs required to effectively treat MDR-TB ranges from three to seven, depending on the drugs and the patient. A literature review of MDR-TB treatment programs reveals that all reported cohorts were treated with four to six drugs (6). The WHO and the Green Light Committee for Second-line Drug Access in MDR-TB Treatment advocate the use of at least four drugs considered to be efficacious (76,116). Since in vitro susceptibility does not correlate perfectly with clinical efficacy, standardized re-treatment regimens often consist of as many as six or seven drugs, at least initially, to ensure that at least four are effective. For example, during the notorious outbreaks of MDR-TB in New York City in the 1980s, an initial regimen of seven drugs was used in order to ensure adequate antimicrobial coverage while awaiting DST studies (117). Many practitioners adhere to the principle that the best opportunity to cure a patient is the current course of treatment (the likelihood of cure decreases with successive courses of treatment). Rather than reserving effective drugs "just in case" the current course of treatment fails, these experts will use every known drug with potential efficacy against a patient's MDR bacilli (69).

Data from drug resistance surveys can play an important role not only in deciding which patients groups should receive empiric MDR-TB treatment but also in the design of standardized re-treatment regimens for those groups. Past history of antituberculous treatment taken by the patient does not always correspond to the resistance pattern of the patient's strain. This is because many cases of primary resistance are not identified until after one or more failed courses of treatment with first-line drugs. In these cases, previous treatment with first-line drugs acts as a screening mechanism for MDR-TB patients and the previous history of TB treatment cannot be relied on to decide the likely resistance pattern. The most common example of this is streptomycin. In many countries, streptomycin resistance is common in MDR strains. Patients who have failed treatment with category I regimens often have resistance to streptomycin even though they have never received it.

In patients who are very likely to have MDR-TB, such as those treated with multiple courses of first-line drugs, data from DST surveillance may help design standardized re-treatment regimens that are likely to include at least four effective second-line drugs. If DST patterns show high rates of resistance to ethambutol or pyrazinamide, additional second-line drugs should be included in the standardized re-treatment regimen. If DST patterns show high rates of resistance to streptomycin and kanamycin, the standardized re-treatment regimen can instead use capreomycin.

In groups with low or moderate rates of MDR-TB, including patients who relapse, return-after-default, and sometimes failures of category I or III treatment regimens, it may be more difficult (if not impossible) to find a single re-treatment regimen that does not deny a large percentage of these patients isoniazid and rifampicin who would in fact benefit from these drugs or unnecessarily expose patients to toxic second-line drugs. If routine use of the WHO category II regimen is not completely safe, a re-treatment regimen including rifampicin and isoniazid and four additional second-line drugs can be designed. Treatment can then be modified after DST results for the individual patient isbreak; available.

Experience in the use of standardized regimens as fully empiric treatment for the entire length of MDR-TB treatment is limited. There have only been three reports to date, from Peru, South Korea, and Bangladesh. Given the low rate of successful outcomes, the programmatic strategies used in the Peruvian and South Korean studies may have been insufficient. The Peruvian study had a cure rate of 48% (and in patients with confirmed MDR-TB the failure rate was 32.2%), which can be attributed in part to regimen design and programmatic problems. A significant percentage of patients (estimated to be 16% in a similar group of patients, unpublished results) were on two or fewer effective drugs since the standard regimen relied heavily on ethambutol and pyrazinamide, both of which had been used extensively in these patients in the past. The injectable drug, which was one of the most bactericidal agents in the regimen, was used for only three months. Other reasons for the program's limited success include the relatively low dosage of ciprofloxacin (1000 mg/day), the untenable costs to the patients of ancillary medicines to treat side effects, and inadequate (low-to-moderate) social support. The late identification of MDR-TB (most patients were not identified until after failure of category II treatment) may have also contributed to the poor outcomes (108). In the South Korean study, first-line DST was used to diagnose patients with MDR and also to choose between one of two standardized re-treatment regimens. The low cure rates in this study are attributable in part to a high default rate (28.9%), likely due to the self-administration of most of the regimen and a lack of support measures to help patients stay in treatment (118). The Bangladesh study documented the best success to date in the use of a standardized regimen, reporting a cure rate of 69%. However, the cohort was small, with only 58 patients, and it is unclear if the seven-drug standardized regimen used for the cohort will be successful in other settings, especially since it included three first-line drugs (119).

Despite their low success in some settings and the limited data on their efficacy, fully standardized regimens are a reasonable alternative in settings where DST is not available or unreliable (108). Even in these settings, DST to isoniazid and rifampicin is strongly recommended. Reliable DST to these drugs will ensure that patients started on MDR-TB re-treatment regimens indeed are infected with MDR-TB strains. DST to additional first-line and second-line drugs can be restricted to surveillance studies and used for the design of standardized re-treatment regimens.

E. Designing an Individualized Regimen

Patients with DST results are increasingly common, even in resource-poor settings. Nonetheless, there are some cautionary points. In reaction to DST results, physicians often make classic management errors, such as adding only one drug to a failing regimen. Such errors can be disastrous both for the patient and for TB control efforts. DST results should complement rather than invalidate other sources of data about the likely efficacy of a specific drug.

If a history of prior antituberculous drug use suggests that a drug is likely to be ineffective, this drug should not be relied on as one of the four core drugs in the regimen even if the strain tests susceptible to it in the laboratory. This is true even for isoniazid and rifampicin. Evidence of clinical or bacteriological treatment failure during a period of regular drug administration is highly suggestive of drug resistance, particularly for isoniazid and rifampicin. As Stewart and Crofton wrote in 1968, "failure while under treatment with the relevant drug must indicate that the drug is no longer suppressing the growth of the patient's bacilli."(120) Patients who continue to be smear- or culture-positive while taking isoniazid and rifampicin should be considered extremely high risk for MDR-TB, irrespective of DST results.

Because of the turnaround time necessary for DST, the patient in question may already have received months of an empiric treatment regimen by the time results become available. The possibility of further acquired resistance during this time must be considered. If there is a high probability of acquired resistance to a drug after the specimen was obtained that gave the DST results, this drug should not be counted as one of the four drugs in the core regimen.

Finally, effective DST interpretation necessitates a high level of confidence in the laboratory performing the tests. If the strain is resistant to a drug in the laboratory, but the patient has never taken the drug and resistance to it is extremely uncommon in the community, laboratory error or the limited specificity of DST for some second-line drugs may be a factor. Some laboratories may report that a strain has a low or intermediate level of resistance to a certain drug. There is very little clinical evidence to support this sort of designation, particularly if the patient previously received the drug as part of DOT.

In the case of inconsistent results or unclear evidence about drug effectiveness, one should follow the dictum "use the medicine, but do not depend on it for success" (121). In short, individualized regimens need to be designed, whenever possible, with at least four medications thought or documented to be efficacious. This may entail a regimen with more than four drugs if the efficacy of one or more of the drugs is unclear or in doubt for any of the reasons discussed above.

Table 5 lists suggested regimens for various DST patterns, with the caveat that this table assumes that patients have never been treated for TB. In re-treatment patients, the history of past TB treatment should also be taken into account. For example, HEZ resistance in a patient who is smear-positive while taking category I is more likely to indicate a laboratory error with respect to rifampicin, rather than true effectiveness of rifampicin. The table also assumes no chance of acquired resistance to additional agents after the specimen was collected that gave the DST results. Finally, the table assumes accessible, reliable, and accurate DST for pyrazinamide. If DST for pyrazinamide is not performed, it cannot be depended upon as being an effective drug in the regimen. In such situations, regimens from Table 5 that assume it to be resistant should be used. Some

Table 5 Suggested Regimens for Drug-Resistant Tuberculosis

Pattern of drug resistance	Suggested regimen[a]	Minimum duration of treatment (months)	Comments
H (±S)	R, Z, and E	6–9	A fluoroquinolone may strengthen the regimen for patients with extensive disease.
H and Z	R, E, and fluoroquinolones	9–12	A longer duration of treatment should be used for patients with extensive disease.
H and E	R, Z, and fluoroquinolones	9–12	A longer duration of treatment should be used for patients with extensive disease.
R	H, E, fluoroquinolones, plus at least 2 mo of Z	12–18	An injectable agent may strengthen the regimen for patients with extensive disease.
R and E (±S)	H, Z, fluoroquinolones, plus an injectable agent for at least the first 2–3 mo	18	A longer course (6 mo) of the injectable agent may strengthen the regimen for patients with extensive disease.
R and Z (±S)	H, E, fluoroquinolones, plus an injectable agent for at least the first 2–3 mo	18	A longer course (6 mo) of the injectable agent may strengthen the regimen for patients with extensive disease.
H, E, Z (±S)	R, fluoroquinolones, plus an oral second-line agent, plus an injectable agent for the first 2–3 mo	18	A longer course (6 mo) of the injectable agent may strengthen the regimen for patients with extensive disease.
H-R	Z, E, injectable agent (for at least first 6 mo), fluoroquinolones, plus one or two oral second-line agents	18–24	One oral second-line agent is sufficient if E and Z susceptibility is well-ascertained. Two oral second-line agents should be used in extensive disease, or if the DST result is questionable (i.e., reported susceptibility to E or Z despite a history of these agents being used in a failing regimen). Surgery, when available, can be considered.
H-R (+/- S) and E or Z	Z, E, injectable agent (for at least first 6 mo), fluoroquinolones, plus two or more oral second-line agents	24	Only use the first-line agents to which the patient is susceptible. Use alternative injectable agent if S resistance present. More than two oral second-line agents should be used in extensive disease or if resistance to E and Z is present or suspected. Surgery, when available, can be considered.

[a] Assumes further acquired resistance is not a factor and laboratory results are reliable.
Source: Adapted from Ref. (122).

clinicians would add pyrazinamide to those regimens because a significant percentage of patients could benefit from the drug.

F. Monitoring the Patient

The systematic and careful monitoring of treatment response (including side effects) is an integral part of the treatment of DR-TB. To establish the baseline mycobacterial burden, sputum specimens for semiquantitative smear and culture should be obtained weekly during the initial part of treatment until conversion is reached (123). The weekly evaluation helps determine when patient isolation can be suspended and allows for an accurate assessment of treatment response. However, programs with very limited laboratory capacity may choose to perform smear and culture monthly until conversion occurs. After conversion, smear and culture should be performed at least every other month while treatment continues. After treatment, smear and culture should be performed twice yearly for two years and thereafter whenever the patient has symptoms suggestive of active TB. Conversion to a negative smear and culture occurs, on average between one and two months (86). Persistence of positive smear or culture past three months after initiating a new regimen should prompt an evaluation of the regimen and the patient's adherence. DST should be repeated on a new specimen.

While bacteriological examination is the main indicator of response to treatment, the patient should also be monitored for weight gain, decrease of cough, absence of fever, and overall clinical progress. Chest radiograph should also be done every three to six months, though radiological signs of improvement will often lag behind bacteriological and clinical indicators. Computerized axial tomography scans better identify cavities that can go unappreciated on chest radiographs. These scans should be done for all patients in whom surgical intervention is a consideration.

DOT is an essential part of the treatment strategy. Clinical and laboratory monitoring for adverse effects depends on the drugs used in the regimen and should be performed according to the information provided in Table 2. Any co-morbid conditions, such as diabetes, HIV, liver disease, alcoholism, etc., may require closer monitoring for side effects. The frequency of adverse effects in 818 patients from five different MDR-TB treatment programs that used DOT is reported in a study by Nathanson et al. (124). The study found that only 2% of patients had to stop treatment completely because of adverse events. Frequent medical encounters with the care provider are essential.

G. Completion of the Injectable Agent (Intensive Phase)

The recommended duration of the injectable agent is guided by smear and culture conversion. The injectable should be continued for a minimum of six months and most practitioners prefer to use the injectable for at least four to six months after the patient first becomes and remains smear- or culture-negative. It is advisable to use an individualized approach and review the patient's cultures, smears, X-rays, and clinical status before stopping the injectable agent. Injections are often extended if extensive lung damage is present. If there is a high level of drug resistance and stopping the injectable could place the patient at risk for failure or early relapse, the injectable can be continued; under extreme circumstances, it can be used throughout the entire treatment.

Intermittent therapy with the injectable agent can be considered for patients who have been on the injectable for a prolonged period of time or when the risk of toxicity becomes a problem. Successful outcomes have been achieved with intermittent dosing (three times a week) of the injectable agent after an initial period of two to three months of daily therapy. However, a high percentage of patients in these cohorts also received surgery, which may have contributed to their successful outcomes (125,126).

H. Length of Treatment

The optimal duration of MDR-TB therapy has not been definitively determined. Generally, it is recommended that treatment lasts for at least 18 to 24 months past culture conversion. In addition to bacteriological results, clinical and radiographic data may be used to determine total treatment duration; treatment for a full 24 months may be indicated in patients with extensive pulmonary damage. The newer generation fluoroquinolones may allow shorter regimens, but to date evidence is lacking and less than 18-month regimens are generally not recommended. Surgical intervention may also allow one to shorten the regimens to less than 18 months in some cases; excellent outcome results from one U.S. treatment center are reported with the use of treatment for 15 to 18 month past conversion when adjuvant surgery was used (126).

I. Surgery in DR-TB

The role of resectional surgery in the management of MDR-TB has not been established through randomized studies. Surgery as an adjunct to chemotherapy for patients with resectable localized disease appears to be beneficial when skilled thoracic surgeons and excellent postoperative care are available (73,126–130). Surgical resection cannot be performed in patients with extensive bilateral disease. While collapse therapy, including thoracoplasty, artificial pneumothorax, and pneumoperitoneum, is commonly used in some parts of the world, we prefer resectional therapy, based on the vast body of experience garnered during the 20th century. There are no clinical trials that directly compare resection to collapse therapy or thoracoplasty; however, case series have shown resectional surgery to be effective and safe under proper conditions (126,131,132).

In settings with limited surgical capacity, patients who remain smear-positive or are resistant to a high number of drugs usually take priority, since they can die without such intervention. General criteria for surgery are localized pulmonary disease, adequate cardiopulmonary reserve, and optimal medical therapy for at least two months. In addition, surgery is often indicated for severe hemoptysis and other pulmonary complications. Even with successful resection, an additional 12 to 24 months of chemotherapy should be given, using the principles of MDR-TB treatment regimen design.

Currently, most resource-limited countries do not have adequate trained staff, materials, or postoperative care to routinely perform surgery on MDR-TB patients. Attempting to perform surgery without adequate expertise, technical capacity, and postoperative care can result in high morbidity and mortality. In addition, surgery should never take the place of, or take priority over, a good chemotherapy program for DR-TB.

J. Treatment of XDR-TB

XDR-TB has been reported in at least 50 countries (see chap. 9), constituting up to 10% of all MDR-TB strains (68,133). It has proven much more difficult to treat than

Table 6 Management Guidelines for a Patient with Documented, or Almost Certain, XDR-TB

1. Use any oral first-line agents that may be effective.
2. Use an injectable agent to which the strain is susceptible and consider an extended duration of use (12 mo or possibly the whole treatment). If resistant to all injectable agents it is recommended to use one the patient has never used before.[a]
3. Use a higher generation fluoroquinolone such as moxifloxacin.
4. Use any bacteriostatic second-line agents (thiamides, cycloserine, terizidone, or PAS) that have not been used extensively in a previous regimen or any that are likely to be effective.
5. Use two or more third-line agents (linezolid, amoxicillin–clavulanate, clofazimine, or clarithromycin).
6. Consider high-dose isoniazid if low-level resistance is documented.
7. Consider adjuvant surgery if there is localized disease.
8. Ensure strong infection control measures.
9. Treat HIV (see chap. 10).
10. Provide comprehensive monitoring (see chap. 11) and full adherence support (see chap. 12).

[a]This recommendation is made because while the reproducibility and reliability of DST to injectables is good, there is little data on clinical efficacy of the test. Options with XDR-TB are very limited and some strains may be affected in vivo by an injectable agent even though they are testing resistant in vitro.
Source: Adapted from Ref. (76).

MDR-TB and extremely difficult in HIV-infected patients (65,68,134,135). Nevertheless, the treatment of XDR-TB is not impossible. Retrospective studies of treatment outcomes of HIV-negative XDR-TB patients have reported cure rates exceeding 50% (136,137). Table 6 summarizes the latest expert consensus on how to manage XDR-TB. There is very limited data on different clinical approaches to XDR-TB and Table 6 is based on WHO recommendations (76).

K. Immune Modulation

For a number of reasons, immune modulation or immunotherapy of the host is an attractive option in the treatment of MDR-TB. First, cure rates could be improved in difficult-to-treat cases. Second, chemotherapeutic regimens might be shortened if adjuvant immunotherapy reduces the time to cure (138). The cytokine γ-interferon has shown the most encouraging results, although most of the studies have been done in patients with a poor chance of recovery by conventional treatment methods (139–143). Interleukin-2 has also been employed, with equivocal results (144). While these modalities are attractive, the evidence to date does not justify their routine use and further investigation in the area of immune modulation is needed.

L. Management of Ultimate Failures

Treatment with second-line drugs is often a patient's last hope for a cure; unfortunately, treatment is not always effective. There is no simple definition for MDR-TB treatment failure. Individualized therapy often consists of a cycle of treatments; if there is no effect, a new plan should be formulated after careful assessment. Often new drugs are added and adjunctive options, most commonly surgery, are entertained.

A single drug should never be added to a failing regimen; if treatment is failing, the best option is to design a new regimen with at least four effective agents. Given the limited number of known antituberculous agents, a wholly new four-drug regimen is often unattainable for patients in whom a regimen of second-line drugs is failing. In these cases, the new regimen should include as many new or potentially efficacious agents as possible. The health care provider should make an extra effort to ensure that patients are taking all their medicines; if care included DOT, the DOT worker should be interviewed. In cases of noncompliance, the contributing conditions should be corrected (i.e., aggressive management of adverse effects) and the response to subsequent therapy observed before treatment failure is declared.

Despite the fact that there is no simple definition for treatment failure, there may come a time when it becomes clear that the treatment is not going to work. Signs indicative of treatment failure include persistent positive smears or cultures past the eighth month of treatment; extensive and bilateral lung disease with no option for surgery; high-grade resistance with no option for adding additional agents; and deterioration in clinical condition, which usually includes weight loss and respiratory insufficiency. The presence of these conditions indicates that cure is highly unlikely.

A number of supportive measures can be implemented once the decision to suspend therapy has been made. Supportive measures include pain control, relief of respiratory insufficiency with oxygen, ongoing nutritional support, and hospitalization or hospice care. Infection control measures should be continued. Some patients can set up home conditions with sufficient space and ventilation along with reliable access to food and other necessities (69). Family members and friends who visit the patient can be provided with personal respirators. When these requisites are in place, there is little risk of further spread. Sanatoria designed for ultimate failures of MDR-TB treatment regimens can also be used for end-of-life care.

Continuing second-line agents when treatment has failed is not recommended because the side effects may add to the suffering at the end of a patient's life in addition to leading to the possible development of XDR-TB strains, which can be transmitted to others. Some experts abandon the less-tolerated and expensive second-line agents and continue the patient on a maintenance program of drugs such as isoniazid, rifampicin, and/or ethambutol (despite the patient being resistant to them) (7). However, there is no firm evidence that this will result in suppression of the bacteria or improve the quality of life. Therefore, we recommend to discontinue all TB medications when no hope for cure remains and to aggressively offer the support measures described above.

M. Drug Adjustment in Renal Insufficiency

Renal insufficiency due to longstanding TB infection or previous aminoglycoside use is not uncommon. Great care should be taken in administering second-line drugs to patients with renal insufficiency and the dose and/or the interval between dosings should

Table 7 Adjustment of Antituberculous Medications in Patients with Renal Insufficiency[a]

Drug	Change in frequency?	Recommended dose[b] and frequency for patients with creatinine clearance <30 mL/min or for patients receiving hemodialysis
Isoniazid	No change	300 mg/day or 900 mg 3×/wk
Rifampicin	No change	600 mg/day or 600 mg 3×/wk
Pyrazinamide	Yes	25–35 mg/kg 3×/wk (not daily)
Ethambutol	Yes	15–25 mg/kg 3×/wk (not daily)
Streptomycin	Yes	12–15 mg/kg 2–3×/wk (not daily)[c]
Capreomycin	Yes	12–15 mg/kg 2–3×/wk (not daily)[c]
Kanamycin	Yes	12–15 mg/kg 2–3×/wk (not daily)[c]
Amikacin	Yes	12–15 mg/kg 2–3×/wk (not daily)[c]
Ciprofloxacin	Yes	1000–1500 mg 3×/wk (not daily)
Ofloxacin	Yes	600–800 mg 3×/wk (not daily)
Levofloxacin	Yes	750–1000 mg 3×/wk (not daily)
Moxifloxacin	No change	400 mg/day
Gatifloxacin	Yes	400 mg 3×/wk (not daily)
Cycloserine	Yes	250 mg/day, or 500 mg/dose 3×/wk[d]
Ethionamide	No change	250–500 mg/day
p-Aminosalicylic acid	No change	4 g 2×/day

[a]The recommended doses are taken from the official joint statement of the American Thoracic Society (ATS), the Centers for Disease Control and Prevention (CDC), and the Infectious Disease Society of America (IDSA) on the Treatment of Tuberculosis (82), except ciprofloxacin, ofloxaxin, moxifloxacin, and gatifloxacin for which the doses are determined from extrapolating data on the recommended renal adjusted doses (91) and to use as close to standard doses as possible to optimize the bactericidal effect of these drugs.
[b]To take advantage of the concentration-dependent bactericidal effect of many antituberculous drugs, standard doses are given unless there is intolerance. For patients on hemodialysis, the medications should be given after hemodialysis on the day of hemodialysis. Data currently are not available for patients receiving peritoneal dialysis. Until data become available, begin with doses recommended for patients receiving hemodialysis and verify adequacy of dosing by using serum concentration monitoring (82).
[c]Caution should be used with injectable agents in patients with renal function impairment because of an increased risk of both ototoxicity and nephrotoxicity (95).
[d]The appropriateness of 250 mg/day doses has not been established. There should be careful monitoring for evidence of neurotoxicity; if possible, measure serum concentrations and adjust regimen accordingly. (82)

be adjusted per Table 7. Sodium salt formulations of PAS may result in an excessive sodium load and may precipitate congestive heart failure in patients with preexisting heart disease worsen fluid retention in patients with renal disease; these formulations should be avoided in such patients. Formulations of PAS that do not include sodium salt (e.g., Jacobus PASER®) can be used without the hazard of sodium retention (121).

N. DR-TB and Diabetes
Patients with immunosuppressive diseases such as diabetes mellitus, vasculitis, long-term corticosteroid therapy, and cancer are at risk for poor outcomes if they develop active

DR-TB. Diabetes, for example, is a common condition in resource-poor settings and may be a risk factor for infection and progression to active TB (145). Diabetic patients who are treated for DR-TB can experience a higher incidence of complications than nondiabetic patients. Gastrointestinal side effects, peripheral neuropathy, and nephrotoxicity can all be potentiated by diabetes. For this reason, improved control of diabetes should be an objective when starting treatment of DR-TB. Creatinine and potassium levels should be monitored more frequently, at least weekly for the first month and then monthly thereafter.

V. DR-TB and HIV

The devastating collision between HIV infection and DR-TB cannot be underestimated. The WHO Fourth Global Report on *Anti-Tuberculosis Drug Resistance* concluded that there was an overall lack of data on HIV serostatus, but in the only two settings with enough HIV-positive cases to examine the relationship, Latvia and Donetsk Oblask, Ukraine, HIV infection was associated with drug resistance and MDR (1). Other data suggests that HIV-positive patients have an increased rate of DR-TB, including MDR-TB (77,78,146,147). There are multiple reports of outbreaks associating MDR-TB and AIDS in New York City (52·148,149) as well as in other parts of the world (150–152). These outbreaks are often associated with delayed diagnosis, extended infectious periods, poor infection control practices, and delayed initiation of appropriate therapy. The development of rifampicin resistance has been associated with HIV therapy. In a case–control study, prior rifabutin use (commonly used as *Mycobacterium avium* prophylaxis), antifungal therapy, and diarrhea were each independently associated with rifampicin monoresistance (153). Finally, numerous studies report dismal outcomes for patients infected with HIV and diagnosed with MDR-TB (51,65,154–157).

HIV testing has become a routine part of TB treatment in many high–HIV-prevalence settings, but should be emphasized in low–HIV-prevalence settings as well. Even in low–HIV-prevalence settings, there may be vulnerable groups with higher rates of HIV infection, who are at increased risk of infection for TB and DR-TB. Routine testing for HIV ensures that patients co-infected with HIV are identified early and evaluated for ART, which can improve DR-TB treatment outcomes.

Given the dire consequences of unaddressed MDR-TB in HIV patients, DST is essential for all HIV-infected individuals diagnosed with TB, especially in settings where drug resistance is common. Prompt diagnosis and initiation of appropriate therapy is particularly critical in patients who are immunocompromised. In a number of retrospective studies of MDR-TB in HIV-positive patients, survival rates were significantly improved if therapy with at least four drugs with in vitro activity was started within one month of diagnosis (7,157,158). In resource-poor settings where access to DST is limited, early diagnosis of DR-TB is a serious problem. In South Africa, for example, DST results showing MDR-TB or XDR-TB may arrive only after the patient has died (159).

There is limited data about the optimal timing of initiation of ART for HIV during MDR-TB treatment. We start ART in all HIV co-infected patients as soon as second-line TB drugs are tolerated, regardless of CD4 count. This practice is based on increasing evidence about the beneficial effect of ART during the treatment of drug-susceptible TB (160). Early initiation of ART must be balanced against risk of immune reconstitution syndrome, confusing side effects, and a higher pill burden. However, anecdotal data from physicians experienced with the management of MDR-TB/HIV co-infection indicates that immune reconstitution syndrome is rare, and that ART is usually well-tolerated compared to second-line antituberculous drugs (161). While it is likely that ART offers improvement in the immune system for patients co-infected with HIV with MDR-TB at any CD4 count, more studies are needed to determine the optimal time to begin ART.

Currently, little is known about drug–drug interactions between anti-TB agents used for DR-TB and ART. There are several known interactions between drugs used to treat HIV and TB and these are summarized below (76):

- **Rifamycin derivatives**—While rifamycin derivatives are not routinely used in DR-TB treatment, they are used in the treatment of rifampicin-sensitive\and monoresistant TB. Guidance on use of rifamycin derivative–based regimens and ART (including with PI-based regimens) is provided in chapter 6.
- **Quinolones and didanosine**—Buffered didanosine contains an aluminum-/magnesium-based antacid and if given jointly with fluoroquinolones may result in decreased fluoroquinolone absorption (162); it should be avoided, but if necessary it should be given six hours before or two hours after fluoroquinolone administration. The enteric-coated (EC) formulation of didanosine can be used concomitantly without this precaution.
- **Ethionamide/prothionamide**—Based on limited information about the metabolism of the thiamides (ethionamide and prothionamide), this drug class may have interactions with antiretroviral drugs. Ethionamide/prothionamide is thought to be metabolized by the CYP450 system, though it is not known which of the CYP enzymes are responsible. Whether doses of ethionamide/prothionamide and/or certain antiretroviral drugs should be modified during the concomitant treatment of DR-TB and HIV is unknown (163).
- **Clarithromycin**—Clarithromycin is a substrate and inhibitor of CYP3A and has multiple drug interactions with protease inhibitors and NNRTIs. If possible avoid the use of clarithromycin in patients co-infected with DR-TB and HIV because of both its weak efficacy against DR-TB and multiple drug interactions.

A reasonable choice for a first-line ART regimen in an MDR-TB patient newly diagnosed with HIV is two nucleoside reverse transcriptase inhibitors (zidovudine or stavudine plus lamivudine) and one nonnucleoside reverse transcriptase inhibitor (efavirenz or nevirapine). It is difficult to make a blanket recommendation for a first-line ART regimen, since many patients may have contraindications for use of one of these drugs, such as peripheral neuropathy or anemia. Other commonly used first-line drugs such as abacavir or tenofovir may be reserved for cases in which zidovudine or stavudine are not tolerated, but further research is needed into the optimal first-line antiretroviral regimens for MDR-TB patients co-infected with HIV.

The management of DR-TB in the presence of HIV co-infection is particularly challenging due to an increased incidence of adverse effects. The reason for this is not well understood, and urgently needs further research, but it is likely to be multifactorial and related to general poor clinical status and the great number of medications that patients are often taking concurrently for treatment of TB, HIV, and opportunistic infections.

Identifying the source of adverse effects in patients receiving concomitant therapy for DR-TB and HIV is difficult. Many of the medications used to treat HIV, DR-TB, and other opportunistic infections have overlapping, or in some cases additive, toxicities. Often it may not be possible to link side effects to a single drug. Furthermore, the risk of drug resistance for ART or TB therapy precludes the typical medical challenge of stopping all medications and starting them one by one. Table 8 (76) lists adverse effects that are common to both antiretroviral and anti-TB drugs.

It should be noted that relatively very little is known about the rates of adverse effects in the concomitant treatment of DR-TB and HIV. Further research is urgently needed into the adverse effects of second-line anti-TB drugs in patients with HIV co-infection. Adverse effects such as hypothyroidism, electrolyte wasting, nephrotoxicity, and peripheral neuropathy may prove to be more common in high–HIV-prevalence settings (161). Given that the current understanding is limited and that the use of drugs with overlapping toxicities is unavoidable at the current time, we recommend more intense monitoring for adverse effects in HIV co-infected patients.

DR-TB in HIV-infected patients is highly lethal and a growing problem in many parts of the world. Realizing the control, diagnosis, and treatment strategies put forth in this chapter are important steps to stem the epidemic of HIV-associated DR-TB.

VI. Factors Associated with Good Treatment Outcomes

With timely and appropriate therapy (including, when appropriate, resectional surgery), MDR-TB can be cured. While not all programs and studies have reported favorable results, promising cure rates of 66% to 100% have been documented in countries with low (United States (126,164,165), Canada (166), New Zealand (167), the Netherlands (168), and Denmark (169) as well as high (South Korea (170), Turkey (171), Hong Kong SAR (172), Peru (86), Bangladesh (119), and Latvia (88)) TB burdens. While no formal randomized controlled studies have been performed, there appear to be a number of factors associated with better MDR-TB treatment outcomes. The three most important factors that result in positive outcomes are (*i*) early diagnosis and treatment initiation, (*ii*) provision of an adequate regimen with a sufficient number of effective drugs, and (*iii*) provision of extensive treatment support, especially in the area of side effect management.

Early diagnosis and prompt entrance into an adequate treatment regimen with second-line drugs are the most critical factors. In particular, cycling patients through repeated ineffective first-line treatment courses is associated with worse outcomes because of increased lung damage and decreased drug efficacy. Furthermore, delays in initiating therapy often result in chronic, cachectic patients who have difficulty tolerating second-line drugs, thus further increasing the likelihood of poor outcomes.

The second critical factor to ensure better outcomes is to treat patients with adequate regimens before resistance patterns worsen. Mitnick et al. demonstrated that resistance to ethambutol and pyrazinamide is associated with poorer outcomes (86). Not being able to use an injectable (173) or a quinolone (126) is also associated with worse outcomes, as is XDR-TB (68). Patients in whom a second-line drug containing regimen failed may be very difficult to cure (173). Therefore, weak re-treatment regimens that have suboptimal cure rates should be avoided. While the optimal number of drugs in a re-treatment regimen has not been determined, the WHO as well as we advocate for at least four drugs (and preferably five at the start of treatment) to which the patient's isolate is considered to be susceptible, with a continuation phase of three to four drugs (76).

Third, extensive treatment support for the DR-TB patient, including DOT and aggressive side effect management, is crucial. Although there is ongoing debate about the necessity of DOT in regular TB treatment, these arguments do not hold for DR-TB.

Table 8 Potential Overlapping and Additive Toxicities of ART and Antituberculous Therapy

Toxicity	Antiretroviral agent	Antituberculosis agent	Comments
Peripheral neuropathy	**D4T, ddI, ddC**	**Lzd, Cs, H,** aminoglyco-sides, Eto/Pto, E	Avoid use of D4T, ddI, and ddC in combination with Cs of Lzd because of theoretically increased peripheral neuropathy. If these agents must be used and peripheral neuropathy develops, replace the ARV agent with a less neurotoxic agent.
Central nervous system (CNS) toxicity	**EFV**	**Cs,** H, Eto/Pto, fluoro-quinolones	Efavirenz has a high rate of CNS side effects (confusion, impaired concentration, depersonalization, abnormal dreams, insomnia, and dizziness) in the first 2–3 wk, which typically resolve on their own. If the CNS side effects do not resolve on their own consider substitution of the agent. At present, there are limited data on the use of EFV with Cs; concurrent use is accepted practice with frequent monitoring for CNS toxicity. Frank psychosis is rare with EFV alone.
Depression	**EFV**	**Cs,** fluoro-quinolones, H, Eto/Pto	Severe depression can be seen in 2.4% of patients receiving EFV.[a] Consider substituting for EFV if severe depression develops. The severe socioeconomic circumstances of many patients with chronic disease can also contribute to depression.
Headache	**AZT, EFV**	**Cs**	Rule out more serious causes of headache such as bacterial meningitis, cryptococcal meningitis, CNS toxoplasmosis, etc. Use of analgesics (ibuprofen, paracetamol) and good hydration may help. Headache secondary to AZT, EFV, and Cs is usually self-limited.
Nausea and vomiting	**RTV, D4T, NVP,** and most others	**Eto/Pto, PAS, H, E, Z,** and others	Nausea and vomiting are common adverse effects and can be managed. Persistent vomiting and abdominal pain may be a result of developing lactic acidosis and/or hepatitis secondary to medications.

Table 8 (*Continued*)

Toxicity	Antiretroviral agent	Antituberculosis agent	Comments
Abdominal pain	**All ART treatment has been associated with abdominal pain**	Eto/Pto, PAS	Abdominal pain is a common adverse effect and often benign; however, abdominal pain may be an early symptom of severe adverse effects such as pancreatitis, hepatitis, or lactic acidosis.
Pancreatitis	**D4T, ddI, ddC**	Lzd	Avoid use of these agents together. If an agent causes pancreatitis suspend it permanently and do not use any of the pancreatitis producing anti-HIV medications (D4T, ddI, or ddC) in the future. Also consider gallstones or alcohol as a potential cause of pancreatitis.
Diarrhea	**All protease inhibitors, ddI (buffered formula)**	Eto/Pto, PAS, fluoro- quinolones	Diarrhea is a common adverse effect. Also consider opportunistic infections as a cause of diarrhea, or clostridium difficile (a cause of pseudomembranous colitis).
Hepatotoxicity	**NVP, EFV, all protease inhibitors (RTV > other protease inhibitors), all NRTIs**	H, R, E, Z, PAS, Eto/Pto, fluo- roquinolones	Also consider TMP/SMX as a cause of hepatotoxicity if the patient is receiving this medication. Also rule out viral etiologies as cause of hepatitis (hepatitis A, B, C, and CMV).
Skin rash	**ABC, NVP, EFV, D4T,** and others	H,R, Z, PAS, flu- oroquinolones, and others	Do not rechallenge with ABC (can result in life threatening anaphylaxis). Do not rechallenge with an agent that caused Steven-Johnson syndrome. Also consider TMP/SMX as a cause of skin rash if the patient is receiving this medication. Thioacetazone is contraindicated in HIV because of life-threatening rash.
Lactic acidosis	**D4T, ddI, AZT, 3TC**	Lzd	If an agent causes lactic acidosis replace it with an agent less likely to cause lactic acidosis.

Table 8 (*Continued*)

Toxicity	Antiretroviral agent	Antituberculosis agent	Comments
Renal toxicity	TDF (rare)	**aminoglycosides, Cm**	TDF may cause renal injury with the characteristic features of Fanconi syndrome, hypophosphatemia, hypouricemia, proteinuria, normoglycemic glycosuria, and in some cases acute renal failure. There is no data on the concurrent use of TDF with aminoglycosides or Cm. Use TDF with caution in patients receiving aminoglycosides or Cm. Even without the concurrent use of TDF, HIV-infected patients have an increased risk of renal toxicity secondary to aminoglycosides and Cm. Frequent creatinine and electrolyte monitoring every 1–3 wk is recommended. Many ARVs and antituberculosis medications need to be dose adjusted for renal insufficiency.
Nephrolithiasis	**IDV**	None	No overlapping toxicities regarding nephrolithiasis have been documented between ART and antituberculosis medications. Adequate hydration prevents nephrolithiasis in patients taking IDV. If nephrolithiasis develops while on IDV, substitute with another protease inhibitor if possible.
Electrolyte disturbances	TDF (rare)	**Cm, aminoglycosides**	Diarrhea and/or vomiting can contribute to electrolyte disturbances. Even without the concurrent use of TDF, HIV-infected patients have an increased risk of both renal toxicity and electrolyte disturbances secondary to aminoglycosides and Cm.
Bone marrow suppression	AZT	**Lzd**, R, Rfb, H	Monitor blood counts regularly. Replace AZT if bone marrow suppression develops. Consider suspension of Lzd. Also consider TMP/SMX as a cause if the patient is receiving this medication. Consider adding folinic acid supplements, especially if receiving TMP/SMX.
Optic neuritis	ddI	**E,** Eto/Pto (rare)	Suspend agent responsible for optic neuritis permanently and replace with an agent that does not cause optic neuritis.

Table 8   (*Continued*)

Toxicity	Antiretroviral agent	Antituberculosis agent	Comments
Hyperlipidemia	**Protease inhibitors, EFV**	None	No overlapping toxicities regarding hyperlipidemia have been documented between ART and antituberculosis medications. Follow WHO ART guidelines for management of hyperlipidemia (160).
Lipodystrophy	**NRTIs (especially D4T and ddI)**	None	No overlapping toxicities regarding lipodystrophy have been documented between ART and antituberculosis medications. Follow WHO ART guidelines for management of lipodystrophy (160).
Dysglycemia (disturbed blood sugar regulation)	**Protease inhibitors**	**Gfx**, Eto/Pto	Protease inhibitors tend to cause insulin resistance and hyperglycemia. Eto/Pto tend to make insulin control in diabetic patients more difficult, and can result in hypoglycemia and poor glucose regulation. Gatifloxacin is no longer recommended by the GLC for use in treatment of TB due to this side effect.
Hypothyroidism	D4T	**Eto/Pto, PAS**	There is potential for overlying toxicity, however evidence is mixed. Several studies show subclinical hypothyroidism associated with HAART, particularly stavudine. PAS and Eto/Pto, especially in combination, can commonly cause hypothyroidism.

Drugs that are more strongly associated with the side effects appear in bold.
[a]Bristol-Myers Squibb, letter to providers, March 2005.
Source: Adapted from Ref. (76).

DR-TB treatment is very difficult and toxic, and patients need full accompaniment throughout treatment to ensure the best outcomes.

There are a number of other factors that may improve patient outcomes, including surgical interventions (discussed in sect. IV.I), drug level monitoring, patient support groups (174), patient incentives, social support, patient and family education, and nutritional supplementation. The extent of these factors on improving cure rates has not been documented.

VII. Summary

DR-TB incidence and prevalence are alarmingly high in many areas of the world and DR-TB exists in all countries (1). DR-TB knows no borders, and even areas where DR-TB is under control are vulnerable (175). DR-TB patients are largely overlooked in many parts of the world, despite the fact that highly effective treatment has been available for over 40 years. To prevent the situation from worsening and to provide much-needed treatment to the hundreds of thousands of prevalent MDR-TB cases, massive financial, technical, and human resources must be mobilized. Within the past decade, the WHO has begun to systematically address DR-TB through the STOP TB strategy (76,176).

DR-TB treatment programs must have adequate protocols and guidelines, qualified personnel, access to microbiological laboratories, constant and reliable supplies of medications, ability to treat side effects, and well-established nutritional and psychosocial support systems. DOT should be used throughout the treatment (177). Regimens consisting of multiple drugs, which are generally more difficult to take, must be administrated for 18 to 24 months. Resectional surgery may be required for certain patients. The convergence of the AIDS and TB epidemics further challenges treatment and infection control efforts.

DR-TB treatment must be integrated into national TB control programs. The faucet of MDR-TB must be turned off—for most areas, this translates to continued efforts and emphasis on DOTS expansion. The quality of first-line drugs must be assured in all countries, as resistance will continue to rise in many areas even with DOTS expansion if drug quality is poor. Improving laboratory capacity will be a significant expenditure: it has been argued that the lack of proper laboratory services is not a matter of affordability, but rather a misguided underestimation of their importance (178).

Incorporating DR-TB prevention and treatment into national health programs will require long-term commitment from governments and international agencies, both in terms of funding and political support. Modest goals and poor strategies will result in hundreds of thousands of deaths as well as maintaining the worldwide persistence of resistant *M. tuberculosis*. At a time when we are aiming to put millions on lifelong HIV therapy (179), arguments against DR-TB treatment that cite high costs and lack of infrastructure no longer hold sway (180). DR-TB must be given proper priority through ambitious goal setting and aggressive, comprehensive prevention, case finding, and treatment.

References

1. World Health Organization. Anti-Tuberculosis Drug Resistance in the World: Fourth Global Report. Geneva, Switzerland, World Health Organization, 2008.
2. Wolinsky E, Reginster A, Steenken W. Drug-resistant tubercle bacilli in patients under treatment with streptomycin. Am Rev Tuberc 1948; 58:335.
3. Medical Research Council. Streptomycin treatment of pulmonary tuberculosis: A Medical Research Council investigation. Brit Med J 1948; 2:769–782.
4. Long ER. The Chemotherapy of Tuberculosis. Baltimore, Maryland: Williams & Wilkins Co., 1958.

5. Partners In Health. DOTS-Plus Handbook: A guide to community based treatment of MDR-TB. Partners In Health (www.pih.org), Harvard Medical School, Bill and Melinda Gates Foundation. 2001.
6. Mukherjee JS, Rich ML, Socci AR, et al. Programmes and principles in treatment of multidrug-resistant tuberculosis. Lancet 2004; 363:474–481.
7. Iseman MD, Huitt GA. Treatment of multidrug-resistant tuberculosis. In: Bastian I, Portaels F, eds. Multidrug-Resistant Tuberculosis. London, UK: Kluwer Academic Publishers, 2000:175–190.
8. Chan ED, Iseman MD. Current medical treatment for tuberculosis. Brit Med J 2002; 325(7375):1282–1286.
9. Farmer PE. Social scientists and the new tuberculosis. Soc Sci Med 1997; 44(3):347–358.
10. Farmer PE, Robin S, Kim JY, et al. Tuberculosis, poverty, and "compliance": lessons from rural Haiti. Sem Respir Infect 1991; 6(4):254–260.
11. Farmer PE. Infections and Inequalities: The Modern Plagues. Berkley, California: University of California Press, 1998.
12. Alangaden G, Kreiswirth BN, Aouad A, et al. Mechanism of resistance to amikacin and kanamycin in *Mycobacterium tuberculosis*. Antimicrob Agents Chemother 1998; 42(5): 1295–1297.
13. Allen BW, Mitchison DA. Amikacin in the treatment of pulmonary tuberculosis. Tubercle 1983; 64(2):111–118.
14. McClatchy JK, Kanes W, Davidson PT, et al. Cross-resistance in M. tuberculosis to kanamycin, capreomycin and viomycin. Tubercle 1977; 58(1):29–34.
15. Cooksey RC, Morlock GP, Crawford JT, et al. Characterization of streptomycin resistance mechanisms among *Mycobacterium tuberculosis* isolates from patients in New York City. Antimicrob Agents Chemother 1996; 40(5):1186–1188.
16. Maranetra KN. Quinolones and multidrug-resistant tuberculosis. Chemotherapy 1996; 45(S2):12–18.
17. Ruiz-Serrano MJ, Alcala L, Bouza E, et al. In vitro activities of six fluoroquinolones against 250 clinical isolates of M. tuberculosis susceptible or resistant to first-line anti-tuberculosis medications. Antimicrob Agents Chemother 2000; 44(9):2567–2568.
18. Alangaden G, Manavathu EK, Lerner SA, et al. Characterization of fluoroquinolone-resistant mutant strains of *Mycobacterium tuberculosis* selected in the laboratory and isolated from patients. Antimicrob Agents Chemother 1995; 39(8):700–1703.
19. Grimaldo ER, Tupasi TE, Rivera AB, et al. Increased resistance to ciprofloxacin and ofloxacin in multidrug-resistant *Mycobacterium tuberculosis* isolates from patients seen at a tertiary hospital in the Philippines. Int J Tuberc Lung Dis 2001; 5(6):546–550.
20. Zhao BY, Pine R, Domagala J, at al. Fluoroquinolone action against clinical isolates of *Mycobacterium tuberculosis*: effects of a C-8 methoxyl group on survival in liquid media and in human macrophages. Antimicrob Agents Chemother 1999; 43(3):661–666.
21. Dong Y, Xu C, Zhao X, et al. Fluoroquinolone action against mycobacteria: effects of C-8 substituents on growth, survival, and resistance. Antimicrob Agents Chemother 1998; 42(11):2978–2984.
22. Lounis N, Ji B, Grosset J. Which aminoglycoside or fluoroquinolone is more active against *Mycobacterium tuberculosis* in mice? Antimicrob Agents Chemother 1997; 41(3):607–610.
23. Tsukamura M. Cross-resistance of tubercle bacilli. Kekkaku 1977; 52(2):47–49.
24. Lefford MJ. The ethionamide susceptibility of East African strains of *Mycobacterium tuberculosis* resistant to thiacetazone. Tubercle 1969; 50(1):7–13.
25. Canetti G. Present aspects of bacterial resistance in tuberculosis. Am Rev Respir Dis 1965; 92(5):687–703.
26. Lefford MJ. The ethionamide susceptibility of British pre-treatment strains of *Mycobacterium tuberculosis*. Tubercle 1966; 47(2):198–206.

27. Canetti G, Kreis B, Le Lirzin M. Current data on primary resistance in pulmonary tuberculosis in adults in France. Second survey of the Centre d'Etudes sur la Resistance Primaire: 1965–1966. Rev Tuberc Pneumol 1967; 31(4):433–474.

28. Lee H, Cho SN, Kim JD, et al. Exclusive mutations related to isoniazid and ethionamide resistance among *Mycobacterium tuberculosis* isolates from Korea. Int J Tuberc Lung Dis 2000; 4(5):441–447.

29. Banerjee A, Dubnau E, Jacobs WR, et al. inhA, a gene encoding a target for isoniazid and ethionamide in *Mycobacterium tuberculosis*. Science 1994; 263(5144):227–230.

30. Chien HP, Yu MC, Luh KT, et al. In vitro activity of rifabutin and rifampin against clinical isolates of *Mycobacterium tuberculosis* in Taiwan. J Formos Med Assoc 2000; 99(5): 408–411.

31. Sintchenko V, Chew WK, Gilbert GL, et al. Mutations in rpoB gene and rifabutin susceptibility of multidrug-resistant *Mycobacterium tuberculosis* strains isolated in Australia. Pathology 1999; 31(3):257–260.

32. Yang B, Koga H, Ohno H, et al. Relationship between antimycobacterial activities of rifampicin, rifabutin and KRM-1648 and rpoB mutations of *Mycobacterium tuberculosis*. J Antimicrob Chemother 1998; 42(5):621–628.

33. Williams DL, Spring L, Collins L, et al. Contribution of rpoB mutations to development of rifamycin cross-resistance in *Mycobacterium tuberculosis*. Antimicrob Agents Chemother 1998; 42(7):1853–1857.

34. Cohn ML, Kovitz C, Oda U, et al. Studies on isoniazid and tubercle bacilli, II. The growth requirements, catalase activities, and pathogenic properties of isoniazid-resistant mutants. Am Rev Tuberc 1954; 70(4):641–664.

35. Iseman MD. A Clinician's Guide to Tuberculosis. Philadelphia, PA: Lippincott Williams & Wilkins, 2000; 333–334.

36. Garcia-Garcia ML, Ponce de Leon A, Jimenz-Corona ME, et al. Clinical consequences and transmissibility of drug-resistant tuberculosis in southern Mexico. Arch Intern Med 2000; 160(5):630–636.

37. Burgos M, DeRiemer K, Small PM, et al. Effect of drug resistance on the generation of secondary cases of tuberculosis. J Infect Dis 2003; 188(12):1878–1884.

38. Simone PM, Dooley SW. Multidrug-Resistant Tuberculosis, 1994. National Center for HIV, STD, and TB Prevention, http://www.cdc.gov/nchstp/tb/pubs/mdrtb/mdrtb.htm. Accessed December 2004.

39. Freiden TR, Sherman LF, Maw KL, et al. A multi-institutional outbreak of highly drug-resistant tuberculosis: epidemiology and clinical outcomes. JAMA 1996; 276(15):1229–1235.

40. Snider DE, Kelly GD, Kilburn JO, et al. Infection and disease among contacts of tuberculosis cases with drug-resistant and drug-susceptible bacilli. Am Rev Respir Dis 1985; 132(1): 125–132.

41. Blower SM, Chou T. Modeling the emergence of the "hot zones": tuberculosis and the amplification dynamics of drug resistance. Nat Med 2004; 10(10):1111–1116.

42. Cohen T, Murray M. Modelling epidemics of multidrug-resistant M. tuberculosis of heterogeneous fitness. Nat Med 2004; 10(10):1117–1121.

43. Gagneux S, Long CD, Small PM, et al. The competitive cost of antibiotic resistance in *Mycobacterium tuberculosis*. Science. 2006; 312(5782):1944–1946.

44. Genewein A, Telenti A, Bernasconi C, et al. Molecular approach to identifying route of transmission of tuberculosis in the community. Lancet 1993; 342(8875):841–844.

45. Small PM, Hopewell PC, Singh SP, et al. The epidemiology of tuberculosis in San Francisco. A population-based study using conventional and molecular methods. N Engl J Med 1994; 330(24):1703–1709.

46. Alland D, Kalkut GE, Moss AR, et al. Transmission of tuberculosis in New York City. An analysis by DNA fingerprinting and conventional epidemiological methods. N Engl J Med 1994; 330(24):1710–1716.

47. Friedman CR, Stoeckle MY, Kreiswirth BN, et al. Transmission of multidrug-resistant tuberculosis in a large urban setting. Am J Respir Crit Care Med 1995; 152(1):355–359.

48. Portaels F, Rigouts L, Bastian I. Addressing multidrug-resistant tuberculosis in penitentiary hospitals and in the general population of the former Soviet Union. Int J Tuberc Lung Dis 1999; 3(7):582–588.

49. Kritski AL, Marques MJ, Rabahi MF, et al. Transmission of tuberculosis to close contacts of patients of multidrug-resistant tuberculosis. Am J Respir Crit Care Med 1996; 153(1):331–335.

50. Centers for Disease Control. Nosocomial transmission of multidrug-resistant TB to health-care workers and HIV-infected patients in an urban hospital— Florida. MMWR Morb Mortal Wkly Rep 1990; 39(40):718–722.

51. Centers for Disease Control. Nosocomial transmission of multidrug-resistant tuberculosis among HIV-infected persons—Florida and New York, 1988–1991. JAMA 1991; 266(11):1483–1485.

52. Edlin BR, Tokars JI, Grieco MH, et al. An outbreak of multidrug-resistant tuberculosis among hospitalized patients with the acquired immunodeficiency syndrome. N Engl J Med 1992; 326(23):1514–1521.

53. Pearson ML, Jereb JA, Frieden TR, et al. Nosocomial transmission of multidrug-resistant *Mycobacterium tuberculosis*: a risk to patients and health care workers. Ann Intern Med 1992; 117(3):191–196.

54. Beck-Sague C, Dooley SW, Hutton MD, et al. Outbreak of multidrug-resistant *Mycobacterium tuberculosis* infections in a hospital: transmission to patients with HIV infection and staff. JAMA 1992; 268(10):1280–1286.

55. World Health Organization. Anti-Tuberculosis Drug Resistance in the World: Report No. 1. Geneva, Switzerland: World Health Organization, 1997.

56. World Health Organization. Global tuberculosis control: surveillance, planning, financing. Geneva, Switzerland: World Health Organization, 2008. WHO/HTM/TB/2008.393.

57. Espinal M. Kim SJ, Suarez PG, et al. Standard short-course chemotherapy for drug-resistant tuberculosis: treatment outcomes in six countries. JAMA 2000; 283(19):2537–2545.

58. Migliori GB, Espinal M, Raviglione MC, et al. Frequency of recurrence among MDR-TB cases "successfully" treated with standardized short-course chemotherapy. Int J Tuberc Lung Dis 2002; 6(10):858–864.

59. Farmer PE, Bayona J, Furin J, et al. The dilemma of MDR-TB in the global era. Int J Tuberc Lung Dis 1998; 2(11):869–876.

60. Farmer PE. Managerial success, clinical failures. Int J Tuberc Lung Dis 1999; 3(5):365–367.

61. Seung KJ, Gelmanova IE, Peremitin GG, et al. The effect of initial drug resistance on treatment response and acquired drug resistance during standardized short-course chemotherapy for tuberculosis. Clin Infect Dis 2004; 39(9):1321–1328.

62. Pasechnikov AD. Medical Director Tomsk Project, Partners In Health, Tomsk, Russia. Personal communication, 2003.

63. Pablos-Mendez A, Gowda DK, Frieden TR. Controlling multidrug-resistant tuberculosis and access to expensive drugs: a rational framework. Bull World Health Organ 2002; 80(6):489–495.

64. Espinal MA. Outbreaks of MDRTB involving HIV-infected patients. In: Bastian I, Portaels F, eds. Multidrug-Resistant Tuberculosis. London, UK: Kluwer Academic Publishers, 2000: 50–51.

65. Gandhi NR, Moll A, Sturm AW, et al. Extensively drug-resistant tuberculosis as a cause of death in patients co-infected with tuberculosis and HIV in a rural area of South Africa. Lancet. 2006; 368(9547):1575–1580.

66. Pillay M, Sturm AW. Evolution of the extensively drug-resistant F15/LAM4/KZN strain of *Mycobacterium tuberculosis* in KwaZulu-Natal, South Africa. Clin Infect Dis 2007; 45(11):1409–1414.

67. The Global MDR-TB and XDR-TB Response Plan 2007–2008. Geneva, Switzerland; World Health Organization, 2007 (WHO/HTM/TB/2007.387).

68. Center for Disease Control. Emergence of *Mycobacterium tuberculosis* with extensive resistance to second-line drugs – worldwide, 2000–2004. MMWR Morb Mortal Wkly Rep 2006; 55(11):301–305.

69. Goble MD. Drug Resistance. In: Friedman LN, eds. Tuberculosis: Current Concepts and Treatment, 2nd ed. New York: CRC Press, 2001:333–376.

70. Kritski AL, Rodrigues de Jesus LS, Andrade MK, et al. Retreatment tuberculosis cases: factors associated with drug resistance and adverse outcomes. Chest 1997; 111(5):1162–1167.

71. Farmer P, Bayona J, Becerra M et al. The dilemma of MDR-TB in the global era. Int J Tuberc Lung Dis 1998; 2(11):869–878.

72. Rigouts L, Portaels F. DNA fingerprinting of *Mycobacterium tuberculosis* do not change during the development of resistance to various anti-tuberculosis drugs. Tuberc Lung Dis 1994; 75(2):160.

73. Iseman MD. Management of multidrug-resistant tuberculosis. Chemotherapy 1999; 45(S2):3–11.

74. Chaulk PC, Kazandjian VA. Directly observed therapy for treatment completion of pulmonary tuberculosis: consensus statement of the public health tuberculosis guidelines panel. JAMA 1998; 279(12):943–948.

75. Farmer PE, Walton DA, Becerra MC. International tuberculosis control in the 21st century. In: Friedman LN, eds. Tuberculosis: Current Concepts and Treatment, 2nd ed. New York: CRC Press, 2001:475–496.

76. World Health Organization. Guidelines for the Programmatic Management of Drug-Resistant Tuberculosis, Emergency Update. Geneva, Switzerland: World Health Organization, 2008.

77. Gordin FM, Nelson ET, Matts JP, et al. The impact of human immunodeficiency virus infection on drug-resistant tuberculosis. Am J Respir Crit Care Med 1996;154:1478–1483.

78. Campos PE, Suarez PG, Holmes KK, et al. Multidrug-resistant *Mycobacterium tuberculosis* in HIV-infected persons, Peru. Emerg Infect Dis 2003; 9(12):1571–1578.

79. Davies AP, Billington OJ, McHugh DA, et al. Comparison of Phenotypic and Genotypic Methods for Pyrazinamide Susceptibility Testing with *Mycobacterium tuberculosis*. J Clin Microbiol 2000; 38(10):3686–3688.

80. Laszlo A. Scientist. Geneva, Switzerland: World Health Organization. Personal communications. November 2004.

81. World Health Organization. Guidelines of Drug Susceptibility Testing for Second-Line Anti-Tuberculosis Drugs in DOTS-Plus Programs; (WHO/CDS/TB/2001.288). Geneva, Switzerland: World Health Organization, 2001.

82. American Thoracic Society/Centers for Disease Control and Prevention/Infectious Diseases Society of America. Treatment of tuberculosis. Am J Respir Crit Care Med 2003; 167(4): 603–662.

83. Kim SJ, Espinal MA, et al. Is second-line anti-tuberculosis drug susceptibility testing reliable? Int J Tuberc Lung Dis 2004; 8(9):1157–1158.

84. Kim SJ. Consultant, Union of Tuberculosis and Lung Disease. Personal communication, 2008.

85. Barnard M, Albert H, Coetzee G, et al. Rapid molecular screening for multidrug-resistant tuberculosis in a high-volume public health laboratory in South Africa. Am J Respir Crit Care Med 2008; 177:787–792.

86. Mitnick C, Bayona J, Palacios E, et al. Community-based therapy for multidrug-resistant tuberculosis in Lima, Peru. N Engl J Med 2003; 348(2):119–128.

87. Farmer PE, Kim JY. Community-based approaches to the control of multi-drug-resistant tuberculosis: Introducing DOTS-Plus. Brit Med J 1998; 317(7159):671–674.

88. Leimane V, Riekstina V, Holtz TH, et al. Clinical outcome of individualised treatment of multidrug-resistant tuberculosis in Lativa: a retrospective cohort study. Lancet 2005; 365: 318–326.

89. Katiyar SK, Bihari S, Prakash S, et al. A randomized controlled trial of high-dose isoniazid adjuvant therapy for multidrug-reisistant tuberculosis. Int J Tuberc Lung Dis 2008; 12(2): 139–145.

90. Laserson KF, Thorpe LE, Leimane V. et al. Speaking the same language: treatment outcome definitions for multidrug-resistant tuberculosis. Int J Tuberc Lung Dis 2005; 9(6): 640–645.

91. Gilbert DN, Moellering RC Jr, Eliopoulos GM, et al. The Sanford Guide to Antimicrobial Therapy, 34th ed. Hyde Park Vermont, USA: Antimicrobial Therapy Inc., 2004:91–92.

92. Shin SS, Furin JJ, Alcántara FV, et al. Hypokalemia among patients receiving treatment for multidrug-resistant tuberculosis. Chest 2004; 125(3):974–980.

93. Peloquin CA, Auclair A. Pharmacology of the second-line antituberculosis drugs. In: Bastian I, Portaels F, eds. Multidrug-Resistant Tuberculosis. London, UK: Kluwer Academic Publishers, 2000:167.

94. Kucers A, Bennett NMck, eds. The Use of Antibiotics, 5th ed. Philadelphia, PA: Lippincott Williams and Wilkins, 1988.

95. Rich ML, ed. Partners In Health. PIH Guide to the Medical Management of Multidrug-Resistant Tuberculosis. Boston, MA: Partners In Health, 2003:107–111.

96. Physician's Desk Reference, 59th ed. USA: Medical Economics, 2005.

97. Ntziora F, Falagas ME. Linezolid for the treatment of patients with mycobacterial infections: a systematic review. Int J Tuberc Lung Dis 2007; 11(6):606–611.

98. Matsumoto M, Hashizume H, Tomishige T, et al. OPC-67683, a nitro-dihydro-imidazooxazole derivative with promising action against tuberculosis in vitro and in mice. PLoS Med 2006; 3(11):e466.

99. Rustomjee R, Diacon AH, Allen J, et al. Early bactericidal activity and pharmacokinetics of the diarylquinoline TMC207 in treatment of pulmonary tuberculosis. Antimicrob Agents Chemother 2008; 52(8):2831–2835.

100. Hu Y, Coates AR, Mitchison DA. Comparison of the sterilising activities of the nitroimidazopyran PA-824 and moxifloxacin against persisting *Mycobacterium tuberculosis*. Int J Tuberc Lung Dis 2008; 12(1):69–73.

101. Wells CD, Cegielski JP, Nelson LJ, et al. HIV infection and multidrug-resistant tuberculosis: the perfect storm. J Infect Dis 2007; 196 (suppl 1):S86–S107.

102. Schaaf HS, Van Rie A, Gie RP, et al. Transmission of multidrug-resistant tuberculosis. Pediatr Infect Dis J 2000; 19(8):695–699.

103. Teixeira L, Perkins MD, Johnson JL, et al. Infection and disease among household contacts of patients with multidrug-resistant tuberculosis. Int J Tuberc Lung Dis 2001; 5: 321–328.

104. Schaaf HS, Gie RP, Kennedy M, et al. Evaluation of young children in contact with adult multidrug-resistant pulmonary tuberculosis: a 30-month follow-up. Pediatrics. 2002; 109(5):765–771.

105. Bayona J, Chavez-Pachas AM, Palacios E, et al. Contact investigations as a means of detection and timely treatment of persons with infectious multidrug-resistant tuberculosis.Int J Tuberc Lung Dis 2003; 7(12 suppl 3):S501–S509.

106. Horne NW, Grant IW. Development of drug resistance to isoniazid during desensitization: a report of two cases. Tubercle 1963; 44:180–182.

107. Heldal E, Arnadottir T, Chacon L, et al. Low failure rate in standardized retreatment of tuberculosis in Nicaragua: patient category, drug resistance and survival of "chronic" patients. Int J Tuberc Lung Dis 2001; 5(2):129–136.
108. Suarez PG, Floyd K, Portocarrero J, et al. Feasibility and cost-effectiveness of standardised second-line drug treatment for chronic tuberculosis patients: a national cohort study in Peru. Lancet 2002; 359(9322):1980–1989.
109. Tuberculosis Research Centre, Chennai, India. Low rate of emergence of drug resistance in sputum positive patients treated with short course chemotherapy. Int J Tuberc Lung Dis 2001; 5(1):40–45.
110. Yoshiyama T, Yanai H, Rhiengtong D, et al. Development of acquired drug resistance in recurrent tuberculosis patients with various previous treatment outcomes. Int J Tuberc Lung Dis 2004; 8(1):31–38.
111. Saravia JC, Appleton SC, Rich ML, et al. Retreatment management strategies when first-line tuberculosis therapy fails. Int J Tuberc Lung Dis 2005; 9(4):421–429.
112. Trébucq A, Anagonou S, Gninafon M, et al. Prevalence of primary and acquired resistance of *Mycobacterium tuberculosis* to anti-tuberculosis drugs in Benin after 12 years of short-course chemotherapy. Int J Tuberc Lung Dis 1999; 3(6):466–470.
113. Quy HT, Lan NT, Borgdorff MW, et al. Drug resistance among failure and relapse cases of tuberculosis: is the standard re-treatment regimen adequate? Int J Tuberc Lung Dis 2003; 7(7):631–636.
114. Enarson DA, Rieder HL, Arnadottir T, et al. Management of Tuberculosis: A Guide for Low Income Countries, 5th ed. Paris, France: International Union Against Tuberculosis and Lung Disease, 2000. http://www.eldis.org/static/DOC11596.htm. Accessed December 2004.
115. World Health Organization. Treatment of Tuberculosis: Guidelines for National Programs, 2nd ed. (WHO/TB/97.220). Geneva, Switzerland: World Health Organization, 1997.
116. Peter Cegielski. Chairperson Green Light Committee for the Access to Second-line Anti-Tuberculosis Drugs; Division of TB elimination, Center for Disease Prevention and Control (CDC). Atlanta, Georgia USA, Personal Communications, Dec 2004.
117. Fischl MA, Daikos GL, Uttamchandani RB, et al. Clinical presentation and outcome of patients with HIV infection and tuberculosis caused by multiple-drug-resistant bacilli. Ann Int Med 1992; 117(3):184–190.
118. Park SK, Lee WC, Lee DH, et al. Self-administered, standardized regimens for multidrug-resistant tuberculosis in South Korea. Int J Tuberc Lung Dis 2004; 8(3):361–368.
119. Van Deun A, Bastian I, Portaels F, et al. Results of a standardised regimen for multidrug-resistant tuberculosis in Bangladesh. Int J Tuberc Lung Dis 2004; 8(5):560–567.
120. Stewart SM, Crofton JW. The clinical significance of low degrees of drug resistance in pulmonary tuberculosis. Am Rev Respir Dis 1964; 89:811–829.
121. Bureau of Tuberculosis Control. Clinical Policies and Protocols, 3rd ed. New York: Department of Health, 1999:58.
122. Drug-resistant tuberculosis: a survival guide for clinicians. San Francisco, Francis J. Curry National Tuberculosis Center and California Department of Health Services, 2004.
123. McCray E, Onorato IM. The interaction of HIV and MDR-TB. In: Bastian I, Portaels F, eds. Multidrug-Resistant Tuberculosis. London, UK: Kluwer Academic Publishers, 2000: 50–51.
124. Nathanson E, Gupta R, Huamani P, et al. Adverse events in the treatment of multidrug-resistant tuberculosis: results from the DOTS-Plus initiative. Int J Tuberc Lung Dis 2004; 8(11):1382–1384.
125. Goble M, Iseman MD, Madsen LA, et al. Treatment of 171 patients with pulmonary tuberculosis resistant to isoniazid and rifampicin. N Eng J Med 1993; 328(8):527–532.
126. Chan ED, Goble M, Iseman MD, et al. Treatment and outcome analysis of 205 patients with multidrug-resistant tuberculosis. Am J Respir Crit Care Med 2004; 169(10):1103–1109.

127. Pomerantz BJ, Cleveland JC, Pomerantz M, et al. Pulmonary resection for multi-drug resistant tuberculosis. J Thorac Cardiovasc Surg 2001; 121(3):448–453.

128. Mishkinis K, Kaminskaite A, Purvanetskene B. Treatment of multidrug-resistant tuberculosis in Santakiskes tuberculosis hospital. [Russian]. Probl Tuberk 2000; (3):9–11.

129. Sung SW, Kang CH, Kim JH, et al. Surgery increased the chance of cure in multi-drug resistant pulmonary tuberculosis. Eur J Cardiothorac Surg 1999; 16(2):187–193.

130. Robinson TD, Barnes DJ. A role for surgery in the management of multi-drug-resistant tuberculosis (MDR-TB). Aust N Z J Med 1998; 28(4):473–474.

131. Potter RT, Laforet EG, Stieder JW. Resectional surgery for pulmonary tuberculosis: analysis of a series of 420 resections performed between 1947 and 1957. Am Rev Respir Dis 1966; 93(1):30–40.

132. Francis RS, Curwen, MP. Major surgery for pulmonary tuberculosis: final report. A national survey of 8232 patients operated on from April 1953 to March 1954 and followed up for five years. Tubercle 1964; 45(S):5–79.

133. XDR TB (Extensively Drug Resistant Tuberculosis): What, Where, How and Action Steps. Geneva, Switzerland: World Health Organization, 2007.

134. Migliori GB, Ortmann J, Girardi E, et al. Extensively drug-resistant tuberculosis, Italy and Germany. Emerg Infect Dis 2007; 13(5):780–782.

135. Jeon CY, Hwang SH, Min JH, et al. Extensively drug-resistant tuberculosis in South Korea: risk factors and treatment outcomes among patients at a tertiary referral hospital. Clin Infect Dis 2008; 46(1):42–49.

136. Mitnick CD, Shin SS, Seung KJ, et al. Extensively drug-resistant tuberculosis: A comprehensive treatment approach. N Engl J Med 2008; 359(6):563–574.

137. Keshavjee S, Gelmanova IY, Farmer PE, et al. Treatment of extensively drug-resistant tuberculosis in Tomsk, Russia: a retrospective cohort study. Lancet 2008; 372(9647):1403–1409.

138. Stanford JL, Grange JM. New concepts for the control of tuberculosis in the twenty first century. J R Coll Physicians London 1993; 27(3):218–223.

139. Condos R, Rom WN, Schluger NW. Treatment of multidrug-resistant pulmonary tuberculosis with interferon-γ via aerosol. Lancet 1997; 349(9064):1513–1515.

140. Smith-Jones PM, Linkesch W, Virgolini I. Interferon-γ for respiratory diseases. Lancet 1997; 350(9076):524.

141. Giosue S, Casarini M, Ameglio F, et al. Minimal dose of aerosolized interferon-α in human subjects: biological consequences and side effects. Eur Respir J 1996; 9(1):42–46.

142. Giosue S, Casarini M, Alemanno L, et al. Effects of aerosolized interferon-α in patients with pulmonary tuberculosis. Am J Respir Crit Care Med 1998;158:1156–1162.

143. Giosue S, Casarini M, Ameglio F, et al. Aerosolized interferon-alpha treatment in patients with multi-drug-resistant pulmonary tuberculosis. Eur Cytokine Netw 2000; 11(1): 99–104.

144. Johnson BJ, Bekker LG, Rickman R, et al. rhuIL-2 adjunctive therapy in multidrug-resistant tuberculosis: a comparison of two treatment regimens and placebo. Tuber Lung Dis 1997; 78(3–4):195–203.

145. Ponce-de-Leon A, Garcia-Garcia L, Garcia-Sancho MC, et al. Tuberculosis and diabetes in southern México. Diabetes Care 2004; 27(7):1584–1590.

146. Small PM, Schecter GF, Goodman PC, et al. Treatment of tuberculosis in patients with advanced human immunodeficiency virus infection. N Eng J Med 1991; 324:289–294.

147. Bradford WZ, Martain JN, Reingold AL, et al. The changing epidemiology of acquired drug-resistant tuberculosis in San Francisco, USA. Lancet 1996; 348:928–931.

148. Frieden TR, Sterling T, Pablos-Mendez A, et al. The emergence of drug-resistant tuberculosis in New York City. N Engl J Med 1993; 328(8):521–526.

149. Coronado VG, Beck-Sague CM, Hutton MD, et al. Transmission of multidrug-resistant *Mycobacterium tuberculosis* among persons with immunodeficiency virus infection in

an urban hospital: epidemiologic and restriction fragment length polymorphism analysis. J Infect Dis 1993; 168(4):1052–1055.

150. Cohn DL, Bustreo F, Raviglione MC. Drug-resistant tuberculosis: review of the worldwide situation and the WHO/IUATLD Global Surveillance Project. Clin Infect Dis 1997; 24(S1):S121–S130.

151. Davies GR, Pillay M, Wilkinson D, et al. Emergence of multidrug-resistant tuberculosis in rural South Africa. Int J Tuberc Lung Dis 1998; 2(11):S327.

152. Ritacco V, Di Lonardo M, Reniero A. Nosocomial spread of human immunodeficiency virus-related multidrug-resistant tuberculosis in Buenos Aires. J Infec Dis 1997; 176(3):637–642.

153. Ridzon R, Whitney CG, McKenna MT, et al. Risk factors for rifampicin mono-resistant tuberculosis. Am J Respir Crit Care Med 1998; 157(6 Pt. 1):1881–1884.

154. Dooley SW, Jarvis WR, Martone WJ, et al. Multidrug-resistant tuberculosis. Ann Intern Med 1992; 117(3):257–259.

155. Multidrug-resistant outbreak on an HIV ward— Madrid, Spain, 1991–1995. MMWR Morb Mortal Wkly Rep 1996; 45(16):330–333.

156. Moro ML, Gori A, Errante I, et al. An outbreak of multidrug-resisitant tuberculosis involving HIV-infected patients of two hospitals in Milan, Italy. AIDS 1998; 12(9):1095–1102.

157. Fischl MA, Uttamchandani RB, Daikos GL, et al. An outbreak of drug-resistant tuberculosis caused by multiple-drug resistant tubercle bacilli among patients with HIV infection. Ann Int Med 1992; 117(3):177–83.

158. Kenyon TA, Ridzon R, Luskin M, et al. A nosocomial outbreak of multidrug-resistant tuberculosis. Ann Int Med 1997; 127: 32–36.

159. Murphy RA. The emerging crisis of drug-resistant tuberculosis in South Africa: Lessons from New York City. Clin Infect Dis 2008; 46:1729–1732.

160. World Health Organization. Antiretroviral therapy for HIV infection in adults and adolescents: Recommendations for a public health approach. Geneva, Switzerland: World Health Organization, 2008.

161. Satti H. Director MDR-TB Project, Partners In Health, Lesotho. Personal communication, 2008.

162. Sahai J, Gallicano K, Oliveras L, et al. Cations in the didanosine tablet reduce ciprofloxacin bioavailability," Clin Pharmacol Ther 1993; 53:292–297.

163. Centers for Disease Control and Prevention (CDC). Managing Drug Interactions in the Treatment of HIV-related Tuberculosis [online]. 2007. Available from URL: http://www.cdc.gov/tb/TB_HIV_Drugs/default.htm.

164. Telzak EE, Sepkowitz K, Alpert P, et al. Multidrug-resistant tuberculosis in patients without HIV infection. N Engl J Med 1995; 333(14):907–911.

165. Narita M, Alonso P, Lauzardo M, et al. Treatment experience of multidrug-resistant tuberculosis in Florida, 1994–1997. Chest 2001; 120(2):343–348.

166. Avendano M, Goldstein RS. Multidrug-resistant tuberculosis: long term follow-up of 40 non-HIV- infected patients. Can Respir J 2000; 7(5):383–389.

167. Cameron RJ, Harrison AC. Multidrug-resistant tuberculosis in Auckland 1988–95. N Z Med J 1997; 110(1041):119–122.

168. Geerligs WA, van Altena R, van her Werf TS, et al. Multidrug-resistant tuberculosis: long-term treatment outcome in the Netherlands. Int J Tuberc Lung Dis 2000; 4(8):758–764.

169. Viskum K, Kok-Jensen A. multidrug-resistant tuberculosis in Denmark 1993–1995. Int J Tuberc Lung Dis 1997; 1(4):299–301.

170. Park SK, Kim CT, Song SD. Outcome of chemotherapy in 107 patients with pulmonary tuberculosis resistant to isoniazid and rifampin. Int J Tuberc Lung Dis 1998; 2(11): 877–884.

171. Tahaoglu K, Torun T, Sevim T, et al. The treatment of multidrug-resistant tuberculosis in Turkey. N Engl J Med 2001; 345(3):170–174.

172. Yew WW, Chan CK, Chau CH, et al. Outcomes of patients with multidrug-resistant pulmonary tuberculosis treated with ofloxacin/levofloxacin-containing regimens. Chest 2000; 117(3):744–751.
173. Mitnick C. Epidemiologist, Partners In Health, Harvard Medical School, Boston USA. Personal communication, 2004.
174. Acha J, Sweetland A. Guia SES para Tratamiento y Manejo de la Tuberculosis Multidrogo Resistente. Lima, Peru: Socios En Salud, 2004.
175. Griffith DE. The United States and worldwide tuberculosis control: a second chance for Prince Prospero. Chest 1998; 113(6):1434–1436.
176. Raviglione MC, Uplekar M. WHO's new Stop TB Strategy. Lancet 2006; 367:952–955.
177. Iseman MD, Cohn DL, Sbarbaro JA. Directly observed treatment of tuberculosis. We can't afford not to try it. N Eng J Med 1993; 328(8):576–578.
178. Heifets LB, Cangelosi GA. Drug susceptibility testing of *Mycobacterium tuberculosis*: a neglected problem at the turn of the century. Int J Tuberc Lung Dis 1999; 3(5):564–581.
179. World Health Organization, The 3 × 5 Initiative. http://www.who.int/3by5/en/. Accessed December 2004.
180. Kim JY, Mate K, Rich ML, et al. From Multidrug-resistant tuberculosis to DOTS expansion and beyond: Making the most of a paradigm shift. Tuberculosis 2003; 83:59–65.

8
Achieving Higher Case Detection and Cure Rates: National Programs and Beyond

KNUT LÖNNROTH, MUKUND UPLEKAR, SALAH OTTMANI, and LÉOPOLD BLANC
Stop TB Department, World Health Organization, Geneva, Switzerland

I. Introduction

Early and effective diagnosis and treatment at low cost are essential for the well-being of individuals with active tuberculosis (TB). Unfortunately, this is not guaranteed for all people with TB today. Poor access to quality services, diagnostic delays, complex and expensive care-seeking paths, and inappropriate treatments, produce poor health outcomes and adverse social and financial consequences for TB patients, as well as for their families and for the wider community (1–4).

As has been discussed in previous chapters (see chaps. 1 and 2), early case detection and high treatment success rates are also essential for reaching epidemiological impact targets for TB control (5–7). High coverage of effective treatment can quickly reduce TB prevalence and death rates. Cutting transmission through early cure of infectious cases is a principle avenue to reduce TB incidence (5,8).

The target for treatment success has now been reached globally. However, great regional variations exist, and many countries report treatment success rates far from the target of 85% (9). Furthermore, a huge number of TB patients are still treated outside national TB programs (NTP), where treatment outcomes are often very poor (10–12). In most countries there is therefore a need to improve treatment and case management practices across the whole health system.

The global case detection target (>70% of estimated incidence of new smear-positive cases), set first for 2000 and then postponed for 2005, has not yet been reached, and the increasing trend has decelerated in the period 2005 to 2007 (9) (Fig. 1).

Furthermore, recent analyses have pointed to the need to *go beyond the 2005 global case detection rate target* and focus more on *early detection* to effectively cut transmission (13) (see chap. 1). Though sputum smear–positive TB is the most infectious form of TB, the risk of transmission in other forms of TB should not be ignored (14–16). Therefore, a major challenge for global TB control is to resume the acceleration seen in the early 2000s of case detection trends for *all types of TB*, and at the same time putting in place strategies that ensure early diagnosis and initiation of effective treatment for *all TB patients* (7).

From both an equity perspective as well as a TB control perspective, it is essential to ensure that the poorest and most vulnerable groups have access to quality diagnosis and treatment (1–3,13,17,18). They are the ones most likely to contract infection, develop disease, have poor treatment outcomes, and experience severe social and economic

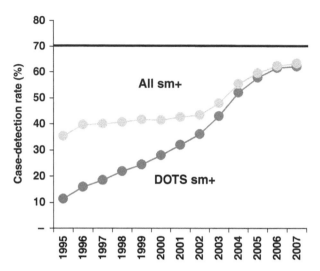

Figure 1   Trend in case-detection rate (DOTS and non-DOTS) for new sputum smear–positive cases, 1995–2007. Horizontal line indicates the 2005 global case detection target (9).

consequences of the disease (3). If TB is not effectively diagnosed and treated among the vulnerable groups, it can perpetuate the epidemic and put the whole population at continuous risk of TB (4). Specific action is therefore required to ensure *equity in access to quality services.* Targeted interventions to reach and support vulnerable groups may be necessary (1,2).

TB is recognized as a grave public health concern globally, especially in low- and middle-income countries. Therefore, TB is included in basic packages of care in the vast majority of countries, and most governments have committed to provide essential TB services free of charge or at highly subsidized costs to the entire population. The conventional service delivery channel for TB diagnosis and treatment under NTP is through selected public health care facilities in the general health system, commonly primary health care facilities and selected hospitals belonging to the department of public health or equivalent. These are essential service delivery channels for TB control. However, it has been demonstrated that such a narrow approach to delivery of TB control interventions is normally insufficient for effective coverage and outreach, since a large proportion of people with TB seek and receive care outside this particular segment of the health system (11,17). All health systems consist of a diverse set of health providers and community and civil society actors engaged in public health action. There is a role for all of them in the fight against TB. Yet, this potential has rarely been fully exploited. Specifically, in many settings there are large parts of both the public and private health care sectors that diagnose and treat large numbers of drug-susceptible as well as drug-resistance TB patients, and at the same time are not being linked to NTPs and thus not necessarily following international standards, nor notifying cases to the health authorities (11). NTPs need to join forces with other partners to find effective service delivery channels (19). They also need to take part in efforts to strengthen the general health system (public as well as private sector), which they need to operate within (20).

This chapter outlines some of the actions that NTPs and their partners may consider for improved TB service delivery, with focus on improved and early case detection and treatment success. The chapter does not discuss in any detail the technical aspects of diagnosis and treatment, which are covered in other chapters of this book.

II. Improving Early Case Detection

A. What is "Case Detection Rate?"

A key performance indicator for NTPs is the so-called "case detection rate." This is in fact not a rate, but a ratio, namely the ratio of the number of TB cases notified and registered for treatment in the country in a year divided by estimated number of incident TB cases in the country in that year (9). Conventionally, this measure is applied to new sputum smear–positive cases only.

The numerator for the case detection rate is usually the number of cases notified and registered for treatment in NTP. This is rarely the same as the number of cases diagnosed with TB in a country, since few NTPs cover all health care institutions. Cases diagnosed outside of NTP, for example, in the private sector or the public sector outside designated NTP facilities, and not referred or notified to NTP, are often not counted and generally unknown to the health authorities, unless there is a comprehensive and well-coordinated notification system in place. This is rarely the case in countries with high TB burden.

Case detection within NTPs may be further subdivided into those registered under DOTS and those treated in NTP but still under other than the internationally recommended principles (21,22). Such disaggregation was particularly important during the decade of DOTS expansion when countries were gradually shifting from non-DOTS to DOTS programs (roughly 1994–2004). However, in recent years, when most NTPs have fully adopted the DOTS strategy, most cases registered under NTP do receive treatment under these basic principles (9) (Fig. 1).

It is important to distinguish between the following elements of case detection: identification of a suspected TB case, diagnosis, notification, and registration for treatment under DOTS, in line with the International Standards of TB Care (ISTC). A TB case can be diagnosed but not notified, or notified but not registered for treatment under DOTS/ISTC. Improving case detection is therefore not only a matter of improving diagnostic quality and outreach, but is also a matter of improving notification and referral mechanisms across the whole health system.

It is also important to recognize that the quality of TB treatment that takes place outside NTPs is normally nonstandardized and often produce poor treatment results (11). Improving case detection by ensuring that all diagnosed patients are notified is not sufficient, unless they are also put on standardized, evidence based, and internationally recommended treatment and case management principles (see section III). The "case detection rate" as currently measured is a useful indicator for this goal (though perhaps not appropriately labeled), as it measures the proportion of the estimated incident cases that are managed under internationally agreed treatment and case management principles (21,22).

B. What is Early Detection?

Early case detection not only implies that patients are detected as early as possible, but also that they are put on appropriate treatment early. The total delay from onset of symptoms to the start of appropriate treatment is thus a main concern. Total delay may be divided into the patient's delay in seeking care and the health system's delay in making the diagnosis and directing the patient to where appropriate treatment can be effectively provided.

Cough more than two to three weeks is normally used as a criteria for TB screening in populations with medium-to-high TB prevalence (23). Diagnosis of sputum smear–positive TB can under optimal conditions be completed in one to two days (not counting all the possible barriers for patients to reach the appropriate place of diagnosis, which are further discussed below). Treatment can start directly after diagnosis. Many sputum smear–positive TB cases can therefore in principle be put on treatment within three to four weeks from onset of symptoms, under normal program conditions.

Diagnosis of smear-negative pulmonary TB and extrapulmonary TB may take much longer, depending on disease presentation and available diagnostic methods. Identification of drug-resistant (DR) TB that requires second- or third-line drug regimens may take up to eight weeks when using traditional diagnostic methods (though it can be substantially accelerated through adoption of liquid culture media and line-probe assays), and is dependent on sufficient lab capacity for drug-susceptibility testing (DST), which is not in place in most high TB burden countries (see chap. 7). Treatment delay of smear-negative TB and DR-TB may therefore be considerable due to technological shortcomings, and what should be considered "too long" depends on the availability of diagnostic tests and the capacity of the health system in a given setting.

Not all people with TB have cough or recognize cough as a symptom that warrants action. Furthermore, several types of access barriers may delay health seeking for those who recognize the need to seek care (24,25). Many studies have documented that the delay to treatment can be extremely long, sometimes ranging from several months to even years (24). There is no internationally agreed maximum acceptable patient delay in seeking care. However, a delay of over one month from onset of symptoms to the first health care action is certainly too long.

C. An Analytical Framework for Early Case Detection

There are several possible reasons for low case detection rate and delayed treatment, including poor understanding of TB and its symptoms in the general population; poor knowledge about where to seek care; poor health service infrastructure; access barriers; poor diagnostic quality; limited human resource for health; poor TB knowledge among health providers; and perverse incentive systems for providers that foster both the use of unnecessary medical technologies and drug treatments, which delay the correct diagnosis and waste resources. Efforts to improve early case detection therefore need to focus on both the demand and supply side. Main avenues to improve early case detection include the following:

1. Improving the quality, outreach, and access to diagnostic facilities (including new diagnostic tools) across the whole health system.
2. Improving referral and notification of cases already diagnosed with TB, but managed outside the NTP.
3. Influencing peoples health-seeking behavior.

A solid analysis of the existing case detection situation is required to devise locally appropriate strategies and prioritize them among possible options. Figure 2 presents a

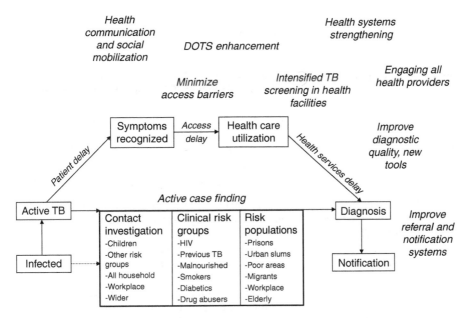

Figure 2 A framework for analysis and action to improve early case detection.

framework for analysis and identification of relevant entry points for improving early case detection.

The upper part of Figure 2 depicts the pathway to diagnosis and treatment based on active care seeking by patients. The steps in this pathway include recognition of symptom by the individual (or caretaker), active health seeking, diagnosis in a health facility, referral to the appropriate place of treatment and/or notification of diagnosis and treatment. This pathway represents what is often called "passive case detection." It is the main approach applied by most NTPs in high TB burden countries.

"Passive" implies that the NTP is not actively looking for cases outside the NTP-affiliated facilities, but waits for people with TB symptoms to approach these facilities.

However, the term may be misleading since this pathway requires a very active and alert health system that has the capacity to identify people who should undergo TB screening once they turn to the health care facility. It requires active strategies for integration of TB diagnosis and treatment throughout the health system. A sufficient health workforce that ensures improved quality of TB diagnostic facilities and case management, is essential. A communication strategy is required to inform people with TB symptoms where to turn for help. In order to attract people to available diagnostic services, it is also essential to make sure that quality treatment is available as well as accessible. A first essential step of any attempt to improve case detection is to ensure that these elements are in place and actively pursued.

The lower part depicts the pathway for "active case finding," implying actions to screen high-risk groups who do not actively seek health care due to TB symptoms. Contact investigation is the first logic extension beyond the "passive case finding" approach. Active screening may also include screening of high-risk populations or clinical risk groups. The latter type of screening among people who actively seek care in a health facility, though not for TB symptoms, conceptually falls somewhere between "passive" and "active" case finding.

The appropriate strategy for improved early case detection depends on the status and nature of the TB epidemic, the performance of the NTP, the capacity of the general health system, and the health-seeking behavior of people with TB symptoms. A careful assessment of the situation with regards to these parameters is therefore required to prepare for local action. The framework in Figure 2 may help identify bottlenecks along the pathways to diagnosis, notification, and treatment initiation. In addition, a good understanding of the TB epidemic is required. Guiding questions for this analysis are listed in Box 1.

Ten Guiding Questions To Identify Approaches for Improved Early Case Detection

1. What is the burden of TB, what are the trends, what are the geographical differences within the country? Is the country moving toward TB elimination? Is the TB epidemic concentrated to certain risk populations only?
2. What is the case-detection gap in the country and in different subgroups?
3. What is the treatment delay and how does it vary between subgroups (gender, age, SES, etc.)?
4. What is the coverage of the NTP? Does it cover all geographical parts of the country? Does it cover essential parts of the health system and all important health providers that diagnose and treat TB?
5. What is the quality of diagnostic services in the NTP-affiliated facilities? How are people with TB symptoms identified and screened?
6. Are people with HIV actively screened for TB? Which other "clinical risk groups" are systematically screened for TB?
7. What are the current policies with regards to contact investigation and active screening for TB outside health facilities? Which are the main risk groups?
8. Where are the missing cases?
   - *By provider*: Which providers are diagnosing and treating TB but not referring/notifying? How many patients are likely to be diagnosed and how many are under treatment with these providers? What is the existing policy and regulation concerning notification of TB cases?
   - *By geographical area*: What is the geographical variation in case detection? Which areas will require special attention?
   - *By risk group*: Which subpopulations have the highest risk of TB? Which groups are underrepresented in the NTP? Which risk factors, risk groups, and risk populations are the most important in the country? Aspects of socioeconomic status and gender?
9. Which are the main access barriers that are contributing to low case detection and delays? How is TB control integrated into the general health system? What are the weaknesses of the general health system that hamper access to quality TB services?
10. What is the level of knowledge and attitude toward TB, TB symptoms, and the NTP in the population? How does the TB stigma affect peoples' health seeking? How do perceptions of quality of care in NTP and elsewhere influence choices?

D. Strategies to Improve Early Case Detection

Depending on findings in an assessment of current case detection gaps and barriers, the following intervention entry points should be considered and prioritized:

DOTS Expansion and Enhancement

Strong political commitment, including sufficient financial support for full coverage and equitable access to evidence-based and quality-controlled TB diagnosis and treatment, is the most important element of a successful national TB control and an essential step toward complete and early case detection. The DOTS strategy (21) clearly defines the appropriate approach to diagnosis, treatment, and case management, as also defined in the ISTC (22). When sufficient resources, infrastructure, and manpower for basic DOTS implementation are not in place, this should be the first priority followed by actions to improve outreach and access to those services.

Intensifying Case-Finding Strategies in Health Care Facilities

Ensure Comprehensive Implementation of Existing Diagnostic Algorithm

This requires that all staff in all parts of the health system are alert and know how to ask patients about TB symptoms and refer them for TB diagnostic tests as per guidelines. This entails training (pre- and in-service) of all health care providers, public and private. Restricting the efforts to improve identification of people with possible TB to the NTP-affiliated facilities only or the specific staff designated for TB care only, misses an opportunity to identify all those cases that seek care elsewhere in the system.

Actively asking all outpatients in primary health care facilities and hospitals for cough (including those who do not mention cough spontaneously) can yield substantial additional number of cases (26–28). Expanding implementation of screening practices may also mean involving nonhealth care staff as symptom surveyors, such as clerks managing the registration in the outpatient department, who may ask a simple question about cough to all attendees and send eligible patients directly to a diagnostic test.

Elaborating the Diagnostic Algorithm for Pulmonary TB

The recommended indication for performing diagnostic test for pulmonary TB is two to three weeks' duration of cough. A shorter recommended duration of cough leads to higher diagnostic sensitivity but lower specificity. Appropriate cutoff depends on both the prevalence of TB in the community (which determines the positive predictive value), as well as the available diagnostic resources. When sufficient diagnostic capacity is available, it will be an advantage to use two weeks as a cutoff point, as it can help increase case detection (29). In principle, any cough of any duration may be used as a screening indication in a high-burden setting. This will maximize sensitivity, but of course many more tests will be performed on people who do not have TB.

Sputum-smear microscopy is the internationally recommended first diagnostic tool for pulmonary TB. The test is effective in quickly identifying those individuals that are most infectious. The overall sensitivity of sputum smear microscopy is however low, whereas specificity is high (30,31). Sensitivity can be improved through use of special techniques such as fluorescent microscopy and bleach techniques (see chap. 4). The definition of smear-positive TB has recently been changed so that it is now sufficient with one positive sputum smear to fulfill criteria for smear-positive TB (31). Adapting this definition means higher sensitivity. Furthermore, when patients can be diagnosed based on the first spot sputum, there is less risk of defaulting during the diagnostic process.

Therefore, the overall case detection may increase and at the same time the diagnosis will be made more quickly and with less resources.

The recommended algorithm for cases that have a negative sputum smear conventionally involves a course of broad-spectrum antibiotics and a follow-up X-ray. This approach minimizes the risk of treating false-positive X-ray-diagnosed TB cases. However, the approach is associated with risk of delay in diagnosis as well as risk of dropout during the diagnostic phase, which is particularly critical for people with TB/HIV coinfection, who are also more likely to present with smear-negative TB (see chap. 6). Good access to high-quality X-ray diagnosis combined with an effective communication strategy that minimizes drop out during the diagnostic phase can potentially improve early case detection of smear negative cases. A diagnosis based on an initial X-ray only has been recommended for people with HIV (32).

Culture, DST, and New Diagnostic Tools

A detailed discussion on culture, DST and new diagnostic tools are provided in chapters 4, 7 and 13. Culture is the gold standard for TB diagnosis, and the method is more sensitive and specific than sputum-smear microscopy. Wide implementation of quality-assured culture services can help increase bacteriologically confirmed case detection. However, the method is expensive and requires an advanced lab network. Conventional culture also takes a long time (up to eight weeks). TB diagnosis would be considerably simplified if and when new sensitive, specific, and cost-effective diagnostic tools, which are also applicable at the point-of-care in field conditions in very poor settings, become available.

Screening People Living With HIV

The Stop TB Strategy emphasizes the need to screen all people with HIV for TB, regardless of symptoms (18,33). The diagnostic algorithm is different for these cases both because smear-negative pulmonary TB is more common in this risk group and because the need to start treatment early is even more critical among people with HIV. Recent experiences show that active screening of people with HIV has made substantial contribution to overall TB case detection in some countries (9,34). The active engagement of HIV/AIDS programs, as well as all health care providers involved in HIV/AIDS care is essential to pursue this approach.

Screening Other Clinical Risk Groups

The risk of TB is also increased among people with smoking-related conditions (35,36), diabetes (37), malnutrition (38), alcoholism (39), and a wide range of other conditions that impair the host defense against TB infection and disease, such as silicosis, malignancies, various systemic immunosuppressant conditions, and treatment with immunosuppressant drugs (40). Table 1 lists estimated relative risk prevalence in TB high-burden countries (HBCs) and corresponding population attributable fractions for selected risk factors. In addition, people who have previously had TB are at a higher risk than then general population to develop active TB. The case finding yield may be high when screening these risk groups in clinical settings, especially if they have TB symptoms. It is a logical part of the individual clinical management of these conditions, at least in high TB burden settings, to screen for TB. However, though a few NTPs have policies to screen these risk groups, no international standards for such screening have been developed. More research

Table 1 The Relative Risk and Population Attributable Fraction for Selected Clinical Risk Factors

	Relative risk for active TB disease (95% confidence intervals)	Weighted prevalence (22 HBCs)	Population attributable fraction
HIV infection	26.7 (20.4–34.9)	0.9%	18%
Malnutrition	3.2 (3.1–3.3)	17.2%	27%
Diabetes	3.0 (1.5–7.8)	3.4%	7%
Alcohol use (>40 g/d)	2.9 (1.9–4.6)	7.9%	13%
Active smoking	2.6 (1.6–4.3)	18.2%	23%

Source: Adapted from Ref. 13.

and documentation is needed on the feasibility, effectiveness, and cost-effectiveness of such approaches, which are required before general recommendations for NTP policies can be developed.

Practical Approach to Lung Health
Respiratory conditions are usually the first or the second leading cause of care seeking in primary health care (PHC) settings. Surveys carried out by WHO in nine countries showed that up to one-third of patients attend PHC facilities for respiratory symptoms (41). Evidence from countries suggest that patients with persistent respiratory symptoms, including TB suspects, are often mismanaged in PHC facilities, and that TB screening among eligible patients is often neglected (42). The Practical Approach to Lung Health (PAL) aims at improving the quality of the management of respiratory patients. It promotes a symptom-based and integrated case management, and seeks to standardize service delivery through the development and implementation of clinical guidelines. PAL is intended to ensure the coordination among different levels of health care and between TB control programs and general health services (43). Country experience has shown that PAL implementation can improve the technical capacities of PHC workers to manage respiratory patients, including TB suspects (44). Data from country pilot sites also suggest that the screening for TB among respiratory patients who meet the definition of a TB suspect increases with PAL (42,45), and that case detection increases as a consequence (46,47). Therefore, PAL is a recommended approach to maximize case detection, especially for middle-income countries.

Minimize Access Barriers, Especially for the Poor and Vulnerable
A basic principle for NTPs is to provide essential diagnostic tests as well as the full treatment course free of charge to patients. Many NTPs aim to decentralize service delivery to ensure access to all patients, including those in remote areas. Nevertheless, it is well recognized that the poorest of the poor, those living in remote rural areas, in conflict zones, and in urban slums that lack basic health care infrastructure often have poor access to quality services (1,2). Disempowered, poorly educated, marginalized, informal, or illegal residents may have great difficulties both in accessing care and in fully availing the available services even if they can reach the appropriate facility. Many turn to informal providers or depend on self-treatment and delay formal health care utilization. Women

seem to face special access barriers in many settings related to, among other things, disempowerment, stigma, and lack of financial resources (48–51).

Guidelines have been developed for NTPs on how to improve access for these groups (2). Many of these actions, such as further decentralization of service delivery, outreach activities, simplification of diagnostic routines, and improved communication with patients, can be pursued by NTP alone. However, much of these activities need to be done in collaboration with actors engaged in general health systems strengthening (20) as well as with civil society and community activists who are engaged in improved health services for the poor and vulnerable (52,53). The guidelines present a step-wise approach, including assessment of specific access barriers and specific vulnerable groups; development of interventions based on the assessment; harnessing of resources for action within and outside NTP and the health sector; and monitoring and evaluation of pro-poor approaches (2). Currently, few NTPs have sufficient information to assess which groups are left out. Indicators and tools for such assessment are under development (54).

Engaging All Health Care Providers

People with TB symptoms utilize a wide range of public and private providers. In many high TB burden countries, the first point of contact for the majority of people with TB, including the poor, is a private provider (private doctors and hospitals, private pharmacies or informal private providers). For example, various studies have shown that the proportion of patients that had turned first to a private provider was 50% in Vietnam (55), 75% in India (56), and 96% in Myanmar (57), and there were only minor differences between the poor and the nonpoor. These providers are normally involved in formal national TB control efforts to a very limited extent; they rarely follow international standards and usually do not notify TB cases to NTP. A similar problem exists in parts of the public health care sector in many countries. Whereas NTP may be fully integrated into PHC, public hospitals, medical colleges, special health insurance-affiliated health facilities, and health facilities belonging to special health services of the armed forces, prison system, police service, etc., may not be linked to the NTP (11).

All the private and public providers that are consulted by people with TB symptoms and who diagnose and/or treat TB, need to be engaged in national TB control efforts in order to ensure early diagnosis, appropriate treatment, and full notification of all TB cases. Guidelines have been developed for the engagement of all health providers through so-called "public–private mix" (PPM) approaches (58). These guidelines are based on documented experiences of such initiatives in over 40 projects in more than 20 countries, and a large body of operational research on initiatives targeting various types of providers in diverse settings (56–63). This research shows that all types of providers can be productively engaged; that case detection (registration for treatment under DOTS/ISTC) can increase between 10% and 50% depending on baseline case detection and intensity of the effort. The PPM approach has been shown to be cost-effective from providers, patients, as well as the society's viewpoint (64,65).

Health Communication and Social Mobilization

If specific awareness about TB, its symptoms, and TB care services are high in the community, this will help ensure that people do not neglect TB symptoms, take appropriate action early, and turn to the right facility for care (53). However, knowledge in itself is not sufficient. People need to believe that the available services offer something valuable at an affordable cost, and they need to be ensured that availing TB services do not come at a social price due to the stigma attached to the disease and/or the offered TB services (1,2,48,66). Any communication strategy to influence the demand side along those dimensions should be based on a good understanding of the current knowledge and attitudes. Therefore, the active engagement of community members and civil society is essential for the planning and execution of an effective strategy.

There is a lot of anecdotal evidence of the value of communication strategies (53) and a few well-documented successes. For example, an educational campaign in Cali, Colombia resulted in 50% increase in case detection, whereas there was no increase in the control areas (67). In Indonesia, community education (as part of a broader community-based TB program) was associated with a tripling of case detection, whereas only a very modest increase (13%) was recorded in the same period in control areas (68).

A powerful way to increase utilization is to ensure that services which are accessible, affordable, and of a high quality are in place. Peoples' health seeking is to a large extent influenced by the experiences and attitudes of their family, local community, and peers. Ensuring client satisfaction is therefore key to successfully communicate to the community about the utility of the available TB services. Cured TB patients can be actively involved to increase awareness in the community and also be formally engaged to identify and refer people with TB symptoms (53).

Contributing to Health System Strengthening

Most NTPs are fully integrated into PHC with respect to diagnosis and treatment of TB. Therefore, the performance of NTP is dependent on the performance of the general health system. Guidelines have been developed for how NTPs can actively contribute to Health Systems Strengthening HSS (20). There is no single key intervention that all NTPs need to pursue. The key point is that NTPs, in order to improve case detection and general performance of the program need to assess weaknesses in the general health system and contribute to addressing them together with other public health programs and relevant stakeholders in the general health system. The WHO health systems strengthening strategy (69) identifies six health systems as building blocks—leadership/governance, financing, health services, health workforce, health information, and medical products—that may be a useful starting point for such analysis. A specific regulatory intervention that can help improve case detection is a disease control law that incorporates compulsory notification of all TB cases. If there are sufficient resources to enforce such a regulation, the number of diagnosed TB cases that are officially accounted for can be substantially increased, which has been recently experienced in China (70).

Active Case Finding
Contact Investigation

A recent systematic literature review of studies assessing the effects of TB contact investigations in low- and middle-income countries has shown that 4.5% of identified household contacts had active TB (8.5% of children less than five years old) (71). The prevalence of bacteriologically confirmed TB was 2.3%.

Recent data collected on routine basis in Morocco have shown that 4% to 8% of TB cases registered annually by the NTP were identified among household contacts. In children less than 10 years of age, approximately 20% of TB cases registered were identified in household contacts (72).

These findings highlight that TB contact investigation can give a high yield of active TB cases, particularly in children. It is not known what proportion of these cases would have been diagnosed anyway, though at a later stage, through "passive case finding." Therefore, though it is plausible that contact investigation would significantly contribute to earlier TB case detection, the contribution in terms of additional number of cases detected is less certain. In many low- and middle-income countries, TB contact investigation is not performed as a routine activity of TB control even if it is included in the national TB control policy and strategy. Often, neither the index cases nor the contacts who should be investigated for TB, are clearly defined in NTP policies. Moreover, the procedures to be used by the NTP services in assessing contacts for TB are often not specified.

Other Active Case Finding Strategies
Mass radiography screening has historically been a standard element of many TB control programs. Even before chemotherapy was available, this was a way to identify TB cases eligible for isolation in TB sanatoria. There are numerous examples of successful screening campaigns covering entire populations that have been effective in identifying additional and previously unknown TB cases (73). Whereas the potential benefit of such an approach is undisputable, the overall experience is that the resources and logistic arrangements required for them render such approaches unfeasible and cost-ineffective as compared to other case-finding approaches (74). Already in the 1960s and 1970s, the WHO Expert Committee on Tuberculosis discouraged mass screening (75).

However, there are several alternatives to mass screening that are more targeted, less resource demanding, and more cost-effective. These include screening of risk groups with high TB exposure, for example, certain health care workers (76), prisoners (77), refugees (78), drug addicts (79), homeless people, slum dwellers, or other identified high-risk populations (1,2). Such screening may be combined with communication strategies to encourage people to approach health facilities if they have TB symptoms (rather than using ambulatory diagnostic units to screen entire communities). There is ample evidence of the feasibility and effectiveness of such approaches for improving case detection and some evidence on shortening of diagnostic delays. However, no rigorous cost-effectiveness analyses have been done to compare these initiatives with passive case finding or with each other (73).

The choice to pursue active case finding approaches, as well as the choice of which approach or combination of approaches to use, should be guided by the local epidemiology (including size and characteristics of various risk groups), capacity of the national program, effectiveness of passive case finding approaches, and available resources (73). Any initiative should include careful monitoring and evaluation of additionality, cost and cost-effectiveness, before scaling up. This would also contribute to the global evidence base on active case finding.

III.   Improving Cure Rates Across the Whole Health System

A.   Improving Case Management Within NTP
Over 50% (12/22) of the TB HBC had treatment success rates below 85% in 2005 cohorts (9). Efforts to improve treatment outcomes are particularly important in those countries, but all countries should strive to optimize success rate and ultimately aim for close to 100% success rate. Default (5%) and death (4%) are the most common of the adverse

treatment outcomes globally, and in several countries the case fatality and default rate are both above 10% (9). A high treatment failure rate is also a problem in several countries, especially where DR-TB is common, whereas a high transfer-out rate is a particular problem in specific settings, such as in urban areas, among migrant workers or nomadic populations.

There are several reasons for poor treatment outcomes and many possible intervention entry points. The areas that require initial attention are the basic DOTS elements, including use of appropriate treatment regimens with quality-assured drugs; continuous drug supply; and sufficient mechanisms for patient support and supervision. Specific interventions should then be guided by an analysis of the dominant type of adverse treatment outcomes, and this may vary considerably within countries and across subgroups.

Case Fatality

High case fatality (death rate among patients on TB treatment) is common in countries with high HIV prevalence, and especially if access to HIV treatment is insufficient and/or collaboration between TB and HIV programs is weak. In such countries, improved HIV/AIDS care and scaled up TB/HIV collaborative activities are essential (see chap. 6). This would rely on good collaboration not only between NTP and HIV/AIDS programs, but also with other governmental and nongovernmental partners involved in TB and HIV care and support.

High prevalence of multidrug-resistant TB can also contribute to high case fatality. In addition, high case fatality may be due to high prevalence of other comorbidities, in which case improved management of these conditions, for example, severe malnutrition, alcoholism, IV drug use, diabetes, psychiatric conditions, (36–40,80) and strengthened collaboration with relevant programs are required. Finally, high death rate may be due to a severe disease status at the time of diagnosis due to late presentation. This requires prompt action so as to reduce treatment delays as has been discussed in the previous section.

Treatment Adherence

Firstly, high default rate is associated with lack of health worker adherence to basic case management principles and insufficient communication and support from health staff to patients. Adequate human and financial resources, as well as sufficient staff training and motivation efforts are required to ensure that patients receive adequate health education, patient-friendly supervision in a supportive environment, and adequate assistance to return to treatment after treatment interruption.

Secondly, access barriers, such as long traveling distances, inconvenient clinic opening hours, and long clinic waiting times contribute to poor treatment adherence. Such barriers are particularly severe for poor people, people in remote areas, daily wage earners, migrants, homeless, and other vulnerable groups (81). Treatment provisions need to be decentralized to the extent possible (82) and made available at the most convenient time and location for the patient. They also need to be provided in a culturally sensitive manner that minimizes stigmatization (2). A range of options exists—beyond facility based treatment in peripheral public health care units—such as community-based treatment supported by a community volunteer, family member, peer in the workplace or equivalent, or treatment by private providers (standardized DOTS) (18,52,58). Engagement of patients, communalities, civil society, nongovernmental organizations, and private sector is essential to achieve this (52,53,58). Such outreach networks can also be effectively deployed to ensure effective tracing and retrieval of patients who interrupt treatment. Active community engagement combined with decentralization of TB services, have been shown to improve treatment outcomes in a highly cost-effective way (52).

Various incentives and enablers packages have been used to further support and motivate patients to complete treatment, including food packages, travel vouchers, financial compensation for missed work, and psychosocial support. Here, too, the engagement of the community and civil society is essential. Several successes have been reported of initiative where incentives and enable packages have been tailored to local conditions. However, the evidence base for specific support packages is still weak (83,84).

Certain patient groups have a high risk of defaulting due to comorbidities that influence their capacity and/or willingness to complete treatment. Alcoholism, illicit drug use, and mental illness can have a very negative impact on adherence (80,85). Such patient groups require special support and, where possible, clinical interventions to treat these comorbidities. However, the evidence base, on feasible and effective approaches to improve TB treatment outcomes through such efforts, is weak.

Initial Default

A special concern in some countries is the high rate of initial default (defaulting after diagnosis but before treatment starts). Depending on recording and reporting practices, such cases may or may not enter into cohort analysis. If not, they are not accounted for in the treatment outcome statistics, but may nevertheless constitute an important problem. For example, in Vietnam, India, and South Africa, between 5% and 14% of diagnosed smear-positive cases were not put on treatment in NTP (86–88). The same access barriers that were discussed above, as well as migration, may explain this phenomenon. Lack of trust in the NTP services or poor communication of health workers during the diagnostic phase, are other possible explanations. In order to minimize initial defaulting, efforts are needed to locally understand the reason for why people intentionally or unintentionally drop out before treatment starts.

Treatment Failure

Where treatment failure rates are high, this may be due to either poor quality of treatment, poor drug quality, poor case management practices, previously poor treatment quality that has generated drug-resistant TB, and/or comorbidities that increase the risk of failure. Chapter 10 discusses the prevention and management of MDR TB. General aspects of good case management are discussed above.

Transfer-Out and Nonevaluated Cases

A few countries still have poor routines for conducting comprehensive cohort analysis even of patients treated within NTPs. However, this reason for unknown clinical treatment results is much more common outside NTPs (see below). With regards to unknown clinical outcome of treatment within NTPs, transfer-out (without reported outcome from the receiving unit) may be a problem especially among patients started on treatment in large health institutions in urban areas and among domestic migrants, such as seasonal workers or nomadic populations. Special attention is required to ensure effective information exchange between health facilities and management units for such cases.

B. Evidence-Based, Quality-Assured TB Management Across the Whole Health System

Most high TB burden countries have put in place mechanisms to ensure that the basic principles for treatment and case management of drug susceptible and drug-resistant TB are followed within the NTP. However, few countries have effective mechanisms to ensure that the same principles are followed in all parts of the public and private health care sectors (11).

The WHO-reported global treatment success of 85% (9) concerns treatment success for TB patients treated under DOTS in NTPs. Since case detection rate was only at about 62% in 2007, it is possible that close to 40% of all cases were treated outside NTPs. Very little information is available about the treatment success rate among those patients since record keeping is poor, notification often nonexisting, and formal cohort analysis not performed. However, research has shown that the treatment success rate is often only about 50% for patients treated in private clinics (10,12). Anecdotal evidence from hospitals not engaged in DOTS programs (public as well as private) suggest that treatment success rate is equally poor there, due to poor mechanisms for ensuring adherence during ambulatory treatment and/or high transfer-out rate. Assuming that the treatment success rate is 50% among 40% of the global TB cases that may be treated outside NTPs, the weighted average treatment success rate globally is currently only about 70%. Poor treatment outcomes are contributing not only to poor health for the individual patients, but also the generation of chronic infectious cases and development of drug-resistant TB. Concerns for improved treatment success rates therefore need to focus on TB treatment across the whole health system.

Engaging All Health Care Providers

As discussed above, evidence-based strategies are available to engage all public and private health care providers in TB control, including measures to ensure that all health care providers are following international standards for TB diagnosis, treatment, and management. Key inputs include provision of quality sputum-smear microscopy, free-of-charge TB drugs from the NTP, and continuous support and supervision of engaged providers and their patients. Experiences from over 20 countries show that treatment success rates above 85% can be achieved as long as the basic DOTS principles are ensured (57).

Many countries are now scaling up the engagement of all care providers in TB care and control (9). However, in most HBCs, there is still a large segment of the health sector that remains unengaged, and a large proportion of patients are still managed outside the NTP under nonstandardized treatments and poor case management principles. Two broad avenues for action are required: first, ambitious scale-up plans for the engagement of all care providers, including promotion of the ISTC. Second, efforts to improve the regulatory environment for TB control, with a special focus on drug regulation.

Regulating Drug Quality and Use Across the Health System

Pharmaceutical manufacturing, import of pharmaceuticals, drug registration, and sales in private retail pharmacy sector are generally poorly regulated in HBCs. In addition, pharmacovigilance and surveillance of drug prescription and use are often weak.

In most countries, first- and second-line TB drugs are available over the counter or against dubious prescriptions from poorly qualified health workers (11,89). TB drug quality is often poor for drugs that are produced from companies that are not prequalified (90). In order to curb the mismanagement of TB and further amplification of TB drug resistance, there is a need to improve the regulation of drug manufacturing, procurement, distribution, prescription, and sales and, more generally, to join national and international efforts to promote rational use of drugs, with focus both on the provider and the user. Such action cannot be pursued by NTPs alone but need to be part of broader health systems strengthening actions together with a range of other stakeholders (20). Nevertheless, NTPs have an important role to advocate the need for drug quality control and restriction of inappropriate use of TB drugs. Some countries have successfully restricted TB drug use to the NTP-affiliated facilities, such as Brazil, Ghana, and Tanzania.

IV. Conclusion

Globally, TB case detection and treatment outcomes have improved substantially in the past decade. Still, much work remains to be done within national programs and beyond. Basic DOTS principles need to be put into place and enhanced, where this has not yet happened. ISTC needs to be adopted universally. In order to achieve this, NTPs need to collaborate actively with all relevant partners within and outside the health system, including civil society and the private sector. The PPM and PAL approaches need to be more actively pursued. TB/HIV collaborative activities and programmatic management of DR-TB need to be strengthened. Poorly functioning general health systems create barriers for TB case detection rate and effective treatment. Therefore, NTPs and technical partners assisting them should join forces with other stakeholders engaged in health systems strengthening, especially to address access barriers for poor and vulnerable groups. Better communication strategies and demand side interventions are required too.

Finally, more research is needed. New tools are required to speed up TB diagnosis and improve treatment success rates. New or renewed avenues for intensified case detection should be explored and assessed, including active screening of selected subpopulations. More research is also needed to develop appropriate strategies for TB screening and TB management among specific TB risk groups.

References

1. WHO. Reaching the poor – challenges for TB programmes in the Western Pacific Region. Manila, Philippines: World Health Organization, 2004. WHO/HTM/TB/2005.352.
2. WHO. Addressing poverty in TB control – options for national TB control programmes. Geneva, Switzerland: World Health Organization, 2005a. WHO/HTM/TB/2005.352.
3. Hanson C, Floyd K, Weil D. Tuberculosis in the poverty alleviation agenda. In: Raviglione M, ed. TB: A Comprehensive International Approach. New York: Informa Healthcare, 2006.
4. Lönnroth K, Jaramillo E, Williams BG, et al. Expanding the global tuberculosis control paradigm – the role of TB risk factors and social determinants. In: Blas E, Sivasankara Kurup A, eds. Priority Public Health Conditions: From Learning to Action on Social Determinants of Health. Geneva, Switzerland: World Health Organization, 2009.
5. Dye C, Garnett GP, Sleeman K, et al. Prospects for worldwide tuberculosis control under the WHO DOTS strategy. Directly observed short-course therapy. Lancet 1998; 352:1886–1891.

6. Maher D, Dye C, Floyd K, et al. Planning to improve global health: The next decade of tuberculosis control. Bull World Health Organ 2007; 85:341–347.
7. Stop TB Partnership. The Global Plan to Stop TB 2006–2015. Geneva, Switzerland: World Health Organization, 2006. WHO/HTM/STB/2006.35.
8. Styblo K, Bumgarner JR. Tuberculosis can be controlled with existing technologies: Evidence. The Hague: Tuberculosis Surveillance Research Unit, 1991.
9. WHO. Global Tuberculosis Control. Geneva, Switzerland: World Health Organization, 2009. WHO/HTM/TB/2009.411.
10. Uplekar M, Juvekar S, Morankar S, et al. Tuberculosis patients and practitioners in private clinics in India. Int J Tuberc Lung Dis 1998; 2:324–329.
11. Uplekar M, Pathania V, Raviglione M. Private practitioners and public health: Weak links in tuberculosis control. Lancet 2001; 358(9285):912–916.
12. Lönnroth K, Thuong LM, Lambregts K, et al. Private tuberculosis care provision associated with poor treatment outcome – a comparative cohort analysis of a semi-private chest clinic and the national tuberculosis control programme in Ho Chi Minh City, Vietnam. Int J Tuberc Lung Dis 2003; 7:165–171.
13. Lönnroth K, Raviglione M. Global Epidemiology of Tuberculosis: Prospects for Control. Semin Respir Crit Care Med 2008; 29:481–491.
14. Behr MA, Warren SA, Salamon H, et al. Transmission of Mycobacterium tuberculosis from patients smear-negative for acid-fast bacilli. Lancet 1999; 353:444–449.
15. Rieder H. What is the role of case detection by periodic mass radiographic examination in tuberculosis control? In: Frieden T, ed. Toman's Tuberculosis, 2nd ed. Geneva, Switzerland: World Health Organization, 2004.
16. Tostmann A, Kik SV, Kalisvaart NA, et al. Tuberculosis transmission by patients with smear-negative pulmonary tuberculosis in a large cohort in the Netherlands. Clin Infect Dis. 2008; 47(9):1135–1142.
17. Raviglione M, Uplekar M. WHO's new Stop TB Strategy. Lancet. 2006; 367:952–955.
18. WHO. The Stop TB Strategy – building on and enhancing DOTS to meet the TB-related Millennium Development Goals. Geneva, Switzerland: World Health Organization, 2006. WHO/HTM/TB2006.368.
19. Uplekar M. Involving private health care providers in delivery of TB care: Global strategy. Tuberculosis 2003; 83:156–164.
20. WHO. Contributing to health system strengthening – Guiding principles for national tuberculosis programmes. Geneva, Switzerland: World Health Organization, 2008. WHO/HTM/TB/2008.400.
21. WHO. WHO Tuberculosis Programme – framework for effective tuberculosis control. Geneva, Switzerland: World Health Organization, 1994. WHO/TB/94.179.
22. Hopewell PC, Pai M, Maher D, et al. International standards for tuberculosis care. Lancet Infect Dis 2006; 6:710–725.
23. Luelmo F. What is the role of case detection in tuberculosis control? In: Frieden T, ed. Toman's Tuberculosis, 2nd ed. Geneva, Switzerland: World Health Organization, 2004.
24. Bassili A, Seita A, Baghdadi S, et al. Diagnostic and treatment delay in tuberculosis in 7 countries of the Eastern Mediterranean Region. Infect Dis Clin Pract 2008; 16:23–35.
25. Storla DG, Yimer S, Bjune GA. A systematic review of delay in the diagnosis and treatment of tuberculosis. BMC Public Health 2008; 8:15.
26. Baily GVJ, Savic D, Gothi GD, et al. Potential yield of pulmonary tuberculosis cases by direct microscopy of sputum in a district of South India. Bull World Health Organ 1967; 37:875–892.
27. Aluoch JA, Swai OB, Edwards EA, et al. Study of case-finding for pulmonary tuberculosis in outpatients complaining of a chronic cough at a district hospital in Kenya. Am Rev Respir Dis 1984; 129:915–920.

28. Sanchez-Perez HJ, Hernan MA, Hernandez-Diaz S, et al. Detection of pulmonary tuberculosis in Chiapas, Mexico. Ann Epidemiol 2002; 12:166–172.

29. Thomas A, Chandrasekaran V, Joseph P, et al. Increased yield of smear positive pulmonary TB cases by screening patients with > or = 2 weeks cough, compared to > or = 3 weeks and adequacy of 2 sputum smear examinations for diagnosis. Indian J Tuberc 2008; 55: 77–83.

30. Harries T. What are the relative merits of chest radiography and sputum examination (smear microscopy and culture) in case detection among new outpatients with prolonged chest symptoms? In: Frieden T, ed. Toman's Tuberculosis, 2nd ed. Geneva, Switzerland: World Health Organization, 2004.

31. WHO. Revision of the case definition for sputum smear positive tuberculosis: Background document. Geneva, Switzerland: World Health Organization, 2008. http://www.who.int/tb/dots/laboratory/policy/en/index.html. Accessed January 15, 2009.

32. WHO. Improving the diagnosis and treatment of smear-negative pulmonary and extrapulmonary tuberculosis among adults and adolescents – Recommendations for HIV-prevalent and resource-constrained settings. Geneva, Switzerland: World Health Organization, 2007. WHO/HTM /TB /2007.379.

33. WHO. Strategic framework to decrease the burden of TB/HIV. Geneva, Switzerland: World Health Organization, 2002b. WHO/CDS/TB/2002.296.

34. Shah NS, Anh MH, Thuy TT, Duong, et al. Population-based chest X-ray screening for pulmonary tuberculosis in people living with HIV/AIDS, An Giang, Vietnam. Int J Tuberc Lung Dis 2008; 12(4):404–410.

35. Lin H, Ezzat M, Murray M. Tobacco smoke, indoor air pollution and tuberculosis: A systematic review and meta-analysis. PLoS Med 2007; 4:X–X

36. Slama K, Chiang CY, Enarson D, et al. Tobacco and tuberculosis: A qualitative systematic review and meta analysis. Int J Tuberc Lung Dis 2007; 11:1049–1061.

37. Stevenson CR, Critchley JA, Forouhi NG, et al. Diabetes and the risk of tuberculosis: A neglected threat to public health? Chronic Illn 2007; 3:228–245.

38. Cegielski P, McMurray DN. The relationship between malnutrition and tuberculosis: Evidence from studies in humans and experimental animals. Int J Tuberc Lung Dis 2004; 8:286–298.

39. Lönnroth K, Williams BG, Stadlin S, et al. Alcohol use as risk factor for tuberculosis disease – a systematic review. BMC Public Health 2008; 8:289.

40. Rieder H. Epidemiologic Basis of Tuberculosis Control. Paris, France: International Union Against Tuberculosis and Lung Disease, 1999.

41. WHO. Respiratory care in primary care services – A survey in 9 countries. Geneva, Switzerland: World Health Organization, 2004. WHO/HTM/TB/2004.333.

42. Me'emary F, Ottmani S, Pio A, et al. Results of the feasibility test of the Practical Approach to Lung Health in Syria. East Mediterr Health J 2009; 15:504–515.

43. WHO. Practical Approach to Lung health (PAL): A primary health care strategy for integrated management of respiratory conditions in people of five years of age and over. Geneva, Switzerland: World Health Organization, 2005. WHO/HTM/TB/2005.351; WHO/NMH/CHP/CPM/CRA/05.3.

44. Erhola M, Brimkulov N, Chubakov T, et al. Development process of the Practical Approach to Lung Health in Kyrgyzstan. Int J Tuberc Lung Dis 2009; 13:540–544.

45. Camacho M, Nogales M, Manjon R, et al. Results of PAL feasibility test in primary health care facilities in four regions of Bolivia. Int J Tuberc Lung Dis 2007; 11:1246–1252.

46. Fairall LR, Zwarenstein M, Bateman ED, et al. Effect of educational outreach to nurses on tuberculosis case detection and primary care of respiratory illness: Pragmatic cluster randomized controlled trial. BMJ 2005; 331:750–754.

47. Zidouni N, Baough L, Laid Y, et al. L'Approche pratique de la Santé respiratoire en Algérie. Int J Tuberc Lung Dis 2009; 13:1029–1037.

48. Diwan V, Thorson A, Winkvist A. Gender and Tuberculosis. NHV Report 1998:3. Gothenburg, Sweden: Nordic School of Public Health, 1998.
49. Gosoniu GD, Ganapathy S, Kemp J, et al. Gender and socio-cultural determinants of delay to diagnosis of TB in Bangladesh, India and Malawi. Int J Tuberc Lung Dis 2008; 12(7): 848–855.
50. TDR. Gender and tuberculosis: Cross-site analysis and implications of a multi-country study in Bangladesh, India, Malawi, and Colombia. TDR Report Series No.3. Geneva, Switzerland: World Health Organization, Special Programme for Research and Training in Tropical Diseases, 2006.
51. Weiss MG, Sommerfeld J, Uplekar M. Social and cultural dimensions of gender and tuberculosis. Int J Tuberc Lung Dis 2008; 12:829–830.
52. WHO. Community contribution to TB care – practice and policy. Geneva, Switzerland: World Health Organization, 2003. WHO/CDS/TB/2003.312.
53. Stop TB Partnership. Advocacy, communication and social mobilization (ACSM) for tuberculosis control: A handbook for country programmes. Geneva, Switzerland: World Health Organization, 2007.
54. Simwaka BN, Benson T, Salaniponi FML, et al. Developing a socio-economic measure to monitor access to tuberculosis services in urban Lilongwe, Malawi. Int J Tuberc Lung Dis 2007; 11:65–71.
55. Lönnroth K, Thuong LM, Linh PD, et al. Utilisation of private and public health care providers among people with symptoms of tuberculosis in Ho Chi Minh City, Vietnam. Health Pol Plan 2001; 16:47–54.
56. Pantoja A, Floyd K, Unnikrishnan KP, et al. Economic evaluation of PPM-DOTS in Bangalore, south India. Part I: Profile and costs of TB patients. Int J Tuberc Lung Dis Accepted.
57. Lönnroth K, Tin-Aung, Win-Maung, et al. Social franchising of TB care through private general practitioners in Myanmar – an assessment of access, quality of care, equity, and financial protection. Health Pol Plan 2007; 22:156–166.
58. WHO. Engaging all health care providers in TB control – guidance on implementing public-private mix approaches. Geneva, Switzerland: World Health Organization, 2006b. WHO/HTM/TB/2006.360.
59. Lönnroth K, Uplekar M, Blanc L. Hard gains through soft contracts – productive engagement of private providers in tuberculosis control. Bull World Health Organ 2006; 84:876–883.
60. Lönnroth K, Uplekar M, Arora VK, et al. Public-Private Mix for Improved TB Control – what makes it work? Bull World Health Organ 2004; 82:580–586.
61. Ambe G, Lönnroth K, Dholakia Y, et al. Every provider counts!: Effects of a comprehensive public-private mix approach for TB control in a large metropolitan area in India. Int J Tuberc Lung Dis 2005; 9:562–568.
62. Dewan PK, Lal SS, Lönnroth K, et al. Public-Private Mix in India: Improving Tuberculosis Control Through Intersectoral Partnerships. BMJ 2006; 332:574–578.
63. Salim MAH, Uplekar M, Declercq E, et al. Turning liabilities into resources: The informal village doctors and TB control in Bangladesh. Bull World Health Organ 2006; 84: 479–484.
64. Floyd K, Arora VK, Murthy KJR, et al. Cost and cost-effectiveness of public and private sector collaboration in tuberculosis control: Evidence from India. Bull World Health Organ 2006; 84:437–445.
65. Pantoja A, Lönnroth K, Lal SS, et al. Economic evaluation of PPM-DOTS in Bangalore, south India. Part II: Cost and cost-effectiveness of intensified efforts. Int J Tuberc Lung Dis Accepted.
66. Lönnroth K, Tran TU, Thuong LM, et al. Can I afford free treatment?: Perceived consequences of health care provider choices among people with tuberculosis in Ho Chi Minh City, Vietnam. Soc Sci Med 2001; 52:935–948.

67. Jaramillo E. The impact of media-based health education on tuberculosis diagnosis in Cali, Colombia. Health Pol Plan 2001; 16:68–73.
68. Becx-Bleumink M, Wibowo H, Apriani W, et al. High tuberculosis notification and treatment success rates through community participation in central Sulawesi, Republic of Indonesia. Int J Tuberc Lung Dis 2001; 5:920–925.
69. WHO. Everybody's Business. Strengthening health systems to improve health outcomes: WHOs Framework for Action. Geneva, Switzerland: Word Health Organization, 2007.
70. Wang L, Liu J, Chin DP. Progress in tuberculosis control and the evolving public-health system in China. Lancet 2007; 369:691–696.
71. Morrison J, Pai M, Hopewell PC. Tuberculosis and latent tuberculosis infection in close contacts of people with pulmonary tuberculosis in low-income and middle-income countries: A systematic review and meta-analysis. Lancet Infect Dis 2008; 8:359–368.
72. Ottmani S, Zignol M, Bencheikh N, et al. TB contact investigations: The results of twelve years of experience of the National TB Programme of Morocco. East Mediterr Health J 2009; 15:494–503.
73. Golub JE, Mohan CI, Comstock GW, et al. Active case finding of tuberculosis: Historical perspective and future prospects. Int J Tuberc Lung Dis 2005; 9:1183–1203.
74. Borgdorff MW, Floyd K, Broekmans JF. Interventions to reduce tuberculosis mortality and transmission in low- and middle-income countries. Bull World Health Organ 2002; 80: 217–227.
75. WHO. WHO Expert Committee on Tuberculosis. Ninth report. WHO Technical Series, No 552. Geneva, Switzerland: World Health Organization, 1974.
76. Menzies D, Joshi R, Pai M. Risk of tuberculosis infection and disease associated with work in health care settings. Int J Tuberc Lung Dis 2007; 11(6):593–605.
77. WHO. Guidelines for the Control of Tuberculosis in Prisons. Geneva, Switzerland: World Health Organization, 1998. WHO/TB/98.250.
78. WHO. Tuberculosis care and control in refugee and displaced populations. Geneva, Switzerland: World Health Organization, 2007d. WHO/HTM/TB/2007.377.
79. WHO. Policy guidelines for collaborative TB and HIV services for injecting and other drug users: An integrated approach. Geneva, Switzerland: World Health Organization, 2008e. WHO/HTM/TB/2008.404.
80. Jakubowiak WM, Bogorodskaya EM, Borisov SE, et al. Risk factors associated with default among new pulmonary TB patients and social support in six Russian regions. Int J Tuberc Lung Dis 2007; 11:46–53.
81. Munro SA, Lewin SA, Smith HJ, et al. Patient adherence to tuberculosis treatment: A systematic review of qualitative research. PLoS Med 2007; 4:e238.
82. Saly S, Onozaki I, Ishikawa N. Decentralized DOTS shortens delay to TB treatment significantly in Cambodia. Kekkaku 2006; 81:467–474.
83. Beith A, Eichler R, Weil D. Performance-based incentives for health: A way to improve tuberculosis detection and treatment completion? Working Paper 122. Washington, DC: The Center for Global Development, 2007.
84. Mookherji S. Evaluating tuberculosis control incentives and enablers in context of scale-up. Evidence and experiences. Draft document. Washington, DC: Management Sciences for Health, 2005.
85. Baddeley A. A systematic literature review to assess the impact of alcoholism on tuberculosis control and strategies to encourage compliance among alcoholic TB patients. (Academic thesis). London, UK: London School of Hygiene and Tropical Medicine, 2008.
86. Botha E, Den Boon S, Verver S, et al. Initial default from tuberculosis treatment: How often does it happen and what are the reasons? Int J Tuberc Lung Dis 2008; 12(7):820–823.
87. Buu TN, Lönnroth K, Quy HT. Initial defaulting in the National TB Programme in Ho Chi Minh City, Vietnam – A survey of magnitude, reasons and actions taken after defaulting. Int J Tuberc Lung Dis 2003; 7:735–741.

88. Sai Babu B, Satyanarayana AV, Venkateshwaralu G, et al. Initial default among diagnosed sputum smear-positive pulmonary tuberculosis patients in Andhra Pradesh, India. Int J Tuberc Lung Dis 2008; 12:1055–1058.
89. Uplekar MW, Shepard DS. Treatment of tuberculosis by private general practitioners in India. Tubercle 1991; 72(4):284–290.
90. Matiru R, Ryan T. The Global Drug Facility: A unique, holistic and pioneering approach to drug procurement and management. Bull World Health Organ. 2007; 85(5):348–353.

9
Antituberculosis Drug Resistance in the World: The Latest Information

ABIGAIL WRIGHT and MATTEO ZIGNOL
Stop TB Department, World Health Organization, Geneva, Switzerland

I. Introduction

The emergence of resistance to antimicrobials is a natural biological occurrence and a response to the selective pressure of the drug. The introduction of every antimicrobial agent into clinical practice for the treatment of infectious diseases in humans and animals has been eventually followed by the detection of isolates of resistant microorganisms, that is, microorganisms able to multiply in the presence of drug concentrations found in hosts receiving therapeutic doses (1). With increasing use and misuse of antibiotics, resistance has emerged in many microorganisms including *Mycobacterium tuberculosis* (2–6). The emergence of drug-resistant *M. tuberculosis* has been associated with a variety of provider, patient, and management factors including poor adherence to treatment (7–9), inappropriate prescription (10,11), irregular drug supply, or poor drug quality (12).

Exposure to a single drug, regardless of the cause, eliminates bacilli susceptible to that drug but permits the multiplication of preexisting drug-resistant mutants (2,3). Resistance developed within the patient because of subtherapeutic doses for any reason is referred to as *acquired resistance*. Subsequent transmission of such bacilli to other persons may lead to a disease that is drug resistant from the outset, an occurrence known as *primary resistance*. The objective of close supervision of treatment based on short-course chemotherapy (SCC), utilizing a combination of antituberculosis (anti-TB) agents including rifampicin, ultimately is to reduce the risk of monotherapy and the subsequent acquisition of drug resistance.

In some countries, management factors may include the lack of a standardized therapeutic regimen and poor program implementation, compounded by frequent or prolonged shortages of drugs, inadequate resources, political instability, or lack of political commitment. Use of anti-TB drugs of unproven quality is an additional concern as is the sale of these medications over the counter and on the black market. Additional management-related factors are associated with increased community transmission of drug resistance: Poor infection control measures in congregate settings is one example.

Patients infected with strains resistant to multiple drugs, particularly to the two most powerful first-line drugs, isoniazid and rifampicin, or multidrug-resistant TB (MDR-TB) are very difficult to cure (13), and the required treatment with second-line drugs is more toxic, lengthy, and expensive. The emergence and spread of drug-resistant TB, particularly MDR-TB, pose a threat to international TB control (14–16).

II. Assessing Anti-TB Drug Resistance in the World

In the early 1990s, several reports were published on the emergence of MDR-TB (17–20), but the populations surveyed were not comparable, and the methods used to quantify the problem were not standardized thus making it difficult to estimate the global magnitude of drug-resistant TB. In 1994, the Global Project on Anti-TB Drug Resistance Surveillance (DRS) was established in order to estimate the global burden of drug-resistant TB worldwide using standardized methodologies so that data could be compared across and within regions (21). The Project aimed to monitor trends in resistance, evaluate the performance of TB control programs, and advise on drug regimens (22). The Supranational TB Reference Laboratory Network (SRLN), a network now consisting of 26 laboratories globally, was developed in order to provide quality assurance to drug-resistance surveys including panel testing before the start of a survey and rechecking of isolates during the survey (23). The Global Project methodology operates on three main principles: (*i*) the survey must be based on a sample of TB patients representative of all cases in the geographical setting under evaluation, (*ii*) drug resistance in survey settings should be clearly distinguished according to the treatment history of the patient (i.e., never treated or previously treated) in order to allow correct interpretation of the data, and (*iii*) laboratory results must be quality assured by a Supranational Reference Laboratory (SRL) (5).

In 2006, a survey conducted by the WHO and Centers for Disease Control established the widespread distribution of isolates of *M. tuberculosis* with resistance to second-line drugs and defined extensively drug-resistant TB (XDR-TB) (6). From 2006, routine drug-resistance surveillance data as well as surveys attempted to ascertain the proportion of XDR-TB among isolates with confirmed MDR-TB in order to develop a better understanding of the global distribution of second-line drug resistance. Because of lack of laboratory capacity to test for second-line drug resistance, the number of countries reporting has been limited (24).

Reports of data from periodic surveys and routine surveillance systems are published approximately every 3 years as most countries require up to 18 months to complete a drug-resistance survey. In this chapter, we have presented data from the fourth global report on anti-TB drug resistance collected between 2002 and 2007, as well as information derived from half a million isolates collected since 1994, in 116 countries and territories representing one half of all notified TB cases. The most recent profile of anti-TB drug resistance globally and regionally as well as the trends in anti-TB drug resistance over time, HIV and drug-resistant TB, and XDR-TB are discussed.

III. Methods for Assessment of Drug Resistance in Tuberculosis

Survey methods are summarized here, while a detailed description can be found in the full report (5,25). For the purposes of analysis, patients are classified as new or previously treated cases. New cases are defined as patients who have never been treated or have received anti-TB treatment for less than one month. These patients are considered to be a proxy for those who have been primarily infected with a drug-resistant strain of *M. tuberculosis*. Previously treated cases are defined as patients who have been treated for TB for one month or more. All newly registered patients with sputum smear–positive pulmonary TB are considered eligible for inclusion, though in many surveillance settings where all TB cases receive culture, all culture positive cases are included regardless of smear result. In the context of standard surveys, sample sizes are based on all new smear-positive cases notified in the previous year and the estimated proportion of rifampicin resistance in this population. In most survey settings, previously treated cases are included during the period of intake for new cases, although some countries develop a separate sample size for these cases, and other countries include all cases during the calendar year. One isolate is examined per TB case. Rechecking of patient treatment history through verification of medical records and patient reinterview is recommended in order to reduce the possibility of misclassification. Country groupings are largely based on the countries' geographical location and, in the case of the countries of the former Soviet Union (FSU), on recent historical and sociocultural characteristics. The main indicators used in all surveys include proportions of cases tested showing (*i*) resistance to any first-line drug; (*ii*) MDR-TB, or resistance to both isoniazid and rifampicin; (*iii*) XDR-TB, or MDR-TB with additional resistance to a fluoroquinolone and a second-line injectable drug.

IV.   Laboratory Methods for Assessment of Drug Resistance in Tuberculosis

Drug-susceptibility tests are performed using the indirect proportion method on Löwenstein–Jensen (L-J) medium (26), the absolute concentration method, the resistance ratio method (27), or the radiometric BACTEC 460 or MGIT 960 methods (28,29). Species other than *M. tuberculosis* are systematically excluded from analysis. Quality assurance is performed by the SRL by sending a panel of isolates prior to the implementation of the survey and later by rechecking a percentage of isolates from patients included in the survey. HIV testing is not a mandatory component of these surveys but HIV serostatus, where available, is included in the analysis.

V.   Approach to Analysis of Data on Drug Resistance in Tuberculosis

Aggregate data reported from settings are entered into a database, built with Microsoft Access^{TM} software. All the data are rechecked during the process of data entry and before starting the analysis, and all data files and epidemiological profiles are returned to the countries for verification. Summary analyses are conducted in STATA (version 9.0, StataCorp LP). For geographical settings reporting more than a single data point since the third report, only the latest data point has been used for the estimation of point prevalence. All tests of significance are two tailed and the α-error is kept at the 0.05 level in all inference procedures. Ninety-five percent confidence intervals (or confidence limits, CLs) are calculated around the proportions and the means. Trend analysis is performed for geographical settings reporting more than two data points since the beginning of the project. Statistical significance of trends is determined through a logistic regression. Where HIV status is a component of surveys or routine surveillance, the association between HIV and drug-resistant TB is evaluated through calculation of an odds ratio to compare proportion of drug resistance in HIV-positive and HIV-negative TB patients. Statistical significance is tested using Fisher's exact test. For analysis of resistance to second-line anti-TB drugs, the denominator used is MDR isolates tested for resistance to at least one fluoroquinolone and one injectable second-line anti-TB drug (required to define XDR-TB) (24). XDR-TB and fluoroquinolone resistance are the two categories reported.

VI. The Global Anti-TB Drug Resistance Situation

The fourth round of the Global Project included data from 83 countries and territories having at least one data point since 2002.[a] The median number of cases tested per setting was 553, but ranged from 5 cases in New Caledonia to 4350 in P.R. China, Hong Kong Special Administrative Region (SAR); 4800 in the United Kingdom; and 10,584 in the United States. Nine countries provided data that did not differentiate between new and previously treated cases.

A. Drug Resistance Among New Cases

Seventy-two countries and two SARs of P.R. China provided data on drug resistance among new cases of TB. Resistance to any drug ranged from 0% (Iceland), 1.4% (95% CLs, 0.6–2.9) in Bosnia and Herzegovina, and 1.5% (95% CLs, 0.6–2.9) in Sri Lanka to 49.2% (95% CLs, 44.4–54.3) in Georgia, 51.2% (95% CLs, 44.1–58.3) in Tashkent, Uzbekistan, and 56.3% (95% CLs, 50.2–62.9) in Baku, Azerbaijan. Thirteen settings reported a prevalence of resistance to any drug of higher than 30%. Sixteen settings reported a prevalence of resistance to isoniazid higher than 15%. All settings with high prevalence of isoniazid resistance were located in countries of the FSU or P.R. China with the exception of Israel and Vietnam. Prevalence of MDR ranged from 0% in Andorra, Cuba, Iceland, Luxembourg, Malta, Slovenia, Spain (Aragon), and Uruguay to 19.4% (95% CLs, 16.5–22.6) in the Republic of Moldova, and 22.3% (95% CLs, 18.5–26.6) in Baku, Azerbaijan. Fourteen settings reported a prevalence of MDR among new cases higher than 6.0%, of which 12 were located in countries of the FSU. The other two settings were provinces in P.R. China (Fig. 1).

B. Drug Resistance Among Previously Treated Cases

There was no resistance reported in Iceland, Israel, and Norway where the number of previously treated cases was very small. In contrast, Baku, Azerbaijan, and Tashkent, Uzbekistan, showed very high prevalences of any resistance—84.4% (95% CLs, 76.9–92.4) and 85.9% (95% CLs, 76.6–92.5), respectively. In sixteen settings, prevalence of any resistance was reported as 50% or higher. No MDR was reported in Denmark, New Zealand, Sri Lanka, or among the preliminary data reported from UR Tanzania. Estonia reported 52.1% (95% CLs, 39.9–64.1%) MDR-TB among previously treated cases; Baku, Azerbaijan, reported 55.8% (95% CLs, 49.7–62.4%); and Tashkent, Uzbekistan, reported 60.0% (95% CLs, 48.8–70.5). The Russian Federation reported data on re-treatment cases in Orel Oblast only. Sixteen settings reported MDR-TB of higher than 25% among previously treated cases. Seven of these settings were located in countries of the FSU (Fig. 2).

VII. Global Estimates of Multidrug-Resistant TB

On the basis of drug-resistance data reported from 116 countries and territories, WHO estimated the proportion of MDR-TB among new, previously treated, and combined TB

---

[a] Two settings in India reported data from 2001. These data have been excluded from the analyses but are included in the annex.

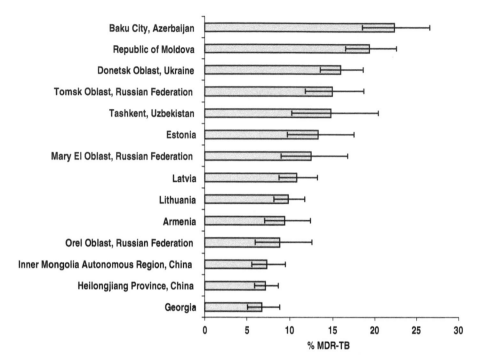

Figure 1   Percent MDR-TB among new TB cases.

cases for a further 69 countries and developed a global estimate of incident MDR-TB cases (5). The estimated number of new TB cases by country was used to calculate the number of MDR-TB cases that occurred among new cases. To estimate the number of previously treated cases, the ratio of notified previously treated cases to notified new cases in 2006 was multiplied by the total number of new cases estimated to have occurred in the same year for each country; therefore, the total number of estimated cases includes estimated re-treatment cases. Estimates were developed using a logistic regression model described in detail elsewhere (30,31).

The global estimated number of incident MDR-TB cases in 2006 is 489,139 (95% CLs, 455, 093–614, 215), which is 4.8% (95% CLs, 4.6–6.0) of the total number of estimated incident TB cases in 2006 in 185 countries (10,229,315).[b] The prevalence of MDR-TB ranged from 0.0% to 28.9%. The median prevalence of MDR-TB among all TB cases was 2.4%, with an interquartile range of 1.4% to 4.2%. Estimates by country can be found in the annexes of the fourth Drug Resistance Surveillance Report (5).

VIII.   Trends in Anti-TB Drug Resistance

Trends were evaluated in 47 countries and territories with 3 or more data points between 1994 and 2007. In low TB prevalence countries conducting continuous surveillance, trends

---

[b] The number of all estimated TB cases includes estimated retreatment cases.

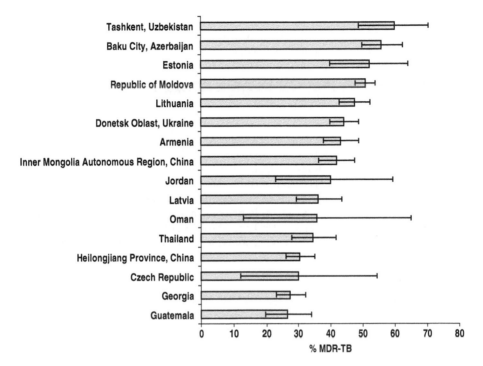

Figure 2 Percent MDR-TB among previously treated TB cases.

were determined in the group of total cases reported. In countries conducting surveys, or where population of previously treated cases tested changed over time, trends were determined in new cases only.

The United States and Hong Kong SAR reported significant reductions in both the proportion of MDR and TB notification rates. In most high-resource countries, such as the UK, France, and Germany, with a low prevalence of TB, trends in MDR were stable. Both Peru and the Republic of Korea reported increases in the proportion of MDR among new cases, but at the same time showed steady declines in TB notification rates followed by recent leveling off. In countries of the FSU there were two scenarios: Two Baltic countries (Estonia and Latvia) showed stable trends in proportions of MDR among new cases, while Lithuania showed a slow but significant increase. All three countries showed a decreasing TB notification rate (5–8% reduction per year). Two oblasts in the Russian Federation (Orel and Tomsk) showed an increase in the proportion of MDR among new cases as well as increases in absolute numbers. Notification rates are declining in both regions but at a slower rate (1–3% reduction per year) than in the Baltic countries.

IX.   The Global XDR-TB Situation

As part of the Global Project, twenty-eight countries or territories reported routine surveillance data on XDR-TB while nine countries reported data from periodic surveys. The majority of countries reporting surveillance data were low–TB-burden countries. Some countries reported data aggregated over a three-year period, and other countries reported over a one-year period. The numbers of MDR cases tested for the appropriate second-line anti-TB drugs are used as a denominator. For this analysis, MDR-TB and XDR-TB cases are not disaggregated by history of the previous treatment. In total, data were reported on 3818 MDR-TB cases, and among those 304 or 7.9% XDR-TB cases were detected. In general, absolute numbers of XDR-TB cases were low in Central and Western Europe, the United States, and African and Asian countries that reported data. The proportion of XDR-TB among MDR-TB in these settings ranged from 0% in 14 settings to 30.9% in Japan. However, this figure represented a total of 17 XDR-TB cases among 55 MDR-TB cases tested for second-line drugs in Japan's nationwide survey. The reporting countries have a relatively low–MDR-TB burden, so this represents few absolute cases. Of the eight countries in the FSU that reported, approximately 10% of all MDR-TB cases were XDR ranging from 4.0% in Armenia to 23.7% in Estonia; and given the underlying burden of MDR-TB, these proportions represent a large absolute number of cases. Since 2002 a total of 55 countries and territories have reported to WHO at least one case of XDR-TB (Fig. 3).

X. The Relationship Between HIV and MDR

Of the seven countries that reported data on drug resistance stratified by HIV status, only Latvia and Donetsk Oblast, Ukraine, reported large enough numbers to allow assessment of the relationship between the two epidemics. MDR was significantly associated with HIV in both Latvia (OR 2.1; 95% CLs, 1.4–3.0) and in Donetsk Oblast (OR 1.5; 95% CLs, 1.1–2.0), and likewise resistance to any TB drug (OR 1.5; 95% CLs, 1.1–2.1 and OR 1.4; 95% CLs, 1.1–1.8 in Latvia and Donetsk Oblast, respectively). However, HIV seronegative and patients with an unknown HIV status were not distinguished in Latvia. From the data reported in Latvia, the proportion of MDR-TB among HIV seropositive cases was shown to be stable over time.

XI. General Considerations

Data available through the WHO Global Project indicate regional and national variation in the magnitude and trends in drug-resistant TB. Countries of the FSU followed by some provinces of P.R. China reported the highest prevalence of resistance. Countries in the Eastern Mediterranean region and South East Asia reported prevalence of resistance on par with estimated global averages. The United States, Western and Central Europe, and the countries of the African region reported the lowest prevalences of MDR-TB. Outliers were identified in all regions, indicating that prevalence of MDR-TB is linked to national TB control performance.

A range of trend scenarios is evident based on the 47 countries that have reported trend information. The majority of settings reporting three or more data points were low TB prevalence settings and showed relatively stable trends with low absolute numbers of MDR-TB. Of these settings, the United States and Hong Kong SAR both with strong political and financial commitment to TB control, reported continued reductions in the prevalence and caseload of MDR-TB. Notably, few high–TB-burden countries were able to report trends, highlighting the difficulty of repeating drug-resistance surveys and the

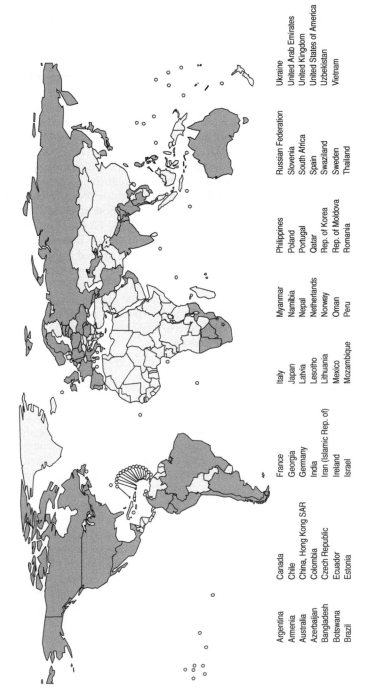

Argentina	France	Myanmar	Russian Federation	Ukraine
Armenia	Georgia	Namibia	Slovenia	United Arab Emirates
Australia	Germany	Nepal	South Africa	United Kingdom
Azerbaijan	India	Netherlands	Spain	United States of America
Bangladesh	Iran (Islamic Rep. of)	Norway	Swaziland	Uzbekistan
Botswana	Ireland	Oman	Sweden	Vietnam
Brazil	Israel	Peru	Thailand	
Canada	Italy	Philippines		
Chile	Japan	Poland		
China, Hong Kong SAR	Latvia	Portugal		
Colombia	Lesotho	Qatar		
Czech Republic	Lithuania	Rep. of Korea		
Ecuador	Mexico	Rep. of Moldova		
Estonia	Mozambique	Romania		

The boundaries and names shown and the designations used on this map do not imply the expression of any opinion whatsoever on the part of the World Health Organization concerning the legal status of any country, territory, city, or area or of its authorities, or concerning the delimitation of its frontiers or boundaries. Dotted lines on maps represent approximate border lines for which there may not yet be full agreement.

Figure 3   Countries reporting at least one XDR-TB case, 2002–2008.

need for strengthening laboratory networks and developing easier methods for surveys. The Russian Federation, Peru, and the Republic of Korea reported increases in MDR-TB. The specific reasons behind the recent increases, particularly in Korea and Peru, two countries with long-term implementation of DOTS, need to be further explored.

The countries of the FSU are facing a serious and widespread epidemic with the highest prevalence of MDR-TB ever reported in 13 years of global data collection. Almost half of all TB cases in countries of the FSU are resistant to at least one drug and one of every five cases of TB will have MDR-TB. In this region, MDR-TB cases have more extensive resistance patterns and the highest prevalences of XDR-TB. Trend data from the Baltic countries likely represent the best scenario for this region with prevalence of MDR-TB among new cases remaining stable and TB notification rates declining. This is likely due to strong political commitment and long-term sustained investment in TB control, optimal management of susceptible and drug-resistant TB cases, and an improving socioeconomic situation. In contrast, the data reported from two Russian oblasts with well-performing TB control programs indicate an alarming situation with increases in both absolute number and prevalence of MDR-TB among new cases and a slowly declining TB notification rate. Although the trend data are based on only two of 89 oblasts in the Russian Federation, national data, not included in this analysis due to nonconforming methodology, support the finding of a nationwide increase in MDR-TB (32). National data showed a 5% annual increase in the prevalence of MDR among new TB cases from 6.7% MDR-TB in 1999 to 9.4% in 2006. The national report acknowledges that in some regions the prevalence of MDR-TB exceeds the prevalence derived from routine reporting. It is expected that routine reporting may underestimate the prevalence due to inadequacies in data collection, laboratory service coverage, or laboratory performance.

The enhancement of TB control in recent years including new legislation to bring policies in line with the Stop TB strategy, the expansion of MDR-TB case management in accordance with international guidelines, and the upgrading of diagnostic services (33) are important steps that have been undertaken. Nevertheless, efforts will have to be considerably accelerated and backed by strong political commitment to have an impact on a growing epidemic of drug-resistant TB. Surveys in 8 of 31 provinces and 2 municipalities in P.R. China over a 10-year period show proportions of resistance only second to countries of the FSU, indicating the presence of a serious drug-resistance problem. Trend data are not yet available from provinces in P.R. China. However, a nationwide survey currently underway will help to develop a national estimate of MDR-TB.

While the magnitude and trends in MDR are epidemiologically important to monitor, estimating the burden of disease is programmatically relevant in shaping policies for screening and treatment. Of the half a million MDR-TB cases estimated to have emerged in 2006, 50% were in India and P.R. China alone. Twenty-seven countries account for 86% of the world's MDR-TB burden. All countries should work toward preventing MDR-TB by optimizing their control and care efforts, and toward managing existing MDR-TB cases by enforcing, screening, and treatment policies for MDR-TB as a matter of priority. To achieve success, countries facing a high prevalence of MDR or high burden of cases will require increased political commitment and international support for development and implementation of these programs.

The widespread reporting of XDR-TB cases indicate that where second-line drugs are used and where cure rates of MDR-TB remain low, XDR-TB will emerge. The magnitude and distribution of XDR-TB is not well-established because of lack of laboratory capacity to test for second-line drug resistance,[c] but the data available in this survey indicate that XDR-TB is currently most severe in countries of the FSU. With continued use of second-line drugs outside of the NTP it is likely that the problem of XDR-TB will grow, and without appropriate laboratory capacity to diagnose rapidly and to treat effectively, the world is ill equipped to manage this emerging specter.

Although few population level data exist on the relationship between HIV and MDR, data from Latvia and Ukraine show that HIV-positive TB cases are significantly more likely to have MDR-TB than HIV-negative TB cases. The data do not allow for determination as to whether the association is related to acquisition or transmission. Nevertheless, the findings have enormous implications for health care systems that should ensure rapid resistance screening and effective clinical management for TB patients living with HIV, as discussed in a recent review paper (34).

Considerable progress has been made in expanding survey coverage, estimating the global burden of MDR-TB, strengthening laboratories, monitoring HIV, and incorporating testing for resistance to second-line drugs. However, the Project has not met some of its initial goals, suggesting a need to revisit the project methods. Primarily as a result of inadequate laboratory capacity, there are still major geographic areas for which there is no information on the burden of drug-resistant TB. In the WHO African region in particular, only 18 of 46 countries had nationwide drug-resistance data and only 8 reported data since 2002. Furthermore, few trend data from high–TB-burden countries are available, thus limiting the possibility of estimating global trends.

If trends are to be determined in high–TB-burden countries, surveys need to be easier to implement. Molecular diagnostics hold the greatest promise for scaling up surveillance rapidly, with a substantial advantage in the reduced laboratory capacity required and the transportation of noninfectious material (35). Understanding of the mutations causing resistance for second-line drugs is currently incomplete. Therefore, use of molecular methods alone would restrict the amount of information obtained to the two most critical anti-TB drugs. However, this would be offset by the shortened time required for screening out the most critical cases (MDR-TB), and phenotypic drug-susceptibility testing (DST) could be undertaken for second-line drugs. Following an expert review of the Global Project, existing international guidelines will be revised in 2009 with new recommendations for both laboratory and survey methods to facilitate more rapid scale-up, but also to better determine trends (36,37). Recommendations include that, at a minimum, periodic representative surveys should be conducted among new TB cases (every three to five years) and continuous surveillance mechanisms should be established among all re-treatment cases (prioritization of subcategories to be identified at country level).

Either phenotypic or genotypic tests could be used for surveillance purposes. At the very least drugs tested should be rifampicin and isoniazid, plus fluoroquinolones, injectable second-line drugs, and ethambutol if the strain is found to be rifampicin resistant. Survey protocols must now be reviewed by an ethical committee or review board.

Transmission dynamics and acquisition of resistance are critical for the prioritization of interventions but are difficult to address in the context of routine surveillance in most settings. Thus, more work is required in the area of coordinated protocol development to address these areas.

---

[c] It is important to note that in settings where only one fluoroquinolone and one injectable drug are tested, XDR-TB rates may be underestimated.

XII. Conclusions

Over the last decade sound standardized TB patient management has been widely implemented and new policies to address TB/HIV and MDR-TB, improved laboratory diagnosis, and the engagement of all health care providers and civil society have been developed, tested, and endorsed. From 2008, DOTS has been implemented in 184 countries, 52 resource-constrained countries are treating MDR-TB according to WHO guidelines, and most countries are beginning to implement the various components of the new Stop TB strategy. The next decade calls for an accelerated scale-up of the Stop TB Strategy, that is, strengthening basic DOTS activities to ensure quality of treatment to prevent acquisition of resistance, rapid diagnosis of resistant cases, and initiation of treatment following international guidelines to prevent further transmission, and broad application of infection control measures, particularly in congregate settings to prevent outbreaks (38). These measures, if implemented widely and effectively, can curb the spreading epidemic of MDR-TB.

Until drug-susceptibility testing is implemented routinely for cases as the standard for diagnosis and surveillance, survey mechanisms will continue to be crucial in determination of trends and in the documentation of the emergence of further resistance to second-line drugs.

References

1. Neu HC. The crisis in antibiotic resistance. Science (New York) 1992; 257(5073):1064–1073.
2. Crofton J, Mitchison DA. Streptomycin resistance in pulmonary tuberculosis. BMJ 1948; 2: 1009–1015.
3. Mitchison DA. Development of streptomycin resistant strains of tubercle bacilli in pulmonary tuberculosis. Thorax 1950; 5:144–161.
4. Canetti G. The J. Burns Amberson lecture. Present aspects of bacterial resistance in tuberculosis. Am Rev Respir Dis 1965; 92:687–703.
5. World Health Organization. Anti-Tuberculosis Drug Resistance in the World: Report 4. Geneva, Switzerland: World Health Organization, 2008. WHO/HTM/TB/2008.394.
6. Centers for Disease Control and Prevention. Emergence of *Mycobacterium tuberculosis* with extensive resistance to second-line drugs—worldwide, 2000–2004. MMWR Morb Mortal Wkly Rep 2006; 55:301–305.
7. Addington WW. Patient compliance: The most serious remaining problem in the control of tuberculosis in the United States. Chest 1979; 76(suppl):741–743.
8. Sumartojo E. When tuberculosis treatment fails. A social behavioral account of patient adherence. Am Rev Respir Dis 1993; 147:1311–1320.
9. Bam TS, Gunneberg C, Chamroonsawasdi K, et al. Factors affecting patient adherence to DOTS in urban Kathmandu, Nepal. Int J Tuberc Lung Dis 2006; 10:270–276.
10. Hopewell PC, Pai M, Maher D, et al. International standards for tuberculosis care. Lancet Infect Dis 2006; 6:710–725.
11. World Health Organization. Treatment of Tuberculosis: Guidelines for National Programmes, 3rd ed. Geneva, Switzerland: World Health Organization, 2003:1–108. WHO/CDS/TB/2003.313.
12. Barnes PF. The influence of epidemiologic factors on drug resistance rates in tuberculosis. Am Rev Respir Dis 1987; 136:325–328.
13. Espinal MA, Laserson K, Camacho M, et al. Determinants of drug-resistant tuberculosis: Analysis of 11 countries. Int J Tuberc Lung Dis 2001; 5:887–893.
14. Dye C, Williams BG. Criteria for the control of drug-resistant tuberculosis. Proc Natl Acad Sci 2000; 97:8180–8185.

15. Dye C, Espinal MA. Will tuberculosis become resistant to all antibiotics? Proc R Soc London B 2001; 268:45–52.
16. Blower SM, Chou T. Modeling the emergence of the 'hot zones': Tuberculosis and the amplification dynamics of drug resistance. Nat Med 2004; 10(10):1111–1116.
17. Ellner JJ, Hinman AR, Dooley SW, et al. Tuberculosis symposium: Emerging problems and promise. J Infect Dis 1993; 168:537–551.
18. Frieden TR, Sterling T, Pablos-Mendez A, et al. The emergence of drug-resistant tuberculosis in New York City. N Engl J Med 1993; 328:521–526.
19. Rastogi N. Emergence of multiple-drug-resistant tuberculosis: Fundamental and applied research aspects, global issues and current strategies. Res Microbiol 1993; 144:103.
20. Sbarbaro JA. TB control in the 21st century [editorial]. Monaldi Arch Chest Dis 1993; 48:197–198.
21. Cohn DL, Bustreo F, Raviglione MC. Drug-resistant tuberculosis: Review of the worldwide situation and the WHO/IUATLD Global Surveillance Project. Clin Infect Dis 1997; 24(suppl 1):S121–S130.
22. World Health Organization. Anti-tuberculosis Drug Resistance in the World. The WHO/IUATLD Global Project on Anti-Tuberculosis Drug Resistance Surveillance. Geneva, Switzerland: World Health Organization, 1997:1–227. WHO/TB/97.229.
23. Laszlo A, Rahman M, Raviglione M, et al. Quality assurance programme for drug susceptibility testing of *Mycobcterium tuberculosis* in the WHO/IUATLD supranational laboratory network: First round of proficiency testing. Int J Tuberc Lung Dis 1997; 1: 231–238.
24. Centers for Disease Control and Prevention. Notice to readers: Revised definition of extensively drug-resistant tuberculosis. MMWR Morb Mortal Wkly Rep 2006; 55:1176.
25. Aziz MA, Wright A, Laszlo A, et al. Epidemiology of antituberculosis drug resistance (the Global Project on Anti-tuberculosis Drug Resistance Surveillance): An updated analysis. Lancet 2006; 368:2142–2154.
26. Canetti G, Froman S, Grosset J, et al. Mycobacteria: laboratory methods for testing drug sensitivity and resistance. Bull World Health Organ 1963; 29:565–78.
27. Canetti G, Fox W, Khomenko A, et al. Advances in techniques of testing mycobacterial drug sensitivity, and the use of sensitivity tests in tuberculosis control programmes. Bull World Health Organ 1969; 41:21–43.
28. Siddiqi S. BACTEC 460TB System. Product and Procedure Manual, 1996. Becton Dickenson and Company, Franklin Lakes, NJ USA 1996.
29. Ruesch-Gerdes S, Pfyffer GE, Casal M, et al. Multicenter laboratory evaluation of the BACTEC MGIT 960 technique for testing susceptibilities of *Mycobacterium tuberculosis* to classical second-line drugs and newer antimicrobials. J Clin Microbiol 2006; 44: 688–692.
30. Zignol M, Hosseini MS, Wright A, et al. Global incidence of multidrug-resistant tuberculosis. J Infect Dis 2006; 194:479–485.
31. Cohen T, Colijn C, Wright A, et al. Challenges in estimating the total burden of drug-resistant tuberculosis. Am J Respir Crit Care Med 2008; 177(12):1302–1306.
32. Ministry of Health and Social Development. Tuberculosis in the Russian Federation, 2006: An Analytical Review of the Main Tuberculosis Statistical Indicators Used in the Russian Federation. Moscow, Russian Federation: Ministry of Health and Social Development. 2007:126. RF/FPHI/RIPP/CTRI/FSIN/WHO.
33. World Health Organization. Global Tuberculosis Control: Surveillance, Planning, Financing. WHO Report 2008. Geneva, Switzerland: World Health Organization, 2008. WHO/HTM/TB/2008.393.
34. Wells C, Cegielski J, Nelson L, et al. HIV infection and multidrug-resistant tuberculosis: The perfect storm. J Infect Dis 2007; 196(suppl 1):S86–S107.

35. Barnard M, Albert H, Coetzee G, et al. Rapid molecular screening for multidrug-resistant tuberculosis in a high-volume public health laboratory in South Africa. Am J Respir Crit Care Med 2008; 177(7):787–792.
36. World Health Organization. Interim Recommendations for the Surveillance of Drug Resistance in Tuberculosis. Geneva, Switzerland: World Health Organization, 2007. WHO/HTM/TB/2007.385.
37. World Health Organization. Interim Policy Guidance on Drug Susceptibility Testing (DST) of Second-line Anti-Tuberculosis Drugs. Geneva, Switzerland: World Health Organization, 2008. WHO/HTM/ TB/2008.392.
38. World Health Organization. The Global MDR-TB & XDR-TB Response Plan 2007–2008. Geneva, Switzerland: World Health Organization, 2007. WHO/HTM/TB/2007.387.

10
Programmatic Control of Multidrug-Resistant Tuberculosis

MICHAEL E. KIMERLING
The Bill and Melinda Gates Foundation, Seattle, Washington, U.S.A.
KITTY LAMBREGTS-VAN WEEZENBEEK
KNCV Tuberculosis Foundation, The Hague, The Netherlands
ERNESTO JARAMILLO
Stop TB Department, World Health Organization, Geneva, Switzerland

I. Introduction

While the importance of drug resistance in the treatment and prevention of tuberculosis (TB) was recognized shortly after the discovery of anti-tuberculous therapy in the 1940s (1), it was not until the early 1990s that multidrug-resistant TB (MDR-TB, defined as resistant to at least isoniazid and rifampicin) was recognized as a public health threat to the control and potential elimination of the disease (2–6). The chief lesson of the first experiences with antituberculous chemotherapy was that monotherapy should never be provided to a TB patient. The experiences with MDR-TB in the 1990s, in the United States and elsewhere, unmasked the important cross-linkages between several concurring threats, each an additive factor for the creation of drug resistance (7,8): lack of financial and political commitment; unprepared public health infrastructures, including inadequate laboratory diagnostic capacities; poor infection control practices in congregate settings including hospitals, prisons, and homeless shelters; lack of community-based treatment plans to provide direct supervision; the rapidly lethal combination of HIV and TB or MDR-TB; and the importance of TB control in poorly resourced, high-burden countries with the generation of drug resistance in these settings. In addition, social barriers to patient adherence to therapy, unsecured supplies of first-line TB drugs, and the use of drugs of poor or unknown quality were also recognized.

When the World Health Organization (WHO) launched the DOTS strategy in 1994, it was developed as a case management system within the broader context of building sustained political commitment, a secure first-line TB drug supply mechanism, decentralized monitoring and evaluation structures, and the prioritization of infectious cases based on smear microscopy. The primary treatment strategy focused on a multidrug chemotherapy regimen using rifampicin—the basis for short-course chemotherapy. The goal was to cure a high proportion of patients while preventing the emergence of drug resistance (9,10). At this time, however, there was very little external non-country support for international TB control efforts, with only approximately USD 16 million available per year (9).

One element of the rollout of the global DOTS strategy was the initiation of the Global Project on Anti-Tuberculosis Drug Resistance Surveillance (DRS) in 1994, cosponsored by the WHO and International Union Against Tuberculosis and Lung Disease

(IUATLD, the Union) (11). The fourth report, released in 2008, includes important trend data (defined as three or more data points) from 48 countries (12). Between 1994 and 2007, the Global Project has produced data from 138 settings in 114 countries and two special administrative regions (Fig. 1). As part of the Global DRS Project, a Supranational Reference Laboratory Network (SRLN) was formed to support standardization of drug-susceptibility testing (DST) with proficiency testing for first- and second-line antituberculous drugs (13). The network currently includes 26 laboratories in 6 WHO regions.

II. The Global Epidemiology of Drug-Resistant TB

The fourth Global Report estimates that the number of *emerged* MDR cases in 2006 was 489,139 (95% CLs: 455,093–614,215), accounting for 4.8% of all TB cases. This estimate has climbed to over 500,000 cases for 2007 (M. Zignol, personal communication, January 2009). Figures 2 and 3 show the proportion of MDR cases identified among new cases (never treated or received anti-TB drugs for less than 30 days) and previously treated cases (received anti-TB drugs for at least 30 days), respectively. While India, P.R. China, and the Russian Federation account for 56% of the global MDR burden, there are 27 high-burden countries that account for approximately 86% of estimated MDR-TB cases. The specific case estimates and numbers of persons expected to be treated in these countries, updated in January 2009, are shown in Table 1 (M. Zignol, personal communication, January 2009).

Trend data are becoming available from an increasing number of countries, primarily outside of the African continent, from developed countries and former Soviet states. These data start to show country variations with emerging patterns that reflect the complex interplay between government and program commitments to innovation in TB control, uptake of new tools, resources, population size, HIV epidemiology, and overall burden of disease. These patterns for new TB cases are as follows (14):

1. MDR-TB is increasing faster than all TB: Russia and Botswana.
2. MDR-TB is decreasing faster than all TB: Hong Kong SAR and Estonia.
3. MDR-TB is decreasing as fast as all TB: Latvia and Lithuania.

In 2006, in response to reports of an outbreak of highly resistant TB with near universal mortality in Tugela Ferry, South Africa (15), the global community defined a subset of MDR-TB known as extensively drug-resistant TB (XDR-TB) at the Task Force meeting called by the WHO in Geneva. This task force developed a global response plan to the evolving MDR/XDR crisis (16). It defined XDR-TB as any *Mycobacterium tuberculosis* strain resistant to isoniazid and rifampicin (which defines MDR-TB) *plus* resistance to any fluoroquinolone and either kanamycin, amikacin, or capreomycin. While XDR is increasingly found wherever MDR-TB is identified, among the MDR data accounted for in the fourth Global Report, XDR accounted for 7.5% of the MDR cases (301 out of 4012) (12).

III. Planning and Implementation for MDR-TB Control: An Expanded Programmatic Framework

The programmatic control of MDR-TB and XDR-TB is a complex public health intervention that normally involves differing public and private partners associated with multiple

Map 1: Global Project coverage, 1994–2007

* Subnational coverage in India, China, Russia, Indonesia.

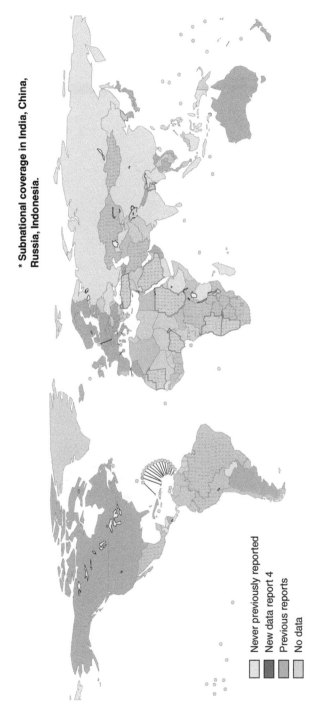

Never previously reported

New data report 4

Previous reports

No data

Figure 1 Map 1 from Report No. 4 of the Global Project (12) shows the coverage of the Drug Resistance Surveillance Project since its inception in 1994. Note the countries where only subnational data are available, including the three highest-burden TB countries (India, P.R. China, Indonesia) that accounted for 41% of the estimated incident TB cases (all forms) in 2006.

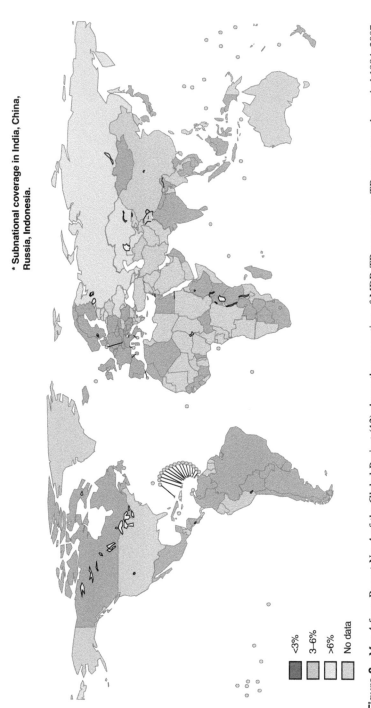

MDR-TB among new TB cases 1994–2007

* Subnational coverage in India, China, Russia, Indonesia.

<3%
3–6%
>6%
No data

Figure 2 Map 4 from Report No. 4 of the Global Project (12) shows the proportion of MDR-TB among *new* TB cases over the period 1994–2007. Note the countries where only subnational data are available, including the three highest burden MDR-TB countries (India, P.R. China, Russia) that accounted for 57% of all estimated MDR cases (pulmonary TB only) in 2006. Note the absence of any data in more than half of the African countries.

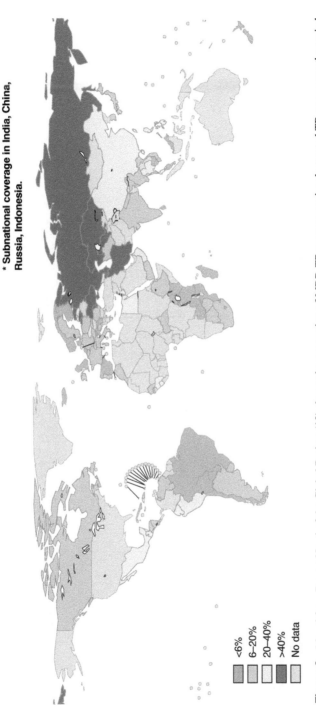

Figure 3 Map 6 from Report No. 4 of the Global Project (12) shows the proportion of MDR-TB among previously treated TB cases over the period 1994–2007. Note the countries where only subnational data are available, including the three highest burden MDR-TB countries (India, P.R. China, Russia) that accounted for 57% of all estimated MDR cases (pulmonary TB only) in 2006. Note the absence of any data in more than half of the African countries.

Table 1 Number of MDR-TB Cases Estimated, Notified, and Expected to be Treated—27 High MDR-TB Burden Countries and WHO Regions

	Estimated cases, 2007			Notified		Expected number of MDR-TB cases to be treated	
	% of all TB cases with MDR-TB	Number of MDR-TB cases	Number of ss+ MDR-TB cases	Number of MDR-TB cases, 2007	% of estimated ss+ MDR-TB cases notified, 2007	2008	2009
1 India	5.4	130,526	99,639	146	0.1	450	900
2 China	7.5	112,348	76,154	79	0.1	388	—
3 Russian Federation	21	42,969	31,397	5,297	17	4,221	9,897
4 South Africa	2.8	15,914	10,708	7,350	69	5,252	—
5 Bangladesh	4.0	14,506	7,694	—	—	150	—
6 Pakistan	4.3	13,218	7,939	—	—	250	250
7 Indonesia	2.3	12,209	6,427	—	—	100	250
8 Philippines	4.6	12,125	6,451	568	8.8	620	1000
9 Nigeria	2.4	11,700	6,934	45	0.6	500	—
10 Kazakhstan	32	11,102	9,540	5568	58	1562	4266
11 Ukraine	19	9,835	5,568	5568	58	—	—
12 Uzbekistan	24	9,450	6,936	484	7.0	334	720
13 DR Congo	2.8	7,336	4,137	82	2.0	523	756
14 Viet Nam	4.0	6,468	4,199	—	—	100	—
15 Ethiopia	1.9	5,979	3,086	145	4.7	45	200
16 Tajikistan	23	4,688	3,286	—	—	—	—
17 Myanmar	4.7	4,181	2,331	600	26	125	150
18 Azerbaijan	36	3,916	3,109	196	6.3	20	—
19 Republic of Moldova	29	2,231	1,656	896	54	466	490
20 Kyrgyzstan	17	1290	813	322	40	—	—
21 Belarus	16	1101	758	870	115	—	—
22 Georgia	13	728	590	269	46	280	540
23 Armenia	17	486	373	125	33	—	—
24 Lithuania	17	464	339	314	93	—	—
25 Bulgaria	12	371	217	82	38	50	—
26 Latvia	14	202	129	98	76	50	120
27 Estonia	20	123	85	80	94	120	100
High MDR-TB burden countries	5.7	435,470	300,496	23,616	7.9	15,676	19,689
AFR	2.4	75,657	45,029	8,841	20	9,337	4,070
AMR	3.2	10,214	7,261	2,522	35	3,670	4,046
EMR	3.8	23,049	14,120	487	3.4	966	707
EUR	17	92,554	67,440	16,062	24	8,414	17,457
SEAR	4.8	173,660	124,826	918	0.7	1,496	1,724
WPR	6.3	135,411	89,926	948	1.1	1,572	1,573
Global	4.9	510,545	348,602	29,778	8.5	25,455	29,577

— Indicates information not available.

Abbreviation: SS, sputum smear.

Source: From Ref. 56.

logistical and technical challenges. There is not a single approach to developing a successful MDR-TB program. On the contrary, each program should be carefully designed based on the epidemiology of drug-resistant TB and health infrastructure within the particular country. As such, the control of drug-resistant TB (DR-TB) is a true framework intervention, in which the framework prescribes the key components of *any* MDR-TB program but allows flexibility for different (locally tailored) approaches to realize and sustain the framework conditions.

The DR-TB framework can be organized around the five components of the DOTS strategy because the underlying principles remain the same (17). However, in the context of this chapter, it is important to stress the issues often under-recognized and of specific importance to addressing drug resistance. There are 10 key areas to consider in the planning and implementation for MDR-TB control:

1. Sustained political and financial commitment.
2. A rational case-finding strategy for drug-resistant TB implemented by all health providers.
3. Laboratory infrastructure for the accurate, timely diagnosis through quality-assured culture and DST, with mechanisms for adoption of new, rapid diagnostics.
4. Treatment strategies and care models for effective case management.
5. Uninterrupted supply of quality-assured second-line drugs (SLD) and drug management.
6. Information systems for monitoring and evaluation.
7. Infection control in all treatment sites.
8. Health education.
9. Human resources development.
10. Special considerations:
    10.1 Ethical considerations.
    10.2 Coinfection with HIV/AIDS.

Each of these components involves more complex and costly operations than those for controlling drug-susceptible TB. Many have argued that for that reason MDR-TB control competes with human and financial resources for "susceptible TB." However, experiences in most countries show the opposite. Addressing DR-TB usually strengthens a national TB control program (18,19), especially regarding the proper classification of patients, case-holding and patient monitoring, recording/reporting mechanisms, infection control, and the centrality of the laboratory as the crossroad for introducing innovation and new diagnostics. Nonetheless, any country embarking on an MDR-TB program should perform a comprehensive situational assessment as to the strengths/weaknesses of their existing TB program and possible causes of drug resistance in their context. Consideration of all components of the TB strategy with a focus on the five core elements of the DOTS component are essential, including all aspects of case management and the quality of first-line drugs (FLD).

The MDR-TB program framework components are discussed below and overlap with relevant chapters of the revised 2008 WHO Guidelines on the programmatic management of drug-resistant TB (17).

A. Sustained Political and Financial Commitment

Political commitment begins with the recognition of MDR-TB as a public health problem coupled with identifying and neutralizing the factors responsible for its development and spread in a particular setting (7,20). Interventions to prevent drug resistance must always be the priority as part of the overall national TB strategy. Addressing DR-TB, therefore, begins with strengthening commitments to effective implementation of the existing basic TB program, which may include important actions across health sectors that fall under different divisions within or between ministries, such as hospitals, laboratory, drug procurement, education, and special populations such as prisoners (16,21). Secondly, sustained political commitment is essential to establish, finance, and maintain the other framework components. It requires both long-term investment and leadership to ensure an appropriate environment for integrating the management of DR-TB into national TB control programs, while reaching out to involve relevant partners such as referral hospitals, medical associations, and academic institutions.

Ensuring an appropriate environment requires many actions: adequate infrastructure, development and retention of human resources, interagency cooperation, enactment of necessary legislation, TB control policies enabling rational implementation of the program, and facilitation of the procurement of quality-assured SLD. Many stakeholders and partners are often involved, including international agencies providing technical assistance and/or human and financial resources. It is of critical importance that the Ministry of Health (MOH) and National TB Program (NTP) become drivers of the process during the planning and preparation phases. Failure to coordinate all national/international partners and the comprehensive planning process brings the risk of an unbalanced and unsustainable MDR-TB program component.

B. A Rational Case-Finding Strategy for Drug-Resistant TB Among All Health Providers

The accurate, timely diagnosis of TB is the backbone of a sound national TB control program and successful treatment outcomes. Therefore, a case-finding strategy to identify those at risk of having drug-resistant TB is essential to preparing any MDR-TB program.

Case-finding strategies may vary depending on the epidemiological situation and local capacity and must be linked to a quality-assured laboratory for culture and DST. In settings with high levels of drug-resistant TB among new cases, as exist in Eastern Europe, one would prefer to offer DST to all TB patients. In regions with low rates of MDR-TB among new cases and limited resources, targeted case finding may be a rational alternative strategy. Targeted case finding requires systematic DST for patient categories at increased risk of drug resistance (Table 2) and the early detection of MDR-TB among those cases failing to respond to treatment. At a minimum, this normally includes previously treated TB cases (re-treatment cases) and contacts of MDR-TB patients. Among previously treated cases, rates of MDR-TB are the highest among patients who have failed one or more treatment episodes and may reach 80%. While MDR-TB rates are usually lower in "relapse cases" and patients returning after default, these depend on many variables and may vary significantly between countries. Therefore, countries should collect representative drug-resistance rates among different re-treatment categories, in order to be able to assess the expected MDR-TB caseload. This is crucial information for MDR-TB program planning

Table 2 Target Groups for DST

Risk factors for DR-TB	COMMENTS
Failure of re-treatment regimens and chronic TB cases	Chronic TB cases are defined as patients who are still sputum smear-positive at the end of a re-treatment regimen. These patients have perhaps the highest MDR-TB rates of any group, often exceeding 80%.
Exposure to a known DR-TB case	Most studies have shown close contacts of MDR-TB patients to have very high rates of MDR-TB. Management of DR-TB contacts is described in chapter 7.
Failure of category I	Failures of category I are patients who while on treatment are sputum smear-positive at month 5 or later during the course of treatment. Not all patients in whom a regimen fails have DR-TB, and the percentage may depend on a number of factors, including whether rifampicin was used in the continuation phase and whether DOT was used throughout treatment. More information on regimen implications for category I failures is given below in this chapter and in chapter 7.
Failure of antituberculosis treatment in the private sector	Antituberculosis regimens from the private sector can vary greatly. A detailed history of drugs used is essential. If both isoniazid and rifampicin were used, the chances of MDR-TB may be high. Sometimes second-line antituberculosis drugs may have been used, and this is important information for designing the re-treatment regimen.
Patients who remain sputum smear-positive at month 2 or 3 of SCC	Many programmes may choose to do culture and DST on patients who remain sputum smear-positive at months 2 and 3. This group of patients is at risk for DR-TB, but rates can vary considerably.
Relapse and return after default without recent treatment failure	Evidence suggests that most relapse and return after default cases do not have DR-TB. However, certain histories may point more strongly to possible DR-TB, for example, erratic drug use or early relapses.
Exposure in institutions that have DR-TB outbreaks or a high DR-TB prevalence	Patients who frequently stay in homeless shelters, prisoners in many countries, and health care workers in clinics, laboratories, and hospitals can have high rates of DR-TB.
Residence in areas with high DR-TB prevalence	DR-TB rates in many areas of the world can be high enough to justify routine DST in all new cases.
History of using antituberculosis drugs of poor or unknown quality	The percentage of DR-TB caused by use of poor-quality drugs is unknown but considered significant. It is known that poor-quality drugs are prevalent in many countries. All drugs should comply with quality-assured WHO standards.

Abbreviation: SCC, short course chemotherapy.

Source: From Ref. 17.

and management. In regions with a significant private/hospital sector contribution to the diagnosis and care of TB patients, strategies to refer treatment failures or others suspected of DR-TB should be devised, including mechanisms for guaranteeing access to a full course of therapy.

C. Laboratory Infrastructure for Accurate, Timely and Quality-Assured Diagnosis with Mechanisms for Adoption of New, Rapid Diagnostics

For the control of drug-resistant TB, quality-assured culture and DST are indispensable. Nonviable cultures, culture contamination, and unreliable DST results have major consequences for both individual patients and the national TB control program. Internal quality control and external quality assurance should therefore be in place, including a link for proficiency testing with a recognized reference laboratory such as one of the WHO-recognized supranational TB reference laboratories (http://www.who.int/tb/challenges/mdr/srl_network_dec08.pdf).

Although countries have been advised to systematically offer free DST to all re-treatment cases, this intervention has not been realized in most settings. This gap reflects the many years of neglect of the TB laboratory component and infrastructure, with prior global efforts focused on smear diagnosis through microscopy. Culture and DST were not considered a priority. A significant move away from complete reliance on microscopy has been occurring since 2006, catapulted in large part by the emergence and spread of MDR/XDR-TB in South Africa and elsewhere. However, the experiences with establishing MDR-TB programs clearly reveal that "placing expensive equipment" does not equate to reliable culture and DST results. Building a functional and sustainable laboratory network requires far more than equipment alone. Conventional culture and DST remain major challenges for laboratory technicians, as labor intensive and complicated standard operating procedures (SOP) need to be strictly adhered to, in order to obtain reliable and reproducible results. Although liquid culture and DST methods are less time consuming, the risk of contamination and the price of the reagents pose other challenges. The recent introduction of rapid molecular-based DST methods, such as the line probe assays (LPA) for the detection of isoniazid (H) and rifampicin resistance, has the potential to greatly facilitate and accelerate the MDR-TB case-finding process but can only be performed presently at the reference-level laboratory. LPA can be used as a screening tool, followed by complete culture and DST only for those patients testing positive (resistant) on the LPA. Such an approach has been piloted successfully and rapid scale-up of their use is increasingly feasible in some regions given the expansion of "PCR labs" worldwide, especially in connection to HIV/AIDS and avian influenza programs.

Beyond DST for FLD, countries increasingly need to establish DST capacity for SLD although the techniques for several SLD are not well-established (13). At a minimum, countries should strive to collect representative SLD-DST data among MDR-TB cases, as these data are crucial for the design of regimens as well as the budgeting and ordering of expensive reserve drugs. In regions with high levels of resistance to SLD, SLD-DST is best offered to all MDR-TB cases. LPA that test for both FLD and key SLD are under development and will be field tested in 2009. Once validated, these will offer major advantages for optimizing both patient management and programmatic planning.

The diagnosis of TB and DR-TB in HIV-infected people is more difficult and may be confused with other pulmonary or systemic infections. HIV-infected persons are more likely to have smear-negative or extrapulmonary TB. The WHO Guidelines recommend clinical algorithms that include the use of chest X-ray and culture to improve the ability to diagnose TB in smear-negative HIV-infected patients. Because of the difficulties in diagnosing TB in HIV-infected patients using conventional tools, and given that unrecognized MDR/XDR-TB is associated with such high mortality, some programs perform culture and DST on all HIV-infected patients with active TB. Programs without facilities or resources to screen all HIV-positive patients for DR-TB should put significant efforts into obtaining them, especially if DR-TB rates are moderate or high. Rapid diagnostic techniques for the HIV-infected TB case could be useful to promptly identify and triage those with DR-TB. In settings documented to have XDR-TB, HIV-infected patients with MDR-TB should also be screened for XDR using liquid media methods or another validated rapid DST technique for second-line injectable agents and a fluoroquinolone (17).

A summary of DST recommendations as noted in the 2008 WHO Guidelines are as follows:

- Patients at increased risk of DR-TB should be screened for drug resistance.
- In the HIV-infected TB patient, whenever possible, perform DST at the start of TB therapy to avoid mortality due to unrecognized DR-TB.
- For the initial screening of DR-TB, use rapid DST methods whenever possible.
- Patients at increased risk of having XDR-TB should be screened for resistance with DST to H, R, second-line injectable agents and a fluoroquinolone.

D. Treatment Strategies and Care Models for Effective Case Management

An appropriate treatment strategy consists of a rational and systematic approach to designing the optimal treatment regimen (see chap. 7), a patient-centered modality for delivering this regimen under direct observation, and early identification and management of adverse drug reactions. Designing an appropriate treatment strategy for a national program (Table 3) requires consideration of all relevant information such as

- representative data on resistance to FLD and key SLD, distinguishing new cases and different types of re-treatment cases;
- history of TB drug use in the country;
- availability of DST to FLD and selected SLS;
- availability of rapid (molecular) DST;
- expected distribution of MDR-TB (scattered MDR-TB cases or "high" MDR-TB caseload);
- health infrastructure and possible DOT modalities;
- human resources for health.

Many countries do not yet have EQA capacity to test for resistance to key SLD. The international WHO policy guidance on SLD-DST was only published in 2008 (13). It assumes that DST to isoniazid, rifampicin, the fluoroquinolones (FQ), and the injectable agents is reliable, but that DST to the other agents is less reliable and basing individualized treatment regimens on DST to these agents should be avoided.

Knowledge of prior use and resistance to FQ and injectable agents is crucial for rational MDR-TB treatment design. This is especially true for Eastern Europe and Asia.

Table 3 Recommended Strategies for Different Programmatic Situations

Patient group	Background susceptibility data[a]	Recommended strategy[b]
New patient with active TB	Resistance *uncommon to moderately common* (i.e., a country where a low to moderate rate of new cases have MDR-TB)	• Start **category I treatment** • Perform DST of at least H and R in patients not responsive to category I[c] • Rapid DST techniques are preferable
	Resistance *common* (i.e., a country where a high rate of new cases have MDR-TB)	• Perform DST of H and R in all patients before treatment initiated • Rapid DST techniques are preferable • Start **category I treatment** while awaiting DST • Adjust regimen to a category IV regimen if DST reveals DR-TB
	Low percentage of failures of category I have MDR-TB *and* Second-line drug resistance is *rare*	• Perform DST of H and R at a minimum in all patients before treatment initiated. IF individual DST not available or long delays likely before results are known, AND ongoing surveillance DST for treatment failures ARE available, base treatment decision on these data. • Rapid DST is preferable • Start **category II treatment** while awaiting DST • Adjust regimen to a category IV regimen if DST reveals DR-TB
Patient in whom category I failed	*High* percentage of failures of category I have MDR-TB *and* Second-line drug resistance is *rare*	• Perform DST of H and R at a minimum in all patients before treatment initiated • Start category IV treatment: **IA–FQ— two group 4 agents, +/– Z**
	High percentage of failures of category I have MDR-TB *and* Second-line drug resistance is *common*	• Perform DST of H, R, IA, FQ before treatment initiated • Start **category IV treatment: IA–FQ— three group 4 agents, +/– Z,** while awaiting DST • Adjust regimen according to DST results if using an individualized approach

Patient in whom category II failed	*High* percentage of failures of category II have MDR-TB *and* Second-line drug resistance is *rare*	• Perform DST of H and R at a minimum in all patients before treatment initiated • Start **category IV treatment: IA–FQ— two group 4 agents, +/– Z,** while awaiting DST • Adjust regimen according to DST results if using an individualized approach
	High percentage of failures of category II have MDR-TB *and* Second-line drug resistance is *common*	• Perform DST of H, R, IA, FQ before treatment initiated • Start **category IV treatment: IA–FQ— three group 4 agents, +/– Z,** while awaiting DST • Adjust regimen according to DST results if using an individualized approach
Patient with history of relapse or patient returning after default	*Low to moderate* rate of MDR-TB in this group of patients is common	• Perform DST of H and R at a minimum in all patients before treatment initiated. IF individual DST not available or long delays likely before results are known, AND ongoing surveillance DST for treatment failures ARE available, base treatment decision on these data. • Start **category II treatment** while awaiting DST • Adjust regimen to a category IV regimen if DST returns DR-TB
Contact of MDR-TB patient now with active TB	*Close* contact with *high* risk of having the same strain	• Perform rapid diagnosis and DST of H and R at a minimum in all patients before treatment starts • Start **category IV treatment** based on the DST pattern and treatment history of the close contact while awaiting DST • Adjust regimen according to DST results
	Casual contact with low risk of having the same strain	• Perform rapid diagnosis and DST of H and R at a minimum in all patients before treatment starts • Start **category I treatment** while awaiting DST • Adjust regimen according to DST results

(Continued)

Table 3 (*Continued*)

Patient with documented MDR-TB	Documented, or almost certain, susceptibility to a FQ and IA	• Start **category IV treatment: IA–FQ— two group 4 agents, +/– Z**
	Documented, or almost certain, susceptibility to FQ Documented, or almost certain, resistance to an IA	• Start **category IV treatment: IA–FQ— three group 4 agents, +/– Z** • Use an IA with documented susceptibility • If the strain is resistant to all IAs, use one for which resistance is relatively rare
	Documented, or almost certain, resistance to a FQ Documented, or almost certain, susceptibility to IA	• Start **category IV treatment: IA–FQ— three group 4 agents, +/– Z** • Use a higher generation FQ (if available)
	Documented, or almost certain, resistance to a FQ and IA	• Start **category IV treatment** for XDR-TB (see chapter 7)
Patient in whom category IV failed or patient with documented MDR-TB and history of extensive second-line drug use.	*Moderate* to *high* rate of XDR-TB in this group of patients	• Perform DST of IA and FQ (and H and R if not already done) before treatment starts • Start **category IV treatment** for XDR-TB (see chapter 7) while awaiting DST • Adjust regimen according to DST results
Patient with documented XDR-TB	Documented resistance to H, R, IA, and FQ	• Start **category IV treatment** for XDR-TB (see chapter 7)

[a]All strategies in this table assume that they will be implemented in resource-constrained areas with limited access to DST. There are no absolute thresholds for low, moderate, or high resistance.

[b]Whenever possible, perform DST of injectable agents (aminoglycosides or capreomycin) and a fluoroquinolone (FQ) if MDR-TB is documented.

[c]Persistently positive smears at 5 months constitute the definition of category I failure; however, some may wish to consider DST earlier based on the overall clinical picture and if the patient is HIV-positive.

Abbreviation: IA, injectable agent.

Source: From Ref. 17.

Fortunately, levels of resistance to these drugs remain low in most African settings, although this situation could change rapidly due to the widespread use of FQ and initiation of MDR-TB treatment programs (22).

Determining a Treatment Strategy for MDR-TB Programs

From a programmatic perspective, standardized regimens offer significant advantages with regard to training, drug forecasting, drug management, recording and reporting, and treatment delivery. In general, standardized regimens also require less specialized medical staff and allow for easier decentralization of care. Unfortunately, there are several misunderstandings about the term "standardized." In this chapter, standardized refers to a "national consensus on the design of MDR-TB treatment regimens taking into account individual or representative drug-resistance data." This essentially means that one country may have only one standardized MDR-TB treatment regimen (for instance based on representative DST data showing very low rates of resistance to SLD), whereas other countries may apply several regimens, ensuring a "standardized response" to treatment in individual patients with different SLD-DST results. For example,

- MDR regimen 1 for patients with full susceptibility to FQ and kanamycin;
- MDR regimen 2 for patients with resistance to FQ, but susceptibility to kanamycin;
- MDR regimen 3 for patients with resistance to kanamycin, but susceptibility to FQ;
- MDR regimen 4 for patients with resistance to both FQ and kanamycin (XDR-TB);
- MDR regimen 5 for patients reporting the use of SLD for which the DST is not considered reliable.

In essence, one can distinguish three *unique options* for programmatic treatment strategies. Each strategy may be rational in one setting and undesirable in another.

1. A standardized regimen based on *representative* DST data to FLD and SLD for all MDR-TB patients and the history of SLD use in the country.
2. Standardized regimens based *on individual* DST results to FLD and SLD.
3. *Individual* regimens designed by *individual* doctors, based on individual DST data and the patient's clinical situation/history.

Example Option 1

In some African countries, such as Tanzania and Benin, SLD have not been available, except for the FQ that are used for other infectious diseases. It means that levels of resistance to SLD other than FQ are likely extremely low and limited to cross-resistance between INH and ethionamide. In such a setting, it is possible to design a safe and effective regimen that is also easy to manage "programwise."

Example Option 2

In Indonesia, by 2007, there were no SLD available in the country except for FQ and kanamycin. In such a setting one would at least require representative data on FQ and kanamycin resistance in MDR-TB patients before deciding on a national strategy to treat MDR-TB. In case levels of resistance to these drugs are extremely low, one could adopt option 1 above. However, if levels of FQ and/or kanamycin resistance are elevated, option 2 is preferable as it offers the opportunity to deliver better individual care for MDR-TB patients but in a standardized manner. This approach will also facilitate SLD forecasting and training of health staff.

Example Option 3

Some settings are characterized by extremely high levels of MDR-TB, a long history of widespread misuse of SLD, and a health structure that emphasizes inpatient TB care by medical specialists. In these settings, the clinical history and knowledge of prior TB drug use is of utmost importance as patients may have taken SLD for which there are not yet reliable DST standards. Examples are certain countries in Eastern Europe. In these settings, option 3 may be preferable and feasible.

An important challenge for any program is the management of the patient between first suspicion and/or confirmation of MDR-TB and the time of availability of full SLD-DST results, where full DST is available. Depending on background resistance rates, it may require very aggressive empiric regimens meant to minimize the risk of amplification of drug resistance. For a standardized empirical regimen that will treat the vast majority of patients with four effective drugs, it is often necessary to use five or six drugs to cover all possible resistance patterns. Therefore, in patients at high risk of MDR-TB, such as patients failing previous treatment, SLD-DST is preferably done simultaneously with FLD-DST. However in most settings, SLD-DST is limited to patients with confirmed MDR-TB. This essentially means that the delay between presenting with symptoms and results of SLD-DST may easily reach three months or more when conventional culture and DST methods are used. The introduction of rapid molecular DST (line probe assays), as discussed above, is a first step to reduce such delays.

Models of Care and Treatment Delivery: Hospitalization and Ambulatory Care Options

When deciding on organization of the treatment delivery for MDR-TB patients, two phases need to be distinguished: the "intensive phase" during which patients will require injections and the "continuation" phase when the patient is only taking oral drugs but likely twice per day. The first phase requires involvement of health staff and/or persons trained in giving injections, whereas during the continuation phase, there are more options for supervision of treatment (workplace, school, family, etc). These two phases need to be distinguished when planning the MDR-TB program.

Given that the comprehensive treatment and care of MDR-TB is a *demanding, relatively complex*, and *costly* activity, national TB control programs are normally not prepared to deliver this intervention, relying on models of care that are either not suitable to the needs of patients, not in line with WHO guidance, or not cost-effective.

The chief *demands* of MDR case management come from the need to (*i*) ensure treatment at least five days a week up to two years duration, including a prolonged initial phase requiring injections up to six months or longer, and (*ii*) deliver directly observed therapy (DOT) using a patient centered approach.

The *complexity* stems from several challenges:

- Second-line anti-TB drugs produce a higher frequency of, and more severe, adverse reactions than first-line anti-TB drugs. Most of the more severe adverse drug reactions occur in the early months of treatment. Poor management of adverse drug reactions contributes significantly to a high treatment default in

MDR-TB cohorts, resulting in lower cure rates and, therefore, a prolonged period of transmission in the community.

- Case management and holding of patients coinfected with HIV is more demanding and complex because of interactions of second-line anti-TB drugs with antiretrovirals and other medical conditions that require hospitalization.
- TB is an airborne disease, therefore, proper infection control measures should be available wherever patients visit or reside, but none of these practices should promote or increase stigmatization of patients.
- Monitoring of the response to treatment is based on culture and not only smear examination.
- Public hospitals and the private health sector, which are quite often the initial, single, or intermittent provider of MDR-TB care, normally do not follow WHO and MOH Guidelines.
- Ethical dilemmas arise from the need to protect community and health care workers from infection while treating patients with respect for human rights and according to local laws.
- Migration due to social, political, or economic reasons results in patients crossing borders of countries with uneven capacities in place to properly manage MDR-TB.

The high *cost* of MDR-TB management is mostly the result of the following:

- Second-line anti-TB drugs: average treatment course for MDR-TB is USD 2500 to 5000.
- Hospitalization: responsible for 30% to 50% of the total cost of MDR-TB treatment in Estonia and Russia (Tomsk Oblast).
- Increased workforce requirement that is necessary to meet the demands for the programmatic management of MDR-TB.
- Reduced income by patients while seeking diagnosis and care and during case-holding, associated with loss or reduction in gainful employment.

Preferred Solutions

Countries have being tackling these three challenges (*demands, complexity*, and *costs* of MDR-TB management) by implementing two different models of care that coexist in many countries: ambulatory/outpatient and hospital based.

A. *Ambulatory or outpatient care* consists of treating patients on an ambulatory basis from the start of treatment and hospitalizing only for medical reasons. The chief advantage of this model is the social acceptability by patients, its lower cost, and the lower risk of nosocomial transmission. The successful implementation of this model depends, to a large extent, on the availability of a (*i*) social support network to promote adherence to treatment through information and education on the disease, psychological counseling, and enablers that address socioeconomic barriers and (*ii*) health care delivery network of primary health care facilities with health workers and other community members properly trained on MDR-TB management living in relative close proximity to the patient. This model has been successfully implemented in countries such as Peru, the Philippines, Nepal, South Korea, and elsewhere (23–25).

B. *Hospital-based care* consists of hospitalizing patients until they become culture negative, which normally occurs during the first three to six months of treatment, followed by treatment on an ambulatory basis. The main advantages of this model are the ease of delivery of DOT and greater potential to interrupt ongoing transmission of infection to household contacts and the general community while the patient remains infectious. This approach simplifies the training requirements of health care workers not familiar with second-line anti-TB drugs. The successful implementation of this model depends to a large extent on the availability of funds and capacity to support hospitalization for long periods, the availability of proper infection control measures in hospital wards, and the implementation of basic ethics and legal principles that guarantee respect for and promotion of human rights. While HIV-positive status does not imply hospitalization, the higher frequency of other medical conditions among those coinfected makes more frequent the need to hospitalize such patients. This model is the one predominately followed by Eastern European and the Baltic countries (26).

Ambulatory care can feature in both models, since hospitalizing a person for two years is not always an option for reasons ranging from costs to social acceptability. Despite the high costs, MDR-TB treatment is cost-effective as measured in cost per Disability Adjusted Life Years averted, both in settings using hospitalization during the initial phase of treatment (Estonia, Tomsk) and in settings treating on an outpatient basis during the full course of treatment (the Philippines, Peru) (27–29). While hospital-based care is significantly more expensive than ambulatory care models, there are no studies that look at the cost-effectiveness of hospital-based care in low-resource settings, nor the mixed-use hospital-ambulatory approaches applied by some programs.

One model is not necessarily superior to the other in terms of achieving comparable treatment outcomes, and some combination of both may coexist to provide optimal care. Depending on patient needs, program capacities, and resources in a given setting, one model, however, may be preferred. In a relatively small-sized country, for example, with plans to treat thousands of cases every year, it is unlikely that there is adequate hospital capacity and a safe environment available to properly treat each patient, making ambulatory care a preferred option early in the treatment cycle. Alternatively, hospitalization may be the preferred choice in the case of HIV infected or severely ill patients during the initial phase of treatment, especially in the absence of social support networks to safeguard treatment adherence, or when primary health care workers properly trained in the management of adverse effects are lacking. Such actions assume that updated infection control standards are being met (see below). In settings with limited or no experience in managing SLD and their side effects, initial hospitalization may serve to build provider competencies and patient-provider trust, especially during the "pilot phase" of any program. Hospitals will also serve as a key referral and follow-up point for community-based care during the continuation phase, working closely with peripheral health units. Even when the health staffs in these peripheral centers are properly trained, given the infrequent number of MDR-TB cases that a single center will likely encounter, they may not be able to maintain their skills due to the limited exposure. Therefore, any MDR-TB program should ensure access to MDR-TB and other specialists, wherever they are located.

Regardless of the selected care model, it is of utmost importance to create an effective *service delivery triangle* between (*i*) hospitals, (*ii*) ambulatory treatment delivery sites/health centers, and (*iii*) laboratories responsible for the monitoring of treatment (for sputum smear, culture, and blood chemistries). In general, a program should consider at least the following factors when developing its MDR-TB model of care:

- Patient's needs and his/her preferred choices to ensure treatment adherence.
- Local laws and ethical standards.
- Engagement of the private sector and (public) hospitals for MDR-TB case management in accordance with international standards, including a cross-referral mechanism.
- Availability of hospitals with infection control measures in place in accordance with WHO Guidelines.
- Estimated number of patients to treat and hospital bed capacity.
- Sufficient funding to establish and maintain the required health care workforce to deliver and/or monitor DOT.
- Burden of HIV among MDR-TB patients to be treated and level of collaboration established with HIV/AIDS control programs.
- Laboratory network capacity to monitor response to treatment during all phases of treatment, whether hospital based or ambulatory.
- Attitudes of caregivers to the different options of care.
- Availability of social support networks to facilitate a patient-centered approach.
- Capacity to educate patients and families on infection control standards at the household level.
- Geographical access to points of MDR-TB care.

E. Uninterrupted Supply of Quality-Assured SLDs and Drug Management

Management of SLD is complex, especially when individualized treatment regimens are used. Most SLD have a short shelf life, global production of quality-assured drugs is limited, and drug registration may be a lengthy and costly process that is not always attractive to drug manufacturers for a given country. If using a standardized regimen approach, DR-TB programs are encouraged to order a limited amount of "reserve" SLD that may not be included in the standard regimen. These drugs are needed to substitute for other drugs under various conditions. For example, a program using a standardized regimen that does not include PAS will need PAS in the following situations: (*i*) patients intolerant or resistant to one of the core "effective" drugs; (*ii*) as part of a "salvage regimen" for those patients that fail the standardized regimen (17).

Steps to secure an uninterrupted drug supply should begin six months or more in advance of the anticipated need, and drug needs must be continuously reevaluated. Countries should use only drugs that are quality assured by a stringent drug regulatory authority recognized by WHO. The drug management cycle comprises six basic elements: drug selection, quantitative assessment of drug requirements, management of procurement, distribution, assurance of drug quality, and rational drug use. Accurate demand forecasting for SLD (i.e., correct quantification of the drug needs for a specific period of time) is one of the elements that guarantees an uninterrupted drug supply. Several additional factors must be considered, including the existing stock, lead time for delivery, buffer stock requirements, and the shelf life of each drug. Shelf lives of SLD are generally shorter than those of FLD, ranging from 18 to 36 months. It is recommended that a buffer stock should be sufficient for a period of two to three times the delivery delay for

SLD. An inventory management system needs to be established to ensure a safety stock, optimize stock movement, and provide an accurate source of information for drug demand forecasting.

To preserve quality, the drugs should be stored and transported by the supplier and the National TB Control Program following "Good Storage Practices" and the recommendations of the manufacturer regarding temperature and humidity (30).

F. Information Systems for Monitoring and Evaluation

Every TB program that develops and integrates the management of DR-TB requires the introduction of a recording and reporting system specifically designed for DR-TB that can be linked to the regular TB "DOTS" recording and reporting system. This is essential for evaluating program performance, identifying operational problems, and assessing treatment effectiveness. The specific characteristics of a DR-TB control program include a recording system with uniquely defined categories for patient registration, culture and DST results, and the monitoring of treatment delivery and response for 24 months. Standard cohort analysis includes both interim indicators and treatment outcomes after two or more years as well as treatment outcomes evaluated by treatment regimen and DST results. The classification of case registration groups and treatment outcome definitions for MDR-TB, developed by WHO and partners, provides a "minimal package" that can be adapted to include country-specific variables relevant for program monitoring (17).

Patients should be assigned to a registration group based on their treatment history. In addition, it is crucial that all programs adhere to internationally determined and mutually exclusive outcome definitions for DR-TB:

- **Cured**—A patient who has completed treatment according to program protocol and has at least five consecutive negative cultures from samples collected at least 30 days apart in the final 12 months of treatment. If only one positive culture is reported during that time, and there is no concomitant clinical evidence of deterioration, a patient may still be considered cured, provided that this positive culture is followed by a minimum of three consecutive negative cultures taken at least 30 days apart.
- **Treatment completed**—A patient who has completed treatment according to program protocol but does not meet the definition for cure because of lack of bacteriological results (i.e., fewer than five cultures were performed in the final 12 months of treatment).
- **Died**—A patient who dies for any reason during the course of MDR-TB treatment.
- **Failed**—Treatment will be considered to have failed if two or more of the five cultures recorded in the final 12 months of therapy are positive, or if any one of the final three cultures is positive. (Treatment will also be considered to have failed if a clinical decision has been made to terminate treatment early because of poor clinical or radiological response or adverse events.
- **Defaulted**—A category IV patient whose treatment was interrupted for two or more consecutive months for any reason without medical approval.
- **Transferred out**—A category IV patient who has been transferred to another reporting and recording unit and for whom the treatment outcome is unknown.

Cohort analyses should be carried out at 24 months, and if needed, repeated at 36 months after the last patient starts treatment. For each treatment cohort, an interim status should be assessed at six months after treatment initiation to monitor program progress. It is recommended that all patients should be analyzed in two different cohorts, depending on the reporting purpose:

- **The treatment cohort** includes only patients who start category IV treatment. It is defined by the date of start of category IV treatment. The purpose is mainly to assess result of treatment and trends over time.
- **The diagnostic cohort** includes patients diagnosed with MDR-TB (identified in the DST Register by date of DST result) during a specific period. The purpose is mainly to assess the number of patients with DR-TB in subgroups and over time. This allows the program to evaluate the delay in treatment start and proportion of patents who started treatment.

G. Infection Control in All Treatment Sites

Well-documented outbreaks of highly drug-resistant strains of TB (31–33) and the high rates of MDR-TB in new cases in Eastern European settings show that transmission of DR-TB is a reality and a public health threat. It is the responsibility of the health services to ensure that everything possible is done to prevent transmission between patients and to staff, starting with a systematic review of current practices in health centers and hospitals managing TB suspects and patients confirmed with DR-TB.

The management of DR-TB does not alter the basic TB infection control strategies and are essentially the same as those to prevent the spread of drug-susceptible TB (34,35). Any infection control plan must address three key elements: administrative controls, environmental or engineering controls, and personal respiratory protection. The administrative controls are the most effective and least expensive, and therefore, have the highest priority in resource-constrained settings.

Specifically, administrative controls include policies and procedures intended to promptly identify TB suspects and infectious cases, and to start them on appropriate therapy, while limiting exposure/transmission to all others. Every institution must develop and implement a site-specific infection control plan. An important aspect of the administrative control measures is the physical separation of patients known or suspected to have TB or DR-TB (especially smear-positive cases) from other patients. The mixing of any TB patient with an HIV-infected patient must also be avoided, especially in clinic settings, waiting areas, hospital wards, or other congregate areas. The risk of transmission to patients and health care workers decreases when community-based ambulatory treatment is established and hospital stays are reduced. Although transmission in the household is likely to have occurred before the diagnosis and start of treatment, ambulatory patients with MDR-TB should be advised to stay at home in "self-isolation" until their sputum culture conversion and avoid contact with susceptible people, such as young children or individuals with HIV infection. Health care workers or volunteers visiting TB patients at home should wear properly fitted personal respirator-type masks. In general, persons with known DR-TB should receive routine care outside of normal HIV care areas.

Environmental (or engineering) controls assume that unsuspected, untreated TB patients will enter hospitals, and that even once identified, they may remain infectious for some period of time after the commencement of TB therapy. Environmental measures include natural and/or mechanical ventilation (air exchange), ultraviolet germicidal irradiation (UVGI), and high-efficiency particulate air filtration. These measures are generally expensive and difficult to maintain. Natural ventilation may be appropriate in some settings (36). In general, it is recommended that budgets for environmental controls have an additional 10% allocated for ensuring future maintenance requirements (P. Jensen, CDC, personal communication, December 2008).

Since administrative and engineering controls may not provide complete protection, persons taking care of patients with DR-TB should wear personal respirators, which are designed to protect the wearer from TB. Surgical masks do *not* offer protection. Patients should also be educated about cough etiquette to cover their mouths when coughing, including the use of (surgical) masks.

H. Health Education

Health education for patients and their families represents a key intervention to reduce defaulting, manage daily side effects, address associated stigma, and improve the quality of life for the patients themselves. Too often the blame for nonadherence is placed upon the patient rather than considering how the health services should properly educate and guide patients throughout the treatment. It is important to consider that many DR cases enrolled on MDR-TB treatment have already "survived" several treatment episodes and thus may not easily be convinced that "this last chance treatment" with all its associated side effects will finally lead to a cure. Also, there are often parallel misunderstandings among family and friends concerning treatment prognosis and infection control. Nonetheless, the supportive role of the patient's family is crucial. The health services are responsible for adequately informing DOT providers in communities and ensuring that health education is provided on a regular basis with materials appropriate to the program and the sociocultural context. Health education materials and methods will vary across settings, ranging from videos and written materials to group education and other literacy sensitive approaches. Former patients working as peer educators have been effectively used in settings to provide health education and, in particular, patient support (37).

I. Human Resources Development

The development of human resources for DR-TB control programs requires careful planning within the national TB control plan. Health authorities cannot simply add a complex intervention like diagnosis and management of DR-TB to the responsibilities of health staff currently implementing basic TB or other disease control programs. The health worker will face many practical and ethical challenges related to MDR-TB management such as stigma, fear of getting infected, drug side effects, and the difficulties for patients to undergo six months of daily injections. The health workers and community volunteers involved, therefore, need sufficient time, motivation, and training to handle their MDR-TB treatment and monitoring assignments (38). After designing the DR-TB program component, all the interventions developed should be "translated" into detailed standard operating procedures, including job descriptions of staff and volunteers at all levels of the program with the focus on the "service delivery triangle" described above (see "Models of Care and Treatment Delivery"). Subsequently, these SOPs should form the basis for the development of training materials and methods, including "training of trainers" materials. Over time, these measures will yield a cadre of capable staff across all categories of personnel involved in the program (hospital, health center, laboratory, pharmaceutical, and management), creating a more sustainable and professional workforce for DR-TB program implementation. Finally, the program management and involved stakeholders should closely monitor the human resources situation and take measures to prevent the unnecessary transfer or loss of experienced staff.

J. Special Considerations

Ethical Considerations

When developing a programmatic response to DR-TB, it is important to consider the ethical and legal issues related to the diagnosis and treatment of drug-resistant disease (including incurable forms) within the broader context of TB control and prevention. This section summarizes the ethical considerations as put forward in the 2008 update of the WHO 2008 Guidelines for the programmatic management of DR-TB (17,39–42).

The promotion of health requires the protection of human rights of vulnerable individuals and those of populations. This is especially important with respect to communicable diseases such as TB. Legislation is an expression of national political commitment. The commitment of governments to sustain TB control is a key component of the national TB prevention and control strategy, and it should be manifested in relevant national legislation and regulations. Legislation expresses and formulates health policies, supports the implementation of public health goals, and sets the foundation for executive action. It also formulates patients' rights and duties, helping them to realize the right to health in terms of health protection and access to care. Legislation must, therefore, provide the legal basis for the implementation of measures proven effective in combating communicable diseases and for the prevention and control of outbreaks, balancing what is justified from the medical viewpoint without unduly compromising individual civil rights and causing needless or unreasonable harm to both patients and the general community.

A patient's right to refuse treatment does not relieve that patient from the duty or responsibility of not doing something that may harm another person or persons. Consequently, a patient who continuously refuses to accept that responsibility may expect actions to curtail their liberty or freedom. Any civil liberty restrictions imposed, however, must be no greater than necessary to protect others, and a patient should have a right of redress if unnecessary restrictions are imposed. A patient who refuses to accept curtailment voluntarily must expect a coercive response from the responsible authorities according to the law. However, such coercion must always be of last resort and used only when all attempts at persuasion, with appropriate offers of support and other measures to encourage and facilitate compliance, have failed to secure a positive response, in line with the five criteria of the Siracusa Principles. (http://www.who.int/tb/features_archive/involuntary_treatment/en/index.html).

Coercive isolation must *never* become a substitute for treatment and access to medical care. Further, all public policies bearing on the well-being of the patient must be compatible and give the patient every incentive to seek and comply with treatment. No government policy should allow the use of isolation as a solution to decrease transmission over treatment, and no patient should be put at an economic or other disadvantage as a direct consequence of accepting treatment or complying with curtailments for the purpose of protecting others. Otherwise, the patient may see that the balance of personal advantage lies with refusing treatment or avoiding compliance with treatment or curtailment.

A particular problem arises when DR-TB treatment has failed and no other options exist for therapy, thereby allowing the disease to continue its natural course. The only course of action at this point may be self-isolation of the patient to prevent transmission to others; however, it cannot be certain how long such a period of isolation will be. Further, it has not been determined at the international level what are to be considered as reasonable measures to ensure that a patient has an acceptable quality of life, given that the reason for isolation is solely the protection of others. Such an "end-of-life" care decision must be provided in a dignified and humane manner, as hospice care is done for cancer patients and others who have entered a terminal disease stage. Interaction with family and friends is fully possible with appropriate infection control measures. The lack of economic and other essential resources, however, may put into doubt the feasibility of such proposed policies and represent a serious commitment on the part of care providers.

In summary, the above-mentioned considerations are intended to serve only as a guide to consider the sometimes delicate balance between the protections of the health of the general population and an individual's (i.e., the patient's) civil and human rights, including access to continued care. All countries should strive for full access to treatment for DR-TB with the establishment of relevant communicable diseases legislation, balancing the safeguards of a patient's rights and those of the community to be protected from TB infection.

Coinfection with HIV/AIDS

The 2008 WHO Programmatic Management Guidelines present a new section on approaching the problem of DR-TB coinfection with HIV/AIDS, which poses especially significant challenges for the prevention, diagnosis, and treatment of MDR and XDR-TB. Several reports have shown high mortality rates among HIV-infected patients with DR-TB (43–46), and even higher mortality in patients coinfected with XDR-TB (15). Therefore, the early recognition and diagnosis of DR-TB and HIV followed by prompt treatment with adequate regimens, sound patient support, and strong infection control measures are all essential components of its management (17,47).

During both the preparation and implementation of the national strategy for the programmatic management of DR-TB, knowledge of the in-country HIV/AIDS situation must be considered and close collaboration with the national HIV/AIDS authorities ensured, according to the WHO framework on collaborative TB/HIV activities (48). Such collaboration represents a top priority for establishing the baseline political commitment to the program. The essential WHO framework recommendations have been adapted to the updated 2008 Guidelines (17), which emphasize the need to

- establish mechanisms for collaboration between HIV and TB programs, if they do not already exist, and involve all key stakeholders in DR-TB/HIV activities;
- perform provider-initiated HIV testing and counseling in all TB suspects;
- use standard algorithms to diagnose pulmonary and extrapulmonary TB;
- use mycobacterial cultures and, where available, newer more rapid methods of diagnosis;
- perform DST at the start of TB therapy to reduce mortality due to unrecognized DR-TB in HIV-infected individuals;

- determine the extent (or prevalence) of TB drug resistance in patients with HIV either through population-based DRS surveys linked to HIV testing or provider-based HIV testing of TB patients;
- Introduce antiretroviral therapy (ART) promptly in DR-TB/HIV patients, according to WHO's ART Guidelines (49);
- consider empirical therapy with second-line anti-TB drugs where rates of MDR-TB are exceedingly high (in accordance with the national DR-TB strategy);
- ensure co-trimoxazole preventive therapy (CPT) as part of a comprehensive package of HIV care to patients with active TB and HIV;
- arrange treatment follow-up by a specialized team with expertise in HIV care and DR-TB management, with special attention to monitoring treatment responses and the overlapping toxicities of ART and DR-TB therapy; specifically, immune reconstitution inflammatory syndrome (IRIS) may complicate therapy and impact mortality rates;
- implement additional nutritional and socioeconomic support;
- ensure effective infection control.

Antiretroviral therapy in HIV-infected TB patients improves survival for both drug-resistant and susceptible disease. Cohorts of patients treated for DR-TB without the benefit of ART have experienced mortality rates greater than 90% (50). However, the high likelihood of adverse effects could compromise the treatment of either HIV or DR-TB if both treatments are started simultaneously. Conversely, undue delay in the start of ART could result in significant risk of HIV-related deaths among patients with advanced disease.

Adverse effects that are common to both antiretroviral and anti-TB drugs are substantial and are detailed elsewhere (17). It should be noted, however, that relatively little is known about the rates of adverse effects in the concomitant treatment of DR-TB and HIV. Therefore, if two drugs with overlapping toxicities are determined to be essential in a patient's regimen, WHO Guidelines currently recommend increased monitoring of adverse effects rather than disallowing a certain combination. For more detailed clinical guidance, see chapter 7.

IV. Scaling Up MDR-TB Management

The revised Global Plan to Stop TB 2006 to 2015 calls on countries to treat 1.6 million MDR-TB cases and achieve universal access to diagnosis and treatment by 2015. This ambitious goal relies on the sustained mobilization of donors, countries, and civil society to build the capacities to ensure care according to the highest standards. While some progress has been achieved to date, the number of patients enrolled on treatment remains far below targets (21,51). Scaling up requires careful, staged planning with an overall focus on building the structures and capacities in a stepwise manner, thereby allowing a "quality-assured" increase in MDR coverage (52). A Green Light Committee–approved program is often the first seed, enabling countries or provinces of large countries to adopt and adapt the WHO Guidelines for the programmatic management in a pilot site initially. The subsequent planning for scaling up follows the same 10 framework components described in section III above. It must incorporate a comprehensive needs assessment that evaluates and identifies the following in each location or area of the country: causes of drug resistance, effectiveness of existing TB control measures, estimated MDR-TB burden, capacities that should be in place to diagnose and treat that burden, existing gaps across the proposed MDR intervention, and a strategy to fill the gaps while making use of the existing structures and capacity.

In addition, there are several key areas to strengthen if not already addressed during the pilot phase of the program to ensure a scalable and sustainable expansion of MDR-TB management:

1. National and legal frameworks that take into account
   * importation of key drugs if not available in the country,
   * duration of use of key drugs beyond normally recommended periods for other diseases,
   * models of care and issues of ensuring adherence to therapy, and
   * needed links across ministries and professional groups to allow optimal care and universal access for all.
2. An authorized (and empowered) coordination committee of decision makers and/or key stakeholders to manage the process and intervene as needed. The committee may function at multiple levels from central to provincial to the level of program implementation.
3. Administrative mechanisms and actions to intervene where existing TB control measures are inadequate after careful evaluation of the effectiveness of program implementation and likely drivers of drug resistance.
4. Validated and recent estimates of the MDR-TB burden.
5. Update of national guidelines and manual of operations, including laboratory, with endorsement from the appropriate committees, professional organizations, and others.
6. Budget and financing sustainability as part of the overall national health strategy.

Since prevention and treatment are two complementary aspects of the strategy for MDR-TB control, the WHO has produced a budgeting tool to facilitate planning while integrating all components of the Stop TB strategy (http://www.who.int/tb/dots/planning_budgeting_tool/en/index.html).

V.   Conclusion and Looking Forward

The globally expanding MDR/XDR-TB epidemic is a reflection of past decades of neglect by national health authorities and the global health community, specifically the failure to invest in and modernize TB control tools and strategies, patient care models, and importantly, scientific and operational research. While progress has been made in the recent years, knowledge gaps in TB have been exposed along the entire continuum of the discovery, development, and delivery platforms (53,54), yielding a situation whereby we currently lack essential products and systems to respond effectively to today's situation. The international community, for its part, has far too long accepted these limitations and restrictions as the status quo. Yet with new sources of global funding available to TB programs and renewed commitments to research that include private–public partnerships, the opportunities for progress have also never been greater.

This chapter has outlined a framework for the programmatic management of MDR-TB and issues central to scaling up the many small-scale pilot programs now being implemented. Looking forward, however, there remain several key challenges and bottlenecks to this mission and the ultimate goal of TB elimination by 2050:

1. Inadequate knowledge about the extent of MDR/XDR, particularly in sub-Saharan Africa, and the lack of representative trend data in most high-burden countries. This lack of data reflects the cumbersome state of current approaches to DRS with the limited diagnostic technology and laboratory network capacity to move from infrequent surveys to routine drug-resistance surveillance and ultimately resistance testing as part of routine care (55).
2. Lack of a clear understanding of the drivers of drug resistance at the population level as well as the relationship between phenotypic and genotypic resistance, particularly with regard to treatment outcomes and markers of disease states. This knowledge is important for future development of diagnostics, drugs, and potential vaccines.
3. Access to and protection of the limited number of quality-assured SLD available for MDR therapy and the challenges ahead to evaluate and incorporate new TB drugs into programs using a "fast track" approach.
4. Maintaining innovation in TB control from the development of new technologies (i.e., point of care diagnostics) to tools for promoting patient adherence such as fixed-dose combinations.
5. An integrated system of care that incorporates all providers, from communities to public health care centers, hospitals, and private providers, to deliver care in all settings and for all populations at risk. This system can only be developed with the training and expansion of a competent workforce to deliver care.

References

1. Mitchison DA. Development of streptomycin resistant strains of tubercle bacilli in pulmonary tuberculosis. Thorax 1950; 5:144–161.
2. Kochi A, Vareldzis B, Styblo K. Multidrug-resistant tuberculosis and its control. Res Microbiol 1993; 144:103–110.
3. Bloch AB, Cauthen GM, Onorato IM, et al. Nationwide survey of drug-resistant tuberculosis in the United States. JAMA 1994; 271(9):665–671.
4. Nunn P, Felten M. Surveillance of resistance to antituberculosis in developing countries. Tuber Lung Dis 1994; 75:163–167.
5. Malin AS, McAdam KPWJ. Escalating threat from tuberculosis: The third epidemic. Thorax 1995; 50(suppl 1):537–542.
6. Frieden TR, Sterling T, Pablos-Mendez A, et al. The emergence of drug-resistant tuberculosis in New York City. N Engl J Med 1993; 328:521–526.
7. Brudney K, Dobkin J. Resurgent tuberculosis in New York City: Human immunodeficiency virus, homelessness, and the decline of tuberculosis control programs. Am Rev Respir Dis 1991; 144:745–749.
8. Frieden TR, Fujiwara PI, Washko RM, et al. Tuberculosis in New York City—turning the tide. N Engl J Med 1995; 333(3):229–233.
9. Raviglione MC, Pio A. Evolution of WHO policies for tuberculosis control, 1948–2001. Lancet 2002; 359:775–780.

10. Dye C, Watt CJ, Bleed DM, et al. Evolution of tuberculosis control and prospects for reducing tuberculosis incidence, prevalence, and deaths globally. JAMA 2005; 293(22):2767–2775.

11. Cohn DL, Bustreo F, Raviglione MC. Drug resistance in tuberculosis: Review of the worldwide situation and WHO/IUATLD's Global Surveillance Project. Clin Infect Dis 1997; 24(suppl 1):S121–S130.

12. World Health Organization. Anti-tuberculosis Drug Resistance in the World. 4th Global Report. The WHO/IUATLD Global Project on Anti-tuberculosis Drug Resistance Surveillance, 2002–2007. World Health Organization. WHO/HTM/TB/2008.394. http://whqlibdoc. who.int/hq/2008/WHO_HTM_TB_2008.394_eng.pdf.

13. World Health Organization. Policy Guidance on Drug-Susceptibility Testing (DST) of Second-Line Antituberculosis Drugs. Geneva, Switzerland: World Health Organization. WHO/HTM/TB/2008.392. http://www.who.int/tb/publications/2008/who_htm_tb_2008_392 .pdf.

14. Dye C. Doomsday postponed? Preventing and reversing epidemics of drug-resistant tuberculosis. Nat Rev Microbiol 2009; 10:81–87.

15. Gandhi NR, Moll A, Sturm AW, et al. Extensively drug-resistant tuberculosis as a cause of death in patients co-infected with tuberculosis and HIV in a rural area of South Africa. Lancet 2006; 368(9547):1575–1580.

16. World Health Organization. The Global MDR-TB & XDR-TB Response Plan, 2007–2008. Geneva, Switzerland: World Health Organization, 2007. WHO/HTM/TB/2007.387.

17. World Health Organization. Guidelines for the Programmatic Management of Drug-Resistant Tuberculosis: Emergency Update 2008. Geneva, Switzerland: World Health Organization, 2008. WHO/HTM/TB/2008.000.

18. Mosneaga A, Yurasova E, Zaleskis R, et al. Enabling health systems in tuberculosis control: Challenges and opportunities for the former Soviet Union countries. In: Coker R, Atun R, McKee M, eds. Health Systems and the Challenge of Communicable Diseases: Experiences from Europe and Latin America. Open University Press, 2008.

19. Keshavjee S, Gelmanova IY, Pasechnikov AD, et al. Treating multidrug-resistant tuberculosis in Tomsk, Russia: Developing programs that address the linkage between poverty and disease. Ann N Y Acad Sci 2008; 1136:1–11. doi: 10.1196/annals.1425.009.

20. Lambregts-van Weezenbeek CSB, Veen J. Control of drug-resistant tuberculosis. Tuber Lung Dis 1995; 76(5):455–459.

21. World Health Organization. Report of the Second Meeting of the WHO Task Force on XDR-TB. Geneva, Switzerland: World Health Organization, 2008. WHO/HTM/TB/2008. 403. http://whqlibdoc.who.int/hq/2008/WHO_HTM_TB_2008.403_eng.pdf.

22. VonGottberg A, Klugman KP, Cohen C, et al. Emergence of levofloxacin-non-susceptible *Streptococcus pneumoniae* and treatment for multidrug-resistant tuberculosis in children in South Africa: A cohort observational surveillance study. Lancet 2008; 371(9618):1108–1113.

23. Kim HJ, Hong YP, Kim SJ, et al. Ambulatory treatment of multidrug-resistant pulmonary tuberculosis patients at a chest clinic. Int J Tuberc Lung Dis 2001; 5(12):1129–1136.

24. Mitnick C, Bayona J, Palacios E, et al. Community-based treatment for multidrug-resistant tuberculosis in Lima, Peru. N Engl J Med 2003; 348(2):119–128.

25. Burgos M, Gonzalez LC, Paz EA, et al. Treatment of multidrug-resistant tuberculosis in San Francisco: An outpatient-based approach. Clin Infect Dis 2005; 40:968–975.

26. Nathason E, Lambregts-van Weezenbeek C, Rich ML, et al. Multidrug-resistant tuberculosis management in resource-limited settings. Emerg Infect Dis 2006; 12(9):1389–1397.

27. Dye C, Floyd K. Tuberculosis. In: Jamison DT, Breman JG, Measham AR, Alleyne G, Claeson M, Evans DB, Jha P, Mills A, Musgrove P, eds. Disease Control Priorities in Developing Countries, 2nd ed. New York: The World Bank and Oxford University Press, 2006:289–309.

28. Suarez PG, Floyd K, Portocarrero J, et al. Feasibility and cost-effectiveness of standardized second-line drug treatment for chronic tuberculosis patients: A national cohort study in Peru. Lancet 2002; 359(9322):1980–1989.

29. Tupasi T, Gupta R, Quelapio M, et al. Feasibility and cost-effectiveness of treating multidrug-resistant tuberculosis: A cohort study in the Philippines. PLoS Med 2006; 3(9):e352.
30. Essential Drugs and Medicines Policy Interagency Pharmaceutical Coordination Group. Operational Principles for Good Pharmaceutical Procurement. Geneva, Switzerland: World Health Organization, 1999. (WHO/EDM/PAR/99.5). http://www.who.int/3by5/en/who-edm-par-99-5.pdf.
31. Beck-Sagu C, Dooley SW, Hutton MD, et al. Hospital outbreak of multidrug-resistant *Mycobacterium tuberculosis* infections: Factors in transmission to staff and HIV-infected patients. JAMA 1992; 268(10):1280–1286.
32. Valway SE, Greifinger RB, Papania M, et al. Multidrug-resistant tuberculosis in the New York state prison system, 1990–1991. J Infect Dis 1994; 170(1):151–156.
33. Escombe AR, Moore DAJ, Gilman RH, et al. The infectiousness of tuberculosis patients coinfected with HIV. PLoS Med 2008; 5(9):e188, 1–11.
34. World Health Organization. Guidelines for the Prevention of Tuberculosis in Health Care Facilities in Resource Limited Settings. Geneva, Switzerland: World Health Organization, 1999. WHO/TB/99.269. http://www.who.int/tb/publications/who_tb_99_269.pdf.
35. World Health Organization. Tuberculosis Infection-Control in the Era of Expanding HIV Care and Treatment: Addendum to WHO Guidelines for the Prevention of Tuberculosis in Health Care Facilities in Resource-Limited Settings. Geneva, Switzerland: World Health Organization, 2007. http://whqlibdoc.who.int/hq/1999/WHO_TB_99.269_ADD_eng.pdf.
36. Escombe AR, Oeser CC, Gilman RH, et al. Natural ventilation for the prevention of airborne contagion. PLoS Med 2007; 4(2):e68, 309–317.
37. Mayho P. The Tuberculosis Survival Handbook, 2nd ed. West Palm Beach, FL: Merit Publishing International, 2006.
38. Furin JJ, Mitnick CD, Shin SS, et al. Occurrence of serious adverse effects in patients receiving community-based therapy for multidrug-resistant tuberculosis. Int J Tuberc Lung Dis 2001; 5(7):648–655.
39. Pinet G. Good practice in Legislation and Regulations for TB Control: An Indicator of Political Will. Geneva, Switzerland: World Health Organization, 2001. WHO/CDS/TB/2001.290. http://whqlibdoc.who.int/hq/2001/WHO_CDS_TB_2001.290.pdf.
40. World Health Organization. European Consultation on the Rights of Patients. 28–30 March 1994. Declaration on the Promotion of Patients' Rights in Europe. Amsterdam, The Netherlands: WHO Regional Office for Europe, 1994. ICP/HLE 121. http://www.who.int/genomics/public/eu_declaration1994.pdf.
41. Regional Office for Europe, World Health Organization; Health Law Section, University of Amsterdam. Promotion of the Rights of Patients in Europe Proceedings of a WHO Consultation. The Hague, The Netherlands: Kluwer Law International, 1995.
42. World Medical Association. World Medical Association Declaration of Helsinki. Ethical Principles for Medical Research Involving Human Subjects. Amended by the 59th WMA General Assembly. Seoul, Korea: World Medical Association, 2008. http://www.wma.net/e/policy/pdf/17c.pdf.
43. Fischl MA, Daikos GL, Uttamchandami RB, et al. Clinical presentation and outcome of patients with HIV infection and tuberculosis caused by multiple-drug-resistant bacilli. Ann Intern Med 1992; 117:184–190.
44. Park MM, Davis AL, Schluger NW, et al. Outcome of MDR-TB patients, 1983–1993. Prolonged survival with appropriate therapy. Am J Respir Crit Care Med 1996; 153(1):317–324.
45. Mannheimer SB, Sepkowitz KA, Stoeckle M, et al. Risk factors and outcome of human immunodeficiency virus-infected patients with sporadic multidrug-resistant tuberculosis in New York City. Int J Tuberc Lung Dis 1997; 1(4):319–325.
46. Telzak EE, Chirgwin KD, Nelson ET, et al. Predictors for multidrug-resistant tuberculosis among HIV-infected patients and response to specific drug regimens. Int J Tuberc Lung Dis 1999; 3(4):337–343.

47. Basu S, Andrews JR, Poolman EM, et al. Prevention of nosocomial transmission of extensively drug-resistant tuberculosis in rural South African district hospitals: An epidemiological modeling study. Lancet 2007; 370(9597):1500–1507.

48. Stop TB Department and Department HIV/AIDS. Interim Policy on Collaborative TB/HIV Activities. Geneva, Switzerland: World Health Organization, 2004. WHO/HTM/TB/2004.330.

49. World Health Organization. Antiretroviral Therapy for HIV Infection in Adults and Adolescents: Recommendations for a Public Health Approach. 2006 revision. Geneva, Switzerland: World Health Organization, 2006. http://www.who.int/hiv/pub/guidelines/artadultguidelines.pdf.

50. Wells CD, Cegielski JP, Nelson LJ, et al. HIV infection and multidrug-resistant: The perfect storm. J Infect Dis 2007; 196(suppl 1):S86–S107.

51. Keshavjee S, Seung K. Stemming the tide of multidrug-resistant tuberculosis: Major barriers to addressing the growing epidemic. A White Paper for the Institute of Medicine of the National Academies, 2008.

52. Shin SS, Yagui M, Ascencios L, et al. Scale-up of multidrug-resistant tuberculosis laboratory services, Peru. Emerg Infect Dis 2008; 14(5):701–708.

53. Cobelens FGJ, Heldal E, Kimerling ME,et al. Scaling up programmatic management of drug-resistant tuberculosis: A prioritized research agenda. PLoS Med 2008; 5(7):e150, 1–6.

54. Peters NK, Dixon DM, Holland SM, et al. The research agenda of the National Institute of Allergy and Infectious Diseases for antimicrobial resistance. J Infect Dis 2008; 197(8):1087–1093.

55. Cohen T, Colijn C, Wright A, et al. Challenges in estimating the total burden of drug-resistant tuberculosis. Am J Respir Crit Care Med 2008; 177:1302–1306.

56. World Health Organization. Global Tuberculosis Control—Surveillance, Planning, Financing. WHO Report 2009. WHO/HTM/TB/2009.411.

11
Programmatic Management of HIV-Associated Tuberculosis

ANTHONY D. HARRIES
International Union against Tuberculosis and Lung Disease, Paris, France, and London School of Hygiene and Tropical Medicine, London, U.K.

PAUL P. NUNN
Stop TB Department, World Health Organization, Geneva, Switzerland

I. Introduction

HIV/AIDS is the modern world's greatest pandemic, and HIV is also the most important risk factor for the development of tuberculosis (TB). This chapter describes recent and updated thinking on how control of TB needs to be adapted to assert and maintain control of TB in high–HIV-prevalence settings, even in the face of rising levels of anti-TB drug resistance in many regions.

II. Global Burden of TB and HIV Infection

Twenty-seven years after first being recognized, HIV has claimed over 25 million lives and created over 13 million orphans. The World Health Organization (WHO) and the Joint United Nations Programme on HIV and AIDS (UNAIDS) estimated that at the end of 2007, the number of adults and children living in the world with HIV/AIDS was 33.2 million, of whom the majority lived in the developing world (1). During that year, 2.5 million people were newly infected with HIV and 2.1 million people died as a consequence of HIV infection. Sub-Saharan Africa, especially southern Africa, bears the brunt of this epidemic. With less than 10% of the world's population, it is the home to 22.5 million people living with HIV/AIDS. During 2007 an estimated 1.7 million adults and children were newly infected with HIV in sub-Saharan Africa and 1.6 million died (76% of the global AIDS deaths for that year). South and Southeast Asia and Eastern Europe with Central Asia house 4.0 and 1.6 million HIV-infected people, respectively.

HIV, by targeting CD4-T-lymphocytes and reducing cellular immune function, is the most important biological driving force behind the current TB epidemic. Not only does HIV increase the risk of reactivating latent *Mycobacterium tuberculosis* (2), but it also increases the risk of rapid TB progression soon after infection or reinfection with *M. tuberculosis* (3). In persons infected with *M. tuberculosis* only, the risk of clinically significant disease within the first one to two years after infection may approach 5%, and it thereafter decreases to reach a fairly stable risk of 0.1% per annum (4). Conversely, in persons coinfected with *M. tuberculosis* and HIV, the annual risk of active TB is much higher. This increased risk is detectable as early as HIV seroconversion, and in the first year of HIV infection the TB incidence doubles (5). As the immune system becomes more compromised, and the CD4-lymphocyte count declines, the risk of active TB further increases to reach levels of between 15% and 20% per annum in patients with CD4 cell counts less than 200 cells/μL (6,7). Recent reports from Donetsk Oblast, Ukraine (8) and Latvia (9) also show a significant association between HIV infection and the risk of multidrug-resistant TB (MDR-TB).

At the population level, the degree of interaction between HIV and *M. tuberculosis* depends on the extent of overlap between the two infections. Based on estimates made for the year 2000, about 25 million people globally are coinfected with HIV and *M. tuberculosis*, of whom 72% live in Africa (10). Among the 9.2 million new cases of TB in 2006, just over 700,000 (7.7%) were HIV positive. As in previous years, the Africa region accounted for 85% of these cases, and in new incident TB cases the HIV-prevalence rate in 2006 was 22% (11). Nine countries in southern Africa (South Africa, Swaziland, Lesotho, Namibia, Botswana, Mozambique, Zambia, Zimbabwe, and Malawi) account for nearly 50% of the global HIV/TB burden, and in Botswana, Malawi, and Swaziland HIV-prevalence rates in incident TB cases are 50% or higher. Most of the remaining HIV-infected TB cases (6%) are in the Southeast Asia region, mainly India. However, data emerging from direct measurement of HIV prevalence among TB patients suggests that many of the current HIV-prevalence estimates in TB patients are likely to be low. For example, the prevalence of HIV among TB patients in Kenya has increased from an estimated 29% in the 2005 cohort to a directly measured 52% in the 2006 cohort (11).

The net result of the HIV/TB interaction is that TB in sub-Saharan Africa has risen faster than in any other region in the world. The WHO Africa region has the highest TB incidence rates in the world (11), although, with HIV-infection rates beginning at last to stabilize or fall, the rise in the number of TB cases is slowing down (12). The high rates of coinfection have three important effects on diagnosis and case finding. First, the high case numbers overload laboratory (and clinical) capacity (see pages 283–284), second, the proportion of all reported pulmonary cases that are smear-negative tends to be higher in countries with higher rates of HIV infection, and, third, an increased proportion of patients with tuberculosis are women aged 15 to 24 years (12). High coinfection rates also complicate management of the disease and high case fatalities reduce treatment success rates (see page 284).

III. Current Interaction Between Tuberculosis and AIDS Programs

Up until the last five years, despite a significant association between the two diseases, there was little formal interaction between TB and AIDS programs, either globally or in most countries. Collaboration has now improved, but to understand why there were previous difficulties and why there has now been a change, it is important to understand the goals, objectives, organizations, and philosophies of the two programs.

A. National Tuberculosis Programs

The overall aim of TB control is to reduce mortality, morbidity, and transmission of the disease, while preventing the development of drug resistance. The main intervention is standardized combination chemotherapy provided under direct observation—at least during the initial phase of treatment—to all TB cases and especially identified sputum smear–positive TB patients, the main sources of infection. The DOTS strategy provides the framework within which this intervention is delivered (13). The five components of the strategy are well known (see also chap. 12). Sustained political commitment is necessary to increase human and financial resources and make TB control a national priority. Access to a quality-assured TB sputum microscopy service is essential for case detection among persons presenting with symptoms of TB, particularly prolonged cough. The provision of standardized short-course chemotherapy for all cases of TB under proper management conditions, including directly observed therapy (DOT), allows the best chance of ensuring a successful treatment outcome. There has to be an uninterrupted supply of quality-assured drugs with proper procurement and distribution systems to ensure cure and to prevent the development of drug-resistant TB. Finally, a standardized recording and reporting system allows the program to be systematically monitored and the identified problems to be corrected.

The DOTS strategy is the first component of the new "Stop TB Strategy," whose vision is a world free of TB and whose goal is to reduce dramatically the global burden of TB by 2015 in line with the Millennium Development Goals (MDGs) and the Stop TB Partnership targets (14). This new strategy, wider than DOTS, was necessary for TB control to evolve to address TB/HIV, expand MDR-TB management, contribute to strengthening health systems, engage all care providers, empower people and communities living with TB, and make the need for research explicit. The key operations needed for the delivery of this new strategy have been presented and discussed in other chapters.

B. National AIDS Programs

The efforts of National AIDS Programs, at least in the high–HIV-burden countries in sub-Saharan Africa, were focused for many years around prevention of HIV (Table 1). The strategies for preventing sexual transmission of HIV have concentrated on the use

Table 1 HIV/AIDS Prevention Activities

Preventing sexual transmission of HIV
- Mass media campaigns
- Education of youth and school children
- Condoms, condom promotion, condom social marketing
- Reducing risky sexual behavior, for example, concurrent sexual networks
- Treatment of sexually transmitted infections
- Male circumcision as a preventive action for HIV-negative men

Preventing mother-to-child transmission of HIV
- Antiretroviral prophylaxis or antiretroviral therapy to HIV-infected eligible pregnant mothers
- Elective cesarean sections (dubious role in sub-Saharan Africa)
- Exclusive breast feeding

Screening of blood for transfusion
- Whole blood rapid testing

Promotion of HIV testing and counseling
- Voluntary counseling and HIV testing (VCT)
- Provider-initiated HIV testing and counseling (PITC)

of condoms, treating sexually transmitted infections, abstinence, and reducing unsafe sexual behavior. Most infected children acquire their HIV from their infected mothers, either during labor or during breast feeding, with rates of mother-to-child transmission of HIV, without any intervention, being estimated at 20% to 40% in sub-Saharan Africa (15). Most efforts in this area have gone into prophylaxis with antiretroviral drugs at or around birth (16). There is a global policy to screen donated blood for HIV. A key factor underpinning any HIV-prevention strategy is accessibility to voluntary counseling and HIV testing (VCT) services, and VCT has been shown to be cost-effective in promoting behavior change and reducing sexual transmission of HIV (17). Unfortunately, during the 1990s, the translation of these HIV-prevention strategies from the research arena into implementation through general health services largely failed, and consequently little impact was made on the global HIV pandemic. The annual estimates reported by UNAIDS on the number of adults and children living with HIV dramatically decreased from 40 million in 2006 to 33 million in 2007 (1), but this downsizing of the pandemic had much more to do with refinements in epidemiological methodology than real trends in the pandemic itself.

Until 2003, little emphasis was paid by AIDS programs to the care and treatment of patients with HIV-related disease and AIDS. However, in 2003, WHO and UNAIDS launched the "3 by 5" initiative, with an ambitious goal of having 3 million people on antiretroviral therapy (ART) in developing countries by the end of 2005 (18). This call to arms happened almost simultaneously with a huge injection of funding for HIV/AIDS prevention and treatment, through the Global Fund to Fight AIDS, Tuberculosis and Malaria (GFATM), the President's Emergency Plan for AIDS Relief (PEPFAR), and the World Bank. Particularly in the hardest hit region of sub-Saharan Africa, impressive efforts were made to provide ART to populations in need. Although the 2005 target was not met, WHO and UNAIDS estimated that by December 2007 over 3 million people from low- and middle-income countries had been placed on treatment, with 2 million coming from sub-Saharan Africa (19).

During this period of ART scale up, the rationale, indications and use of cotrimoxazole (CTX) preventive therapy for HIV-infected adults and children also received well deserved, renewed attention with several publications of efficacy in African countries where background resistance rates to the antibiotic are high (20,21). Previously the adoption of CTX, especially in Africa, was slow because of lack of good evidence of effectiveness throughout the region, concerns about resistance to the drug in commonly occurring pathogens, and possible consequences for the treatment of malaria in countries where sulfadoxine-pyrimethamine is used because of shared mechanisms of action and resistance patterns. That position has now changed, and CTX preventive therapy is correctly perceived as a useful adjunct to treatment that, in addition to reducing morbidity and mortality by 20% to 40% (20,21), can be used in settings that have yet to access ART or in patients whose CD4-lymphocyte counts are too high for initiation of ART.

Thus, TB and AIDS programs were kept apart by the prevention–treatment divide until 2003. The emphasis on treatment for AIDS and the emergence of MDR-TB and extensively drug resistant TB (XDR-TB) in the context of HIV infection has since uncovered common ground between National TB Programs and National AIDS Programs. HIV-infected patients with TB are potential clients for ART programs, although this has been taken full advantage of in only a few countries. Within ART programs, it has been rapidly recognized (not surprisingly) that TB is one of the commonest potentially fatal conditions that occurs, and there is a common and shared interest for both programs to lower mortality rates. From a management perspective, the experience of decentralizing anti-TB treatment to fairly remote health facilities acts as a model for the decentralization of ART. The appallingly high case fatality rates from successive outbreaks of MDR-TB among HIV-infected persons (22) culminated in the emergence of XDR-TB in Tugela Ferry, KwaZulu Natal, South Africa, where 52 (98%) of 53 cases died, the median time to death being 15 days: all of those tested were HIV infected (23). This event spotlighted the gaping hole in infection control for airborne diseases in health care facilities, emphasized the weaknesses in basic TB control and laboratory services, and was a tipping point not only in South Africa itself, but also at the global level (24). HIV programs recognized that TB represented an "Achilles' heel" for ART programs, and began work that resulted in April 2008 in international recommendations for action in infection control, intensified case finding for TB and isoniazid preventive therapy—the so-called three I's (25).

C. Association Between HIV and TB
HIV adversely affects TB control by creating problems with programmatic delivery and patient management (Table 2).

Programmatic Delivery
In many high-burden HIV/TB countries, TB case notifications have risen dramatically over the last 10 to 15 years, plateauing at levels 500% higher than baseline. There are three important comments to make about this upsurge in TB burden. First, most countries have seen a time lag between rising adult HIV prevalence and rising TB cases, and when HIV-prevalence rates have stabilized TB notifications have continued to rise to plateau seven or eight years later. This phenomenon is explained by the fact that most HIV-infected people start with a CD4-lymphocyte count of about 1000 cells/μL. This declines by 100 to 120 cells/μL every year until it reaches 180 cells/μL, which is the median level for developing TB (26). This means that if HIV infection is controlled and HIV prevalence starts to fall, it may take seven or eight years for TB case notifications to similarly fall. Second, as HIV prevalence rises, the number of TB patients who are women (particularly young women) also increases (12). Third, the increased number of cases inevitably means an increased number of TB suspects, and this may lead to a breakdown in diagnostic logistics--algorithms are not followed as shortcuts are taken; there are stock-outs of sputum containers as demand fails to keep pace with supply; more

Table 2 Adverse Effects of HIV on TB Programmatic Control and Patient Management

Effects on TB program delivery	Effects on patient management
• Increased TB case notifications, especially of smear-negative TB	• More difficult diagnosis especially of smear-negative PTB and disseminated TB
• "Hot spots" of TB transmission in congregate settings	• Increased morbidity and mortality
• Creation of stigma	• Increased rates of recurrent TB
• Illness and death in the health care workforce	• Facilitation of the spread of drug-resistant TB

Abbreviations: HIV, human immunodeficiency virus; TB, tuberculosis; PTB, pulmonary tuberculosis.

smears have to be prepared and examined which in turn can lead to an increase in false-negative sputum smear rates. Thus, paradoxically as TB case burden rises, case detection rates for smear-positive PTB may decline.

Subsumed within the general HIV/TB epidemic, there are hot spots of TB transmission in places where HIV-infected persons and those with TB come closely together—prisons, refugee camps, boarding schools, health facilities, and of course in the homes of index smear-positive PTB patients. Prisons especially seem to be centers for the amplification of anti-TB drug resistance. The issue of stigma is hard to drive away, and the perceived association between HIV and TB among the community and patients means that patients with TB may be reluctant to seek care resulting in delayed diagnoses, poor treatment outcomes, and increased transmission of infection. Health care delivery is weakened, with staff at all levels, including those from TB programs, being absent from work because of illness, attending funerals, or dying as a result of AIDS (27).

Patient Management

HIV makes the diagnosis of TB more difficult. As the immune system becomes more compromised, granuloma formation decreases, and the pattern of TB shifts from typical smear-positive, cavitary, upper lobe pulmonary disease to atypical smear-negative, infiltrative, lower lobe pulmonary disease, or extrapulmonary disseminated disease. The diagnosis of smear-negative PTB in adults and children is especially problematic in resource-poor facilities, particularly when patients with culture-positive PTB present with normal chest radiographs (28). However, recent guidelines on the empirical diagnosis and management of patients with smear-negative TB will go some way to assist front-line workers with this difficult problem (29).

Case fatality rates increase as the HIV prevalence in TB patients rises (30). The causes are many and include late presentation of tuberculosis and HIV-related nontuberculous bacterial infections such as *Salmonella typhimurium* and the pneumococcus, parasitic infections especially toxoplasmosis, Kaposi's sarcoma, lymphoma, and the HIV wasting syndrome (31). Case fatality rates in sub-Saharan Africa range from 10% in smear-positive pulmonary TB patients to 40% to 50% in smear-negative pulmonary TB patients and are even higher in HIV-associated MDR- and XDR-TB cases (23). These high death rates challenge the credibility of TB control programs among health-care workers, patients, and the wider community. Adverse effects of anti-TB drugs also appear to be more common among HIV-infected patients, of which the potentially fatal cutaneous hypersensitivity reactions to thioacetazone are the best known (32) and have given rise to the WHO's recommendation that this drug not be used in patients known, or suspected, to be HIV infected (33).

If patients complete treatment satisfactorily, the rates of recurrent TB are much higher in HIV-infected patients compared with HIV-negative patients (34). This adversely affects TB control. The additional cases add to the burden of TB, and management is more complicated and expensive as many patients need to be treated with a re-treatment regimen. Finally HIV facilitates the spread of drug-resistant TB, as exemplified by the emergence of XDR-TB in KwaZulu Natal, South Africa (23).

Effects on Global TB Control: Past, Present, and Future

During the first decade of DOTS expansion unprecedented progress was achieved worldwide. In 2006, 184 countries were using DOTS, and 31.8 million people had been treated under DOTS between 1995 and 2006. During the same period the global case detection rate for smear-positive cases rose from 15% to 61%, the treatment success rate rose from 77% to 85% and global TB incidence stabilized (11). Unfortunately, progress in the African region was less marked: the case detection rate reaching only 46% and the treatment success rate 76%. The principal reason for the lack of progress in Africa was the interaction between HIV and TB: the high case burden and resulting stigma of HIV/TB reduced case detection rates and the high case fatality impacted on treatment success. Weak health systems and insufficient numbers of trained staff were unable to redress the balance.

In 2000, the MDGs were adopted by the United Nations General Assembly, and the Stop TB Partnership set additional goals, namely, to halve the prevalence and death rates from TB by 2015 compared with 1990 levels. Using the old DOTS approach and with current progress, this goal is thought to be unachievable unless due attention is paid to the HIV/TB epidemic in Africa and drug-resistant TB in Eastern Europe, China, and India (9,11). With this in mind, the Stop TB Partnership developed a new 10-year Global Plan to Stop TB, 2006 to 2015 (35), backed by the new WHO Stop TB Strategy (14). The plan has six main themes, the second of which includes management of HIV/TB. The total plan is budgeted at US $56 billion for country level implementation, of which US $6.7 billion is earmarked for TB/HIV (36). To understand the formulation of the policy and strategy to control HIV/TB within this global plan, it is necessary to revisit the thoughts and development that underpinned this approach.

IV. Development of Policy, Strategy, and Guidelines To Decrease the Burden of TB/HIV

While HIV is seen as having deleterious effects on TB control, TB is also one of the commonest causes of morbidity throughout the course of HIV disease and is one of the leading causes of death in HIV-positive adults living in resource-poor countries (37,38). Thus, it is essential for TB and AIDS programs to collaborate in order to reduce the burden of disease in their patients. The slogan "two diseases, one patient" captures the essence of this philosophy. TB and HIV programs have to share mutual concerns: minimizing the impact of HIV should be a priority for TB control, and TB care and prevention should be priority concerns for HIV/AIDS programs. The first steps exploring collaborative approaches to HIV and TB service delivery were through the ProTEST projects undertaken at subdistrict level in Malawi, Zambia, and South Africa (39). These provided valuable lessons from the field that paved the way for a more informed international policy, strategy, and guideline development, which took place between 2002 and 2004 (40–42).

Three main principles underpinned the development of the TB/HIV policies and guidelines. First, after small-scale operational research projects, national programs insisted on a sense of urgency in the development of policy. TB/HIV policy therefore had to include the capacity to go rapidly to national scale on the basis of what was currently known. The policy would need to adjust as more evidence became available—"learning by doing." Second, policy should be centered on patients, that is, all services likely to be needed by patients with TB and/or HIV infection should, ultimately, be available at the same place and at the same time provided there are appropriate safeguards against transmission of TB from infectious patients to those most susceptible. Third, TB/HIV activities should, in no sense, form a separate program, but rather, they should add

HIV-related activities to National Tuberculosis Programs (NTPs) and TB-related activities to the National AIDS Control Programs (NACPs).

The guidelines (41) for implementing collaborative TB and HIV program activities reflected the lessons learnt from TB/HIV field sites with additional experience from comprehensive TB/HIV health services and interventions. With the strategic framework addressing *what can be done* and the Guidelines addressing *how things can be done*, an interim global policy was produced in 2004 describing *what should actually be done* to decrease the joint burden of TB and HIV (42). While there is good evidence for the cost-effectiveness of the DOTS strategy and several HIV-prevention measures, the evidence for collaborative TB/HIV activities is limited and is still being generated in different settings. For this reason, an interim policy document was developed to be continuously updated to reflect new evidence and best practices. The global policy does not call for the institution of a new specialist or independent disease control program, but rather enhanced collaboration between TB and AIDS programs.

V. Decreasing the Burden of TB/HIV

The policy goal is to decrease the burden of TB and HIV in populations affected by the two diseases. The objectives of the collaborative TB/HIV activities are as follows: (*i*) to establish mechanisms for collaboration between the two programs, (*ii*) to decrease the burden of TB in people living with HIV/AIDS, and (*iii*) to decrease the burden of HIV in TB patients. The collaborative activities needed to achieve these objectives are shown in Table 3.

A. The Mechanisms for Collaboration

Both programs need to create a joint national TB and HIV coordinating body, to work also at regional/district and local levels and oversee the direction and implementing of joint activities. In Eastern Europe and countries of the Former Soviet Union (FSU), TB/HIV administrative orders, or *prikaz*, will need to be promulgated to mandate the new activities.

Table 3   The 12-Point Policy Package Recommended Collaborative TB/HIV Activities

Establish the mechanism for collaboration
- Set up a coordinating body for TB/HIV activities effective at all levels
- Conduct surveillance of HIV prevalence among tuberculosis patients
- Carry out joint TB/HIV planning
- Conduct monitoring and evaluation

Decrease the burden of tuberculosis in people living with HIV/AIDS
- Establish intensified tuberculosis case finding
- Introduce isoniazid preventive therapy
- Ensure tuberculosis infection control in health care and congregate settings

Decrease the burden of HIV in tuberculosis patients
- Provide HIV testing and counseling, and link with HIV prevention
- Introduce cotrimoxazole (CTX) preventive therapy
- Ensure HIV/AIDS care and support
- Introduce HIV-prevention methods
- Provide antiretroviral therapy to HIV-infected TB patients

The TB and HIV/AIDS programs require joint strategic planning to collaborate successfully and systematically. Either they may work together to produce joint TB/HIV plans, or they may introduce TB/HIV components into each of the national TB and national AIDS control plans. These plans should be realistic and sufficiently resourced in terms of capacity building, finances, sustainable and effective commodity and supply mechanisms, effective advocacy and communication, and community involvement. The expansion of laboratory facilities and implementation of infection control (see below) require a joint and unified effort of both programs. Collaborative activities need to be monitored. TB programs, through their already well-tried and experienced system of quarterly monitoring, recording, and reporting, need to now incorporate HIV parameters (numbers HIV tested, HIV-positive, started on CTX and started on ART), and HIV programs need to reflect TB parameters in their recording and reporting mechanisms. Finally, operational research is an effective way of determining the most efficient way of implementing collaborative activities, and should be an integral part of any development plan (43).

Surveillance of HIV prevalence in TB patients is essential to program planning, implementation, and effective TB/HIV collaboration, and HIV testing also provides the entry point for delivery of ART. Guidelines on how to conduct surveillance have been published, and include (*i*) periodic cross-sectional surveys, (*ii*) sentinel surveys (using TB patients as a sentinel group within the general HIV sentinel surveillance system), and (*iii*) data from routine HIV testing and counseling of TB patients (44). The last option is the goal to aim for, where resources are sufficient.

B. Decreasing the Burden of Tuberculosis in People Living with HIV/AIDS

Intensified TB case finding comprises screening for symptoms and signs of TB in settings where HIV-infected people are concentrated. Intensified case finding includes the active identification of TB among patients with HIV in care settings, among household contacts, and if resources permit among other groups at high risk of HIV such as those living in congregate settings (e.g., prisons, workers' hostels, police and military barracks). Simple questionnaires and diagnostic algorithms to identify patients with TB should be administered to those known to be HIV infected. Whether chest X-rays should form part of the minimum essential investigations for the identification of asymptomatic tuberculosis in HIV-infected people remains unresolved (45). With the massive scale up of ART programs, particularly in the Africa region, attention needs to be paid to the identification of patients about to start ART who are staged as eligible for treatment based on symptoms and signs of weight loss and fever (WHO clinical stage 4). Tuberculosis may be an important cause of the "HIV wasting syndrome" (37), and how to best identify underlying TB in resource-limited settings should be a high research priority. Extending active TB case finding to household members can identify many cases of undiagnosed HIV and TB, and these efforts should interlink in order to also identify those in need of isoniazid preventive therapy (46). Whether intensified case finding is best placed under HIV programs or TB programs or a combination of the two is not clear, but what is clear is that the activity is feasible and potentially very rewarding.

The provision of isoniazid preventive therapy (IPT), linked particularly to counseling and HIV testing, is used to prevent the progression of latent *M. tuberculosis* to active disease. Several randomized trials in HIV-infected persons have shown that IPT can reduce the incidence of TB by approximately 60% (47), and a recent study in South Africa showed that in children the reduction in incidence of TB is also associated with a decrease in mortality (48). Protection against TB can last from 18 months to 4 years (49,50). The lack of long-term protection may be due to repeated infections of TB that occur in persons with HIV, especially those severely immunosuppressed living in high–TB-prevalence communities. Isoniazid is as effective and appears safer than rifampicin-containing regimens (and pyrazinamide-containing regimens) and is the preferred drug. However, IPT requires several steps to be taken, including identification of HIV-positive subjects, screening to exclude active TB, and provision of information to promote adherence.

Unfortunately, the widespread routine implementation of this effective intervention outside of efficacy or feasibility studies has been very poor. The reasons given are several, and chief among them is the fear of creating drug resistance if IPT is inadvertently given to a patient with subclinical or undiagnosed TB and the lack of guidance about who should take responsibility for the prevention package. Recently, there have been strong calls that HIV programs should take the lead in implementation, and link IPT to TB screening. HIV programs should systematically and routinely screen HIV-infected individuals and classify them as having no evidence of active TB (in which case they need IPT), evidence of active TB (in which case they need anti-TB treatment), or indeterminate (in which case they remain under observation) (51). Delivery and monitoring of IPT needs incorporation into programs of HIV care and support, which, prior to patients starting ART, would include CTX preventive therapy, regular measurements of CD4 counts and follow-up support.

Studies in Haiti and South Africa have found that post-treatment isoniazid in HIV-infected patients significantly reduces the rate of recurrent TB (52,53). This intervention has also yet to find a place in the routine management of TB. If the main mechanism of recurrence is reinfection, which appears to be the case in HIV-infected individuals who develop recurrent TB several months after completing treatment, then isoniazid may need to be given for life. Outside of ART clinics where it would be possible to deliver post-treatment isoniazid, there are no structures yet set up for delivering and monitoring this intervention.

TB infection control is of crucial importance, especially for the highly immunosuppressed patients, who in the absence of effective control measures, can acquire highly resistant tuberculosis strains in health care facilities (54) and has been in the spotlight recently as a result of transmission of XDR-TB in South Africa (23). Transmission of drug-sensitive TB, however, occurs at much greater magnitude than that of drug-resistant TB, and the control of both types of infection in outpatient and inpatient health facilities and in HIV clinics themselves is very challenging. Tuberculosis infection control guidelines exist (Table 4) and are in the process of being revised. However, infection control activities are rarely implemented (55). Health facilities should all have a TB infection control plan, that is incorporated into a wider Universal Infection Control Plan that deals also with blood-borne pathogens, and should ensure that activities that can make a difference are implemented such as educating patients about cough hygiene, ensuring maximal natural ventilation, separating patients with suspected or diagnosed TB from other HIV-infected patients, and so on.

Antiretroviral therapy in its own right is a good TB preventive measure, and massive scale up of ART should lead to a reduction in incidence and prevalence of TB. Studies in

Table 4 Tuberculosis Infection Control in Health Care Settings

---

Administrative measures
  • Early recognition, diagnosis, and treatment of pulmonary TB suspects
  • Separation of pulmonary TB suspects from others
  • Separation of pulmonary TB cases from others
Environmental protection
  • Maximizing natural ventilation
  • Using ultraviolet radiation (if applicable)
Personal protection
  • Protection of HIV-positive persons from possible exposure to TB
  • Offering isoniazid preventive therapy and antiretroviral therapy

---

South Africa, have shown firstly that rates of TB are significantly reduced in HIV-positive patients on ART compared with HIV-positive patients not on ART (6), and secondly that the longer a patient is on effective ART the lower the annual risk of developing TB (56). However, rates of TB still remain substantial in patients on ART and are much higher than those observed in HIV-negative populations (57,58). The reasons for this are unclear but may relate to incomplete immune restoration of TB-specific immune responses on ART or poor adherence to the medication. Data from Brazil confirm the benefit of ART on its own and IPT on its own, but importantly, show that ART and IPT together result in a highly significant synergistic decline in risk of active TB (59). Implementers need to work on how best to combine ART and IPT with maximum benefit and minimum risk of side effects.

C. Decreasing the Burden of HIV in TB Patients

The provision of HIV testing and counseling (HTC) in TB patients, using rapid tests, is indicated for several reasons: (a) establishment of the diagnosis of HIV, (b) a gateway to an adjunctive package of HIV clinical treatment and care, and (c) prevention of onward transmission of HIV, through disclosure, HIV testing of partners, reduction in risky behaviors, harm-reduction measures for TB patients when injecting drug use is a problem, screening and treating sexually transmitted infections and preventing unintended pregnancies and mother-to-child transmission (60). The recommended approach, now referred to as Provider-Initiated (opt-out) Testing and Counseling (61), dictates that health care workers request and perform an HIV test as an integral part of the clinical interaction, unless the patient specifically declines, and a higher priority is placed on posttest rather than pretest counseling, particularly if the patient is HIV-positive. In various country reports, provider initiated HIV testing for TB patients appears feasible and acceptable and can be associated with high rates of uptake (11,62).

  CTX-preventive therapy is an integral part of the WHO TB/HIV interim policy and is promoted by WHO and UNAIDS for the prevention of several bacterial and parasitic infections in eligible adults and children living with HIV/AIDS in Africa (63). The first randomized controlled study from Cote d'Ivoire demonstrated a 48% reduction in mortality in HIV-infected TB patients given CTX compared with placebo (64). Despite the proven efficacy, the routine use of CTX remained minimal for reasons discussed earlier, but in the last few years further clinical trials, even in areas where there are high rates of bacterial resistance, have established the efficacy of this intervention in both adults and children (20,21). Other concerns have also been allayed. A household study in Uganda provided reassuring evidence that use of CTX did not lead to an increase in bacterial resistance of CTX among family members (65), and a study in Mali showed that CTX in children aged 5 to 15 years was associated with excellent protective efficacy against malaria and did not select for sulfadoxine-pyrimethamine–resistant parasites (66).

Access to HIV care and support, including good clinical management of opportunistic infections and malignancies, nursing care, nutritional support, home care, and palliative care, is feasible and helps generate synergies and collaboration between TB and HIV/AIDS programs.

The provision of ART to HIV-positive TB patients is the intervention that should have the most significant impact on improving quality of life and reducing death rates in HIV-positive patients. In the industrialized world, ART has transformed AIDS from a fatal infectious disease into one that is chronic and manageable. The scale up of ART in developing countries was greatly facilitated five years ago by the production of cheap, generic, fixed dose combinations of two nucleoside reverse transcriptase inhibitors (NRTI; either stavudine–lamivudine or zidovudine-lamivudine), and one non-nucleoside reverse transcriptase inhibitor (NNRTI; nevirapine or efavirenz) to be used as first-line regimens. Second-line regimens use various combinations of NRTI with protease inhibitors. The early indications from well-run clinics in the developing world, and particularly in Africa where the HIV/AIDS burden is greatest, point to similar treatment efficacy of these first-line regimens in both adults and children compared with the industrialized world (67,68). However, as numbers of patients starting ART continue escalating, it is apparent that patient retention in large African programs is less than desirable, with loss to follow-up and death being the major causes of attrition (69). Unless active attempts are made to address the dire human resource shortages across the African region, unless better ways are found to get patients on to ART at an earlier stage than currently happens, unless outbreaks of MDR- and XDR-TB can be prevented in ART clinics, and unless improved ways of tracing defaulters are found, the credibility of ART as a cost-effective measure to treat HIV/AIDS in resource-poor settings will come under scrutiny and threat.

WHO Guidelines on eligibility to ART specify that patients in WHO clinical stage 4 can start ART regardless of CD4 count, and those in WHO clinical stage 3 can start ART if the CD4 count is less than 350 cells/μm. Furthermore, if no CD4 counting capability exists, as is often the case in peripheral hospitals, then patients in WHO clinical stage 3 can start ART based on clinical criteria (70,71). HIV-infected TB patients are thus all potentially eligible for ART because patients with pulmonary TB (and children with TB lymphadenitis) are classified in WHO clinical stage 3 and patients with extrapulmonary TB in WHO clinical stage 4 (70,71). With the scale up of ART, there is every reason to expect that ART will reduce TB case fatality rates and the risk of recurrent TB in coinfected patients. Despite these expectations, the combination of anti-TB drugs with ART drugs, both first and second line, is not easy, and the difficulties encountered in the field have resulted in less patients accessing ART than expected. The issues around combined therapy are shown in Table 5, and are briefly discussed below.

The optimal time to start ART in coinfected TB patients is not known with arguments for early as well as delayed therapy. Current WHO Guidelines provide recommendations about when to start ART in relation to CD4 cell counts or when CD4 counts are unavailable (Table 6) (70). In practice, many TB patients are commenced on ART after the two-month

Table 5 Implementation Issues Around Delivery of Combined Antituberculosis and Antiretroviral Therapy to HIV-Infected TB Patients

- Timing of antiretroviral therapy in relation to antituberculosis treatment, with advantages and disadvantages for early as well as delayed treatment
- Additive adverse drug effects from antituberculosis drugs and antiretroviral therapy drugs
- Drug–drug interactions, particularly between rifampicin and non-nuceloside reverse transcriptase inhibitors (nevirapine and efavirenz) and protease inhibitors
- Pill burden and adherence to therapy
- Development of immune reconstitution inflammatory syndrome (IRIS)
- Where to provide antiretroviral therapy and antituberculosis treatment to patients who are dually infected—in separate clinics or in the same clinic?
- The need for adjunctive cotrimoxazole preventive therapy and/or isoniazid preventive therapy

initial phase of anti-TB treatment because of fears of pill burden, additive side effects, and the immune reconstitution inflammatory syndrome (IRIS). The problem with delayed initiation of ART is that many deaths occur during the first two months of TB treatment (30), thus reducing the potential benefit of ART in reducing case fatality rates. Data from South Africa favor much earlier initiation of ART in terms of survival benefit, particularly in patients with stage 4 disease and CD4 counts less than 100 cells/μL (57,72). However, early initiation of ART will undoubtedly be associated with an increase incidence of IRIS (73), and although the evidence to date suggests that this is not associated with excess mortality, it will nevertheless complicate patient management.

Drug–drug interactions complicate combined therapy. Rifampicin reduces levels of efavirenz, nevirapine and protease inhibitors by induction of hepatic enzymes, and there is obvious concern that subtherapeutic drug levels might lead to HIV drug resistance

Table 6 WHO Recommendations About When To Start ART in TB Patients

CD4 cell count	ART recommendations	Timing of ART in relation to start of TB treatment
CD4 < 200 cells/mm^3	Recommend ART[a]	Between 2 and 8 wk (in initial phase of TB treatment)[b]
CD4 between 200 and 350 cells/mm^3	Recommend ART	After 8 wk (in continuation phase of TB treatment)
CD4 > 350 cells/mm^3	Defer ART[c]	Reevaluate the patient at 8 wk and at the end of TB treatment
Not available	Recommend ART[d]	Between 2 and 8 wk

[a] An efavirenz (EFV)-containing regimen is the preferred first-line regimen. Alternative first-line regimens include nevirapine (NVP) and triple NRTI [based on tenofovir (TDF) or abacavir (ABC)] regimens.
[b] ART should start as soon as TB treatment is tolerated, particularly in patients with severe immunosuppression.
[c] ART should be started if other non-TB stage 3 or stage 4 events are present.
[d] For some TB diagnoses that generally respond well to anti-TB therapy (e.g., lymph node TB, uncomplicated pleural effusion), deferral of ART should be considered.
Source: Adapted from Ref. 70.

and treatment failure. In first-line ART, efavirenz is the recommended NNRTI (except in women of child-bearing years) because the reduction in levels is less than those seen in nevirapine. However, both NNRTIs have a broad therapeutic index, and experience has shown that patients receiving standard dosages concurrently with rifampicin have good clinical, immunological, and virological outcomes (57), although these are better with efavirenz than nevirapine (74). In second-line ART, ritonavir-boosted protease inhibitors must be used, but much higher levels of ritonavir have to be used than normal and this can lead to severe hepatotoxicity (75). ART should improve the prognosis of HIV-related drug resistant TB, although there are no data to confirm this. Second-line anti-TB drugs are associated with considerable adverse effects, which overlap with those of ART drugs, although the absence of rifampicin from the regimens does simplify the issue to some extent. Some of the difficulties with these current drug–drug interactions may be resolved through use of triple or quadruple NRTI regimens or rifabutin, a less potent inhibitor of hepatic enzymes than rifampicin. At the moment none of these options has made its way into routine implementation.

There appears to be added benefit in combining ART with CTX preventive therapy. Early six-month ART mortality may be reduced, and gains in life expectancy may occur if both treatments are initiated together (76,77). However, the type of ART regimen used with CTX may be an important detail, as stavudine-lamivudine-nevirapine creates no additive adverse effects, while zidovudine may have added hematological side effects with CTX.

The final issue is where to deliver combined treatment. In most cases, TB treatment is given through TB clinics while ART is given through HIV-care and treatment clinics, creating logistic and financial difficulties for coinfected patients. Although the concept of "one-stop" shops where both treatments are administered together in the same clinic is attractive, hurdles about work overload, risks of TB transmission, and lack of good infrastructure need to be overcome if this is to become reality.

D.   Thresholds for Starting Recommended HIV/TB Collaborative Activities

Unlike many other HIV-related opportunistic infections, TB can occur at all levels of immune status. Thus, countries in any HIV-epidemic state and with intersecting epidemics of TB and HIV should consider implementing collaborative TB/HIV activities as indicated in Table 7 (42). HIV prevalence among TB patients is the most sensitive and reliable indicator for when to start collaborative activities, but in the absence of these data, the national HIV-prevalence rate can be used.

VI.   Current Progress and the Future

The current global monitoring system to assess progress in HIV/TB activities relies on information provided by countries to the WHO. In some areas there is evidence of progress. The number of countries that report TB/HIV collaboration has risen from 11 in 2002 to 102 in 2006 (11). Other data on TB/HIV activities in relation to Global TB/HIV targets is shown in Table 8. The rate of HIV testing in TB patients has risen dramatically, but with most other interventions the progress in implementation is lagging far behind the global targets, and at this rate it is very unlikely that the Stop TB targets for 2015

Table 7 Thresholds for Countries To Start Recommended Collaborative TB/HIV Activities

Criteria	Recommended collaborative TB/HIV activities
Countries in which the national adult HIV-prevalence rate is at or above 1% OR In which the national HIV prevalence among TB patients is at or above 5%	Undertake all collaborative activities listed in Table 4
Countries in which the national adult HIV-prevalence rate is below 1% AND In which there are administrative areas with an adult HIV-prevalent rate of 1% or more	Undertake all collaborative activities listed in Table 4 for the administrative areas with adult HIV rate of 1% or more In other parts of the country implement a. joint national TB/HIV planning, particularly with respect to surveillance of HIV prevalence in TB patients b. measures to decrease the burden of TB in people living with HIV/AIDS by intensified TB case finding, isoniazid preventive therapy, and TB infection control in health care and congregate settings
Countries in which the national adult HIV-prevalence rate is below 1% AND In which there are no administrative areas with an adult HIV-prevalent rate of 1% or more	Implement a. joint national TB/HIV planning, particularly with respect to surveillance of HIV prevalence in TB patients b. measures to decrease the burden of TB in people living with HIV/AIDS by intensified TB case finding, isoniazid preventive therapy, and TB infection control in health care and congregate settings

Source: Adapted from Ref. 42.

will be met. A number of important actions have to happen to reverse this situation. New earmarked funds for HIV/TB activities from agencies such as PEPFAR and the GFATM must be applied for and, more importantly, flow down to where they are needed for the implementers on the ground and for infrastructure development and improved laboratory capability. With the dire shortage of skilled human resources especially in the hard-hit areas of Africa, there is an urgent need to embrace WHO's new human resource initiative of "treat, train, retain" which aims to treat HIV-infected health workers with ART, train many more health workers, and retain those who might consider leaving for "greener pastures" or who have reached (an arbitrary) retirement age. Perhaps more controversially, new

Table 8 Progress Against Collaborative TB/HIV Targets in the Global Plan To Stop TB, 2006–2015

Activity	Global plan target for the year 2006	Country reports for the year 2006[a] (as % of target)
Number of HIV-infected persons actively screened for tuberculosis	11,000,000	314,000 (2.8)
Number of eligible HIV-infected persons offered isoniazid preventive therapy	1,200,000	27,000 (2.2)
Number of tuberculosis patients tested and counseled for HIV	1,600,000	687,000 (43)
Number of HIV-positive tuberculosis patients started on co-trimoxazole	500,000	147,000 (29)
Number of HIV-positive tuberculosis patients started on antiretroviral therapy	220,000	66,000 (30)

[a]Values have been rounded to nearest thousand.
Source: Adapted from Ref 11, (based on updated numbers from country reports).

policies also advise shifting tasks to less skilled cadres of health worker (78). To make health facilities safe for those with HIV infection, to prevent reactivation of TB, and to improve their treatment outcomes, HIV programs must work with general health facilities and start to take on and incorporate TB control activities into their programs (51). HIV programs need to be involved with the diagnosis and treatment of TB, advocate and push for rapid TB diagnostic tests, conduct operational research around the optimal ways to get ART to coinfected patients including decentralization of services to the periphery, and launch educational efforts in partnership with the community to reduce TB transmission. There is evidence that this is beginning to happen. The HIV Department of WHO is spearheading the "three I's" (infection control, intensified case finding, and isoniazid preventive therapy), and has already stated that these activities fall under the remit of HIV programs. This bold international leadership now needs to be heeded at national and grassroots level.

Although great strides have been made with scaling up HIV testing and counseling services, in sub-Saharan Africa nearly 80% of HIV-infected adults are still unaware of their HIV status and more than 90% are unaware of their partners' status (79). Such lack of knowledge is a denial of the human right to health as these adults cannot benefit from HIV prevention, care, and treatment, or from other interventions, which are of proven efficacy for reducing HIV transmission and HIV-related morbidity and mortality. TB control programs in high–HIV-prevalent areas have a unique opportunity to take a lead in implementing provider-initiated HIV testing and counseling, and at the same time to work toward a supportive social policy and legal framework that maximizes positive outcomes and minimizes potential harms to patients. As TB control services are often decentralized to primary level facilities and health centers, TB programs should take a proactive stance to raise community awareness about HIV/AIDS and promote the rights of people living with HIV/AIDS and the benefits of knowing and disclosing one's HIV status. Confidentiality and privacy must be respected, and health facilities should develop codes of conduct so that their health care workforce avoid stigmatizing and discriminating against patients on the basis of HIV status. By setting good examples of practice, TB programs can assist in the formulation and implementation of policies and laws that protect the HIV-infected patient.

At the international level, principles of equity and justice also oblige the richer countries of the world to continue increasing their development aid budgets, even when their own economies are not performing well. Furthermore, the "new" problems, such as climate change and rising food costs, should not encourage aid agencies to switch funding away from the "old," but unfinished, agenda of communicable disease control, such as HIV and TB control. The global institutions, the GFATM, the World Bank, UNAIDS, and WHO, have a particular role to continue to advocate for adequate funding against these epidemics—until the job is finished.

References

1. UNAIDS. AIDS epidemic update. December 2007. UNAIDS/07.27E/JC1322E.
2. Selwyn PA, Hartel D, Lewis VA, et al. A prospective study of the risk of tuberculosis among intravenous drug users with human immunodeficiency virus infection. N Engl J Med 1989; 320:545–550.
3. Daley CL, Small PM, Schecter GF, et al. An outbreak of tuberculosis with accelerated progression among persons infected with the human immunodeficiency virus. N Engl J Med 1992; 326:231–235.
4. Enarson DA, Rouillon A. The epidemiological basis of tuberculosis control. In: Davies PDO, ed. Clinical Tuberculosis, 2nd ed. London, U.K.: Chapman and Hall Medical, 1998.
5. Sonnenberg P, Glynn JR, Fielding K, et al. How soon after infection with HIV does the risk of tuberculosis start to increase? A retrospective cohort study in South African gold miners. J Infect Dis 2005; 191:150–158.
6. Badri M, Wilson D, Wood R. Effect of highly active antiretroviral therapy on incidence of tuberculosis in South Africa: A cohort study. Lancet 2002; 359:2059–2064.
7. Antonucci G, Girardi E, Raviglione MC, et al. Risk factors for tuberculosis in HIV-infected persons. A prospective cohort study. The Gruppo Italiano di Studio Tuberculosi e AIDS (GISTA). JAMA 1995; 274:143–148.
8. Dubrovina I, Miskinis K, Lyepshina S, et al. Drug-resistant tuberculosis and HIV in Ukraine: A threatening convergence of two epidemics? Int J Tuberc Lung Dis 2008; 12:756–762.
9. The WHO/IUATLD Global Project on Anti-tuberculosis Drug Resistance Surveillance. Anti-Tuberculosis Drug Resistance in the World. Report No. 4. Geneva, Switzerland: World Health Organization, 2008. WHO/HTM/TB/2008.394.
10. Corbett EL, Watt CJ, Walker N, et al. The growing burden of tuberculosis. Global trends and interactions with the HIV epidemic. Arch Intern Med 2003; 163:1009–1021.
11. World Health Organization. Global Tuberculosis Control 2008. Surveillance, Planning, Financing. Geneva, Switzerland: World Health Organization, 2008. WHO/HTM/TB/2008 .393.
12. Dye C. Global epidemiology of tuberculosis. Lancet 2006; 367:938–940.
13. World Health Organization. Treatment of Tuberculosis. Guidelines for National Programmes, 3rd ed. Geneva, Switzerland: World Health Organization, 2003. WHO/CDS/TB/2003.313.
14. The Stop TB Strategy: Building on and enhancing DOTS to meet the TB-related Millennium Development Goals. Geneva, Switzerland: World Health Organization, 2006. WHO/HTM,STB, 2006.368.

15. Working Group on Mother-To-Infant Transmission of HIV. Rates of mother-to-infant transmission of HIV-1 in Africa, America, and Europe: Results from 13 perinatal sites. J Acquir Immun Defic Syndr Retrovirol 1995; 8:506–510.

16. Guay LA, Musoke P, Feling T, et al. Intrapartum and neonatal single-dose nevirapine compared with zidovudine for the prevention of mother-to-child transmission of HIV-1 in Kampala, Uganda: HIVNET 012 randomised trial. Lancet 1999; 354:795–802.

17. Sweat M, Gregorich S, Sangiwa G, et al. Cost-effectiveness of voluntary HIV-1 counselling and testing in reducing sexual transmission of HIV-1 in Kenya and Tanzania. Lancet 2000; 356:113–121.

18. World Health Organization. Treating 3 Million by 2005: Making It Happen: The WHO Strategy. Geneva, Switzerland: World Health Organization, Joint United Nations Programme on HIV/AIDS, 2003.

19. World Health Organization, UNAIDS and UNICEF. Towards Universal Access. Scaling up Priority HIV/AIDS Interventions in the Health Sector. Geneva, Switzerland: Progress Report 2008.

20. Chintu C, Bhat GJ, Walker AS, et al. Cotrimoxazole as prophylaxis against opportunistic infections in HIV-infected Zambian children (CHAP): A double-blind randomized placebo-controlled trial. Lancet 2004; 364:1865–1871.

21. Nunn A, Mwaba P, Chintu C, et al.; for the UNZA-UCLMS Project LUCOT Collaboration. Role of co-trimoxazole prophylaxis in reducing mortality in HIV infected adults being treated for tuberculosis: Randomised clinical trial. BMJ 2008; 337:220–223.

22. Wells CD, Cegielski JP, Nelson LJ, et al. HIV infection and multidrug-resistant tuberculosis—the perfect storm. J Infect Dis 2007; 196:S86–S107.

23. Gandhi NR, Moll A, Sturm W, et al. Extensively drug-resistant tuberculosis as a cause of death in patients co-infected with tuberculosis and HIV in a rural area of South Africa. Lancet 2006; 368:1575–1580.

24. Report of the Meeting of the WHO Global Task Force on XDR-TB, Geneva, Switzerland, 9–10 October 2006. WHO/HTM/TB/2007.375. Available at: http://whqlibdoc.who.int/hq/2007/WHO_HTM_TB_2007.375_eng.pdf. Accessed August 24, 2009.

25. STOP-TB Partnership. TBHIV May 2008 Bimonthly Newsletter. WHO HIV and TB Departments issue joint call for TB to be seen as intrinsic part of HIV care. Geneva: Switzerland: World Health Organization, 2008:4.

26. Nunn P, Williams B, Floyd K, et al. Tuberculosis control in the era of HIV. Nat Rev 2005; 5:819–826.

27. Hongoro C, McPake B. How to bridge the gap in human resources for health. Lancet 2004; 364:1451–1456.

28. Colebunders R, Bastian I. A review of the diagnosis and treatment of smear-negative pulmonary tuberculosis. Int J Tuberc Lung Dis 2000; 4:97–107.

29. World Health Organization. Improving the Diagnosis and Treatment of Smear-Negative Pulmonary and Extrapulmonary Tuberculosis Among Adults and Adolescents: Recommendations for HIV-Prevalent and Resource-Constrained Settings. Geneva, Switzerland: World Health Organization, 2007.

30. Diul MY, Maher D, Harries AD. Tuberculosis case fatality rates in high HIV prevalence populations in sub-Saharan Africa. AIDS 2001; 15:143–152.

31. Nunn PP, Brindle R, Carpenter L, et al. Cohort study of HIV infection in tuberculosis patients, Nairobi, Kenya: Analysis of early (6 months) mortality. Am Rev Respir Dis 1992; 146: 849–854.

32. Nunn P, Kibuga D, Gathua S, et al. Cutaneous hypersensitivity reaction due to thiacetazone in HIV-1 seropositive patients treated for tuberculosis. Lancet 1991; 337:627–630.

33. WHO. Severe hypersensitivity reactions among HIV-seropositive patients with tuberculosis treated with thioacetazone. Wkly Epidemiol Rec 1992; 67:1–3.

34. Korenromp EL, Scano F, Williams BG, et al. Effects of human immunodeficiency virus infection on recurrence of tuberculosis after rifampicin-based treatment: An analytic review. Clin Infect Dis 2003; 37:101–112.
35. World Health Organization. The Global Plan To Stop TB 2006–2015. Stop TB Partnership. Geneva, Switzerland. 2006.
36. Floyd K, Pantoja A. Financial Resources required for tuberculosis control to achieve global targets set for 2015. Bull World Health Organ 2008; 86:568–576.
37. Lucas SB, De Cock KM, Hounnou A, et al. Contribution of tuberculosis to slim disease in Africa. BMJ 1994; 308;1531–1533.
38. Corbett EL, Churchyard GJ, Charalambos S, et al. Morbidity and mortality in South African gold miners: Impact of untreated HIV infection. Clin Infect Dis 2002; 34: 1251–1258.
39. World Health Organization. Report of a "Lessons Learnt" Workshop on the Six PROTEST Pilot Projects in Malawi, South Africa and Zambia. Geneva, Switzerland: World Health Organization, 2004. WHO/HTM/TB/2004.336.
40. World Health Organization. Strategic Framework to Decrease the Burden of TB/HIV. Geneva, Switzerland: World Health Organization, 2002. WHO/CDS/TB/2002.296. WHO/HIV_AIDS/2002.2.
41. World Health Organization. Guidelines for Implementing Collaborative TB and HIV Programme Activities. Geneva, Switzerland: World Health Organization, 2003. WHO/CDS/TB/2003.319. WHO/HIV/2003.01.
42. World Health Organization. Interim Policy on Collaborative TB/HIV Activities. Geneva, Switzerland: World Health Organization, 2004. WHO/HTM/TB/2004.330. WHO/HTM/HIV/2004.1.
43. Salaniponi FML, Harries AD, Nyirenda TE, et al. TB Research. Putting Research into Policy and Practice: The Experience of the Malawi National Tuberculosis Control Programme. Geneva, Switzerland: The Communicable Disease Cluster of the World Health Organization, 1999. WHO/CDS/CPC/TB/99.268.
44. World Health Organization. Guidelines for HIV Surveillance Among Tuberculosis Patients, 2nd ed. Geneva, Switzerland: World Health Organization, 2004. WHO/HTM/TB/2004.339. WHO/HIV/2004.06. UNAIDS/04.30E.
45. Chintu C, Mwaba P. Is there a role for chest radiography in identification of asymptomatic tuberculosis in HIV-infected people? Lancet 2003; 362:1516.
46. Wood R, Middlekoop K, Myer L, et al. Undiagnosed tuberculosis in a community with high HIV prevalence: Implications for tuberculosis control. Am J Respir Crit Care Med 2007; 175:87–93.
47. Wilkinson D, Squire SB, Garner P. Effect of preventive treatment for tuberculosis in adults infected with HIV: Systematic review of randomised placebo controlled trials. BMJ 1998; 317:625–629.
48. Zar HJ, Cotton MF, Strauss S, et al. Effect of isoniazid prophylaxis on mortality and incidence of tuberculosis in children with HIV: Randomised controlled trial. BMJ 2007; 334:136. Epub 2006. Nov 3.
49. Johnson JL, Okwera A, Hom DL, et al. Duration of efficacy of treatment of latent tuberculosis infection in HIV-infected adults. AIDS 2001; 15:2137–2147.
50. Quigley MA, Mwinga A, Hosp M, et al. Long-term effect of preventive therapy for tuberculosis in a cohort of HIV-infected Zambian adults. AIDS 2001; 15:215–222.
51. Havlir DV, Getahun H, Sanne I, et al. Opportunities and challenges for HIV care in overlapping HIV and TB epidemics. JAMA 2008; 300:423–430.
52. Fitzgerald DW, Desvarieux M, Severe P, et al. Effect of post-treatment isoniazid on prevention of recurrent tuberculosis in HIV-1-infected individuals: A randomised trial. Lancet 2000; 356:1470–1474.

53. Churchyard GJ, Fielding K, Charalambous S, et al. Efficacy of secondary isoniazid preventive therapy among HIV-infected South Africans: Time to change policy? AIDS 2003; 17:1–8.
54. Andrews J, Gandhi N, Moodley P, et al. Exogenous re-infection with multidrug- and extensively drug-resistant TB among TB/HIV co-infected patients in rural South Africa. 15th Conference on Retroviruses and Opportunistic Infections, Boston, Massachusetts, USA, 2008, Abstract #143.
55. Harries AD, Hargreaves NJ, Gausi F, et al. Preventing tuberculosis among health workers in Malawi. Bull World Health Organ 2002; 80:526–531.
56. Lawn SD, Badri M, Wood R. Tuberculosis among HIV-infected patients receiving HAART: Long term incidence and risk factors in a South African cohort. AIDS 2005; 19:2109–2116.
57. Lawn SD, Myer L, Bekker LG, et al. Burden of tuberculosis in an antiretroviral treatment programme in sub-Saharan Africa: Impact on treatment outcomes and implications for tuberculosis control. AIDS 2006; 20:1605–1612.
58. Moore D, Liechty C, Ekwaru P, et al. Prevalence, incidence and mortality associated with tuberculosis in HIV-infected patients initiating antiretroviral therapy in rural Uganda. AIDS 2007; 21:713–719.
59. Golub JE, Saraceni V, Cavalcante SC, et al. The impact of antiretroviral therapy and isoniazid preventive therapy on tuberculosis incidence in HIV-infected patients in Rio de Janeiro, Brazil. AIDS 2007; 21:1441–1448.
60. Bunnell R, Mermin J, De Cock KM. HIV prevention for a threatened continent. Implementing positive prevention in Africa. JAMA 2006; 296:855–858.
61. WHO and UNAIDS. HIV/AIDS Programme. Strengthening Health Services to Fight HIV/AIDS. Guidance on Provider-Initiated HIV Testing and Counselling in Health Facilities Geneva, Switzerland. May 2007. ISBN 978 92 4 159556 8.
62. Odhiambo J, Kizito W, Njoroge A, et al. Provider-initiated HIV testing and counseling for TB patients and suspects in Nairobi, Kenya. Int J Tuberc Lung Dis 2008; 3(suppl):S63–S68.
63. World Health Organization. Guidelines on cotrimoxazole prophylaxis for HIV-related infections among children, adolescents and adults. Recommendations for a public health approach. Geneva, Switzerland: World Health Organization, 2006. Available at: http://www.who.int/hiv/pub/guidelines/ctx/en/index.html. Accessed February 20, 2008.
64. Wiktor SZ, Morokro MS, Grant AD, et al. Efficacy of trimethoprim-sulphamethoxazole prophylaxis to decrease morbidity and mortality in HIV-infected patients with tuberculosis in Abidjan, Cote d'Ivoire: A randomised controlled trial. Lancet 1999; 353:1469–1474.
65. Mermin J, Lule J, Ekwaru JP, et al. Cotrimoxazole prophylaxis by HIV-infected persons in Uganda reduces morbidity and mortality among HIV-uninfected family members. AIDS 2005; 19:1035–1042.
66. Thera MA, Sehdev PS, Coulibaly D, et al. Impact of trimethoprim-sulfamethoxazole prophylaxis on falciparum malaria infection and disease. J Infect Dis 2005; 192:1823–1829.
67. Calmy A, Pinoges L, Szumilin A, et al; Medecins sans Frontieres. Generic fixed-dose combination antiretroviral treatment in resource-poor settings: Multicentric observational cohort. AIDS 2006; 20:1163–1169.
68. Sutcliffe CG, van Dijk JH, Bolton C, et al. Effectiveness of antiretroviral therapy among HIV-infected children in sub-Saharan Africa. Lancet Infect Dis 2008; 8:477–489.
69. Rosen S, Fox MP, Gill CJ. Patient retention in antiretroviral therapy programs in sub-Saharan Africa: A systematic review. PLoS Med 2007; 4:e298.
70. World Health Organization. Antiretroviral therapy for HIV infection in adults and adolescents: Recommendations for a public health approach. 2006 Revision. Available at: http://www.who.int/hiv/pub/guidelines/artadultguidelines.pdf. Accessed February 20, 2008.
71. World Health Organization. Antiretroviral therapy for HIV infection in infants and children: Towards universal access. Recommendations for a public health approach. 2006 Revision. Available at: http://www.who.int/hiv/pub/guidelines/art/en. Accessed February 20, 2008.

72. Lawn SD, Wood R. When should antiretroviral treatment be started in patients with HIV-associated tuberculosis in South Africa? S Afr Med J 2007; 97:412–415.
73. Lawn SD, Myer L, Bekker LG, et al. Tuberculosis-associated immune reconstitution disease: Incidence, risk factors and impact in an antiretroviral treatment service in South Africa. AIDS 2007; 21:335–341.
74. Boulle A, van Cutsem G, Cohen K, et al. Outcomes of nevirapine- and efavirenz-based antiretroviral therapy when coadministered with rifampicin-based antitubercular therapy. JAMA 2008; 300:530–539.
75. McIlleron H, Meintjes G, Burman W, et al. Complications of antiretroviral therapy in patients with tuberculosis: Drug interactions, toxicity and immune reconstitution inflammatory syndrome. J Infect Dis 2007; 196(suppl 1):S63–S75.
76. Lowrance D, Makombe S, Harries A, et al. Lower early mortality rates among patients receiving antiretroviral treatment at clinics offering cotrimoxazole prophylaxis in Malawi. J Acquir Immune Defic Syndr 2007; 46:56–61.
77. Goldie SJ, Yazdanpanah Y, Yosina E, et al. Cost effectiveness of HIV treatment in resource-poor settings—the case of Cote d'Ivoire. N Eng J Med 2006; 355:1141–1153.
78. Samb B, Celletti F, Holloway J, et al. Rapid expansion of the health workforce in response to the HIV epidemic. N Engl J Med 2007; 357:2510–2514.
79. Bunnell R, Cherutich P. Universal HIV testing and counseling in Africa. Lancet 2008; 371:2148–2150.

12
WHO's Stop TB Strategy: Progress and Prospects

MUKUND UPLEKAR, DIANA WEIL, and MARIO C. RAVIGLIONE
Stop TB Department, World Health Organization, Geneva, Switzerland

"In addressing the TB epidemic, including drug-resistant TB and HIV-associated TB, the world faces a human rights and health imperative: universal access to early and effective diagnosis, treatment, and cure for TB disease is essential to save lives and prevent transmission. Guided by the vision of the UN MDG 6 TB-related targets and by the mandate of strengthening health systems within the context of comprehensive universal primary health care for all, WHO must work with countries to implement the Stop TB Strategy and the Global Plan to Stop TB."

WHO Strategic and Technical Advisory Group for Tuberculosis, 2008

I. Introduction

Since the passage of the 1991 World Health Assembly (WHA) resolution declaring tuberculosis (TB) as a global public health emergency, the progress in global TB control has been steady (1). In 1994, the internationally recommended TB control strategy, later named DOTS, was launched (2). The DOTS framework was subsequently expanded in 2002 to better address the prevailing constraints to global TB control (3). On World TB Day, March 24, 2006, WHO launched a comprehensive Stop TB Strategy, developed with the engagement of a range of stakeholders and endorsed by the Stop TB Partnership as well as the WHA (4,5). The Stop TB Strategy is built on the foundation of DOTS and underpins the Global Plan to Stop TB, 2006 to 2015 (6,7). Since its launch, the strategy has been adopted and implemented widely by countries including all with a high burden of TB. By the end of 2007, nearly 40 million patients had been treated under the DOTS approach. Where DOTS had been provided, treatment success has steadily increased from 77% in 1994 to 85% in 2006. TB detection under DOTS increased from an estimated 11% in 1995 to an estimated 63% in 2007. However, in the past two years, the earlier acceleration has come to an end and the case detection rate is stagnating (8).

This chapter describes the Stop TB Strategy (Table 1) and also summarizes the progress made since its launch. The section below outlines the current challenges to global TB control and the opportunities to address them effectively. Section III presents the goals and the targets of the Stop TB Strategy. The major part of this chapter, section IV, details the six components of the Strategy including recent achievements under each component. On the basis of the recent experience in implementation of the Strategy and to help amplify and clarify the objectives, WHO, in late 2008, has adopted some revision of components and subcomponents of the Stop TB Strategy. Section V presents approaches

Table 1   The Stop TB Strategy at a Glance

Vision	A TB-free world
Goal	To dramatically reduce the global burden of TB by 2015 in line with the Millennium Development Goals and the Stop TB Partnership targets
Objectives	• Achieve universal access to quality diagnosis and patient-centered treatment
	• Reduce the human suffering and socioeconomic burden associated with TB
	• Protect vulnerable populations from TB, TB/HIV, and drug-resistant TB
	• Support development of new tools and enable their timely and effective use
Targets	• MDG 6, Target 8: halt and begin to reverse the incidence of TB by 2015
	• Targets linked to the MDGs and endorsed by Stop TB Partnership
	2015: reduce prevalence of and deaths due to TB by 50%
	2050: eliminate TB as a public health problem

Components of the strategy and implementation approaches

1. Pursue high-quality DOTS expansion and enhancement
    a. Secure political commitment, with adequate and sustained financing
    b. Ensure early case detection and diagnosis through quality-assured bacteriology
    c. Provide standardized treatment with supervision and patient support
    d. Ensure effective drug supply and management
    e. Monitor and evaluate performance and impact
2. Address TB/HIV, MDR-TB, and the needs of poor and vulnerable populations
    a. Scale up collaborative TB/HIV activities
    b. Scale up prevention and management of multidrug-resistant TB (MDR-TB)
    c. Address the needs of TB contacts and of poor and vulnerable populations
3. Contribute to health system strengthening based on primary health care
    a. Help improve health policies, human resource development, financing, supplies, service delivery, and information
    b. Strengthen infection control in health services, other congregate settings and households
    c. Upgrade laboratory networks and implement the Practical Approach to Lung Health (PAL)
    d. Adapt successful approaches from other fields and sectors, and foster action on the social determinants of health
4. Engage all care providers
    a. Involve all public, voluntary, corporate, and private providers through Public–Private Mix (PPM) approaches
    b. Promote use of the International Standards for Tuberculosis Care
5. Empower people with TB and communities through partnership
    a. Pursue advocacy, communication, and social mobilization
    b. Foster community participation in TB care, prevention, and health promotion
    c. Promote use of the Patients' Charter for Tuberculosis Care
6. Enable and promote research
    a. Conduct program-based operational research
    b. Advocate for and participate in research to develop new diagnostics, drugs, and vaccines

to measuring the progress and the impact of the Stop TB Strategy and related efforts to control TB. The chapter ends with concluding remarks in section VI.

II. Challenges and Opportunities

The concerted global efforts to control TB for over a decade have had an important impact on reducing morbidity and mortality. Estimated prevalence and death rates per 100,000 population declined from 296 (1990) to 206 (2007) and from 29 (1990) to 26 (2007), respectively (8). Although TB prevalence and mortality rates are apparently falling, recent trends suggest that the Stop TB Partnership targets of halving 1990 prevalence and death rates by 2015 are unlikely to be met globally. In the past two years, the earlier acceleration in detection has come to an end and the case detection rate is now stagnating (9). Particularly, urgent action is needed where the epidemic worsened dramatically in the late 20th century, notably in Africa but also in Eastern Europe. Sub-Saharan Africa has to face the challenge of managing the rapid rise in TB cases produced by the HIV epidemic, often in places where the human resources and health services are already overburdened. In Eastern Europe, the socioeconomic crisis that followed the dismantling of the Soviet Union in the early 1990s and related impoverishment of public health systems contributed to rising incidence and prevalence of TB, including multidrug-resistant TB (MDR-TB). Asia also demands serious attention, as it bears two-thirds of the global TB case burden. India, P.R. China, and Indonesia rank first, second, and third among countries worldwide in estimated cases. An emerging HIV epidemic and MDR-TB also present important challenges in Asia. In all settings, identifying and reaching all those in need of care, especially the poorest among the poor, pose a major challenge. Related to this, efforts to improve TB care and control must progress as an integral part of strengthening primary health care (PHC)–based health systems as a whole. At the same time, bringing down incidence and mortality at a much faster pace, fully tackling HIV among TB patients, preventing and treating MDR-TB, and, ultimately, eliminating TB—all depend heavily on the discovery and introduction of new diagnostics, drugs, and vaccines.

WHO and Stop TB partners have developed approaches to overcome some of today's major constraints to TB control. These include focused policy to expand use of newer diagnostic tools and impact measurement (10); public–private mix (PPM) strategies aimed at engaging all care providers, public and nonstate, and partnerships with patients and affected communities in TB care and control (11,12); innovative mechanisms such as the Global Drug Facility (GDF) and the Green Light Committee (GLC) to improve access to quality-assured, affordable drugs for well-designed programs in resource-poor settings (13,14). The collaborative activities that need to be implemented by both TB and HIV/AIDS programs via primary care facilities have been defined (15), and strategies to prevent and manage MDR-TB have been developed and are beginning to be rolled-out (16). New product development partnerships and academic research initiatives have created the first serious pipeline of new diagnostics, drugs, and vaccines to take the world from 19th to mid-20th century technology into the 21st century—albeit far later than for other urgent concerns such as HIV. Partnerships are being developed across and within countries and among a wide array of stakeholders to respond to health system and disease-control challenges. The recent emergence of extensively drug-resistant TB (XDR-TB) has stimulated a new energy in facing TB as a health security threat—an unfortunate wake-up call to the world that moderate advances in facing this age-old disease are not enough (17). Far more bold interventions on insufficient and unsafe public health practice and far more rigorous action in research were needed long before and must be taken up now (18).

Investments in TB have grown dramatically in the last five years, with more rich country attention to development, and the creation of the Global Fund to fight AIDS, TB, and Malaria ("The Global Fund") and UNITAID (see below) offer innovation in the sources and modalities of international financing for disease control efforts. Yet, the resource improvements fall far shy of the needs outlined in the Global Plan to Stop TB, 2006 to 2015, especially the interventions required to address TB/HIV and MDR/XDR-TB (7).

III. Goals and Targets

The Stop TB Strategy responds to a vision of a world free of TB. The goal of the Stop TB Strategy is to dramatically reduce the global burden of TB by 2015 in line with the Millennium Development Goals (MDGs) and the Stop TB Partnership targets, and to achieve major progress in the research and development of new tools needed for TB elimination. The Stop TB Strategy has four major objectives, which are designed to achieve the goal. These are

1. to achieve universal access to high-quality diagnosis and patient-centered treatment for all people with TB;
2. to reduce the human suffering and socioeconomic burden associated with TB;
3. to protect vulnerable populations from TB, TB/HIV, and MDR-TB; and
4. to support development of new tools and enable their timely and effective use.

Targets for TB control have been established by the WHA (1), by the United Nations as part of the MDGs (19), and by the Stop TB Partnership (7). The Stop TB Strategy is designed to achieve these targets. The WHA targets for 2005 were not met globally by all countries, although the Western Pacific region as a whole and 26 countries worldwide did achieve the 70% case detection and 85% treatment success rate levels required. The aim beyond 2005 is now to maintain or exceed 85% treatment success and move toward full care detection. The MDG target relevant to TB (Goal 6, Target 8) is "to have halted and begun to reverse incidence by 2015" (19). The interpretation of Target 8 is that the incidence rate of all forms of TB should be falling by 2015. TB indicators have been defined for MDG 6, Target 8. These are TB prevalence and death rates and the proportion of cases detected and successfully treated under DOTS (Table 2).

The Stop TB Partnership has endorsed two epidemiological targets related to the MDGs: to decrease 1990 TB prevalence and death rates by 50% by 2015 (7) (Table 2). Achievement of these "impact" targets globally requires sustained progress in implementation, which in turn requires all of the TB care and control innovations already tested and yet more innovation ahead—else the Stop TB Partnership commitment to eliminate TB as a public health problem by 2050 will not be viable.

Table 2 Millennium Development Goal, Targets, and Indicators for TB and the Stop TB Partnership Targets

Millennium Development Goal 6
Goal: Combat HIV/AIDS, malaria, and other diseases
Target 8: Have halted by 2015 and begun to reverse the incidence of malaria and other major diseases
Indicator 23: Prevalence and death rates associated with tuberculosis
Indicator 24: Proportion of tuberculosis cases detected and cured under DOTS
Stop TB Partnership Targets
By 2005: At least 70% of people with infectious TB will be diagnosed (under the DOTS strategy) and at least 85% cured
By 2015: The global burden of TB (disease prevalence and deaths) will be reduced by 50% relative to 1990 levels; specifically, this means reducing prevalence to 155 per 100, 000 per year or lower and deaths to 14 per 100,000 per year or lower by 2015 (including TB cases coinfected with HIV); the number of people dying from TB in 2015 should be less than approximately 1 million, including those coinfected with HIV
By 2050: The global incidence of TB disease will be less than 1 case per million population per year

IV. Components of the Stop TB Strategy

Tackling TB effectively requires addressing all the risk factors that make individuals vulnerable to being infected with TB and to developing the disease. It also means reducing the adverse effects of the disease including its social and economic consequences. Stopping TB must, therefore, be seen within the framework of country-owned strategies to reduce poverty, advance development, and strengthen health systems. Therefore, the Stop TB Strategy must be aligned with other strategies and partnerships to address poverty and face all major public health challenges. The main focus of the Stop TB Strategy is on the risk factors that can be directly addressed through use of currently available tools for diagnosis, treatment, and prevention of TB as well as the improved tools that are likely to become available in the near future through research and development. The Stop TB Strategy builds on DOTS while also broadening its scope to address remaining constraints and current challenges in TB control. The six components of the Stop TB Strategy are as follows:

1. Pursue high-quality DOTS expansion and enhancement;
2. Address TB/HIV, MDR-TB, and the needs of poor and vulnerable populations;
3. Contribute to health system strengthening based on PHC;
4. Engage all care providers;
5. Empower people with TB and communities through partnership; and
6. Enable and promote research.

The application of the Strategy has demonstrated that the implementation stage and speed for each of the components of the Strategy will vary depending on the socioeconomic situation, TB epidemiology, the health services landscape, and the soundness of DOTS implementation to date. In promoting the Stop TB Strategy within different country contexts, some observations have been made with regard to its formulation. The first two components provide the technical core of the strategy, while the rest offer approaches that will enhance the scope, effectiveness, and impact of the technical components. Also, the first element of the first component—to secure political commitment to TB care and control, with adequate and sustained financing—is essential for the success of the overall strategy not only for basic DOTS efforts.

The paragraphs below describe each component of the Stop TB Strategy with reference to progress in its implementation.

A.   Pursue High-Quality DOTS Expansion and Enhancement

The five elements of DOTS are well established. To address known implementation constraints and challenges, further strengthening of the basic elements of the DOTS approach is required along the following lines.

Secure Political Commitment to TB Care and Control, with Adequate and Sustained Financing

Clear and sustained political commitment by national governments to TB care and control efforts is the backbone of the response in all settings and essential for the whole Stop TB Strategy to be taken forward. The nature of governance and the structure of public health systems notwithstanding, a stewardship function to support TB control efforts through PHC is needed. A national TB program (NTP) with a central unit that establishes norms and policies, supports intermediate and district management, builds capacity, fosters partnerships, solves problems, helps innovation, and provides monitoring and evaluation of services is critical. A medium-term strategic plan for TB control is also needed, with clear process and impact indicators. The Global Plan to Stop TB, 2006–2015, provides a guide for such national plans with benchmarks of progress toward 2015 targets under varying regional scenarios (7). The medium-term plan should be integrated within a national health plan and within poverty reduction and development frameworks. The plan should address technical and financial requirements and promote accountability for results at all levels of the health system. Partnerships with the many potential contributors will help improve TB care in terms of access, equity, and quality. Care can be TB-specific and integrated with broader disease control and other priority public health interventions. Political commitment should be backed-up by national legislation on TB prevention, care, and control (20). This legislation can lay out the ethical and rights-based principles for protection from the risk of infection, access to diagnosis and care, responsibility and accountability for actions, and results by health authorities and all service providers. The plan must be supported by adequate and sustained financing with increasing domestic resources complemented by external funding, where necessary. WHO data collection and analysis of national TB control financing over recent years suggest that there has been substantial recent growth in national financing for TB control in low and middle-income countries as well as in international financing, most notably from the Global Fund. However, new resources are helping to meet more core needs of DOTS implementation, with a greater proportional funding gap in meeting the needs for TB/HIV and MDR-TB investments, as well as advocacy, communications, and social mobilization efforts.

Even with adequate financing, critical deficiencies in the health workforce in the public sector will likely impede progress in many low- and middle-income countries, especially in Africa. Overall, structural and financial changes are required to improve the availability, distribution, and motivation of human resources for health to enable an adequate response to all health MDGs (21–24). Changes are needed also to strengthen other health system "building blocks" as noted under the third component of the Stop TB Strategy. A number of global partnerships, including the International Health Partnership and Related Initiatives (IHP+), aim to strengthen coherent national health strategies and harmonize support for these strategies from various sources under compacts among governments, donors, and other partners (25). The Global Health Workforce Alliance is addressing means to overcome some of the major constraints to human resources development, such as reducing the brain drain, reforming civil service payment structures, developing new performance-based incentive structures for geographical and service-level staffing balance, and building preservice and in-service capacity (26).

Ensure Early Case Detection and Diagnosis Through Quality-Assured Bacteriology

Effective reduction of morbidity, mortality, and transmission of TB depends on accurate and early detection of persons with TB symptoms and their diagnostic screening. The recommended method of TB diagnosis is bacteriology, first using sputum-smear microscopy, and also culture and drug-sensitivity tests when indicated. The latter are crucial for diagnosis and monitoring of smear-negative and drug-resistant TB cases.

Access to quality-assured sputum-smear microscopy means that health services with properly equipped laboratories and well-trained personnel need to be widely available and accessible. This will require additional investments in the public health laboratory network, including a national TB reference laboratory, in many countries. The laboratory network should be based on the following principles: adoption of national standards in accordance with international guidelines, decentralization of diagnostic services while maintaining high proficiency levels, continuous interaction between members at various levels of the network, and functional internal and external quality management including supervision.

Culture and drug-sensitivity testing services should be introduced as quickly as possible as well as periodic surveys or continuous surveillance of the prevalence of drug resistance. This means that national and subnational reference laboratories need urgent upgrading in most countries. Referral facilities are also needed to improve diagnosis of sputum smear-negative TB, diagnosis of TB among HIV-positive patients and children, and monitoring of patients with drug-resistant disease. The introduction of new diagnostic tools recommended by WHO, such as culture using liquid media, and line probe assays for rapid genetic identification of drug resistance will be essential for efficient response to diagnostic needs and will take planning and investment to introduce and to scale-up access (27). Maintaining the quality of the laboratory network depends on regular training, supervision and support, and motivation of laboratory staff. Existing public and private laboratories should be used optimally. Generally weak laboratory capacity in face of the need to scale up MDR-TB response poses a great challenge to many NTPs. A Global Laboratory Initiative (GLI) has been established by the WHO and the Stop TB Partnership to strengthen capacity and support mobilization of technical and financial assistance for this challenging process (28). The GLI is already enabling access to new diagnostic tools by working with partners such as the Foundation for Innovative New Diagnostics (FIND), a product development partnership (29), and with UNITAID—an innovative financing mechanism based largely on the generation of financing for HIV, TB, and malaria commodities through airline taxation by selected countries (30).

Ensuring early and complete case detection requires greater attention for a variety of reasons. Firstly, monitoring of the TB epidemic clearly indicates recent stagnating TB case detection at just above 60%. Ways to increase case detection and sustain it must be identified and implemented rapidly. This translates into the need to progressively shift from detection of TB cases among people presenting symptoms spontaneously to health services toward a more active detection effort. To be productive and cost-effective, such active search for cases should be focused especially on the highly vulnerable populations. Secondly, since most of the disease transmission occurs before a TB case is diagnosed and put on treatment, detecting not just more cases but detecting them early enough is important to achieve an impact on the TB epidemic. New approaches should aim at achieving both early and complete case detection. Thirdly, application of new WHO policies on optimization of the number of sputum smears and use of liquid culture could now help in increasing the speed and quality of case detection (27). Enhancing "case detection" will require context-specific approaches for early identification of those with suspected disease, and improving "case diagnosis" will require choosing the diagnostic technique and technology to be employed.

Provide Standardized Treatment with Supervision and Patient Support

The mainstay of TB control is organization and administration of standardized treatment countrywide for all adult and pediatric TB. In all cases, WHO's most recent recommendations in published guidelines on patient categorization and management should be followed (31). These guidelines emphasize the use of the most effective, standardized, short-course regimens and of fixed-dose combinations (FDCs) to facilitate adherence and prevent the risk of acquiring drug resistance. WHO guidelines are also available for management of patients with drug-resistant TB (15).

Supervision and patient support remain the cornerstone of DOTS-based care. Staff responsible for delivery of TB care should identify and address factors that may make patients interrupt or stop treatment. Supervised treatment assists patients in taking their drugs regularly and in completing the treatment, thus helping to achieve cure, prevent development of drug resistance, and, by reducing transmission, protect general public from contracting the disease. Supervision of treatment is meant to ensure adherence on part of both: the providers (in giving proper care and detecting treatment interruption) and the patients (in taking regular treatment). It must be carried out in a context-sensitive and patient-friendly manner. Depending on the local conditions, supervision may be undertaken at a health facility, in the workplace, in the community, or at home. A treatment supporter must be identified for each TB patient: a person acceptable to and chosen by the patient and trained and supervised by health services to guarantee regular intake of drugs by the patient. Patient and peer support groups can help further to promote adherence to treatment.

Locally appropriate measures should be consciously undertaken to identify and address physical, financial, social and cultural, as well as health system barriers, to access TB treatment services. Particular attention should be paid to the poorest and most vulnerable groups. Examples of appropriate actions include providing free diagnosis and treatment, expanding treatment outlets in the poor rural and urban settings, involving providers and treatment supporters in the community that practice and reside close to where patients live, and offering psychological, social, and legal support. Also useful are treatment enablers that can compensate for the indirect costs of care and enable adherence, efforts to explicitly address gender issues, improve staff attitudes, enhance communication and social mobilization, and support patient and community groups to help create demand and avail quality-assured support and services. It is essential that these approaches are based on ethical principles where the needs, rights, capabilities, and responsibilities of patients, their families, and their communities are all addressed.

Factors such as the type of drug regimen (daily or intermittent), the type of drug formulation (FDCs or separate drugs), as well as characteristics of the patient should be considered in organizing patient supervision. Use of Directly Observed Treatment (DOT) as a method of supervision recommended by WHO has been a subject of lengthy debates and controlled trials, thanks to the exaggerated attention paid solely to the literal act of watching patients while swallowing pills, rather than viewing it as an integral and essential part of any patient support package designed to guarantee the full course of treatment and remove any obstacles that may make treatment onerous for patients (32,33). Direct supervision of the taking of each dose of drugs is indispensable in the treatment of, for example, patients with psychosocial problems, prison inmates, or patients receiving second-line anti-TB drugs. As TB is a public health problem and its transmission poses a risk to the community, facilitating and ensuring regular intake of all the drugs by the patient for the complete duration is a responsibility of the health care staff and of the national TB program, but it does not mean that health workers must be the supervisors. The whole purpose of undertaking DOT would be lost if it limits access to care, turns patients away from treatment, or adds to their hardships. The emergence and spread of MDR and XDR-TB further reinforces the absolute necessity of helping a TB patient not to miss any drug doses. Many country TB programs now have considerable experience in identifying adherence promotion strategies that work or do not work and tailoring treatment supervision to a given context. TB programs should continue to strengthen patient supervision and support with the goal of achieving complete access to a full course of treatment, full treatment adherence, and patient satisfaction with care.

Ensure Effective Drug Supply and Management

An uninterrupted and sustained supply of quality-assured anti-TB drugs are fundamental to TB control. For this purpose, an effective drug procurement, distribution, and management system is essential and should be provided through the essential drug-supply system if it exists, as part of PHC. Anti-TB drugs should be available free of charge to all TB patients, both because many patients are poor and TB treatment has benefits that extend to society as a whole—successful treatment prevents disease transmission. Legislation related to drug regulation should be in place and use of anti-TB drugs by all providers should be strictly monitored. The use of FDCs of proven bioavailability and innovative packaging, such as blister packs and patient kits, can help improve drug supply logistics as well as drug administration, reduce nonadherence to treatment, and prevent development of drug resistance. The GDF and the GLC meant for access to second-line anti-TB drugs offer support to secure financing and procurement of quality-assured anti-TB drugs at competitive prices and also facilitate access to strengthen their drug management capacity (13,14). The GDF is governed by WHO on behalf of the Stop TB Partnership and utilizes an independent procurement agent which directly procures first-line anti-TB drugs with GDF resources or those of the recipient country or a third party, a donor agency for example (13). The GLC is managed by WHO and vets proposals for MDR-TB case management and then enables access to concessionally priced second-line drugs and technical assistance for implementation (14). The establishment of UNITAID has been a major step in resolving gaps in financing for anti-TB drugs, especially pediatric formulations and second-line drugs for MDR-TB treatment (30).

Since the launch of the Stop TB Strategy, availability of quality-assured and affordable anti-TB drugs has improved. For example, the prequalification process for pediatric formulations of FDCs has been accelerated via mechanisms including pooled procurement by the GDF, the involvement of UNITAID, and provision of technical assistance from the WHO prequalification project. Despite progress, drug shortages continue to occur in all regions at both central and peripheral levels. Better monitoring and management of drug supply and distribution are still required (9). Improving supply systems is among the major stated concerns for health system strengthening efforts in general.

Monitor and Evaluate Performance and Impact

Establishing a reliable system to monitor and evaluate TB performance and impact is vital. This system needs to be embedded within overall national health information systems, and it depends on regular communication between the central and peripheral levels. The system must encompass standardized recording of individual patient data, including information on case detection by category for quarterly case notification, and on treatment outcomes, which are then used to compile quarterly treatment outcomes in cohorts of patients. These data, when compiled and analyzed, can be used at the facility level to monitor treatment outcomes, at the facility and the district level to identify local problems as they arise, and at a provincial or national level to ensure support and secure consistency of TB control across geographical areas. Lastly, data are used nationally and internationally to evaluate the performance of each country and for epidemiological surveillance. Regular program supervision should be carried out to verify the quality of information and to address performance problems.

Increasingly, countries have additional information at their disposal, including results of sputum culture, results of drug sensitivity tests, and HIV test results. WHO has recently developed and shared with countries a revised framework for TB recording and reporting (34). This system incorporates recording of additional data that should be routinely collected to enable monitoring of the implementation of the Stop TB Strategy. Countries have also begun to revise their recording and reporting systems to reflect the various components and subcomponents of the Stop TB Strategy. Many countries are beginning to shift to electronic and internet-based recording and reporting systems, which is assisting with increased speed of data collection and review and depth of analysis.

To make the best use of data at all levels, many countries will need to do more to train staff in the analysis and interpretation of data as well as in the use of computer software that can greatly facilitate this work. As electronic recording systems become more widely available, consideration should be given to storing individual patient data, which will make it possible to not only carry out more detailed analyses using aggregated data but also raise the need for increased care in maintaining confidentiality of information.

In view of the need for each country to assess the progress of its control efforts toward achieving established national or global targets, a number of approaches to impact measurement have been recommended (35). While the definitive tool would be to monitor incidence trends through routine well-functioning surveillance systems, disease prevalence surveys and death registration systems (or verbal autopsy where those are not in place) are also useful methods to assess the burden. Each country should plan impact measurement, which is of increasing importance in designing national programs, in mobilizing and justifying financial resources for program operations and in reviewing and revising strategies.

B. Address TB/HIV, MDR-TB, and the Needs of Poor and Vulnerable Populations

Scale Up Collaborative TB/HIV Activities

By suppressing the immune response, HIV promotes the progress of recent and latent infection due to *Mycobacterium tuberculosis* to active TB. It also increases the rate of recurrent TB. The HIV epidemic has caused a substantial increase in the proportion of TB cases that have smear-negative pulmonary and extrapulmonary TB. HIV-positive smear-negative pulmonary TB patients have inferior treatment outcomes and higher early mortality compared with HIV-positive smear-positive pulmonary TB patients. In the long term, only effective control of the HIV epidemic will reverse the associated increase in TB incidence. However, until then, interventions to reduce HIV-related TB morbidity and mortality need to be implemented (35).

WHO has published a policy document on collaborative TB/HIV activities (15). This is a twelve-point policy package incorporating three broad categories: establishing the mechanisms for collaboration, decreasing the burden of TB in people living with HIV/AIDS, and decreasing the burden of HIV in TB patients. The second category is focused on efforts that can be taken up principally under the guidance of HIV programs and partners through primary care facilities and is referred to as the *three I's*: intensified case finding, isoniazid preventive therapy, and infection control. Special attention has been given to the scale-up of these interventions in Africa and to high-level commitment by governments and partners to support the full TB/HIV policy package (36). A Ministerial Forum on the theme was organized at the UN in June 2008, under the leadership of the UN Special Envoy to Stop TB (37). UNAIDS, PEPFAR, and the Global Fund, among others, are expanding their efforts on TB/HIV work. In several African countries, including Malawi, Rwanda, and Kenya, remarkable progress has been made in expanding access to HIV testing for TB patients, reaching more than three-fourths of their patients (9). This trend is being repeated in other countries now and the challenge ahead is ensuring easy access to care for those testing positive for HIV and those HIV-infected persons testing positive for TB infection and other diseases. Far more work still needs to be done to enable universal access to antiretroviral therapy for qualifying TB patients and to pursue all of the three *I's*.

Scale Up Prevention and Management of MDR-TB

Global surveillance of anti-TB drug resistance indicates that it is present everywhere and that it is especially prevalent in countries of the former Soviet Union and some provinces of P.R. China. The highest ever reported levels of MDR-TB disease (up to 20% of all new patients in some former Soviet countries) were published in the 2008 WHO Report on *Anti-Tuberculosis Drug Resistance in the World* (17). This report also documented the rising number of countries (more than 50 by late 2008) with reported cases of XDR-TB, a more lethal form of MDR-TB that is more difficult and more costly to treat. Evidence from Southern Africa suggests that where XDR-TB is introduced into congregate settings, like health centers and hospitals with significant numbers of immunocompromised individuals such as those infected with HIV, the consequences can be severe with extremely high mortality. Once introduced, XDR-TB can stretch low-income country capacity to provide adequate public health protection and patient care (38).

In the areas where MDR-TB has reached alarming levels, TB cannot be controlled if MDR-TB prevention and management are not explicitly addressed, alongside strong basic DOTS services. This means that special attention is given to infection control, early screening and diagnosis for drug-resistant TB, and adequate and appropriate treatment of MDR-TB. Detection and treatment of all forms of drug-resistant TB should eventually be an integral part of NTP activities. Although this may be challenging, experience shows that it strengthens the program's overall capacity to implement TB control measures. The key actions to prevent and control drug-resistant TB include a comprehensive care framework including models of care for different levels of the health system, patient support, a reliable supply of diagnostics and drugs, and measures to improve the guidance and regulation of MDR-TB treatment by all health care providers, including hospitals, clinics, private practitioners, and community-based treatment supporters.

Management of MDR-TB under programmatic conditions is feasible, effective, and cost-effective when implemented in the context of a well-functioning TB control program and based on WHO's policy guidelines on the programmatic management of MDR-TB (16).

The GLC reviews project and programmatic proposals for the initiation and scale-up of programmatic management of MDR-TB and enables access to second-line drugs for approved efforts (14). GLC-approved projects have now been initiated in 60 countries. However, in the 27 countries estimated by WHO to have the heaviest burdens of MDR-TB, few have national plans devised for full national scale-up of MDR-TB response. In the next few years, it will be imperative for all to be working urgently in building the support and capacity needed to mount such responses.

Address the Needs of TB Contacts, and of Poor and Vulnerable Populations

TB programs need to pay specific attention through focused approaches and activities to TB contacts and to all poor and vulnerable populations who face a higher risk of contracting TB, barriers to accessing care, and problems in adhering to treatment. Guidance on identifying and managing contacts of TB patients, at home and outside, needs to be provided to all countries. Contact tracing results in early case detection and treatment as well as provision of preventive therapy where appropriate. There may be significant challenges in establishing contact tracing and follow up mechanism in health systems with limited human resources. The well-established but widely underutilized intervention of contact tracing deserves systematic implementation by NTPs in high-burden countries (HBCs).

Populations that are more vulnerable to contract TB include the very poor; women and children; malnourished persons; smokers, alcoholics, and injecting drug users; persons with comorbidities such as diabetes; prison populations; internally displaced persons and refugees; migrating workers and others working in ill-ventilated and congested workplaces; indigenous people; and specific ethnic groups and other marginalized populations. Special situations requiring extra attention for the design of TB prevention and treatment efforts include unexpected population movements such as political unrest, war, natural disaster, and other conditions causing refugee movements. In these circumstances, there may be a disruption of social networks. In all these contexts, there is also the imperative to help ensure that ethics and human rights tenets are supported, as the populations and communities of concern may also be those that lack voice and other means to ensure that their rights are upheld and advanced.

TB services need to adapt to address the specific needs of high-risk groups and to support TB prevention and control in special situations (39–43). NTPs must not lose the sight of the fact that TB is primarily a disease of poverty and it is often the poorest and the most vulnerable who have problems in availing services meant for them. Ministries of Health should ensure that TB diagnosis and drugs are free of charge, that the density of services near the poorest populations is adequate, and that the local communities are effectively engaged to make care and health promotion more accessible to the poor.

In the face of stagnating TB case detection in spite of wide coverage and implementation of basic DOTS services, focused action is needed to reach the most vulnerable through targeted strategies and to ensure that NTPs collaborate with all partners working to meet other health and development needs of these populations.

C.   Contribute to Health System Strengthening Based on PHC

Strengthening health systems is now seen as an urgent prerequisite for achieving all the health MDGs. There is a recognition that disease control responses have helped build commitments in the health sector and toward system strengthening, but the demands are great. There are new partnerships and high-level cooperation to help build momentum for the scale-up of health interventions while also improving the human resources and supportive systems that enable delivery of health services and outcomes. WHO has called for a renewal of commitment to PHC principles as a guiding framework in improving systems and outcomes (44). This is why coherent contributions by national TB programs to these processes are important and will benefit the program as well as the whole system. The section below presents the core elements of this component of the Stop TB Strategy.

Help Improve Health Policies, Human Resource Development, Financing, Supplies, Service Delivery, and Information

Health system strengthening is defined as "improving capacity in some critical components of health systems, in order to achieve more equitable and sustained improvement across health services and outcomes." TB control programs and their partners should participate actively in country-led and global efforts to improve the "building blocks" of systems, which include leadership and governance, the health workforce, health financing, medical products and technologies, service delivery, and information (45). Health system strengthening also means working across all levels of systems and with all actors in the public sector, nonstate sector, civil society, and communities. This includes efforts to improve sector strategies and plans, align all efforts with these plans, increase coherent implementation of the plans, monitor performance to achieve health outcomes, and help devise, test, and share new ways of working. The top concerns today include increasing the predictability and sustainability of health financing; implementing key means to retain, expand, and improve the capabilities of the health workforce; and reinforce PHC to support universal health coverage and the MDGs. WHO guidelines produced in 2002 to help orient and align TB control efforts within health system reforms are still highly relevant today (46), and a new guide to how programs can contribute has been developed (47). NTPs and partners should help to reduce any duplication or distortions caused in local systems by the rapid scaling up and/or expanded financing for TB efforts and help to build coordination across disease-specific initiatives.

Strengthen Infection Control in Health Services, Other Congregate Settings and Households

The emergence and spread of drug-resistant TB has provided a pointed reminder to address infection control measures seriously and systematically. There have been a number of well-documented outbreaks of TB, including MDR and XDR-TB, that have occurred in health care facilities (48–51). There is also good evidence that incidence of TB in congregate settings and households exceeds the incidence among the general population. Particularly, the high frequency of HIV infection in many health care facilities and the concern of the spread of drug resistant TB make infection control an issue of paramount importance.

TB infection control (TB-IC) is a combination of control measures: (a) managerial activities (e.g., planning), (b) administrative controls (e.g., separation of patients), (c) environmental controls (e.g., ventilation), and (d) use of personal protective equipment (e.g., respirators). All are aimed at minimizing the risk of TB transmission within populations. It is critical that each control measure is implemented in a patient-centered approach. Evidence shows that implementation of these measures reduces transmission of TB in health care facilities (52). This in turn decreases transmission of TB among patients, health workers, and visitors, and thereby can avert TB cases and deaths. All facilities, public and private, caring for TB patients and for persons suspected of having TB should implement the TB-IC measures. TB-IC should complement general infection control efforts and those targeting other airborne infections.

To date, only very few countries have strategies to implement TB-IC interventions. TB-IC strategies require coordinated efforts of multiple stakeholders not only within ministries of health, justice, infrastructure, etc., but also through engagement with civil society and technical partners. The multisectoral nature of interventions makes TB-IC a challenge and addressing it requires both political commitment and coordination at higher levels across relevant ministries. The best combination of controls will be informed by local programmatic, climatic, and socioeconomic conditions.

The updated WHO policy on TB-IC provides guidance on what to do and how to prioritize TB IC at national level. While the focus of the recommendations is on health facilities, the document also provides guidance on preventing TB transmission in congregate settings and households (53).

Upgrade Laboratory Networks, and Implement the Practical Approach to Lung Health

Strengthening laboratory networks and implementing the Practical Approach to Lung Health (PAL) offer opportunities to help strengthen systems while also pursuing specific TB prevention, diagnosis, and care objectives. Both areas of work aim to improve core clinical and public health practice through innovation in the efficient use of the health workforce, infrastructure, and technologies.

The GLI (28), noted above, provides one launch pad to support national public health laboratory networks by, among other roles, providing norms, standards, and practical guidance for the use of new diagnostic tools and facilitating technical assistance coordination and support for development of system-wide laboratory strengthening plans as part of sector strategies. Today, disease-specific initiatives may offer one of the best avenues for financing laboratory service delivery and improvements. Improving TB laboratory capacity will address major barriers in overall laboratory systems, including infrastructure, supply chain management, and human resource development. Fundamental to this work, therefore, is NTP collaboration with and support to public health laboratory leadership and staff.

PAL is among the innovations initiated within the TB control community that can strengthen the health system as a whole. Pulmonary TB often manifests as a cough, and persons with TB symptoms first present themselves to primary care services as undefined respiratory patients (54). By linking TB control activities to proper management of all common respiratory conditions, TB programs and staff implementing DOTS services at local level can help to improve the efficiency and quality with which care is provided. PAL aims at improving the quality of the management of respiratory patients in PHC settings. It is a patient-centered approach to diagnosis and treatment of common respiratory illnesses encountered in PHC. It promotes a symptom-based and integrated management system and seeks to standardize service delivery through the development and implementation of clinical guidelines. PAL is intended to ensure the coordination among different levels of health care and between TB control programs and general health services. Implementing PAL can improve TB case detection and also enhance the quality of care for common respiratory illnesses (55).

PAL has been initiated in more than 35 countries and is being scaled up within the PHC network in approximately 10 countries. However, technical capacities to support countries to implement PAL activities need to be developed at global and regional levels. Countries where PAL is at the expansion phase need to generate data on routine basis to show the impact of this approach on the integration of respiratory care in PHC, the management of TB suspects, TB detection, and drug consumption.

Adapt Successful Approaches from Other Fields and Sectors, and Foster Action on the Social Determinants of Health

To respond to all six elements of the Stop TB Strategy, TB programs and their partners can adapt approaches that have been applied in other priority public health fields and even in other sectors, and build further on some of the common systems that are already in place. This may include, for example, further integration of TB-control activities within the community and PHC outreach pursued in maternal and child health programs, social mobilization along the lines used by HIV/AIDS programs and partners, regulatory actions that have been used in tobacco control, innovations for human resources development offered by the wider education field, logistics innovations offered in a range of other fields, or financing initiatives and methods to reach the poorest that have been set up for financing vaccine development and immunization services. It can also include further collaboration with broader information platforms (household surveys, etc.) to advance TB surveillance and program monitoring. Effective integration of delivery systems depends on testing, adapting, scaling up, and evaluating common approaches.

There are a range of social determinants of TB exposure, disease and treatment outcomes. There is increasing documentation of the nature and scope of some of these TB-related determinants, but far more needs to be done to stimulate "upstream" and "downstream" actions to eliminate these risk factors and/or reduce their impact (56). The WHO and partners are now acting to more explicitly and urgently address social determinants and resulting equity concerns, through promoting "health for all policies" across sectors. NTPs must be aware of the global and local evidence, help contribute to improving the knowledge base, and act to influence change. Some actions can be taken by NTPs themselves through their own monitoring and evaluation, policy and programmatic guidance, and related capacity building of the health workforce, patients, and communities. Many of these steps can and should be taken in collaboration with others.

D. Engage All Care Providers

Involve All Public, Voluntary, Corporate, and Private Providers Through PPM Approaches

In most settings, patients with symptoms suggestive of TB seek care from a wide array of health care providers within and outside the public sector TB services. These may include private clinics operated by formal and informal practitioners and institutions owned by the public, private, voluntary, and corporate sectors (e.g., general and specialty public hospitals; nongovernmental organizations (NGOs); faith-based organizations (FBOs); prison, military, and railway health services; and health insurance organizations). These non-NTP providers may serve a large proportion of TB symptomatic patients while not always applying recommended TB management practices or reporting their cases to NTPs. Some settings have large private and NGO/FBO sectors, while others have public sector providers (such as general and specialty hospitals) that operate outside the structure of NTPs. Evidence suggests that failure to involve all care providers used by TB symptomatic patients hampers case detection, delays diagnosis, causes improper diagnosis as well as inappropriate and incomplete treatment, increases drug resistance, and places a large and unnecessary financial burden on patients (57–59).

WHO has produced guidelines on how to engage all care providers in TB control (11). The feasibility, effectiveness, and cost-effectiveness of involving different types of care providers using a PPM approach have been demonstrated (60,61). NTPs should aim to engage all care providers in DOTS implementation to help achieve the TB control targets, improve access to care, standardize the quality of TB care across providers, and save costs of care for patients. Priority should be given to identifying and setting up collaboration with health care providers who diagnose and treat a large number of TB patients and suspects and are used by the poor sections of the population. The major limiting factors in working with individual private providers have been their large number and weak organization. An efficient way of engaging with private practitioners would be through professional associations. NTPs should engage with professional associations to involve individual providers in TB control. Where they are weak, it would be worthwhile to help develop capacity of such organizations to contribute effectively to TB care and control.

Promote Use of the International Standards for TB Care

The *International Standards for Tuberculosis Care* (ISTC) have been formulated based on a wide global consensus of appropriate practices in TB diagnosis and treatment (62,63). They should be actively promoted and used to help engage all care providers in DOTS implementation and are particularly complementary to the PPM approaches described above. The standards of care are evidence based. They can be used to secure a broad base of support for TB control efforts from NTPs and professional, medical, and nursing societies, academic institutions, NGOs/FBOs, and HIV-focused organizations. They can also help to create peer pressure to encourage providers to conform to the principles and serve as a basis for preservice and in-service training (62,63). Early experience in using the ISTC as an advocacy and technical tool to foster collaboration between NTPs and professional associations has been encouraging.

Making involvement of all care providers an essential component of the Stop TB Strategy has stimulated countries to embark on initiating and scaling up locally appropriate strategies to systematically engage diverse providers operating outside the scope of NTPs. All HBCs have explicit policies to help implement PPM programs; many countries have begun scaling up and over a dozen of them have funds from the Global Fund for this purpose. In 2007, for example, private providers in Pakistan contributed about a quarter of all smear-positive cases notified in the country. In the Philippines, in the areas where PPM activities are being implemented (and where one-third of the country's population lives), approximately 13% of TB cases were reported through PPM units operated by diverse for-profit, voluntary, educational, and corporate institutions. PPM approaches are also being extended to TB/HIV and MDR-TB implementation. Weak capacities in both public and private sector remain a major constraint to scale up PPM. To help address this partly, for the first time in October 2008, representatives of national professional associations from 22 HBCs joined NTP managers to discuss collaborative ways to make rapid progress with wide application of ISTC.

E.   Empower People with TB, and Communities Through Partnership

One of the greatest gains in global health in the last decade has been the active creation of new partnerships among a wide range of stakeholders. Many partnerships and resulting collaborative initiatives and financing mechanisms are mentioned in several sections of this paper. One area where partnership has particular significance and resonance is in the area of empowering those affected by disease and communities, particularly the most vulnerable. The process of empowerment requires strong actions taken by the target groups themselves as well as supportive efforts and solidarity provided by NTPs and other partners.

Pursue Advocacy, Communication, and Social Mobilization

In the context of wide-ranging partnerships for TB control, advocacy, communication, and social mobilization can help build greater commitment to, and effectiveness in, fighting TB. Advocacy is intended to secure support of key constituencies in relevant local, national, and international policy discussions and is expected to prompt greater accountability from governmental and international actors. Communication is concerned with informing and enhancing knowledge among the general public and people with TB and empowering them to express their needs and take action. Encouraging providers, at the same time, to be more receptive to expressed concerns and views of people with TB and community members will make TB services more responsive to actual needs. Social mobilization is the process of bringing together all feasible and practical intersectoral allies to raise people's knowledge of, and demand for, quality TB care and health care in general to assist in the delivery of resources and services and to strengthen community participation for sustainability (64). Advocacy, communication, and social mobilization efforts in TB control should be linked with overarching efforts to promote public health and social development.

Foster Community Participation in TB Care, Prevention and Health Promotion

Community participation in TB care, prevention, and health promotion implies establishing a working partnership between the health sector and the community, especially poor and vulnerable populations in general and TB patients, current as well as cured, in particular. Enabling people with TB and communities to be informed about TB, to enhance general awareness about the disease and to share responsibility for their health can lead to effective patient empowerment and community participation, by increasing the demand for health services and bringing care closer to the community. For this purpose, TB programs should provide support to frontline health workers and involve communities to help create an empowering environment by, for instance, facilitating setting up of patient groups, encouraging peer education and support, and linking with other community-level partnerships and local initiatives. Programs and health workers should intervene under the notion of subsidiarity, where they aim to provide support that complements and supplements that offered by the community and does not aim to duplicate or supplant action where the community already has capacity. Community volunteers also need regular support, motivation, instruction, and supervision. Evidence shows that community-based TB care is cost-effective compared to hospital-based care and other ambulatory care models (65,66). Community involvement in planning, implementation, monitoring, and evaluation is essential to sustain community TB initiatives. WHO has recently published evidence-based guidelines to help countries scale up community TB care and prevention. The overall principles outlined here are presented in depth in that publication (12).

Promote Use of the Patients' Charter for TB Care

Developed by patients from around the world, the Patients' Charter outlines the rights and responsibilities of people with TB and complements the *International Standards for Tuberculosis Care* intended for health care providers (67). It is based on the principles of various international and national charters and conventions on health and human rights. It also addresses some of the underlying ethical principles that are critical in public health, primary care practice, and research. It aims to empower people with TB and the communities and make the patient–provider relationship mutually beneficial. The charter sets out the ways in which patients, communities, health care providers, and governments can work as partners and help enhance the effectiveness of health services in general and TB care in particular. The charter provides a useful tool to guide action to achieve greater involvement of people in TB care. There is urgent work to be done to support efforts in countries to adopt and respond to the principles, given varying degrees of development and organization of their health systems.

F. Enable and Promote Research

Conduct Program-Based Operational Research

The Stop TB Strategy consolidates DOTS implementation and involves the implementation of several new approaches to tackle challenges facing NTPs and those affected by TB. To put them into practice, program-based operational research should be a core component of NTP work. Designing and conducting locally relevant operational research can help identify problems, determine workable solutions, test them in the field, and plan for scale up. For this purpose, collaboration between program managers and researchers is essential. Acquiring basic skills in identifying and addressing issues related to program operations and performance can help program managers to initiate operational research in collaboration with researchers and academia. This can then help to sustain and strengthen TB control efforts by expanding existing activities and introducing new strategies effectively. For this purpose, sustainable partnerships and networks need to be established for productive collaboration on operational research. Also joint projects should be considered within wider networks of those working on "research for health" (68).

Advocate for and Participate in Research to Develop New Diagnostics, Drugs, and Vaccines

Existing tools for prevention and treatment of TB make standard TB care demanding for both patients and their care providers. The tools include a century-old, tedious, and weakly sensitive smear microscopy test for diagnosis (although it is the best method available today to identify highly infectious cases), and a relatively long "short-course" chemotherapy with several drugs. A truly effective vaccine is lacking. The need to rely on these tools has substantially hindered the pace of progress in global TB control. Increasing advocacy and voiced demand from countries in most need of improved tools is critical to help enable financing and conduct more basic research and development for TB prevention, care, and control. The Stop TB Partnership's Working Groups on New Diagnostics, Drugs, and Vaccines are helping increased understanding of the needs and growth of the pipelines in all fields through innovative public–private product development partnerships. TB programs should actively encourage and participate in this process. In addition to advocating for research and capacity building for research in developing nations, NTPs and their national research counterparts can help enable and speed up the field testing of new products and prepare for swift adoption and roll out of new tools as they become available.

The Stop TB Partnership sponsors a subgroup on "Retooling," which signifies the process of planning for guidelines and tools revision, capacity building, and stakeholder engagement needed to successfully and rapidly adopt new tools into national TB control efforts. The subgroup involves a wide range of stakeholders such as program staff, civil society, researchers, product developers, research and program donors, and technical assistance providers. The subgroup is helping by providing guidance tools to help foster this process (69). One example is that checklists are available to help ease the planning process for introducing liquid culture methods at country level (70).

V. Measuring Global Progress and Impact

A. Measurement of Program Outcomes and Impact on Burden of Disease

The Stop TB Strategy is designed to achieve the MDG and related Stop TB Partnership targets (explained in section "Goals and Targets") as well as to stimulate regular monitoring to assess the progess toward targets. Table 3 shows the indicators that apply for each of the targets and how they can be measured.

Table 3   Selected Indicators for Monitoring TB Programs

Indicator	Target	Measurement
Prevalence of disease—number of people per 100,000 population who have TB disease at a given time	Halve 1990 prevalence rate by 2015	Cross-sectional surveys (preferably), or estimated from incidence and duration of disease (approximate)
Incidence of disease—number of new cases of TB disease (all forms) per 100,000 population per year	Incidence rate in decline by 2015	Longitudinal surveys, or from case notifications (where complete)
Mortality rate—number of TB deaths (all forms) per 100,000 population per year	Halve 1990 mortality rate by 2015	From vital registration (where complete), verbal autopsy surveys, or from incidence and case fatality rates (approximate)
Case detection rate—number of new smear-positive cases notified in 1 yr divided by the annual incidence	at least 70% by 2005	From notification data and estimates of incidence
Treatment success rate—percentage of new smear positive TB cases registered for treatment that are cured or complete treatment	at least 85% by 2005	Routinely collected data on cohorts of patients undergoing treatment

The MDG and related Stop TB Partnership targets include three impact indicators, that is, indicators to measure the reduction in burden of disease: incidence, prevalence, and death rates. TB incidence rates can be estimated through longitudinal population-based surveys or from notification data where these are complete. TB prevalence rates can be measured through cross-sectional population-based surveys and also from the product of estimated incidence and duration of disease. Mortality rates can be estimated from vital registration records, from verbal autopsy studies, or from the product of estimated incidence and case fatality rates. Countries should consider carrying out surveys of disease prevalence over the next 10 years in order to measure the change in burden, though it should be borne in mind that such surveys are costly and logistically complex. Incidence should be monitored regularly using routine indicators or proxies.

The other two targets relate to the performance and quality of TB control programs: the case detection rate and the treatment success rate.

In assessing trends in the total burden of TB and the quality of TB control efforts, it is worth taking into account, where possible, factors such as the age and sex of the patients, the level of MDR-TB, and the prevalence of HIV, all of which may affect case detection and treatment outcomes. In addition subnational assessments are useful to detect variations in performance and outcomes in different settings.

As more countries develop better systems for collecting health information routinely, it should be possible to assess the state of the epidemic and the quality of control using annual TB surveillance data, together with data from vital registration. To complement and check the quality of routine surveillance data, it will be important to carry out population-based surveys of disease prevalence or infection. The WHO Task Force on TB impact measurement has recommended a set of epidemiological criteria to guide selection of countries that should undertake prevalence of disease surveys during the period up to 2015 (35). Of the 57 countries that meet the criteria, 30 have plans to carry out a national or subnational survey.

B. Financing for TB Control

Achieving the MDG and Stop TB Partnership targets will require increased, predictable, and sustained financing for TB control, as reflected in Component 1 of the Stop TB Strategy. Financing of TB control needs to be monitored and evaluated at subnational, national, and international level to document trends in NTP budgets, available funding for these budgets, funding gaps, expenditures, and total TB control costs (total TB control costs include costs reflected in NTP budgets plus costs associated with using general health services staff and infrastructure). A consistent categorization of budget line items and funding sources should be used to allow analysis of changes over time. These categories may be modified periodically, for example, to reflect the introduction of a major new source of funding or when a major shift in strategy alters the line items for which it is relevant to collect data. WHO collects financial data through a questionnaire, which is sent to all countries annually. These data are analyzed and presented in the annual WHO report on global TB control.

Some of the key indicators that are relevant to financial monitoring and evaluation of TB control include the annual NTP budget requirement, the NTP budget per patient treated, the percentage of the NTP budget that is funded, the percentage of the NTP budget that is funded by the government (including loans), the percentage of available funding that is spent, the total annual cost of TB control, the cost per patient treated, and the cost per patient successfully treated. Unlike the outcome and impact indicators described above, national and international targets for financing have not been established. Nevertheless, monitoring changes over time is useful and should be undertaken regularly. WHO has recently prepared a planning and budgeting tool to help countries develop costed plans in line with the global targets (71). Workshops conducted subsequently have supported over 50 countries including 15 HBCs to use the tool for plan development. These costed TB plans can then be embedded with national health strategies and national budgets. In times of financial crisis, when reductions in financing and increased vulnerability can have serious public health consequences, it is particularly critical to have well-costed disease control plans, along with strong monitoring mechanisms of program efficiency, outcomes, and impact.

VI. Conclusion

The Stop TB Strategy comprehensively addresses the problem of TB. It is equipped with the lessons from DOTS implementation, field-tested approaches to tackle current challenges, early experiences of implementing the components beyond DOTS, renewed efforts in developing new tools, and a strong Stop TB Partnership of all stakeholders. The Strategy also provides the basis and the context for the Global Plan to Stop TB,

2006–2015 (7). This inclusive plan exploits the various synergies and new approaches and carries an estimated cost of US $67 billion over 2006 to 2015, US $56 billion for implementation and the rest for research. The strength of global efforts to control TB lies in the coordinated and collaborative efforts of the Stop TB Partnership. With a clear global strategy and related global plan, the framework is in place for unprecedented efforts in TB control over the next six years. Experience to date shows that adopting all components of the Strategy takes significant coordination and stewardship capacity of National TB Programs and full implementation will require substantial resources. Although funding is rising, more is needed if we are to achieve the MDG and the Stop TB Partnership targets for TB control and set ourselves on the path toward elimination of this ancient scourge of humanity.

References

1. World Health Organization. Forty-Fourth World Health Assembly. Geneva, Switzerland: WHO, 1991. WHA44/1991/REC/1.
2. World Health Organization. Framework for Effective Tuberculosis Control. Geneva, Switzerland: WHO, 1994. WHO/TB/94.179.
3. World Health Organization. An expanded DOTS Framework for Effective Tuberculosis Control. Geneva, Switzerland: WHO, 2002. WHO/CDS/TB/2002.297.
4. Raviglione MC, Uplekar MW. WHO's new Stop TB Strategy. Lancet 2006; 367: 952–955.
5. World Health Organization. Sixtieth World Health Assembly. Geneva, Switzerland: WHO, 2007. WHA60/2007. Available at: http://www.who.int/gb/ebwha/pdf_files/WHASSA_WHA60-Rec1/E/reso-60-en.pdf. Accessed January 14, 2009.
6. Dye C, Maher D, Weil D, et al. Targets for global tuberculosis control. Int J Tuberc Lung Dis 2006; 10(4):460–462.
7. Stop TB Partnership and WHO. Global Plan to Stop TB 2006–2015. Actions for Life—Towards a World Free of Tuberculosis. Geneva, Switzerland: WHO, 2006. WHO/HTM/STB/2006.35.
8. World Health Organization. Global Tuberculosis Control—Surveillance, Planning, Financing, WHO Report 2009. Geneva, Switzerland: WHO. 2009.
9. World Health Organization. Global Tuberculosis Control—Surveillance, Planning, Financing, WHO Report 2008. Geneva, Switzerland: WHO, 2008. WHO/HTM/TB/2008.393.
10. World Health Organization. Report of the Eighth Meeting of the Strategic and Technical Advisory Group for Tuberculosis (STAG-TB). Geneva, Switzerland: WHO, 2008.
11. World Health Organization. Guidance on Implementing Public-Private Mix for DOTS. Engaging All Health Care Providers To Improve Access, Equity and Quality of TB Care. Geneva, Switzerland: WHO, 2006. WHO/HTM/TB/2006.360.
12. World Health Organization. Community Involvement in Tuberculosis Care and Prevention. Towards Partnerships for Health. Guiding Principles and Recommendations Based on a WHO Review. Geneva, Switzerland: WHO, 2008. WHO/HTM/TB/2008.397.
13. World Health Organization. Ten Million Treatments in Six Years—GDF Achievements Report. Geneva, Switzerland: WHO, 2007. WHO/HTM/STB/2007.40.
14. World Health Organization. Report of the Annual Meeting of the Green Light Committee (GLC) of the Working Group on MDR-TB of the Stop TB Partnership. Geneva, Switzerland: WHO, 2008. WHO/HTM/TB/2008.409.
15. World Health Organization. Interim Policy on Collaborative TB/HIV Activities. Geneva, Switzerland: WHO, 2004. WHO/HTM/TB/2004.330.
16. World Health Organization. Guidelines for the Programmatic Management of Drug-Resistant Tuberculosis. Geneva, Switzerland: WHO, 2008. WHO/HTM/TB/2008.402.

17. World Health Organization. WHO/IUATLD Global Project on Anti-tuberculosis Drug Resistance Surveillance. Anti-tuberculosis Drug Resistance in the world. Geneva, Switzerland: WHO, 2008. Report no. 4, WHO/HTM/TB/2008.394.

18. Raviglione MC. Facing extensively drug-resistant tuberculosis—a hope and a challenge. N Engl J Med 2008; 359(6):638–638.

19. United Nations Statistics Division. Millennium indicators database. Available at: http://unstats.un.org/unsd/mi/mi_goals.asp. Accessed January 13, 2009.

20. World Health Organization. Good Practice in Legislation and Regulations for TB Control: An Indicator of Political Will. Geneva, Switzerland: WHO, 2001. WHO/CDS/TB/2001.290.

21. World Health Organization. Human Resources Development for TB Control: Report of a Consultation Held on 27–28 August 2003. Geneva, Switzerland: WHO, 2004. WHO/HTM/TB/2004.340.

22. World Health Organization. Check-list for the Review of Human Resource Development Component of National Plans to Control Tuberculosis. Geneva, Switzerland: WHO, 2005. WHO/HTM/TB/2005.354.

23. World Health Organization. The World Health Report 2006: Working Together for Health. Geneva, Switzerland: WHO, 2006.

24. World Health Organization. Planning the Development of Human Resources for Health for implementation of the stop TB strategy—A Handbook. Geneva, Switzerland: WHO, 2008. WHO/HTM/TB/2008.407.

25. International Health Partnership and Related Initiatives 2007, IHP+. Available at: http://www.internationalhealthpartnership.net. Accessed December 18, 2008.

26. Global Health Workforce Alliance. World Health Organization, 2009. Available at: http://www.who.int/workforcealliance/en/. Accessed January 14, 2009.

27. World Health Organization. New Technologies for Tuberculosis Control: A Framework for Their Adoption, Introduction and Implementation. Geneva, Switzerland: WHO, 2007. WHO/HTM/STB/2007.40.

28. Global Laboratory Initiative (GLI). World Health Organization. Available At: http://www.who.int/tb/dots/laboratory/gli/en/index.html. Accessed January 12, 2009.

29. Foundation for Innovative New Diagnostics (FIND). Delivering on the promise: Five years of progress towards more effective diagnostic tests for poverty-related diseases. Available at: http://www.finddiagnostics.org/news/resources/delivering_on_the_promise_sep08.pdf. Accessed February 15, 2009.

30. UNITAID. Innovative Financing for health the air tax-A journey to access. December 2008. Available At: http://www.unitaid.eu/images/stories/unitaiden.pdf. Accessed February 15, 2009.

31. World Health Organization. Implementing the Stop TB Strategy: A handbook for National Tuberculosis Control Programmes. Geneva, Switzerland: WHO, 2008. WHO/HTM/TB/2008.401.

32. Volmink J, Garner P. Directly observed therapy for treating tuberculosis. Cochrane Database Syst Rev 2003; 1:CD003343.

33. Volmink J, Matchaba P, Garner P. Directly observed therapy and treatment adherence. Lancet 2000; 355(9212):1345–1350.

34. Norval PY, Heldal E, L'Herminez R, et al. Revising the tuberculosis recording and reporting information system. Int J Tuberc Lung Dis 2008; 12(3)(suppl 1):17–19.

35. Dye C, Bassili A, Bierrenbach AL, et al. Measuring tuberculosis burden, trends, and the impact of control programmes. Lancet Infect Dis 2008; 8(4):233–243. Epub 2008 Jan 16.

36. Nunn P, Williams B, Floyd K, et al. Tuberculosis control in the era of HIV. Nat Rev Immunol 2005; 5:819–826.

37. Stop TB Partnership. First HIV/TB Global Leaders' Forum held at UN Headquarters. STOP TB News. July 2008. Available at: http://www.stoptb.org/resource_center/assets/documents/STBNEWSJULY08.pdf. Accessed January 13, 2009.

38. Andrews JR, Shah NS, Gandhi N, et al. Multidrug-resistant and extensively drug-resistant tuberculosis: Implications for the HIV epidemic and antiretroviral therapy rollout in South Africa. J Infect Dis 2007; 196(suppl 3):S482–S490.

39. World Health Organization. Addressing Poverty in Tuberculosis Control: Options for National TB Control Programmes. Geneva, Switzerland: WHO, 2005. WHO/HTM/TB/2005.352.

40. World Health Organization. Tuberculosis Care and Control in Refugee and Displaced Populations: An Interagency Field Manual, 2nd ed. Geneva, Switzerland: WHO, 2007. WHO/HTM/TB/2007.377; WHO/CDS/DCE /2007.2.

41. Coninx R. Tuberculosis control in complex emergencies. Bull World Health Organ 2007; 85:637–640.

42. Gayer M, Connolly MA. Tuberculosis control in refugee and displaced populations. In: Raviglione MC, ed. Reichman and Hershfield's Tuberculosis: A Comprehensive, International Approach, 3rd ed. Part B. New York: Informa Healthcare USA, Inc., 2006:907–919.

43. World Health Organization. Tuberculosis Control in Prisons: A Manual for Programme Managers. Geneva, Switzerland: WHO, 2000. WHO/CDS/TB/2000.281.

44. World Health Organization. The World Health Report 2008: Primary Health Care Now More Than Ever. Geneva, Switzerland: WHO, 2008.

45. World Health Organization. Everybody's Business—Strengthening Health Systems To Improve Health Outcomes. WHO's Framework for Action. Geneva, Switzerland: WHO, 2007.

46. World Health Organization. Contributing to Health System Strengthening: Guiding Principles for National Tuberculosis Programmes. Geneva, Switzerland: WHO, 2008. WHO/HTM/TB/2008.400.

47. World Health Organization. Expanding DOTS in the Context of a Changing Health System. Geneva, Switzerland: WHO, 2003. WHO/CDS/TB/2003.318.

48. World Health Organization. Tuberculosis Infection Control in the Era of Expanding HIV Care and Treatment. Addendum to WHO Guidelines for the Prevention of Tuberculosis in Health Care Facilities in Resource-Limited Settings, 1999. Geneva, Switzerland: WHO, 2006.

49. Frieden TR, Sterling T, Pablos-Mendez A. The emergence of drug-resistant tuberculosis in New York City. N Engl J Med. 1993; 328(8):521–526.

50. Moro ML, Gori A, Errante I, et al. An outbreak of multi drug-resistant tuberculosis involving HIV-infected patients of two hospitals in Milan, Italy. Italian Multidrug-Resistant Tuberculosis Outbreak Study Group. AIDS 1998; 12(9):1095–1102.

51. Gandhi NR, Moll A, Sturm AW, et al. Extensively drug-resistant tuberculosis as a cause of death in patients co-infected with tuberculosis and HIV in a rural area of South Africa. Lancet 2006; 368:1575–1580.

52. Harries AD, Hargreaves NJ, Gausi F, et al. Preventing tuberculosis among health workers in Malawi. Bull World Health Organ 2002; 80:526–531.

53. World Health Organization. WHO policy on TB infection control in health-care facilities, congregate settings and households. Geneva, Switzerland: WHO, 2009. WHO/HTM/TB/2009.419.

54. World Health Organization. Practical Approach to Lung Health (PAL). Manual on Initiating PAL Implementation. Geneva, Switzerland: WHO, 2008. WHO/HTM/TB/2008.410.

55. Ottmani S, Mahjour J. The practical approach to lung health strategy for integrated respiratory care. In: Raviglione MC, ed. Reichman and Hershfield's Tuberculosis: A Comprehensive International Approach, 3rd ed. Part B. New York: Informa Healthcare USA, Inc., 2006: 1059–1081.

56. World Health Organization. Commission on social determinants of health. Social determinants of tuberculosis. In: Blas E, ed. Social Determinants of Health and Public Health Programmes. Report of the Priority Public Health Conditions Knowledge Network. Geneva, Switzerland: WHO, 2008.

57. Lönnroth K, Tin-Aung, Win-Maung,et al. Social franchising of TB care through private general practitioners in Myanmar—an assessment of access, quality of care, equity, and financial protection. Health Policy Plan 2007; 22:156–166.

58. Uplekar M. Involving private health care providers in delivery of TB care: Global strategy. Tuberculosis 2003; 83:156–164.

59. Lönnroth K, Uplekar M, Arora VK, et al. Public-private mix for DOTS implementation: What makes it work? Bull World Health Organ 2004; 82(2):580–586.

60. Pantoja A, Lönnroth K, Lal SS, et al. Economic evaluation of public-private mix for TB, India. Part I Int J Tuberc Lung Dis 2009, 13(6):695–704.

61. Pantoja A, Floyd K, Unnikrishnan KP, et al. Economic evaluation of public-private mix for TB, India. Part II Int J Tuberc Lung Dis 2009, 13(6):705–712.

62. Hopewell PC, Pai M. Tuberculosis, vulnerability and access to quality care. JAMA 2005; 293:2790–2793.

63. Hopewell PC, Pai M, Maher D, et al. International standards for tuberculosis care. Lancet Infect Dis 2006; 6:710–725.

64. World Health Organization, Stop TB Partnership. Advocacy, Communication and Social Mobilization (ACSM) for Tuberculosis Control: A Handbook for Country Programmes. Geneva, Switzerland: WHO, 2007.

65. Okello D, Floyd K, Adatu F, et al. Cost and cost-effectiveness of community-based care for tuberculosis patients in rural Uganda. Int J Tuberc Lung Dis 2003; 7(9)(suppl 1):S72–S79.

66. World Health Organization. Community Contribution to TB Care: Practice and policy. Geneva, Switzerland: WHO, 2002. WHO/CDS/TB/2002.318.

67. Patient's charter for Tuberculosis care. World Care Council, 2006. Available at: http://www. imaxi.org/pdf/PatientsCharterEN2006.pdf. Accessed January 13, 2009.

68. The Lancet. The Bamako call to action: Research for health. Lancet 2008; 372(9653):1855.

69. World Health Organization, Stop TB Partnership. Engaging Stakeholders for Retooling TB Control. Geneva, Switzerland: WHO, 2008.

70. Stop TB Partnership. Checklist of key actions for the use of liquid media for culture and drug susceptibility testing (DST). Retooling Task Force – February 2008. http://www.stoptb.org/retooling/assets/documents/Retooling%20Task%20Force%20-%20Liquid%20Culture-DST%20Checklist%20-%20Feb2008.pdf. Accessed January 13, 2009.

71. Floyd K, Pantoja A. Financial resources required for tuberculosis control to achieve global targets set for 2015. Bull World Health Organ. 2008; 86(7):568–576.

13

New Diagnostics for Tuberculosis: Status of Development

MARK D. PERKINS and RICHARD J. O'BRIEN
Foundation for Innovative New Diagnostics (FIND), Geneva, Switzerland

I. Introduction

The continuing epidemics of HIV-associated tuberculosis (TB) and multidrug-resistant (MDR) TB have radically changed thinking on the need for new TB control tools. The much-publicized outbreak of extensively drug-resistant (XDR) TB among HIV-infected patients in KwaZulu-Natal, South Africa, in 2006 with rapid progression of disease and high mortality (1) has accelerated this process, pointing to the urgent need for rapid drug-susceptibility testing (DST) integrated into TB control programs. Earlier it had been widely assumed that the most commonly available diagnostic tool, acid-fast bacillus (AFB) microscopy, when properly applied was sufficient for the diagnosis of the most infectious cases, who often were also critically ill and in need of treatment. In addition, it was thought that TB treatment services should be strengthened before increasing case finding in order to avoid the creation of a large pool of poorly treated, potentially drug-resistant cases. Thus, the diagnostic focus of the World Health Organization (WHO) DOTS strategy was appropriately on improving the quality of smear microscopy through training and quality assurance programs.

Over the past decade this thinking has shifted, and now in response to the growing problems of MDR and XDR-TB, WHO and its partners have called for greatly enhanced global capacity for mycobacterial culture and DST as well as for implementation of rapid methods for screening MDR-TB (2). This massive scale-up is thought to require that up to 2000 new culture-capable TB laboratories be established and 10,000 new laboratory workers be trained by 2015. Although a daunting task, recent developments have suggested that much might be achieved within the next decade. Several member organizations of the Stop TB Partnership, notably WHO, the U. S. Centers for Disease Control and Prevention (CDC), FIND (the Foundation for Innovative New Diagnostics), and the American Society for Microbiology (ASM) have established the Global Laboratory Initiative (GLI) that is housed within WHO (3). In recognition of its importance, the GLI was designated as a full Stop TB Working Group in November 2008. The focus of GLI is on development of technical laboratory guidelines, coordination of laboratory technical assistance, and training programs to address the current deficit in laboratory personnel.

While the cost of the needed increase in global TB laboratory capacity is estimated to be as high as $2.5 billion, more resources are becoming available to address this need. The U. S. President's Emergency Plan for AIDS Relief (PEPFAR) has committed to spend $4.0 billion on TB control in its TB/HIV focus countries from 2009 to 2013 (4). Much of this effort will be directed to improving the diagnosis of TB, including MDR-TB, in HIV-infected persons through enhanced laboratory capacity. In 2007, FIND, together with the Ministry of Health of Lesotho, WHO, and Partners in Health, demonstrated that it is possible to introduce modern, rapid methods for TB and MDR-TB case detection in a low-income setting in a very short period of time (5). In 2008, GLI, FIND, and the WHO Global Drug Facility received a $26 million grant from UNITAID to provide modern TB diagnostics to laboratories in 16 MDR-TB priority countries that will increase the current MDR-TB global diagnostic capacity from 2% to 15% in three years (6). Many national TB programs (NTPs) are now including support for TB laboratory strengthening in their Global Fund applications.

While funding for the development of new TB diagnostics remains suboptimal, the situation has been improving. Groups such as Médecins Sans Frontières (MSF) and the Treatment Action Group (TAG) have stepped up advocacy efforts for increasing funding for research on new TB diagnostics. FIND has accelerated its work on MDR-TB diagnostics and has assisted WHO to establish a process through which it issues evidence-based policy recommendations for the implementation of new TB diagnostics in low- and medium-income countries. In 2007, data and lessons learned from FIND's large-scale demonstration projects of automated TB liquid culture and DST assisted in the development of WHO policy on these systems (7). The Stop TB Partnership's Retooling Task Force subsequently issued detailed guidance to assist countries in implementing these systems (8). In 2008, WHO issued guidelines on the use of line-probe assay (LPA) for the rapid detection of MDR-TB (9), again assisted by FIND through its demonstration projects of LPAs that it had accelerated as part of the MDR-TB and XDR-TB Global Response Plan.

The prospects for new TB diagnostics, importantly simplified molecular tests for case detection and diagnosis of drug-resistant TB that can be decentralized to microscopy centers, and for highly accurate point-of-care (POC) tests that can be used in even more peripheral settings have never been better. In this chapter, we will outline in more detail the need for new diagnostics, list the impediments to progress in this area and how they are being addressed, and review the current developmental pipeline of new diagnostics.

II. The Need for New TB Diagnostics

As noted above, the primary TB diagnostic technology promoted in the DOTS strategy, sputum AFB smear microscopy, addresses the limited need to identify and treat the most infectious TB cases. However, the technology requires well-maintained equipment and trained technicians who should spend up to 15 minutes examining a single sputum smear before recording it as negative. The original DOTS diagnostic strategy calls for a patient with suspected pulmonary TB to provide three sputum specimens over two days and return on a third day to receive results. In an average developing country setting, 10 patients with suspected TB are screened to identify a single case. Thus, under optimal conditions one technician would spend an entire day examining AFB smears to diagnose a single patient with AFB smear-positive TB. However, such human resources are seldom available and so the quality of smear microscopy is usually wanting. This process is burdensome for the patients as well, and in some settings the dropout rate even from this limited diagnostic process is significant (10). Recent changes in WHO policy allow for the examination of only two sputum specimens in the settings of high workload (11), and work is ongoing to attempt to decrease patient dropout by examination of both the smears on the same day. Despite these measures to facilitate rapid microscopic diagnosis, the method remains inherently cumbersome and only partially sensitive.

By definition, microscopy cannot identify patients with paucibacillary pulmonary TB that may constitute half or more of those with pulmonary disease. Patients whose sputum smears are negative often undergo additional diagnostic procedures, including chest radiograph and a trial of broad-spectrum antibiotics. Facilities for mycobacterial culture, the cornerstone of TB diagnosis in industrialized countries, are generally not available. Thus, during this slow and complex diagnostic process, many patients drop out or are misdiagnosed, resulting in both under- and overtreatment. Diagnosis of other forms of paucibacillary TB, notably extrapulmonary disease and childhood TB, is at least as difficult.

There has been a significant increase in the incidence of AFB smear-negative pulmonary TB in countries where both TB and HIV are prevalent. This increase in smear-negative cases strains already overloaded laboratories, while also eroding the predictive value of microscopy. For a number of reasons, HIV-positive, smear-negative pulmonary TB patients have inferior treatment outcomes, including higher mortality rates, than do HIV-positive, smear-positive pulmonary TB patients and HIV-negative TB patients (12). In the absence of an easily applied diagnostic test that is more sensitive than AFB smear microscopy, diagnostic algorithms that include a trial of broad-spectrum antibiotics have been recommended. However, these algorithms lack sensitivity and specificity, and it is believed that during the evaluation process that may take up to one month under routine program conditions, many HIV-infected patients die before TB treatment is begun. In fact, autopsy studies have found disseminated TB in 40% to 60% of HIV-infected people in TB endemic countries, many of whom were undiagnosed prior to death (13,14). Outbreaks of drug-resistant TB in HIV-infected cohorts reported in the United States in 1991 (15) and in South Africa 15 years later (1) with high and rapid mortality underscored the lethality of untreated or mistreated TB in patients with advanced immunocompromise (Table 1 and Fig. 1) and thus the urgency of early diagnosis. They also highlight the need for rapid and effective detection of drug resistance to guide therapy in settings where MDR-TB is prevalent.

The emergence of drug-resistant strains of *Mycobacterium tuberculosis* is proving to be one of the most formidable obstacles faced by national TB programs. Random mutations in the bacterial DNA that occur at low but predictable rates confer resistance to individual anti-TB drugs. The growth of such mutants can be controlled by the other drugs

Table 1 High Mortality in HIV-Associated MDR-TB Outbreaks in U.S. Facilities, 1990–1992

Facility	HIV infection (%)	Mortality (%)	Median interval TB Dx to death (wk)
Hospital A	93	72	7
Hospital B	100	89	16
Hospital C	95	77	4
Hospital D	91	83	4
Hospital E	14	43	4
Hospital F	82	82	4
Hospital I	100	85	4
Hospital J	96	93	4
Prison system	98	79	4

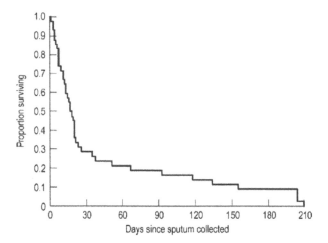

Figure 1   High mortality in HIV-associated XDR TB cases in KwaZulu-Natal, 2005–2006.

used in recommended treatment regimens within the DOTS approach. However, improper or inadequate treatment permits these mutants to grow unchecked, resulting in treatment failure with the emergence of drug-resistant TB and in the subsequent transmission of these resistant strains. Amplification of resistance, that is, acquired resistance to additional drugs may occur with further ineffective treatment. This has led to the worldwide development and spread of MDR-TB. This form of TB is significantly more difficult to treat than drug-susceptible TB in large part because the necessary second-line drugs are more expensive, must be administered for a longer period of time, are less effective, and are often associated with more severe side effects than the standard first-line anti-TB drugs.

In response to the emergence of MDR-TB, the WHO adopted the DOTS-Plus treatment strategy for MDR-TB in 1998. Despite the recommendation of this program and the establishment of the Green Light Committee (GLC), which grants the programs' access to discounted second-line anti-TB drugs, the management of MDR-TB cases and controlling the spread of resistance remain serious public health concerns throughout the world. It is estimated that there are about 500,000 incident cases of MDR annually and that China and India bear 50% of the global burden (16).

Although well-functioning DOTS and MDR-TB management programs are critical for the control of MDR-TB, these strategies are hindered by the difficulty and length of time required to diagnose drug-resistant TB. Conventional DST is a slow process, requiring culture of mycobacteria from clinical specimens, followed by comparative growth evaluation after exposure to the drug in a solid media such as Löwenstein–Jensen (LJ) media. This process can take two to six months during which time patients with drug-resistant infections are often treated inappropriately for drug-susceptible TB. The resultant delay in proper treatment may adversely affect treatment outcome and contribute to the transmission of drug-resistant TB. Thus, it is imperative that concerted efforts are made to develop and implement rapid methods for the diagnosis of both paucibacillary and drug-resistant forms of TB.

Although of less relevance to developing countries, improved tests for the diagnosis of latent TB infection (LTBI) are needed in settings where the incidence of active disease is low and identification and treatment of patients with LTBI is an important control strategy. The limitations of the tuberculin skin test (TST) are well known. Recently, two tests based on release of interferon-gamma from sensitized lymphocytes have been developed and are being marketed in industrialized countries (17,18). It is expected that these tests will gradually come to replace the TST in these settings. However, the role and optimal use of these tests in low-income countries are yet to be defined.

III. Obstacles to TB Diagnostic Development and How They Are Being Addressed

The primary role of the private sector in technology development has resulted in prioritization of products that are likely to be profitable, often to the exclusion of poverty-associated diseases. Insufficiently attractive private markets have inhibited large-scale commercial interest in the development of better TB diagnostics that would be appropriate for public sector use in developing countries. Funding for research and development in TB is largely dominated by public sector funding from national governments and their research institutes and by private philanthropic organizations such as the Bill and Melinda Gates Foundation (BMGF) and the Wellcome Trust. A report from G-FINDER, an organization tracking resource flows for work on neglected diseases, found that roughly $400 million was spent on TB R&D in 2007. Of this, only 8%, or around $35 million, was invested in diagnostics. About 80% of TB R&D funding came from public sources, notably the U.S. National Institutes of Health (NIH), with the Bill and Melinda Gates Foundation being the second largest contributor (19).

Most of the TB R&D funds spent by the NIH are dedicated to basic science and to advancing our understanding of host and pathogen biology during TB infection and disease. Such advances may lead to insights into novel approaches to TB diagnosis. However, such funding rarely provides for assay development or commercialization and does not specifically target work on technologies that are appropriate for developing world settings.

Mindful of the failure of market forces to drive the development of technologies for impoverished populations and of the need for a focus on product development, in the mid-1990s a new group of nonprofit agencies emerged, often with instrumental funding from the Rockefeller Foundation and the Bill and Melinda Gates Foundation, which worked in partnership with the private sector to harvest their product development capacity and put it to use for public good. More than two dozen of such Product Development Partnerships (PDP) have been established, including three with substantial programs in TB vaccines (the Aeras Global TB Vaccine Foundation), drugs [the Global Alliance for TB Drug Development (GATB)], and diagnostics (FIND). The creation of FIND has provided a mechanism to move promising diagnostic technologies that may be stalled because of lack of funding through the development pipeline.

FIND seeks to identify the most promising product candidates and accelerate the process of development, testing, approval, distribution, and incorporation into routine public health policy. Although motivated by the desire to create new public goods, FIND has many of the attributes of a private company, pursuing a clear business plan and using

Stage of development	Concept-ualization	Project planning	Develop-ment	Evaluation	Regulatory	Marketing	Postmarket
Usual commercial activity	Identification of market needs.	Identification of technology platform and reagents. Business plan.	Prototype development and analytic validation.	Clinical trials.	Regulatory submission.	Manufacturing, advertising, education, and distribution.	Product support, training, quality control.
Obstacle to development	Lack of visible market. Needs not expressed by the public sector. No perceived return on investment.	Basic science incomplete, lack of proven technology. Intellectual property (IP) risk.	Lack of access to reference clinical materials and disease specific expertise.	No access to patients, and limited contacts or experience in developing world trials.	Diverse, non-rationalized regulatory requirements. Lack of agreed performance goals for HBCs.	Public sector suspicion of industry. Wide diversity in settings of use.	Poor infrastructure in widely distributed market.
Public sector input	Clarify medical need, settings of use, & desired specifications. Describe public sector market.	Identify targets and reagents. Finance R&D and manage IP and contracts to protect public and commercial partners.	Provide reference clinical materials and reduce investment risk with technical support and reagent access.	Run regulatory-quality trials in experienced sites in high-prevalence settings of intended use.	Clarify criteria for success with Health Ministries technical agencies. Interact with DEC regulators.	Demonstrate effectiveness in programmatic settings. Provide evidence to normative agencies and donors.	Assist in scale-up in TB control programs and survey test performance. Catalyze training and infrastructure support.

Figure 2 Public sector support to facilitate commercial development of tests for disease-endemic countries. HBC, high burden country; DEC, disease endemic country.

rigorous scientific criteria to identify priority product candidates. FIND partners with public and private sector research teams to drive the development of products strictly designed for use in disease-endemic settings under contractual agreements that manage intellectual property, device design, and manufacturing in a way that maximizes afford-ability. Using industry-style project management, FIND provides public sector support to overcome obstacles that block commercial development of the types of assays that are needed, as shown schematically in Figure 2 above.

Technologies that are successfully shepherded through the R&D pathway and reach the stage of a manufactured, design-locked prototype are evaluated in well-controlled clin-ical settings using populations of intended final use. In the past, diagnostic evaluations, which are analogous to phase III clinical trials of a new drug, have often been undertaken without regard to the standards that are well-accepted for clinical therapy trials. Problems that have plagued published diagnostic studies include failure to include representative patients with and without TB, inappropriate choice of the reference standard for diagnosis, observational biases because of failure to blind readers to both clinical and laboratory results, and absence of valid statistical methods to analyze study results (20). Fortunately, a recent initiative to bring rigor to studies of diagnostic tests has gained widespread accep-tance, especially among editors of biomedical research journals (21). The requirement for adherence to the STARD initiative (Standards for Reporting of Diagnostic Accuracy) for consideration for publication of diagnostic trials should result in a much higher quality of diagnostic test research reported in the medical literature. A Diagnostics Evaluation Expert Panel (DEEP), convened jointly by FIND and the UNICEF, UNDP, World Bank, and WHO Special Program for Research and Training in Tropical Diseases (TDR), is working to further set methodologic standards for the design and execution of trials to evaluate diagnostic tests for infectious diseases (22).

Studies of new tests for active TB are best evaluated in the population of intended use, that is, in patients with signs and symptoms of TB. These studies would include mycobacterial culture on solid and liquid media and careful assessment, with clinical and microbiologic follow-up, of culture-negative patients who may have paucibacillary TB. Test sensitivity should be based on a gold standard that includes patients with culture-negative disease and test specificity on those patients with signs and symptoms of TB found not to have disease after careful assessment and follow-up.

A critical component of FIND's strategy is large-scale demonstration projects of technologies that have been proven to perform well in carefully controlled studies. In these projects, newly proven tests are incorporated into routine laboratory and program settings to assess their ease of implementation, acceptance, and impact on such factors as morbidity, mortality, and disease transmission and, importantly, cost. Data from these studies can be used by internationally recognized technical bodies such as WHO and the International Union Against Tuberculosis and Lung Disease (UNION) to guide policy on test use and by Ministries of Health and Finance and nongovernmental organizations working on TB to make decisions about test purchase and implementation. Finally, guaranteeing access to new tests by those most in need can be facilitated by distribution networks such as through UNITAID or the Global Drug Facility that have been established to assist national TB programs in access to high-quality TB drugs and other products. GLI and its partners are working to strengthen TB laboratory services in the developing world, so that promising new tools do not flounder for lack of infrastructure to support their use.

IV. Priorities for Diagnostics Development

As TB is detected in clinical settings that vary widely, multiple types of diagnostics are needed. For the public sector, the priority diagnostics are those that would have the greatest impact on case finding, on interruption of transmission, and on decrease in morbidity and mortality from TB.

The diagnostic priorities for TB control are summarized in Figure 3. The order of these priorities is based on (*i*) the number of individuals that would directly benefit by an improved tool, (*ii*) the importance of specific populations (such as smear-positive patients) to disease control efforts, and (*iii*) the degree of medical benefit that new technologies could offer over existing tests.

Detection of active TB is the highest priority and requires differentiating the 9 million new cases of TB from over 10 times as many individuals who have other similar symptoms due to other conditions (23). For simplicity, these calculations are generally based on the annual number of incident cases and not the number of prevalent cases, though clinics will obviously see a mixture of both. The number of prevalent cases, which includes those already diagnosed and currently on therapy, those with chronic untreatable disease, and those with undetected disease, may be twice as large as the number of incident cases.

Extrapulmonary and pediatric TB, though less common, are both lethal and especially difficult to diagnose using the technologies currently available in disease-endemic countries. The need for improved DST methods that could be used to direct drug therapy (using more expensive and more toxic second-line drugs for multidrug-resistant cases) is ranked above the need for DST surveillance tools not because the latter use is not important but because existing DST technologies, although slow, are generally adequate for this purpose.

The need for new diagnostic tests for LTBI is of less relevance for global TB control efforts for the near term. However, new tests may facilitate surveys to determine the annual

Purpose	Test indications	Target population size
Case detection	• Detect pulmonary TB with high bacterial load (SS+)	100–200 million
	• Detect pulmonary TB with low bacterial load (SS−, Cx+)	100–200 million
	• Detect extrapulmonary and pediatric TB	5–50 million
Drug-susceptibility testing	• Detect MDR-TB for treatment	10 million
	• Detect MDR-TB for surveillance	100,000
Latent TB infection	• Detect LTBI for surveillance	Unknown
	• Detect LTBI for treatment	Test dependent

Figure 3   TB diagnostic priorities.

risk of infection (ARI) that currently rely on TST. In addition, improved diagnostics for LTBI in HIV-infected persons may become more important as HIV/AIDS care programs expand to include provision of isoniazid preventive therapy.

As for most health interventions, patient access will be at least as important in determining the overall impact of a given diagnostic test as are its specific performance characteristics. Tests that are so complex that they can only be used at referral laboratories will have a much lower impact than those that are widely accessible at lower levels of the health system such as a local health clinic. The vast majority of TB patients first seek care at peripheral health clinics where microscopy services are often not available. Thus, tests that could replace microscopy, especially if they were simple enough to be used at the local clinics, would reach the greatest number of patients. Such tests would also have the greatest impact by providing rapid access to correct treatment and thus reducing both morbidity and transmission of TB.

In an idealized health system such as represented in Figure 4, the types of TB testing carried out at each level would match the services intended to be provided there. Thus, national reference laboratories would support the laboratory network both through appropriate supervision and the provision of reference methods necessary for both quality control and assurance. District or regional referral laboratories would work to resolve complex cases or detect those that could not be detected with the diagnostics available more peripherally. The bulk of diagnostic work would be carried out in the local health care facilities. In many health systems, diagnostic services at peripheral health centers are scarce and much of the microbiologic confirmation of disease today occurs at district laboratories. This is largely due to the complexity of the current diagnostic tools. Simplifying these technologies would allow testing at a more appropriate local level and significantly facilitate the diagnostic process.

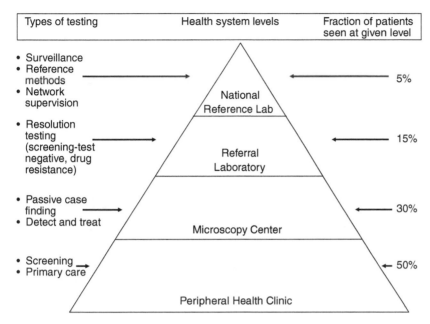

Figure 4   Diagnostic needs at levels of the health system.

For these reasons, the bulk of public sector investment in TB diagnostics, including that of FIND, is targeting the development of rapid, simple, POC testing methodologies that could allow in-clinic TB testing and, where possible, immediate initiation of appropriate therapy. The basic characteristics of such a test is defined below in a *customer requirement document* such as used by the diagnostic industry to capture the product needs of the end user. As in the example of customer requirement document below for testing in primary care settings, clinical performance targets as well as other required features, such as ease of use and robustness, for a given use indicator are described.

A.   Customer Requirement Document

B.   Product: TB Diagnostic Test, Peripheral Clinic Level

Intended Use

Detection of active infection with *M. tuberculosis*. This is presently accomplished via AFB smear, which is relatively insensitive even for pulmonary disease; by clinical examination and X-ray, which is relatively nonspecific; or (more rarely) by culture, which takes four to –six weeks. The primary goal is to provide a test system with sensitivity and specificity equal to or better than microscopy, but at a much faster time-to-result. This test system must work properly in HIV-infected patients from high-endemic countries for TB.

Feature	Desired	Minimum	Comments
A. Workflow			
1. Sample			
1.1. Sample type	Sputum, skin, breath, urine	Sputum, skin, breath, blood, serum, urine	Should work with at least one of the mentioned sample types
1.2. Sample preparation	None	Simple, 1–2 step procedure, <30 min	Includes sample preparation and readout
2. Time-to-result	<10 min	<1 wk, if sensitivity equal to culture	
3. Instrumentation	None	None, or small, maintenance-free single device; only sample addition needed	
4. Additional equipment required	None	Only robust equipment with minimal maintenance (>3 mo between maintenance); no balance, HEPA filter, temperature control, etc., needed	
5. Biosafety	No need for biosafety cabinet; no special disposal needs	No need for biosafety cabinet	
B. Performance			
1. Diagnostic sensitivity	>75% of culture-positive patients >95% of smear-positive patients	>90% smear-positive cases (if significantly easier than microscopy) and >40% smear-negative cases detected	Determined in an adult population of symptomatic individuals with and without HIV or parasitic coinfection
2. Diagnostic specificity	>98%, with no nontuberculous mycobacteria (NTM) cross-reactivity	>97% overall, with some false positives in clinically important NTM infections	Determined in TB suspects confirmed not to have TB by negative microscopy and culture on two specimens AND either improvement without TB

C. Product design

1. Stability/storage requirements			
1.1. Kit stability	24 mo storage at 35°C, 70% humidity, including transport stress (48 hr at 50°C)	12 months storage at 35°C, 70% humidity, including transport stress (48 hr at 50°C)	treatment OR confirmation of an alternate cause of symptoms; must not require exclusion of patients with prior BCG-vaccination, TB exposure, NTM infection, cured TB or HIV infection
1.2. Reconstituted reagents stability	Ready-to-use reagents, no reconstitution	8 hr at 4°C	Cannot require packaging configuration mandating high unit manufacturing costs
2. Calibrators	Fixed cutoff	No more than 1 calibrator	
3. Controls	Full-process positive control and negative control	Positive control, negative control	Full-process positive must include lysis process where appropriate
4. Determinations per "reconstituted reagent unit"	Ready-to-use units, no reconstitution	Opened package lasts 2 wk at 4°C	
5. Result capturing and documentation	Yes	No	
6. Instrument design	Option for battery operation (if electricity required); instrument can be used also for testing of other infections	115/220V AC operates at 35°C	
7. Training and education needs	<1 hr, nurse level	<2 day high school diploma or equivalent	

V. Diagnostics in the Pipeline

A. Low Cost, Manual Systems for Rapid Culture and DST: Far from Obsolete

Microbiologic isolation and identification of *M. tuberculosis* from a diagnostic specimen remains the reference standard for the diagnosis of TB. Until now, in many developing countries culture capability was limited to a single reference laboratory that supported periodic surveys, for example, drug resistance surveys, and research studies. Most of these laboratories used solid culture media, most commonly Löwenstein-Jensen, for case detection and indirect drug-susceptibility testing. These methods are slow, requiring up to six to–eight weeks for culture and three months for DST results to be available.

Automated liquid culture and DST systems are widely used in industrialized countries, as the shorter time to detection (half of that for solid culture) and increased sensitivity for mycobacterial isolation, especially from paucibacillary specimens, are important advantages (24). However, because of increased cost and increased technical complexity for specimen processing and potentially high rates of bacterial contamination and isolation of nontuberculous mycobacteria (NTM) of no clinical significance, these systems were rarely used in the public health laboratories in low-income countries. This situation is now changing. A negotiated agreement between FIND and Becton Dickenson (BD) allowed for preferential pricing for its automated liquid culture and DST system (MGIT) that significantly reduces the costs close to those for testing on solid media. In addition, the development of the MPT64 antigen detection strip made species identification from positive cultures simple and inexpensive. These advances and the clinical data associated with FIND studies supported WHO endorsement of liquid culture with rapid species identification and DST (7). Countries that are developing national TB laboratory strengthening plans now often incorporate these systems into their plans, ideally first at the national reference level and then decentralized to regional laboratories as appropriate.

At the same time as these commercial liquid culture and DST systems are being widely implemented, there continues to be great interest in lower-cost systems. The microscopic observation drug susceptibility (MODS) assay uses essentially the same media as that in the MGIT system but inoculates cultures in 24-well tissue culture plates with both drug-free and drug-containing wells (25). Mycobacterial growth is detected by visualization of cording colonies with an inverted light microscope. As with MGIT culture, the somewhat laborious and expensive N-acetyl-L-cysteine/NaOH sputum processing method is used, but otherwise material costs are low. If the culture plates are sealed and identification of *M. tuberculosis* is based on detection of slow growth with cording colonies, that is, no culture manipulation is needed for species identification or further DST, the work can be preformed in a BSL-2 laboratory. Otherwise, a BSL-3 laboratory is needed to ensure adequate biosafety. The largest published study of MODS conducted by Moore and colleagues in Peru found that MODS had higher sensitivity for TB detection than automated liquid culture and somewhat shorter time-to-detection (25). Moreover, in contrast to automated liquid culture, there was little difference in time-to-positivity for smear-negative and smear-positive sputum specimens. Accuracy for detection of rifampin resistance was excellent and for isoniazid resistance reasonably good, but poor for resistance to ethambutol and streptomycin. Several funding agencies, such as Wellcome Trust and the U.S. Agency for International Development, are now supporting additional studies of MODS to standardize testing and address operational issues in programmatic implementation.

FIND is supporting the evaluation of a similar system, the MDR-XDR TB Color Test, developed by C. Evans, who is also working in Peru. This system utilizes a single-step decontamination step, which is done in the specimen collection cup, and utilizes low-cost chemicals and does not require centrifugation. The processed specimen is inoculated directly onto a selective thin-layer chromogenic agar plate that is then sealed, so that biosafety concerns are no greater than those for AFB smear examination. The agar plate has four colored quadrants: one drug-free and the others containing isoniazid, rifampin, and ciprofloxacin. Detection of *M. tuberculosis* is based on the development of visible dark colonies with microscopic confirmation of morphology. In an unpublished study, the sensitivity of the Color Test was comparable to that of MODS (with concentrated specimens) and significantly higher than that of the culture of concentrated specimens on thin-layer agar (C. Evans, personal communication e-mail, May 5, 2008). Accuracy for direct detection of MDR-TB, compared to direct MODS testing, was good. This system has great appeal because of simplified specimen processing and potential for implementation at a lower level of the high system where only an incubator and a light microscope would be needed. Work is now underway to optimize the testing format, identify a manufacturer for production of high-quality tests, and execute large-scale and rigorous test evaluations.

VI. Molecular Testing for Case Detection and MDR Screening: The Coming Revolution

Molecular methods, in particular nucleic acid amplification tests (NAATs), have demonstrated high specificity and sensitivity approaching that of culture for the diagnosis of pulmonary TB (26–28). Results from these assays are available within a day, compared with four to six weeks for culture results on solid media. However, the cost and moderate complexity of NAATs have limited their widespread use, even in industrialized countries. Studies of NAAT use in developing countries have produced mixed results, with widely variable performance (29). There are data, however, suggesting that such assays might be more cost-effective than AFB smear examination when patient costs are included (30). It may be possible to dramatically simplify NAAT technology by using isothermal amplification methods with visual readout (31) and by engineering the sputum processing steps to provide a relatively inexpensive, handheld device. FIND is partnering with Eiken Chemical Co., Ltd., on the development of such a system using its LAMP (Loop-Mediated Isothermal Amplification) technology.

FIND selected this technology out of the numerous alternative molecular amplification platforms based in part on considerations of intellectual property and corporate commitment, but primarily because of the specific advantages of the method that make it particularly suitable for the development of a robust application useful in developing countries (32). This technology uses isothermal amplification, which removes the need for a thermocycler, in a closed tube, which reduces the chance of false-positive results from workspace contamination with amplified DNA. It is a very rapid reaction, with results available in less than 45 minutes, and, critically, generates results (based on turbidity and fluorescence) that can be seen with the naked eye. FIND has signed a joint development agreement with Eiken that gives royalty-free access to the technology to the public sector of developing countries and is working with Eiken to develop a version of the assay that can be used at the microscopic level by technologists with no molecular experience. To date work has advanced through several prototypes with the current test system having only three plastic devices and a single instrument, a heating block. Testing has been simplified, now requiring only 11 steps, that is, fewer than those for AFB microscopy. The performance of TB-LAMP prototypes suggests that the technology may have the potential to revolutionize diagnostic care at microscopy center.

Even more advanced in development are rapid, molecular tests for TB drug resistance based on detection of mutations in the genome that confirm drug resistance, for example, *rpoB* for rifampin and *katG* and *inhA* for isoniazid. One commercial test, the INNO-LIPA Rif. TB assay (Innogenetics), is an LPA that uses multiplex PCR amplification and reverse hybridization to identify *M. tuberculosis* complex and mutations to the *rpoB* gene in culture isolates and has been available for more than 10 years (33). In a large study of rapid tests for MDR-TB in Peru supported by FIND and WHO/TDR, this test also had excellent performance when applied directly to AFB smear-positive sputum specimens (FIND, unpublished data).

A second commercial LPA, the MTBDR*plus* test (Hain Lifescience, GmbH), has more recently been developed that also includes probes for *katG* and *inhA* and can be used on culture isolates or AFB smear-positive sputum specimens. In preparation for large-scale demonstration studies of this test in MDR-TB settings, FIND together with the Medical Research Council of South Africa and the National Health Laboratory Service, evaluated the test in over 500 smear-positive sputum specimens from MDR-TB at-risk patients (34). The results indicated that the test performed better than conventional liquid culture and DST, in terms of time-to-detection (results in 1–2 days compared with 60 days), number of valid test results (97% compared to 90%), accuracy for MDR-TB diagnosis (99% sensitivity and 100% specificity with conventional culture and DST as reference standard). In a subsequent demonstration study in South Africa that enrolled over 20,000 MDR-TB suspects, test performance was similar, and a detailed costing analysis found that the cost per valid test result was 60% lower for the LPA compared to MGIT culture and DST on solid media (FIND, unpublished data). These results, together with published data on laboratory performance studies (35), enable WHO to endorse LPAs for MDR-TB screening in low-income settings (9). With the potential to substantially reduce the need for routine culture and DST for MDR-TB screening, it is expected that these tests can play a critical role in addressing the MDR-TB crisis.

As LPAs are somewhat complex to perform and require highly skilled personnel for accurate testing, decentralizing LPAs beyond reference laboratories is currently not feasible in most low-income countries. To bring rapid molecular testing for MDR-TB closer to the microscopy level, FIND is partnering with Cepheid on the development of an application for TB and rifampin-resistance detection on its GeneXpert platform. This system is self-contained, fully integrated, and automated platform that combines onboard sample preparation with real-time PCR amplification and detection. The system is designed to purify, concentrate, detect, and identify targeted nucleic acid sequences, delivering results in less than 100 minutes directly from unprocessed samples. Because the system is self-contained, there is no need for a biosafety cabinet and technician training is minimal. In preliminary studies, sensitivity and TB detection was nearly 100% for AFB smear-positive, culture-positive specimens and 70% to 80% for smear-negative, culture-positive specimens, with high test specificity (FIND, unpublished data). Sensitivity and specificity for rifampin resistance has been high.

VII. POC Tests: The Ultimate Revolution

The ability to diagnose disease and deliver care in the same setting at the same time decreases dropout and improves outcomes. The convenience for the patient and the potential for cost savings in the health system is driving the development of so-called POC tests for a variety of conditions and pushing the creation of new testing platforms. Such tests have obvious advantages for developing country use, obviating the need for strong laboratory infrastructure at the community level. Rapid lateral flow immunochromatographic tests (like pregnancy tests) were developed for malaria some 15 years ago and have now been put into widespread use, with some 70 million tests performed a year in developing countries, and largely replacing microscopy in many settings. For health workers and patients, such a test for TB would be a huge advance.

The phrase "point-of-care" implies that testing and treatment are done at the same place. For some diseases, including HIV and TB, the treatment location is likely to be at a referral center. This has implications for the design and use of rapid tests for TB. For example, a highly sensitive test with relatively poor specificity might still be useful as a screening test at the community level to refer patients for confirmatory testing, or to rule out TB in suspects at the primary care level. Alternatively, if a very simple dipstick test were developed tomorrow that could detect TB from urine, for example, with specificity high enough to prompt therapy, it would not be given to mobile community health workers along with sacks of therapeutics. Instead, it would be integrated into existing TB control networks but would allow the extension of treatment centers to progressively lower levels of the health system, reducing delays in care and improving access.

The attractions of POC testing are obvious, but to date no effective POC test for TB has been developed. Why is this? Successful development of a POC test requires (*i*) the existence of a pathogen-specific substance or analyte or diagnostic immune response (the target) and (*ii*) a simple methodology that can detect the target in the concentrations at which it is found in human samples (testing platform). The most widely used POC platform is the lateral flow immunochromatographic test, which is both easy to use and easy to manufacture. Unfortunately, there is no currently known TB analyte that is present, at concentrations detectable by lateral flow tests, in the body fluids of a sufficient number of TB patients to use for clinical testing. A number of protein and nonprotein mycobacterial molecules, including lipoarabinomannan (LAM), are currently being targeted by public and commercial research groups hoping to develop an antigen detection test. Such a test might have the obvious advantage of high specificity, lack of dependence on host immunity, and correlation with bacterial or disease burden. Unfortunately, TB antigens tend to be found in very low concentrations in body fluids such as urine and serum, and the complexity of sputum makes it intractable for use in simplified membrane-based assays. Detection of antibodies to TB is more straightforward, and dozens of lateral flow tests that detect antibodies to TB proteins have been developed and are currently being sold into private markets but none of these yet have performance adequate for routine programmatic use (36).

On the other hand, there are TB analytes that can be readily detected on more complex testing platforms. For example, mycobacterial nucleic acids are targeted by a number of commercial and noncommercial tests, and mycolic acids or other TB-specific lipids can be detected with sophisticated chromatography systems. The platforms used for these systems are not readily adapted for POC use, though substantial work is underway in this area.

The options for the development of a successful POC test for TB, then, are to identify readily detectable TB biomarkers that can be used as targets for existing POC test platforms, or to develop new testing platforms that are able to detect low-abundance or complex molecules in a way simple enough to be used outside of the laboratory. Though a full discussion of this work is beyond the scope of this chapter, a number of research groups have active programs addressing one or both prongs of the problem, and there is the expectation that within five years assays will be launched that can meet the needs of at least some TB control programs in developing countries.

VIII.   LTBI Diagnosis: Do IGRAs Have a Role in Low-Income Settings?

Two interferon-gamma release assays (IGRAs) assays for the diagnosis of LTBI have been commercialized and are undergoing further development to make the application more feasible in field settings (37). These are the QuantiFERON-TB Gold In-Tube test, a whole blood IGRA from Cellestis, Inc., and the T-Spot.TB test, an Enzyme-linked immunosorbent spot (ELISPOT) assay from Oxford Immunotech, Inc. These assays use the proteins ESAT-6 and CPF-10 from a section of the mycobacterial genome designated RD1 for being a "region of deletion" from *Mycobacterium bovis* BCG. Such RD1 genes are also absent from most strains of nontuberculous mycobacteria. Thus, the specificity of these tests compared to that of the TST that uses purified protein derivative (PPD) is high, especially in persons with prior BCG vaccination. Study data also suggest that these assays are as, or more sensitive than, the TST, especially in immunocompromised persons, including HIV-infected persons. In low-incidence countries where testing for LTBI and treating infected persons at high risk of progression to active TB is an important component of TB control, guidelines on the use of IGRAs, either to supplement or replace the TST, have been issued (38–40). It is widely expected that with time IGRAs will replace the TST in screening for LTBI.

However, test performance and the utility of such tests in countries with a high burden of TB is not yet clear. Research priorities addressing these questions are underway, focusing on testing in HIV-infected persons and childhood TB contacts (41), persons for whom both WHO and the Union recommend IPT. Critically important in these studies is the question of the predictive value of a positive IGRA for subsequent development of TB. There are a few data suggesting that in low-incidence settings, for TB contacts, IGRAs may be a more accurate predictor of future TB than the TST (42).

Early attempts to use these and other specific antigens as skin test reagents, while showing some promise in animal models, have not succeeded in human studies. However, more recent studies of ESAT-6 suggested that it might have better performance characteristics than the current PPD-TST (43). However, interest in new, specific TSTs has been tempered with the advent of the IGRAs.

IX.   Conclusions

The last few years has seen substantial progress in the development of improved tools for TB detection, and in the strengthening of laboratory systems for their use, but for the majority of patients, access to those tests and those laboratory systems is still limited. Global TB control is at a crossroad. Nearly two decades after the introduction of the WHO DOTS strategy, its successes and limitations have never been more apparent.

The basic elements of sound TB control are largely in place throughout the world. However, further advancement to meet the challenges posed by the HIV epidemic and the widespread emergence of MDR-TB will not be possible without both the expansion of diagnostic capabilities beyond AFB microscopy and the implementation of new diagnostic technologies. These needs, and the opportunities for significant progress to meet them, have been captured in both the new WHO's Stop TB Strategy (44), which enhances DOTS, and the Stop TB Partnership's Global Plan for 2006 to 2015 (45). The network to implement the elements of the plan related to diagnostics led by FIND and its partners is in place. It is now up to the world at large to see that this plan is implemented with adequate support. If it is, ten years from now we will be able to plan for global elimination of human TB. If not, we will likely be mired in an expanding, out-of-control epidemic caused by a pathogen, where breathing becomes a high-risk behavior. The choice is ours.

References

1. Gandhi NR, Moll A, Sturm AW, et al. Extensively drug-resistant tuberculosis as a cause of death in patients co-infected with tuberculosis and HIV in a rural area of South Africa. Lancet 2006; 368:1575–1580.
2. World Health Organization. The Global MDR-TB and XDR-TB Response Plan. Geneva: World Health Organization, 2007. WHO/HTM/TB/2007.387.
3. Global Laboratory Initiative (GLI). http://www.who.int/tb/dots/laboratory/gli/en/index.html. Last Accessed January 16, 2009.
4. U.S. President's Emergency Plan for AIDS Relief (PEPFAR). http://www.america.gov/st/texttrans-english/2008/July/20080731114623eaifas0.1355707.html. Last Accessed January 16, 2009.
5. Foundation for Innovative New Diagnostics (FIND). http://www.finddiagnostics.org/activities/lp/index.shtml. Last Accessed January 26, 2009.
6. Expanding and accelerating access to diagnostics for patients at risk of MDR-TB. http://www.unitaid.eu/en/Expanding-and-accelerating-access-to-diagnostics-for-patients-at-risk-of-MDR-TB.html. Last Accessed August 21, 2009.
7. The use of liquid medium for culture and DST. http://www.who.int/tb/dots/laboratory/policy/en/index3.html. Last Accessed January 16, 2009.
8. Checklist of key actions for the use of liquid media for culture and drug susceptibility testing (DST). http://www.stoptb.org/retooling/assets/documents/Retooling%20Task%20Force%20-%20Liquid%20Culture-DST%20Checklist%20-%20Feb2008.pdf. Last Accessed January 16, 2009.
9. World Health Organization (WHO). Molecular line probe assays for rapid screening of patients at risk of multidrug resistant tuberculosis (MDR-TB). http://www.who.int/tb/dots/laboratory/lpa_policy.pdf. Last Accessed January 16, 2009.
10. Squire SB, Belaye AK, Kashoti A, et al. 'Lost' smear-positive pulmonary tuberculosis cases: Where are they and why did we lose them? Int J Tuberc Lung Dis 2005; 9:25–31.
11. World Health Organization (WHO). New WHO policies. http://www.who.int/tb/dots/laboratory/policy/en/index.html. Last accessed August 21, 2009.
12. Hargreaves NJ, Kadzakumanja O, Whitty CJ, et al. 'Smear-negative' pulmonary tuberculosis in a DOTS programme: Poor outcomes in an area of high HIV seroprevalence. Int J Tuberc Lung Dis 2001; 5:847–854.
13. Pronyk PM, Kahn K, Hargreaves JR, et al. Undiagnosed pulmonary tuberculosis deaths in rural South Africa. Int J Tuberc Lung Dis 2004; 8:796–799.
14. Gutierrez EB, Zanetta DM, Saldiva PH, et al. Autopsy-proven determinants of death in HIV-infected patients treated for pulmonary tuberculosis in Sao Paulo, Brazil. Pathol Res Pract 2002; 198:339–346.

15. Centers for Disease Control. Nosocomial transmission of multidrug-resistant tuberculosis among HIV-infected persons—Florida and New York, 1988–1991. JAMA 1991; 266(11):1483–1485.

16. World Health Organization. Anti-tuberculosis Drug Resistance in the World. Fourth Global Report. WHO/IUATLD Global Project on Anti-Tuberculosis Drug Resistance Surveillance 2002–2007. Geneva: World Health Organization, 2008.

17. Ewer K, Deeks J, Alvarez L, et al. Comparison of T-cell-based assay with tuberculin skin test for diagnosis of *Mycobacterium tuberculosis* infection in a school tuberculosis outbreak. Lancet 2003; 361:1168–1173.

18. Ferrara G, Losi M, Meacci M, et al. Routine hospital use of a new commercial whole blood interferon-gamma assay for the diagnosis of tuberculosis infection. Am J Respir Crit Care Med 2005; 172:631–635.

19. Moran M, Guzman J, Ropars AL, et al. G-FINDER 2008. Neglected Disease Research and Development: How much are we really spending? London, United Kingdom: The George Institute for International Health, 2009.

20. Small P, Perkins MD. More rigour needed in trials of new diagnostic agents for tuberculosis. Lancet 2000; 356(9235):1048–1049.

21. Bosssuyt PM, Reitsma JB, Bruns DE, et al. Towards complete and accurate reporting of studies of diagnostic accuracy: The STARD Initiative. Clin Chem 2003; 49:1–6.

22. Banoo S, Bell D, Bossuyt P, et al; DEEP Working Group. Guidelines for the evaluation of diagnostic tests for selected infectious diseases. Nat Rev Microbiol 2006; 4(suppl 12):520–532.

23. World Health Organization. Global Tuberculosis Report 2004. Geneva: World Health Organization, 2004.

24. Dinnes J, Deeks J, Kunst H, et al. A Systematic Review of Rapid Diagnostic Tests for the Detection of Tuberculosis Infection. Health Technol Assess 2007; 11:1–314.

25. Moore DA, Evans CA, Gilman RH, et al. Microscopic-observation drug-susceptibility assay for the diagnosis of TB. N Engl J Med 2006; 355:1539–1550.

26. Shamputa IC, Rigouts L, Portaels F. Molecular genetic methods for diagnosis and antibiotic resistance detection of mycobacteria from clinical specimens. APMIS 2004; 112:728–752.

27. Huggett JF, McHugh TD, Zumla A. Tuberculosis: amplification-based clinical diagnostic techniques. Int J Biochem Cell Biol 2003; 35:1407–1412.

28. Woods GL. Molecular techniques in mycobacterial detection. Arch Pathol Lab Med 2001; 125:122–126.

29. Suffys P, Palomino JC, Cardoso Leao S, et al. Evaluation of the polymerase chain reaction for the detection of *Mycobacterium tuberculosis*. Int J Tuberc Lung Dis 2000; 4:179–183.

30. van Cleeff M, Kivihya-Ndugga L, Githui W, et al. Cost-effectiveness of polymerase chain reaction versus Ziehl-Neelsen smear microscopy for diagnosis of tuberculosis in Kenya. Int J Tuberc Lung Dis 2005; 9:877–883.

31. Iwamoto T, Sonobe T, Hayashi K. Loop-mediated isothermal amplification for direct detection of *Mycobacterium tuberculosis* complex, *M. avium*, and *M. intracellulare* in sputum samples. J Clin Microbiol 2003; 41:2616–2622.

32. Boehme CC, Nabeta P, Henostroza G, et al. Operational feasibility of using loop-mediated isothermal amplification for diagnosis of pulmonary tuberculosis in microscopy centers of developing countries. J Clin Microbiol 2007; 45:1936–1940.

33. Morgan M, Kalantri S, Flores L, et al. A commercial line probe assay for the rapid detection of rifampicin resistance in *Mycobacterium tuberculosis*: A systematic review and meta-analysis. BMC Infect Dis 2005; 5:62.

34. Barnard M, Albert H, Coetzee G, et al. Implementation of rapid molecular screening for multi-drug resistant tuberculosis in a high volume public health laboratory in South Africa. Am J Respir Crit Care Med 2008; 177:787–792.

35. Ling DI, Zwerling AA, Pai M. GenoType MTBDR assays for the diagnosis of multidrug-resistant tuberculosis: A meta-analysis. Eur Respir J 2008; 32(5):1165–1174.
36. WHO/TDR. Laboratory Evaluation of 19 Commercially Available Tests for the Diagnosis of Tuberculosis (Diagnostics evaluation series, 2). Geneva: World Health Organization, 2008. http://www.who.int/tdr/publications/tdr-research-publications/diagnostics-evaluation-2/pdf/diagnostic-evaluation-2.pdf. Last Accessed August 21, 2009.
37. Pai M, Zwerling A, Menzies D. Systematic review: T-cell-based assays for the diagnosis of latent tuberculosis infection: an update. Ann Intern Med 2008; 149:177–184.
38. Centers for Disease Control and Prevention. Guidelines for using the QuantiFERON®-TB Gold Test for detecting *Mycobacterium tuberculosis* infection, United States. MMWR Recomm Rep 2005; 54(RR-15):49–55
39. Updated recommendations on interferon gamma release assays for latent tuberculosis infection. Can Commun Dis Rpt 2008; 34:1–13.
40. Drobniewski F, Cobelens F, Zellweger J-P. Use of Gamma-interferon assays in low- and medium-prevalence countries in Europe: A consensus statement of a Wolfheze Workshop organised by KNCV/EuroTB, Vilnius Sept 2006. Euro Surveill 2007; 12(No 7):4–6.
41. Pai M, Dheda K, Cunningham J, et al. T-cell assays for the diagnosis of latent tuberculosis infection: Moving the research agenda forward. Lancet Infect Dis 2007; 7:428–438.
42. Diel R, Loddenkemper R, Meywald-Walter K, et al. Predictive value of a whole blood IFN-gamma assay for the development of active tuberculosis disease after recent infection with *Mycobacterium tuberculosis*. Am J Respir Crit Care Med 2008; 177:1164–1170.
43. Arend SM, Franken WP, Aggerbeck H, et al. Double-blind randomized Phase I study comparing rdESAT-6 to tuberculin as skin test reagent in the diagnosis of tuberculosis infection. Tuberculosis (Edinb) 2008; 88:249–261.
44. Raviglione MC, Uplekar M. WHO's new StopTB Strategy. Lancet 2006; 367:952–955.
45. Stop TB Partnership and World Health Organization. Global Plan to Stop TB 2006–2015. Geneva, Switzerland: World Health Organization, 2006. WHO/HTM/STP/2006.35.

14

New Drugs for Tuberculosis

ANN GINSBERG and MELVIN SPIGELMAN
Global Alliance for TB Drug Development, New York, New York, U.S.A.

I. Introduction

The need for new, improved drugs for the treatment of tuberculosis (TB) is growing ever more urgent. Although the treatment of active, drug-sensitive, pulmonary tuberculosis is potentially 95% to 98% effective under ideal conditions (1), cure rates in the field are often significantly lower (2), and recently identified extensively drug-resistant (XDR) strains of *Mycobacterium tuberculosis* (3) are only 50% to 70% curable under the best of conditions (4). In some situations, particularly in HIV-positive individuals, XDR-TB has been reported to be close to 100% incurable (5). New TB drugs and improved TB treatment regimens are required to (*i*) shorten and simplify treatment of active, drug-sensitive disease; (*ii*) provide shorter, safer, more effective, and lower-cost treatment alternatives for multidrug-resistant (MDR) and XDR-TB; (*iii*) remove obstacles to effective treatment of TB in HIV-positive individuals; and (*iv*) shorten treatment of latent TB infection (LTBI). The following sections examine each of these pressing needs in turn.

II. Treatment of Drug-Sensitive, Active Tuberculosis

The current recommended treatment regimens for drug-sensitive, active pulmonary TB are lengthy (lasting a minimum of six months) and complex (typically requiring adminis-tration of four drugs daily during the first two months and two drugs during the remaining four months) (6,7). A key component of the World Health Organization's Stop TB Strat-egy, DOTS has at its core the direct observation by trained personnel of patients taking their TB medications to ensure compliance and prevent development of drug resistance. These features, although key to treatment success, render TB therapy burdensome and labor-intensive to deliver effectively, as well as difficult for patients to adhere to (current TB treatment has been discussed in detail in chap. 5). As a result, many patients do not receive adequate treatment, inhibiting control of the global TB epidemic and enabling the development and spread of drug-resistant strains of *M. tuberculosis*. Components of the current regimens, primarily the rifamycins, have the added disadvantage of interacting with antiretroviral therapy (ART) [primarily protease inhibitors (PIs) and nonnucleoside reverse transcriptase inhibitors (NNRTIs); (8,9) see also section V., below, and chap. 6], a significant problem given the high incidence and prevalence of HIV/*M. tuberculosis* coinfection. The primary goal in improving treatment of active TB is to deliver to all patients (irrespective of HIV status) more efficacious, safer agents, and regimens that will shorten and simplify the therapeutic course. Attaining this goal will decrease the burdensome nature of the treatment regimen for both patients and health care systems and increase rates of successful treatment completion while lowering rates of treatment default and loss to follow-up.

III. Treatment of MDR-TB and XDR-TB

Drug-resistant TB is a man-made scourge resulting originally from inappropriate or incomplete treatment of patients with active disease. Factors contributing to the development of drug resistance include inadequate treatment programs, drug shortages, poor quality drugs and lack of adherence to prescribed regimens, creating conditions that select for *M. tuberculosis* strains resistant to the currently used drugs. Even more worrisome is that, in some high-burden settings, the prevalence of drug-resistant disease is now sufficiently high that primary resistance (due to direct transmission of MDR/XDR-TB strains) is also becoming a significant issue among new patients (5).

Streptomycin, the first anti-TB drug identified, was introduced for use in 1944; by 1946, cases of streptomycin-resistant TB had been reported in patients receiving streptomycin as monotherapy under clinical trial conditions (10), and by 1948 in patients treated under field conditions (11). To be classified as MDR-TB, a strain must be resistant to at least isoniazid and rifampicin. In the latest WHO/International Union Against Tuberculosis and Lung Disease (IUATLD)-sponsored global surveillance of drug resistance (12), a global mean of 2.9% of newly diagnosed cases were found to be MDR-TB. XDR-TB strains are defined as resistant to at least isoniazid, rifampicin, plus any fluoroquinolone, and any of the injectable second-line drugs (amikacin, kanamycin, and capreomycin) (13). By June 2008, XDR-TB had been identified in 49 countries (14). Treatment of MDR-TB mostly relies on drugs that are less effective and more toxic than first-line therapy, as well as up to 110-fold more expensive overall (15–17). The choice of drugs for treatment of XDR-TB is even more limited and unsatisfactory. To significantly improve treatment of MDR- and XDR-TB, novel drugs that are affordable as well as safe and effective against these strains must be developed.

To contain the spread of MDR- and XDR-TB, a combination of appropriate and effective treatment of drug-sensitive cases with careful introduction of novel, second-line drugs for treatment of drug-resistant cases must be instituted. This approach is necessary both to prevent further emergence of resistance to known drugs and to protect new drugs from the development of resistance (18). Prospective, randomized, controlled trials of novel MDR-TB treatment regimens pose significant challenges, but may also represent a relatively short timeline to regulatory approval for an MDR-TB indication, based on using six-month sputum conversion rates as an efficacy endpoint and assuming the ability to enroll into such trials at a reasonable rate (19,20). Two novel compounds are currently in clinical development for an MDR-TB indication: J&J's (Tibotec) diarylquinoline, TMC207, and Otsuka Pharmaceuticals' nitroimidazo-oxazole (OPC67683) (see section VIII). Current MDR- and XDR-TB treatment regimens are based on anecdotal evidence and retrospective cohort studies, rather than on data from randomized clinical trials. Clearly, a more systematic and robust development program for novel agents should benefit future patients with drug-resistant TB.

As can be seen in the later descriptions, except for the rifamycins and fluoroquinolones, all classes and agents in the current pipeline of compounds being developed for treatment of active TB have novel mechanisms of action relative to current first- and second-line TB drugs and therefore have the potential to be effective against MDR- and XDR-TB.

IV.   Treatment of Active TB in Individuals Infected with HIV

In 2006, 7.2% of all new TB cases were in HIV-positive individuals, and 12% of the estimated 1.7 million TB deaths in 2006 were attributable to HIV (2). WHO estimates that one-third of the 40 million people currently infected with HIV are coinfected with *M. tuberculosis*. Up to half of the people living with HIV/AIDS develop active TB, and TB speeds HIV progression, so effective therapy of TB in these individuals is crucial. Unfortunately, the rifamycins, and particularly rifampicin, induce certain cytochrome P450 enzymes (CYP3A4 and CYP2C8/9, and to a lesser extent, CYP2C19 and CYPD6) that are involved in the metabolism of key nonnucleoside reverse transcriptase inhibitors (NNRTIs) used in ART. Therefore, concomitant use of rifampicin with ART can lead to decreased serum levels of these drugs. PIs and NNRTIs can also affect the P450 system, thereby altering serum levels of rifampicin. These drug–drug interactions complicate the treatment of TB in individuals with HIV/AIDS, making the treatment of these individuals difficult to manage, particularly in many high-burden settings. In addition, both isoniazid and nucleoside reverse transcriptase inhibitors can cause peripheral neuropathy, leading to enhanced toxicity if these are used together. Therefore, a priority for treatment of HIV/*M. tuberculosis* coinfected patients is to develop novel drugs for TB treatment with an enhanced safety profile, and in particular, without clinically significant cytochrome P450 interactions.

V.   Treatment of Latent TB Infection

Based primarily on the results of tuberculin skin test surveys, an estimated 2 billion people are infected with *M. tuberculosis* (21). Current recommended treatment of LTBI to prevent later reactivation consists of six to nine months of isoniazid in HIV-positive individuals. Because of the long duration of therapy and potential for hepatic toxicity, nonadherence with the regimen is a significant problem. There are also significant operational barriers to implementing such a regimen on a scale widespread enough to eradicate this enormous reservoir of future disease. Shorter and more intermittent regimens have been tested and are used under some conditions but have demonstrated significant rates of adverse effects, including hepatic toxicity and joint pain, and those that contain rifamycin pose difficulties for administration in HIV-positive persons taking antiretroviral medications (22,23). New drugs are needed to shorten the LTBI treatment course while maintaining efficacy and ensuring tolerability, as well as suitability for HIV-positive individuals. As the prevalence of MDR- and XDR-TB increases, so does the prevalence of drug-resistant latent TB infections, creating an increasing need for LTBI regimens based on novel drugs. One major hurdle in the search for new drugs for the improved treatment of LTBI is the lack of understanding of the underlying mechanisms of chronic, asymptomatic (latent) infection. However, recent investigations are beginning to make inroads in understanding potential mechanisms. For example, evidence is accumulating that latent *M. tuberculosis* infections demonstrate some characteristics of biofilms (24,25), and modern imaging techniques are helping to elucidate the replication behavior of mycobacteria in chronic infections (26).

VI. Drug Development Process

The process of drug development is frequently described as advancing compounds through a "pipeline" which begins with Discovery and proceeds through Preclinical or Nonclinical Development (including in vitro and in vivo animal testing) to Clinical Development (human testing, typically divided into phases I, II, and III).[a] If the clinical data warrant, compounds are then registered with regulatory agencies for the desired indication. Registration is generally followed by "postmarketing" trials known as phase IV studies, to investigate further how a drug is functioning in terms of safety and/or efficacy in the marketplace, and potentially to explore new indications or combinations. In reality, drug development is a highly iterative process. Results from one stage of development most often inform additional studies still being designed and executed in an "earlier" stage, either for that compound or for a "next generation" compound in the same chemical class for the same or a similar indication.

VII. The Current Global Tuberculosis Drug Portfolio

Current first-line TB drugs were discovered between the 1940s and 1960s, and since then no new classes of drugs have been registered for TB treatment. Even the current second-line classes of anti-TB agents were identified in the 1950s to 1980s. TB drug development languished in the ensuing decades both due to the misperception or hubris that the TB "problem" had been solved and due to a lack of adequate market incentive to spur private sector investment in TB drug R&D. Since 2000, however, a combination of public and private sector efforts, often in collaboration, have created a growing pipeline of new drugs being explored specifically for their potential utility in the treatment of drug-sensitive and drug-resistant TB. While a small number of these drugs belong to classes that have already been approved for TB therapy, such as the rifamycins, most belong to chemical classes that have never been approved for a TB indication. The classes now represented in the pipeline that are discussed in some detail below include the fluoroquinolones, diarylquinolines, nitroimidazoles, pyrroles, diamines, oxazolidinones, macrolides, riminophenazines, and long-acting rifamycins. Several compounds in development have completely novel mechanisms of action and therefore hold the greatest potential for improving treatment of drug-resistant as well as drug-sensitive TB.

A. Fluoroquinolones

Two late-generation fluoroquinolones are in advanced clinical testing for the treatment of active TB. Although there are few clinical data to support their use other than anecdotal reports, during the past decade fluoroquinolone antibiotics have become a key class of "second-line" drugs for treating patients infected with MDR strains of *M. tuberculosis*.

---

[a] The phases I, II, and III are typically defined as follows (see: http://www. clinicaltrials.gov/ct/info/):

Phase I trials: researchers test an experimental drug or treatment on a small group of people (20–80) for the first time to evaluate its safety, determine a safe dosage range, and identify side effects.

Phase II trials: the experimental study drug or treatment is given to a larger group of people (100–300) to see if it is effective and to further evaluate its safety.

Phase III trials: the experimental study drug or treatment is given to large groups of people (1,000–3,000) to confirm its effectiveness, monitor its side effects, compare it to commonly used treatments, and collect information that will allow the experimental drug or treatment to be used safely.

Only recently, however, have these drugs begun to be actively considered for the treatment of drug-susceptible disease. In part, this is because the few randomized, controlled trials of fluoroquinolones for drug-susceptible TB that were conducted in the past did not demonstrate any benefit. The publication by the Tuberculosis Research Centre, Chennai, India, in 2002, of a clinical trial with ofloxacin-containing regimens restimulated interest. This trial unfortunately did not include a standard control group, but rather randomized patients with newly diagnosed pulmonary TB to one of four ofloxacin-containing regimens (27). Rates of sputum–culture conversion to negativity at two months, an endpoint that correlates well under appropriate conditions with relapse rates following TB treatment (28), ranged from 92% to 98%. This was in comparison to an expected rate of approximately 75% with the standard four-drug treatment (29). In patients randomized to three months of daily isoniazid, rifampicin, pyrazinamide, and ofloxacin or three months of daily isoniazid, rifampicin, pyrazinamide, and ofloxacin followed by twice weekly of isoniazid and rifampicin for one or two months, relapse rates during the two years following completion of treatment were 8%, 2%, and 4%, respectively. These results suggest that fluoroquinolones have the potential to shorten the duration of TB treatment regimens.

Subsequent data from the mouse model also indicate that fluoroquinolones may be able to significantly shorten treatment regimens for active TB. Of the more recently developed fluoroquinolones, the two most potent against *M. tuberculosis* in vitro and in animal models are moxifloxacin and gatifloxacin. An evaluation of fluoroquinolones in an in vitro model of persistent *M. tuberculosis* infection indicated that moxifloxacin might have the greatest sterilizing potential among this class of drugs (30).

Jacques Grosset and colleagues at Johns Hopkins University recently conducted a series of studies of moxifloxacin in mouse models of acute *M. tuberculosis* infection, which have also contributed to the interest in this drug. The initial study, in which infected mice were treated for one month with one of several fluoroquinolones, found that moxifloxacin had the greatest bactericidal activity, comparable to that of isoniazid, the most potent bactericidal drug in early bactericidal activity (EBA) studies. A second study suggested that moxifloxacin also had potent sterilizing activity and might substantially improve the efficacy of the once-weekly rifapentine treatment (31). A third study surprisingly demonstrated that a combination of rifampicin, pyrazinamide, and moxifloxacin had substantially greater sterilizing activity than not only the standard regimen but also than the standard regimen plus moxifloxacin (32). The results of two small EBA studies have demonstrated that moxifloxacin has bactericidal activity superior to that of rifampicin and perhaps comparable to that of isoniazid (33,34).

Moxifloxacin and gatifloxacin are both currently in phase III clinical development. Both are dose limited by potential for prolongation of the cardiac QT interval at higher doses. Other fluoroquinolone class effects pertinent to both drugs include rare instances of severe liver toxicity and tendinopathies. Studies of gatifloxacin are being conducted by a product development team supported by the United Nations Children's Fund (UNICEF), United Nations Development Program (UNDP), World Bank, WHO, Special Program for Research and Training in Tropical Diseases, and the European Commission. A phase II study reported by this team randomized newly diagnosed patients to one of three fluoroquinolone-containing regimens (ofloxacin, moxifloxacin, or gatifloxacin) in combination with isoniazid, rifampicin, and pyrazinamide during the first two months of treatment (35). This study compared the rate of decrease of *M. tuberculosis* in serial sputum samples (serial sputum colony counts or SSCC) during the first eight weeks of therapy and demonstrated that moxifloxacin substituted for ethambutol in the standard first-line regimen appeared superior to gatifloxacin, ofloxacin, or ethambutol during the early phase of a biexponential fall in colony counts, and that moxifloxacin and gatifloxacin caused significant and similar increases in the rate of *M. tuberculosis* clearance during the late phase of the biexponential clearance curve ($p = 0.002$). Substitution of ofloxacin for ethambutol during the first eight weeks of therapy had no effect on SSCC. The same team is currently conducting a phase III, randomized, open label trial of a four-month gatifloxacin-based regimen (two months of gatifloxacin, rifampicin, isoniazid, and pyrazinamide, followed by two months of gatifloxacin, rifampicin, and isoniazid) versus six months of standard, four-drug, first-line therapy in five African countries. Enrollment was stopped in the fourth quarter of 2008, somewhat shy of the originally intended 2070 patients. Patients are to be followed for a total of two years for safety and efficacy. Gatifloxacin development for TB has also been hampered by reports of dysglycemia in some elderly and diabetic patients taking gatifloxacin for other indications (36).

In addition to the SSCC trial noted earlier, investigators have recently completed three phase II trials of moxifloxacin-based regimens in the treatment of adult, pulmonary, drug-sensitive TB: (*i*) the United States Centers for Disease Control and Prevention's (CDC) TB Trials Consortium (TBTC) conducted TBTC Study 27 (37), a randomized, double-blind study of two months of isoniazid, rifampicin, pyrazinamide, and either moxifloxacin or ethambutol (each regimen administered either thrice weekly or five times per week), comparing sputum conversion rates at the end of eight weeks of treatment as the primary efficacy endpoint. The regimens gave statistically indistinguishable sputum conversion rates at eight weeks, irrespective of the frequency of dosing, but the moxifloxacin-containing regimens had a somewhat faster mean time to sputum negativity than the ethambutol-containing regimens (38). (*ii*) Johns Hopkins University investigators and colleagues at Clementino Fraga Filho Hospital in Rio de Janeiro, Brazil conducted a phase II study of similar design except that it was open label and tested only five-days-a-week dosing (39). In this study, the moxifloxacin-containing two-month regimen resulted in a higher proportion of patients converting their sputum to negative at eight weeks of treatment than the ethambutol-containing regimen did (85% vs. 68%; $p = 0.02$) (40). (*iii*) TBTC Study 28, the TBTC evaluated the safety and eight-week sputum conversion rates of rifampicin, pyrazinamide, ethambutol, and either moxifloxacin or isoniazid doses five times per week (41). In this study the moxifloxacin- and isoniazid-containing regimens gave similar sputum conversion rates at eight weeks (42).

Based on results of these four phase II studies, which together indicated that during the two-month, intensive phase of first-line TB treatment, moxifloxacin is well tolerated and at least as efficacious as either ethambutol or isoniazid, moxifloxacin is now undergoing phase III clinical evaluation. The safety and efficacy of two different four-month regimens are being compared in a noninferiority design to the six-month standard, first-line treatment regimen for adult, pulmonary, drug-sensitive TB: one regimen substitutes moxifloxacin for ethambutol in the intensive phase and then adds it to isoniazid and rifampicin during a two-month continuation phase, and the other regimen substitutes moxifloxacin for isoniazid in the intensive phase and then adds it to rifampicin during a two-month continuation phase. This randomized, double-blind study is intended to enroll 800 patients in each of the three treatment arms. The goal, if the results are supportive, is to register one or both four-month, moxifloxacin-based regimens as a first-line treatment for adult, pulmonary TB. If successful, this is likely to represent the first truly novel approved treatment for TB in over thirty years.

B. Diarylquinolines

Another novel, potent class of compounds, the diarylquinolines, are being investigated by Tibotec/Johnson & Johnson and the Global Alliance for TB Drug Development for their utility in TB therapy (43). The lead compound, TMC207 (also known as R207910), is active in vitro against both drug-sensitive and drug-resistant strains of *M. tuberculosis* (MIC 0.06 μg/mL). Strains tested include those resistant to a wide variety of commonly used drugs including isoniazid, rifampicin, streptomycin, ethambutol, pyrazinamide, and the fluoroquinolones. Although TMC207 is active in vitro against other mycobacteria, including *Mycobacterium smegmatis*, *M. kansasii*, *M. bovis*, *M. avium*, and *M. fortuitum*, the compound is not active against a variety of gram-positive and gram-negative organisms such as *Nocardia asteroides*, *Escherichia coli*, *Streptococcus aureus*, *Enterococcus faecium*, or *Haemophilus influenzae*. Of note, two resistant *M. smegmatis* isolates were not cross-resistant to a wide range of antibiotics, including the fluoroquinolones.

Based on gene sequences of drug-resistant mutants, the mechanism of action of TMC207 has been demonstrated to be inhibition of the proton pump of adenosine triphosphate (ATP) synthase. Point mutations that conferred resistance to TMC207 were identified in both *M. tuberculosis* and *M. smegmatis*. In three independent mutants, the only gene commonly affected encoded atpE, a part of the F0 subunit of ATP synthase. Two point mutations were identified, one in *M. smegmatis* and one in *M. tuberculosis*. Further transformation studies confirmed the importance of the atpE gene in the mechanistic pathway of TMC207 (43). Additional genetic, biochemical, and binding assays confirmed ATP synthase to be the target of TMC207 (44). Recently, the drug has been demonstrated to be active against nonreplicating as well as actively replicating bacilli (45).

Pharmacokinetic studies in mice have shown rapid absorption with extensive tissue distribution in at least liver, kidney, heart, spleen, and lung. Of note, half-lives ranged from 28.1 to 92 hours in tissues and from 43.7 to 64 hours in plasma. One contribution to the relatively long half-life appears to be slow redistribution from the tissue compartments. TMC207 has also demonstrated significant in vivo activity in mouse models of both established and nonestablished disease. In the nonestablished disease model mice were treated for four weeks, starting the day after inoculation. In this setting, a once weekly dose of 12.5 mg/kg was almost as efficacious as 6.5 mg/kg given five times per week. At 12.5 and 25 mg/kg, TMC207 was more efficacious than isoniazid at 25 mg/kg administered five days per week. In the established disease model, treatment was begun 12 to 14 days after *M. tuberculosis* inoculation. In combination studies, the substitution of TMC207 for any of the three commonly used drugs (isoniazid, rifampicin, and pyrazinamide) had greater efficacy than the standard regimen of isoniazid, rifampicin, and pyrazinamide. The combination of either TMC207 and isoniazid and pyrazinamide, or TMC207 and rifampicin and pyrazinamide, resulted in negative spleen and lung cultures after eight weeks of therapy (46). Recently, studies of the once-weekly therapy in the established infection model demonstrated that a once-weekly TMC207, rifapentine, pyrazinamide regimen administered for only two months cleared the lungs of bacilli in 9 out of 10 mice and was significantly more efficacious than the once-weekly TMC207 monotherapy or any of the other combination regimens tested, thereby suggesting the potential for developing a significantly shorter and simpler regimen than the current standard of care (47). In another recent study, mice treated with four months of a regimen consisting of TMC207, isoniazid, rifampin and pyrazinamide had relapse rates similar to those of mice treated with six months of standard isoniazid, rifampin and pyrazinamide therapy (97).

TMC207 has also been tested in phase I pharmacokinetic and safety studies in healthy volunteers. A single oral administration of TMC207 at doses ranging from 10 to 700 mg revealed the drug to be well absorbed, with peak serum concentrations at about five hours. The pharmacokinetics were dose-proportional over the range studied. A multiple ascending dose study (once-daily doses of TMC207 at 50, 150, and 400 mg per day for 14 days) was then performed in healthy volunteers. Accumulation was observed with a doubling of the area under the time-concentration curve (AUC) on the 14th day compared to day one; steady state was not achieved by day 14 due to a long terminal elimination half-life (48). Of note, the average observed AUCs were greater than those that achieved optimal activity in the established infection in the mouse. A drug–drug interaction study conducted in healthy volunteers demonstrated that rifampicin decreases the AUC of TMC207 by approximately 50%, presumably resulting from enhanced metabolism of TMC207 by CYP3A4 in the presence of rifampicin, a known inducer of this enzyme (49). Safety evaluations in phase I studies revealed only mild or moderate adverse events with the majority considered only possibly related to the study drug.

A phase II, randomized, open-label, extended EBA study was conducted in South Africa in which TMC207 was dosed at 25 mg, 100 mg, or 400 mg per day for seven days in newly diagnosed, adult, smear-positive, pulmonary TB patients; control patients received either 600 mg per day of rifampicin or 300 mg per day of isoniazid (15 patients per arm). The study showed that starting at approximately Day 4 of dosing, 400 mg per day of TMC207 caused a detectable decrease in sputum colony-forming units (CFUs) relative to pretreatment levels. Lower doses of TMC207 had no detectable effect. Steady state levels of TMC207 were not achieved by Day 7 of dosing. The drug appeared to be well tolerated in this population (50). TMC207 was further evaluated for activity, safety, and tolerability in stage 1 of a randomized, double-blind, phase IIb study in newly diagnosed MDR-TB patients. In stage 1 of this study, either TMC207 or a placebo was administered to MDR-TB patients in addition to a five-drug MDR-TB regimen during the first two months of treatment. TMC207 was dosed at 400 mg per day for two weeks followed by 200 mg three times per week for six weeks. As determined by liquid culture in the MGIT system, 47.5% of patients receiving TMC207 vs. 8.7% of patients receiving placebo in addition to the background MDR-TB regimen, converted their sputum culture to negative at 8 weeks of treatment ($p = 0.003$) (51). In addition, the drug appeared to be well tolerated in these patients, and there were no serious adverse events judged related to the study drug, although some prolongation of the QT interval, when corrected with Fridericia's formula (QTcF), was observed. Stage 2 of this study is currently recruiting; in this stage, newly diagnosed and newly recruited MDR-TB patients will receive TMC207 (same dosing regimen as stage 1) or placebo, in a randomized, double-blind fashion, in addition to a five-drug background MDR-TB treatment regimen for six months. All patients will then continue treatment on an appropriate background MDR-TB regimen for the remainder of their treatment course. The primary efficacy endpoint for stage 2 is sputum conversion rate at six months. The results to date suggest that TMC207 has significant potential for improving MDR-TB therapy. A possible role for the drug as part of a novel, multidrug regimen for drug-sensitive tuberculosis remains to be evaluated.

C. Nitroimidazoles

Two compounds within the nitroimidazole class are currently under investigation as potential anti-TB drugs. These are the nitroimidazo-oxazine, PA-824, being developed by the public–private partnership, Global Alliance for TB Drug Development (TB Alliance; www.tballiance.org), and the dihydroimidazo-oxazole, OPC-67683, being developed by Otsuka Pharmaceutical Company. Each of these compounds can trace its history back to at least the 1970s, when Ciba-Geigy studied a series of nitroimidazoles for their potential as radiosensitizing drugs. These compounds were subsequently discovered to have antimicrobial activity, including activity against *M. tuberculosis*. However, when the lead compound (CGI-17341) was found to be mutagenic in the Ames assay, Ciba-Geigy stopped development of the class.

PA-824

In the 1990s, PathoGenesis, a small biotechnology company, modified the ring structure of the nitroimidazoles that Ciba-Geigy had developed, and thereby discovered the nitroimidazo-oxazines (also referred to in earlier literature as nitroimidazopyrans). From more than 700 novel compounds tested, PA-824 (2-nitro-6, 7-dihydro-5H-imidazo [2, 1-b] (1,3) oxazine) was found to be both nonmutagenic and the most active against *M. tuberculosis* in a murine infection model (52). The development of PA-824 was stopped, however, when Chiron (now Novartis) purchased PathoGenesis in 2000. Soon thereafter, the TB Alliance secured an exclusive license agreement from Chiron that granted the TB Alliance worldwide rights to PA-824 and the other nitroimidazole derivatives that had been discovered by PathoGenesis. Since this agreement, the TB Alliance has been developing PA-824.

The preclinical evaluation of PA-824 revealed in vitro and in vivo activity against *M. tuberculosis*. In vitro studies showed that the minimum inhibitory concentration (MIC) of PA-824 against a variety of drug-sensitive TB isolates is in the range of ≤ 0.015 to 0.25 mg/mL. The activity is highly selective, with potent activity only against Bacille Calmette–Guérin (BCG) and *M. tuberculosis* of the mycobacterial species tested, and without significant activity against a broad range of gram-positive and gram-negative bacteria (with the exception of *Helicobacter pylori* and some anaerobes). Perhaps of even greater significance is the finding in anaerobic culture that PA-824 has activity against nonreplicating bacilli, indicating its potential for activity against persisting organisms and shortening treatment duration. PA-824 is also active against strains of *M. tuberculosis* with known resistance to standard TB therapies, indicating a novel mechanism of action (52).

PA-824 also demonstrates pronounced in vivo activity. Pathogenesis tested PA-824 in a mouse model of TB, employing an *M. tuberculosis* reporter strain expressing firefly luciferase. At oral doses of 25, 50, and 100 mg/kg daily in mice for 10 days, PA-824 significantly reduced *M. tuberculosis* levels in both spleen and lung compared to controls and demonstrated a linear dose response. Longer term mouse studies with PA-824 at 50 mg/kg/d demonstrated reductions in bacillary lung burden similar to isoniazid at 25 mg/kg/d, with all mice treated with PA-824 surviving while all untreated control animals died by day 35. In a guinea pig aerosol infection model, daily oral administration of PA-824 at 37 mg/kg/d for 35 days also produced reductions of *M. tuberculosis* counts in lungs and spleens comparable to those produced by isoniazid (52). Mouse model studies by Grosset, Nuermberger, and colleagues have shown that the minimum effective dose of PA-824 (defined as the minimum dose that prevents the development of gross lung lesions and splenomegaly) is 12.5 mg/kg/d, and that the minimum bactericidal dose of PA-824 (defined as the minimum dose that reduces the lung colony forming unit counts by 99%) is 100 mg/kg/d (53).

Although, as noted earliler, PA-824 appears to have a novel mechanism of action, the exact target is not known. The compound appears to inhibit both protein and lipid synthesis but does not affect nucleic acid synthesis. There is a resultant accumulation of hydroxymycolic acid with a concomitant reduction in ketomycolic acids, suggesting inhibition of an enzyme responsible for the oxidation of hydroxymycolate to ketomycolate (52,54). Interestingly, PA-824 is a prodrug that undergoes activation via an F420-dependent mechanism. Mutations in the gene encoding the F420 enzyme (*fgd*) are responsible for some instances of PA-824 resistance identified in vitro (54). One hypothesis is that PA-824 undergoes nitroreduction, producing highly reactive intermediates, including nitrous oxide, which interacts with multiple intracellular targets (55). Several other drugs used in TB treatment are also prodrugs, including isoniazid, pyrazinamide, and ethionamide (a second-line TB drug).

When tested in the Ames assay, both with and without S9 activation, PA-824, unlike the Ciba-Geigy lead compound, CGI-17341, has shown no evidence of mutagenicity. Furthermore, chromosomal aberration, mouse micronucleus, and mouse lymphoma tests have all been negative, confirming no evidence of genotoxic potential for the compound. Of importance also are the in vitro findings that PA-824 neither inhibits nor is metabolized by major P450 enzyme isoforms, indicating a low potential for drug–drug interactions with the presently used AIDS antiretrovirals (56).

Pharmacokinetic studies of PA-824 in rats indicate excellent tissue penetration. Total exposure in lung for example, as measured by AUC is approximately twofold higher than exposure in plasma.

The TB Alliance filed an IND for development of PA-824 in April 2005, and since then has performed a number of safety, tolerability, and pharmacokinetic phase I trials in healthy volunteers to better understand this drug's potential. These studies demonstrated that PA-824 has a pharmacokinetic profile consistent with once daily or less frequent oral dosing in humans, and appears to be safe and well tolerated in this population (98,99). Most recently, PA-824 was evaluated in an extended EBA study in newly diagnosed, adult, sputum smear-positive, TB patients in South Africa, which demonstrated that PA-824 has a substantial and (at doses of 200 to 1200 mg per day) an equivalent ability to kill *M. tuberculosis* in patient sputa over a 14-day period when given as monotherapy (57). The next planned clinical trial is a second extended EBA study, to further define an appropriate clinical dose to take into late-stage development, evaluating doses of 200 mg per day and below. This study initiated enrollment in South Africa in the third quarter of 2009.

OPC-67683

The dihydroimidazo-oxazole, OPC-67683, is a newly synthesized nitroimidazole under development by Otsuka Pharmaceutical Company for the treatment of TB. Currently in phase II of clinical development in MDR-TB patients, Otsuka has reported that the compound has extremely potent in vitro antimicrobial activity against *M. tuberculosis*, with MICs against multiple clinically isolated TB strains ranging from 0.006 to 0.024 µg/mL

(58). As with PA-824, OPC-67683 shows no cross-resistance with any of the currently used first-line TB drugs, thereby also most likely indicating a novel mechanism of action. Based on their relatively similar chemical structure, it is likely that the mechanisms of action of PA-824 and OPC-67683 will prove to be the same.

In a chronic infection mouse model, the efficacy of OPC-67683 is superior to that of the currently used TB drugs. In these experiments, the effective plasma concentration was 0.100 μg/mL, which was achieved with an oral dose of 0.625 mg/kg, confirming the remarkable in vitro potency of OPC-67683.

Phase I studies were completed and the drug was well tolerated. An ongoing phase II study is evaluating the efficacy and safety of OPC-67683 compared to placebo when each is added to a standardized MDR-TB treatment regimen for the first two months of treatment. The study is currently enrolling at ten sites in six countries with an enrollment goal of 430 participants (59). Little additional information on the clinical development of this compound is publicly available.

D. Pyrroles

Another class of compounds being investigated for TB therapy is the pyrroles. First described in 1998 by Diedda et al. (60) as having antimycobacterial activities, the most potent compound was designated BM212. MICs for BM212 ranged between 0.7 and 1.5 μg/mL against several strains of *M. tuberculosis*. The MICs for strains resistant to the commonly used antitubercular drugs were similar to those for sensitive strains, most likely indicating a novel mechanism of action. However, no mechanism of action has yet been elucidated for this class of compounds. Some non-TB mycobacterial strains also appeared to be sensitive to BM212, albeit with MICs higher than for *M. tuberculosis*.

A novel pyrrole compound, LL3858, discovered by Lupin Limited, is currently in clinical development for TB (61). Limited information on this compound is publicly available; however, the compound has been reported by Lupin to have submicromolar MICs and significant efficacy in a mouse model of TB. In combination with currently used anti-TB drugs, LL3858 reportedly sterilized the lungs and spleens of infected animals in a shorter timeframe than with conventional therapy. The compound has been evaluated in phase I single- and multiple-dose ascending dose studies in human volunteers in India and is currently awaiting regulatory approval for a phase IIa proof-of-concept study (62).

E. Diamines

SQ109, an adamantan-ethane-diamine, is under development by Sequella, Inc. for its potential use in the treatment of TB. Although originally conceived as a second-generation improvement of the first-line TB drug, ethambutol, its structural dissimilarity to ethambutol and potential differences in its intracellular target(s) suggest that it may be a truly novel antimycobacterial agent and not simply an ethambutol analog.

A diverse combinatorial library of compounds with the 1, 2-diamine pharmacophore of ethambutol was synthesized and tested for activity against *M. tuberculosis* (63). After a series of sequential in vitro and in vivo tests, SQ109 was ultimately identified as the most potent compound in the series and was subjected to pharmacokinetic (PK)/pharmacodynamic (PD) testing.

In vitro studies of SQ109 revealed an MIC against *M. tuberculosis* in the range of 0.1 to 0.63 mg/mL, with 99% inhibition of *M. tuberculosis* growth in macrophages at its

MIC. The compound is also active against MDR strains of *M. tuberculosis* in vitro, and *M. tuberculosis* demonstrates a relatively low mutational frequency for developing resistance to SQ109 (2.18×10^{-9}). In vivo mouse studies showed a reduction of 2 to 2.5 log in CFU counts in lung and spleen with enhanced antimycobacterial activity when used in combination with rifampicin and isoniazid (rapid-mouse model and chronic-infection model).

Although the mechanism of action of SQ109 appears to be that of a cell wall inhibitor because it induces, like other cell wall-targeting antibiotics (ethambutol, isoniazid, ethionamide, and thiacetazone), the Rv0341 promoter, the specific target of SQ109 is not yet clearly defined (64).

The pharmacokinetic profile of SQ109 (65) is interesting in that the oral bioavailability of the drug in mice is only 4%. However, SQ109 distributes into lungs and spleen at concentrations exceeding the MIC, and therefore the relatively low overall oral bioavailability of this drug may not represent a hindrance to the drug's use. Cytochrome P450 reaction phenotyping suggests exclusive involvement of CYP2D6 and CYP2C19 in SQ109 metabolism. Incubation of SQ109 with human, mouse, dog, and rat microsomes suggests similar metabolism of the drug in all tested species.

An IND for clinical development of SQ109 was filed by Sequella, Inc. with the U.S. FDA in August 2006. Since that time it has been evaluated in a single ascending dose, phase I study in healthy volunteers at doses from 5 mg to 300 mg. It demonstrated linear pharmacokinetics in the dose range studied and a half-life of approximately 60 hours after a single 300 mg dose (66).

F. Oxazolidinones

The oxazolidinones, a relatively new class of antimicrobial agents, exert their antimicrobial effect by inhibiting protein synthesis and by binding to the 70S ribosomal initiation complex (67,68). They have a relatively broad spectrum of activity, including anaerobic and gram-positive aerobic bacteria as well as mycobacteria (69,70). The class was initially discovered at DuPont in the 1970s (71,72).

The first and thus far the only oxazolidinone to be approved is linezolid. Although not approved for use in TB, linezolid has in vitro activity against *M. tuberculosis*. Of the oxazolidinones that have been evaluated for their activity in in vivo systems, the most active appears to be PNU-100480, with efficacy similar to that of isoniazid or rifampicin (70).

Because of the clinical availability of linezolid, it has been used sporadically in patients with MDR-TB and demonstrates biologic activity as evidenced by sputum–culture conversion (73). However, with relatively long-term use in MDR-TB patients, there are emerging reports of peripheral and optic neuropathy (74). NIAID is currently evaluating linezolid in XDR-TB patients in South Korea in an open label, randomized, two arm trial (75), and the CDC is planning a one-period, double-blind, single-center pharmacokinetic study of linezolid in patients with MDR or XDR-TB (76).

Linezolid's neuropathic side effects will likely require careful monitoring if it becomes more commonly used in the treatment of MDR-TB.

Recently, investigators from Johns Hopkins University and Pfizer, Inc. presented promising data on a novel oxazolidinone with improved potency against *M. tuberculosis* compared to linezolid in a mouse infection model: PNU-100480 (PNU) (77). Whereas linezolid is primarily bacteriostatic in the mouse model, PNU demonstrated both bacteri-cidal and sterilizing activity, and more rapid clearance of bacilli from the lungs of mice in various three- and four-drug combinations with rifampicin, moxifloxacin, isoniazid, and pyrazinamide than the standard three-drug combination of rifampicin, isoniazid, and pyrazinamide. Adding PNU to a standard rifampicin, isoniazid, and pyrazinamide com-bination therapy in the mouse, shortened treatment by one to two months. This novel compound deserves further careful evaluation in vivo for safety and efficacy.

G. Macrolides

The macrolides, potent inhibitors of protein synthesis, bind to the 50S ribosomal subunit of bacteria at the peptidyl transferase center formed with 23S rRNA; they may also block formation of the 50S subunit in growing cells. Macrolides therefore have the potential to add a novel mechanism of action to TB combination therapy, and thereby also hold the promise of being equally effective against MDR-TB and drug-sensitive TB. The macrolides, known to be orally active, have also proven to be safe and well-tolerated when used for non-TB indications. Key for TB treatment, they also tend to exhibit high levels of intracellular activity and extensive distribution into the lungs. This class of antibiotics has therefore recently been evaluated as potential TB therapy at the Institute for Tuberculosis Research at the University of Illinois at Chicago, in conjunction with the TB Alliance.

Erythromycin, a natural product isolated from *Streptomyces erythreus* in the 1950s, represents the first-generation macrolides. It has proven to be effective in treatment of infections caused by gram-positive bacteria, but its use is hampered by its short serum half-life and by its side effects on gastric motility. This latter characteristic, due to marked acid lability, causes gastrointestinal discomfort. Second-generation macrolides, including azithromycin, clarithromycin, and roxithromycin, were successfully developed by blocking the acid degradation pathway of erythromycin. Although they have little activity against *M. tuberculosis*, many of the second-generation antibiotics have proven to be potent against *M. avium* and *M. leprae*. Second-generation macrolides also demonstrate good potency against other mycobacterial pathogens, including *M. kansasii*, *M. xenopi*, and *M. marinum*.

Unfortunately, gram-positive cocci have developed significant levels of resistance to the second-generation macrolides, primarily via two mechanisms: efflux pathways (encoded by *mef* genes) and ribosome modification (due to activity of methyl transferases encoded by *erm* genes). Third-generation macrolides, represented primarily by members of the ketolide class, have been developed to overcome this resistance. Telithromycin, the first commercially available third-generation macrolide, is more potent than clar-ithromycin against mycobacteria, including *M. tuberculosis*, *M. bovis*, BCG, *M. avium*, *M. ulcerans*, *M. paratuberculosis*, *M. africanum*, and *M. simiae* (78).

Recent work at the University of Illinois at Chicago by Scott Franzblau and col-leagues to develop even more potent macrolides for the treatment of TB involved modify-ing various substituents on the macrolide scaffold to enhance potency while maintaining low toxicity and avoiding key resistance mechanisms and drug–drug interactions. Unfor-tunately, more potent macrolides were not identified in this project. To the best of the authors' knowledge, no new macrolides are currently under investigation for TB treat-ment. Clarithromycin, however, is used off-label as part of a multidrug regimen to treat some patients with MDR- and XDR-TB (4,79,80).

H. Riminophenazines

Clofazimine is the prototype riminophenazine, a class of drugs that may inhibit mycobacterial respiration; the precise mechanism of action has not yet been elucidated. Clofazimine is used in treatment of leprosy, another mycobacterial disease, and occasionally as a second-line drug in the treatment of MDR- and XDR-TB. It has significant potency in vitro and in the mouse model (81), but its use is hampered primarily by its long half-life in humans (82) and its propensity to accumulate in the subcutaneous adipose tissue, together causing a long-lasting, red discoloration of the skin in patients treated for an extended period with the drug. Efforts are currently underway by the TB Alliance in collaboration with the Institute of Materia Medica and the Beijing Tuberculosis and Thoracic Tumor Research Institute in Beijing, P.R. China to identify a new generation of riminophenazines that will improve on clofazimine's tolerability profile, while maintaining or even enhancing its efficacy against TB.

I. Long-Acting Rifamycins

Rifampin has probably had the greatest impact of any drug on shortening the duration of therapy for active TB disease. However, even rifampicin-based regimens must be administered for at least six months for optimal effectiveness, usually daily for the first two months of therapy and then three to seven days a week for the ensuing four months. Regimens based on more intermittently delivered dosing have proven to be less efficacious and have demonstrated higher rates of acquired rifampicin resistance in HIV-infected patients. Therefore, several other rifamycin derivatives with significantly longer serum half-lives than rifampicin's (which is two to four hours) have been evaluated in intermittent regimens. Rifabutin, with a terminal half-life of 36 hours, was the first to enter clinical testing (83). The initial trials tested its potential role in prophylaxis for MAC infection in HIV-positive individuals (84). Rifabutin was approved for MAC prophylaxis in the United States and for the treatment of TB in several other countries, but it is now utilized primarily as a rifampicin substitute in patients for whom rifampicin-based drug–drug interactions are problematic (85). It is not recommended for use as part of intermittent regimens in patients with advanced immunosuppression due to associated high rates of acquired rifamycin resistance in these individuals (83).

Rifalazil, a second long-acting rifamycin derivative, has an even longer half-life than rifabutin (approximately 60 hours), demonstrates relatively high potency against *M. tuberculosis* in animal-infection models (86), and has a relatively low potential for drug–drug interactions (87). In phase I tolerability studies, however, rifalazil (50 mg single dose) was associated with unacceptably high rates of a "flu-like" syndrome (88). This dose-limiting side effect may be due to cytokine release, as it is associated with increased interleukin-6 serum levels. Once-weekly rifalazil did not demonstrate significant antimycobacterial activity in an EBA study (at relatively low doses: 10 and 25 mg) when administered with isoniazid for two weeks (89). There is the potential that rifalazil analogs could be identified with a better tolerability profile and low potential for enzyme induction, but there are no currently active programs investigating such compounds for TB treatment.

The best studied of the long-acting rifamycins has been rifapentine, a cyclopentyl-substituted rifampicin with a half-life of 14 hours to 18 hours in healthy adults. Following a 600 mg dose, serum levels in excess of the MIC persist beyond 72 hours, suggesting the potential for intermittent administration. Daniel et al. reported that in mice, a once weekly continuation phase of rifapentine and isoniazid for four months following a standard two-month induction phase with daily isoniazid, rifampicin, and pyrazinamide was as effective as standard therapy given daily for six months (90). This work stimulated the large phase III trial that was begun by the CDC in 1995 (known as TBTC Study 22).

Study 22 randomized adults with newly diagnosed, drug-susceptible pulmonary TB to a four-month (16-week) continuation phase regimen of either once-weekly rifapentine–isoniazid or twice-weekly rifampicin–isoniazid following a standard two-month induction phase (91). Early in the trial, however, a high rate of relapse with acquired rifampicin-monoresistance was found among HIV-positive patients assigned to the rifapentine arm, and enrollment of HIV-positive patients was stopped (92).

The results of this study, along with other rifapentine data, led to the approval of rifapentine for the treatment of TB in the United States and to a recommendation for the use of a once-weekly rifapentine–isoniazid continuation phase regimen for HIV-negative adults with drug-susceptible, noncavitary TB and negative acid-fast bacilli (AFB) smears at two months (7). However, rifapentine-based treatment is not recommended either for those with cavitary disease or concomitant HIV infection. Experimental studies have also suggested that weekly rifapentine and isoniazid for as short a period as three months may provide effective treatment for LTBI (93). Therefore, in 2002 the CDC embarked on an ambitious study, intended to randomize 8000 patients with LTBI to either weekly rifapentine–isoniazid for 12 weeks or daily isoniazid for nine months. This study is now expected to complete in 2010 (94).

Interest has also recently been rekindled in the potential of high-dose rifapentine to shorten therapy of drug-sensitive, active TB. Nuermberger and colleagues published data from the mouse aerosol-infection model (95) demonstrating that a daily or thrice weekly rifapentine (at 10 mg/kg or 15 mg/kg, respectively), moxifloxacin, pyrazinamide regimen sterilizes the lungs of mice (i.e., produces relapse-free survival) in three months compared to six months for the standard rifampicin, isoniazid, pyrazinamide regimen. However, the potential for use of high dose rifapentine-based regimens in humans will require a careful evaluation of safety, tolerability, and pharmacokinetics, as well as efficacy, in appropriate animal toxicity studies and subsequent clinical trials. A recent phase I study (96) demonstrated that rifapentine metabolic autoinduction produces moderate decreases in both moxifloxacin and rifapentine plasma exposures when the drugs are co-administered and may result in rifamycin hypersensitivity syndrome in a subset of patients. However, if appropriate, safe, well-tolerated regimens can be defined, rifapentine has the potential to make a substantial contribution to shortening the duration of therapy for drug-sensitive TB.

VIII.   Future Prospects in TB Drug Development

Ten years ago, the pipeline of novel TB drugs was virtually nonexistent. Now it is reinvigorated and growing, with at least seven drugs currently in clinical testing for drug-sensitive and/or MDR-TB. There is also a more robust Discovery-stage portfolio now than has existed in many decades, targeting a wide variety of *M. tuberculosis* enzymes and pathways. These Discovery efforts are focused to a significant degree on mycobacterial functions and novel targets that are believed essential to cell survival during slow- or nonreplicating persistence. The results of such efforts should be new, antituberculosis drugs that shorten therapy of both drug-sensitive and drug-resistant TB. More efficient development of these novel TB drugs and identification of optimized treatment regimens will require enhanced clinical trial site capacity in high-burden TB settings and validated surrogate markers of drug efficacy to speed clinical testing. The lack of TB drug development over the past several decades means that few clinical trial sites in TB-endemic regions are experienced in the conduct of registration-quality TB drug trials and little effort has gone into identification and validation of biomarkers for TB drug development. New paradigms are also needed to speed clinical development of novel regimens for both drug-sensitive and drug-resistant TB. The current approaches of substituting a new drug for one of the current drugs (for drug-sensitive TB) or adding a new drug to what is already typically a five-drug regimen (for drug-resistant TB) are too slow and unwieldy to satisfy the urgent medical need for improved TB treatments.

References

1. Fox W, Ellard G, Mitchison DA. Studies on the treatment of tuberculosis undertaken by the British Medical Research Council tuberculosis units, 1946–1986, with relevant subsequent publications. Int J Tuberc Lung Dis 1999; 3(10)(suppl. 2):S231–S279.
2. World Health Organization. Global Tuberculosis Control 2008 – Surveillance, Planning, Financing. WHO Report 2008. Geneva, Switzerland: World Health Organization. WHO/HTM/TB/2008.393.
3. U.S. Centers for Disease Control and Prevention (CDC). Emergence of *Mycobacterium tuberculosis* with extensive resistance to second-line drugs-worldwide, 2000–2004. MMWR Morb Mortal Wkly Rep 2006; 55:301–305.
4. Mitnick CD, Shin SS, Seung KJ, et al. Comprehensive treatment of extensively drug-resistant tuberculosis. N Engl J Med 2008; 359:563–574.
5. Andrews JR, Gandhi NR, Moodley P, et al. Tugela Ferry Care and Research Collaboration. Exogenous reinfection as a cause of multidrug-resistant and extensively drug-resistant tuberculosis in rural South Africa. J Infect Dis 2008; 198(11):1582–1589.
6. World Health Organization. Treatment of Tuberculosis: Guidelines for National Programmes, 3rd ed. Geneva, Switzerland: World Health Organization, 1993. WHO/CDS/TB/2003.313.
7. American Thoracic Society/Centers for Disease Control and Prevention/Infectious Diseases Society of America. Treatment of tuberculosis. Am J Respir Crit Care Med 2003; 167:603–662.
8. Burman WJ. Issues in the management of HIV-related tuberculosis. Clin Chest Med 2005; 26(2):283–294.
9. Ginsberg AM. Novel Treatment strategies for TB patients with HIV coinfection. In: Kaufmann S, van Helden P, eds. Tuberculosis Handbook, Vol. 3. Weinheim, Germany: Wiley-VCH, 2008:213–225.
10. Youmans GP, Williston EH, Feldman WH, et al. Increase in resistance of tubercle bacilli to streptomycin; a preliminary report. Proc Staff Meet Mayo Clin 1946; 21:126–127.
11. Crofton J, Mitchison DA. Streptomycin resistance in pulmonary tuberculosis. Br Med J 1948; 2:1009–1015.
12. World Health Organization. Anti-tuberculosis Drug Resistance in the World. Fourth Global Report 2008. Geneva, Switzerland: World Health Organization. WHO/HTM/TB/2008.394.
13. U.S. Centers for Disease Control and Prevention (CDC). Emergence of *Mycobacterium tuberculosis* with extensive resistance to second-line drugs—worldwide, 2000–2004. MMWR Morb Mortal Wkly Rep 2006; 55:301–305 [revised definition: MMWR Morb Mortal Wkly Rep 2006; 55:1176].
14. http://www.who.int/tb/challenges/xdr/xdr_map_june08.pdf. Accessed December 2008.
15. Moore-Gillon J. Multidrug-resistant tuberculosis: This is the cost. Ann N Y Acad Sci 2001; 953:233–240.
16. Dye C, Williams BG, Espinal MA, et al. Erasing the world's slow stain: Strategies to beat multidrug-resistant tuberculosis. Science 2002; 295:2042–2046.
17. Costa JG, Santos AC, Rodrigues LC, et al. Tuberculosis in Salvador, Brazil: Costs to health system and families. Rev Saude Publica 2005; 39(1):1–7.

18. Espinal MA. The global situation of MDR-TB. Tuberculosis 2003; 83:44–51.
19. Mitnick CD, Castro KG, Harrington M, et al. Randomized trials to optimize treatment of multidrug-resistant tuberculosis. PLoS Med 2007; 4(11):e292.
20. Sacks LV, Behrman RE. Developing new drugs for the treatment of drug-resistant tuberculosis: A regulatory perspective. Tuberculosis (Edinb) 2008; 88(suppl. 1):S93–S100.
21. http://www.who.int/mediacentre/factsheets/fs104/en/index.html. Accessed November 2008.
22. American Thoracic Society, Centers for Disease Control and Prevention. Targeted tuberculin testing and treatment of latent tuberculosis infection. Am J Respir Crit Care Med 2000; 161(suppl):S221–S247.
23. Gordin F, Chaisson RE, Matts JP, et al. Rifampin and pyrazinamide vs. isoniazid for prevention of tuberculosis in HIV-infected persons: An international randomized trial. JAMA 2000; 283:1445–1450.
24. Ojha AK, Baughn AD, Sambandan D, et al. Growth of Mycobacterium tuberculosis biofilms containing free mycolic acids and harbouring drug-tolerant bacteria. Mol Microbiol 2008; 69(1):164–174.
25. Lenaerts AJ, Hoff D, Aly S, et al. Location of persisting mycobacteria in the Guinea pig model of tuberculosis revealed by R207910. Antimicrob Agents Chemother 2007; 51:3338–3345.
26. Muñoz-Elías EJ, Timm J, Botha T, et al. Replication dynamics of *Mycobacterium tuberculosis* in chronically infected mice. Infect Immun 2005; 73(1):546–551.
27. Tuberculosis Research Centre. Shortening short course chemotherapy: A randomized clinical trial for treatment of smear positive pulmonary tuberculosis with regimens using ofloxacin in the intensive phase. Ind J Tuberc 2002; 49:27–38.
28. Mitchison DA. Assessment of new sterilizing drugs for treating pulmonary tuberculosis by culture at 2 months. Am Rev Respir Dis 1993; 147:1062–1063.
29. Tuberculosis Research Centre. A controlled clinical trial of oral short-course regimens in the treatment of sputum-positive pulmonary tuberculosis. Int J Tuberc Lung Dis 1997; 1(6):509–517.
30. Hu Y, Coates AR, Mitchison DA. Sterilizing activities of fluoroquinolones against rifampin-tolerant populations of *Mycobacterium tuberculosis*. Antimicrob Agents Chemother 2003; 47:653–657.
31. Lounis N, Bentoucha A, Truffot-Pernot C, et al. Effectiveness of once-weekly rifapentine and moxifloxacin regimens against *Mycobacterium tuberculosis* in mice. Antimicrob Agents Chemother 2001; 45:3482–3486.
32. Nuermberger EL, Yoshimatsu T, Tyagi S, et al. Moxifloxacin-containing regimen greatly reduces time to culture conversion in murine tuberculosis. Am J Respir Crit Care Med 2004; 169:334–335.
33. Gosling RD, Uiso LO, Sam NE, et al. The bactericidal activity of moxifloxacin in patients with pulmonary tuberculosis. Am J Respir Crit Care Med 2003; 168:1342–1345.
34. Pletz MW, De Roux A, Roth A, et al. Early bactericidal activity of moxifloxacin in treatment of pulmonary tuberculosis: A prospective, randomized study. Antimicrob Agents Chemother 2004; 48:780–782.
35. Rustomjee R, Lienhardt C, Kanyok T, et al. Gatifloxacin for TB (OFLOTUB) study team. A Phase II study of the sterilizing activities of ofloxacin, gatifloxacin and moxifloxacin in pulmonary tuberculosis. Int J Tuberc Lung Dis 2008; 12(2):128–138.
36. Park-Wyllie LY, Juurlink DN, Kopp A, et al. Outpatient gatifloxacin therapy and dysglycemia in older adults. N Engl J Med 2006; 354:1352–1361.
37. TBTC Study 27: Moxifloxacin vs Ethambutol for TB Treatment. www.clinicaltrials.gov.
38. Burman WJ, Goldberg S, Johnson JL, et al. Moxifloxacin versus ethambutol in the first 2 months of treatment for pulmonary tuberculosis. Am J Respir Crit Care Med 2006; 174(3):331–338. Epub 2006 May 4.
39. Moxifloxacin As Part of a Multi-Drug Regimen For Tuberculosis. www.clinicaltrials.gov.

40. Conde MB, Efron A, Loredo C, et al. Moxifloxacin versus ethambutol in the initial treatment of tuberculosis: a double-blind, randomised, controlled, Phase 2 trial. Lancet 2009; 373(9670):1183–1189.
41. TBTC Study 28: Moxifloxacin Versus Isoniazid for TB Treatment. www.clinicaltrials.gov.
42. Dorman SE, Johnson JL, Goldberg S, et al. Substitution of moxifloxacin for isoniazid during intensive phase treatment of pulmonary tuberculosis: Study 28 of the Tuberculosis Trials Consortium. Am J Resp Crit Care Med 2009; 180(3):273–280.
43. Andries K, Verhasselt P, Guillemont H, et al. A diarylquinoline drug active on the ATP synthase of *Mycobacterium tuberculosis*. Science 2005; 307:223–227.
44. Koul A, Dendouga N, Vergauwen K, et al. Diarylquinolines target subunit c of mycobacterial ATP synthase. Nat Chem Biol 2007; 3(6):323–324. Epub 2007 May 13.
45. Koul A, Vranckx L, Dendouga N, et al. Diarylquinolines are bactericidal for dormant mycobacteria as a result of disturbed ATP homeostasis. J Biol Chem 2008; 283(37):25273–25280. [Epub 2008 Jul 14.]
46. Ibrahim M, Andries K, Lounis N, et al. Synergistic activity of R207910 combined with pyrazinamide against murine tuberculosis. Antimicrob Agents Chemother 2007; 51(3):1011–1015. [Epub 2006 Dec 18.]
47. Veziris N, Ibrahim M, Lounis N, et al. Once-weekly R207910-containing regimen exceeds activity of the standard daily regimen in murine tuberculosis. Am J Respir Crit Care Med 2008. [Epub ahead of print as doi:10.1164/rccm.200711-1736OC.]
48. McNeeley D. Open Forum on Key Issues in TB Drug Development, London, U.K., 2006. Available at: http://www.kaisernetwork.org/health_cast/uploaded_files/McNeeley,_David_ (12–12)_TMC207.pdf. Accessed December 2008.
49. Lounis N, Gevers T, Van Den Berg J, et al. Impact of the interaction of R207910 with rifampin on the treatment of tuberculosis studied in the mouse model. Antimicrob Agents Chemother 2008; 52(10):3568–3572. [Epub 2008 Jul 21.]
50. Rustomjee R, Diacon A, Allen J, et al. Early bactericidal activity and pharmacokinetics of the investigational diarylquinoline TMC207 in treatment of pulmonary tuberculosis. Antimicrob Agents Chemother 2008; 52:2831–2835.
51. Diacon AH, Pym A, Grobusch M, et al. Interim analysis of a double-blind, placebo-controlled study with TMC207 in patients with multi-drug resistant (MDR) tuberculosis. In: 48th Annual ICAAC/IDSA 46th Annual Meeting, Washington, D.C., Oct 23–28, 2008; Abstract B-881b.
52. Stover CK, Warrener P, VanDevanter DR, et al. A small-molecule nitroimidazopyran drug candidate for the treatment of tuberculosis. Nature 2000; 405:962–966.
53. Grosset J, Nuermberger E, Yoshimatsu T, et al. The nitroimidazopyran PA-824 has promising activity in the mouse model of TB. Am J Respir Crit Care Med 2004; 169(suppl):A260.
54. Manjunatha UH, Boshoff H, Dowd CS, et al. Identification of a nitroimidazo-oxazine-specific protein involved in PA-824 resistance in *Mycobacterium tuberculosis*. Proc Natl Acad Sci U S A 2006; 103(2):431–436. [Epub 2005 Dec 30.]
55. Singh R, Manjunatha UH, Boshoff HI, et al. PA-824 kills nonreplicating *Mycobacterium tuberculosis* by intracellular NO release. Science 2008; 322(5906):1392–1395.
56. Global Alliance for TB Drug Development, personal communication, December 2008.
57. Ginsberg A, Diacon A, Dawson R, et al. Abstracts of Presentations. In: 48th Annual ICAAC/IDSA 46th Annual Meeting, Washington, D.C., Oct 23–28, 2008. Abstract B-881a. Extended Early Bactericidal Activity (EBA) of PA-824, a Novel Drug for Tuberculosis Treatment.
58. Sasaki H, Haraguchi Y, Itotani M, et al. Synthesis and antituberculosis activity of a novel series of optically active 6-nitro-2,3-dihydroimidazo[2,1-b]oxazoles. J Med Chem 2006; 49(26):7854–7860.
59. Personal Communication: Dr. Lawrence Geiter, Otsuka Pharmaceutical Company, December 2, 2008.

60. Diedda D, Lampis G, Fioravanti R, et al. Bactericidal activities of the pyrrole derivative BM212 against multidrug-resistant and intramacrophagic *M. tuberculosis* strains. Antimicrob Agents Chemother 1998; 42:3035–3037.
61. Arora SK, Sinha N, Sinha RK, et al. Synthesis and in vitro anti-mycobacterial activity of a novel anti-TB composition LL4858. In:44th Annual Interscience Conference on Antimicrobial Agents and Chemotherapy (ICAAC), Washington, D. C., Oct 30–Nov 2, 2004; Abstract F-1115–2004.
62. Personal communication: Dr. Rajender Kamboj, President, Novel Drug Discovery & Development, Lupin Limited, Pune, India to Stop TB Partnership Working Group on New Drugs, 30 September 2008.
63. Lee R, Protopopova M, Crooks E, et al. Combinatorial lead optimization of (1, 2)-diamines based on ethambutol as potential antituberculosis preclinical candidates. J Comb Chem 2003; 5:172–187.
64. Boshoff HI, Myers TG, Copp BR, et al. The transcriptional responses of *M. tuberculosis* to inhibitors of metabolism: Novel insights into drug mechanisms of action. J Bio Chem 2004; 279:40174–40184.
65. Jia L, Tomaszewski JE, Hanrahan C, et al. Pharmacodynamics and pharmacokinetics of SQ109, a new diamine-based antitubercular drug. Br J Pharmacol 2005; 144:80–87.
66. Horwith G, Einck L, Protopopova M, et al. Abstract of Presentation. In: 45th IDSA Annual Meeting, San Diego, C. A., Oct 4–7, 2007.
67. Birmingham MC, Rayner CR, Meagher AK, et al. Linezolid for the treatment of multidrug-resistant, gram-positive infections: Experience from a compassionate use program. Clin Infect Dis 2003; 36c:159–168.
68. Eustice DC, Feldman PA, Zajac PA, et al. Mechanism of action of DuP 721: Inhibition of an early event during initiation of protein synthesis. Antimicrob Agents Chemother 1988; 32:1218–1222.
69. Slee AM, Wuonola MA, McRipley RJ, et al. Oxazolidinones, a new class of synthetic antibacterial agents: In vitro and in vivo activities of DuP 105 and DuP 721. Antimicrob Agents Chemother 1987; 31:1791–1797.
70. Cynamon MH, Kelmens SP, Sharpe CA, et al. Activities of several novel oxazolidinones against *M. tuberculosis* in a murine model. Antimicrob Agents Chemother 1999; 43:1189–1191.
71. Gregory WA, Brittelli DR, Wang C-LU, et al. Antibacterials, synthesis and structure-activity studies of 3-aryl-2-oxooxazolidines. 2. The "A" Group. J Med Chem 1990; 33:2569–2578.
72. Gregory WA, Brittelli DR, Wang C-LJ, et al. Antibacterials, synthesis and structure-activity studies of 3-aryl-2-oxooxazolidinones. 1. The "B" Group. J Med Chem 1989; 32:1673–1681.
73. Dworkin F, Winters SS, Munsiff C, et al. Use of linezolid in treating multidrug-resistant tuberculosis in New York City. Am J Respir Crit Care Med 2004; 169(suppl):A233.
74. Bressler AM, Zimmer SM, Gilmore JL, et al. Peripheral neuropathy associated with prolonged use of linezolid. Lancet Infect Dis 2004; 4:528–531.
75. Linezolid to Treat Extensively-Drug Resistant Tuberculosis. www.clinicaltrials.gov.
76. Linezolid Pharmacokinetics (PK) in Multi-Drug Resistant (MDR)/Extensively-Drug Resistant (XDR) Tuberculosis. www.clinicaltrials.gov.
77. Williams K, Stover CK, Brickner S, et al. The oxazolidinone PNU-100480 has strong bactericidal and sterilizing activity in the murine model of tuberculosis (TB). Abstracts of Presentations. In: 48th Annual ICAAC/IDSA 46th Annual Meeting Washington D.C., Oct 23–28, 2008.
78. Rastogi N, Goh KS, Berchel M, et al. In vitro activities of the ketolides telithromycin (HMR 3647) and HMR 3004 compared to those of clarithromycin against slowly growing mycobacteria at pHs 6.8 and 7.4. Antimicrob Agents Chemother 2000; 44:2848–2852.
79. Chan E, Iseman M. Current medical treatment for tuberculosis. Br Med J 2002; 325:1282–1286.

80. Di Perri G, Bonora S. Which agents should we use for the treatment of multidrug-resistant *Mycobacterium tuberculosis*? J Antimicrob Chemother 2004; 54:593–602.
81. Van Rensburg CEJ, Jooné GK, Sirgel FA, et al. In vitro investigation of the antimicrobial activities of novel tetramethylpiperidine-substituted phenazines against *Mycobacterium tuberculosis*. Chemotherapy 2000; 46:43–48.
82. Nix DE, Adamb RD, Auclair B, et al. Pharmacokinetics and relative bioavailability of clofazimine in relation to food, orange juice and antacid. Tuberculosis 2004; 84(6):365–373.
83. O'Brien RJ, Lyle MA, Snider DE Jr. Rifabutin (ansamycin LM 427): A new rifamycin-S derivative for the treatment of mycobacterial diseases. Rev Infect Dis 1987; 9:519–530.
84. Nightingale SD, Cameron DW, Gordin FM, et al. Two controlled trials of rifabutin prophylaxis against *Mycobacterium avium* complex infection in AIDS. N Engl J Med 1993; 329, 828–833.
85. Centers for Disease Control and Prevention. Updated guidelines for the use of rifabutin or rifampin for the treatment and prevention of tuberculosis among HIV-infected patients taking protease inhibitors or nonnucleoside reverse transcriptase inhibitors. Morb Mortal Wkly Rep 2000; 49:185–189.
86. Klemens SP, Cynamon MH. Activity of KRM-1648 in combination with isoniazid against *Mycobacterium tuberculosis* in a murine model. Antimicrob Agents Chemother 1996; 40:298–301.
87. Mae T, Hosoe K, Yamamoto T, et al. Effect of a new rifamycin derivative, rifalazil, on liver microsomal enzyme induction in rat and dog. Xenobiotica 1998; 28:759–766.
88. Rose L, Vasiljev KM, Adams P, et al. Safety and pharmacokinetics of PA-1648, a new rifamycin in normal volunteers. Am J Respir Crit Care Med 1999; 159(suppl):A495.
89. Dietze R, Teixeira L, Rocha LM, et al. Safety and bactericidal activity of rifalazil in patients with pulmonary tuberculosis. Antimicrob Agents Chemother 2001; 45:1972–1976.
90. Daniel N, Lounis N, Ji B, et al. Antituberculosis activity of once-weekly rifapentine-containing regimens in mice. Long-term effectiveness with 6- and 8-month treatment regimens. Am J Respir Crit Care Med 2000; 161:1572–1577.
91. Tuberculosis Trials Consortium. Rifapentine and isoniazid once a week versus rifampin and isoniazid twice a week for treatment of drug-susceptible pulmonary tuberculosis in HIV-negative patients: A randomised clinical trial. Lancet 2002; 360:528–534.
92. Vernon A, Burman W, Benator D, et al. Acquired rifamycin mono-resistance in patients with HIV-related tuberculosis treated with once-weekly rifapentine and isoniazid. Lancet 1999; 353:1843–1847.
93. Chapuis L, Ji B, Truffot-Pernot C, et al. Preventive therapy of tuberculosis with rifapentine in immunocompetent and nude mice. Am J Respir Crit Care Med 1994; 150:1355–1362.
94. TBTC Study 26: Weekly RFP/INH for 3 no. vs. Daily INH for 9 mo. for the Treatment of LTBI. www.clinicaltrials.gov.
95. Rosenthal IM, Zhang M, Williams KN, et al. Daily dosing of rifapentine cures tuberculosis in three months or less in the murine model. PLoS Med 2007; 4(12):e344.
96. Dooley K, Flexner C, Hackman J, et al. Repeated administration of high-dose intermittent rifapentine reduces rifapentine and moxifloxacin plasma concentrations. Antimicrob Agents Chemother 2008; 52(11):4037–4042.
97. Ibrahim M, Truffot-Pernot C, Andries K, et al. Sterilizing activity of R207910 (TMC207) containing regimens in the murine model of tuberculosis. Am J Respir Crit Care Med. 2009 Jul 16. [Epub ahead of print].
98. Ginsberg AM, Laurenzi MW, Rouse DJ, et al. Safety, tolerability, and pharmacokinetics of PA-824 in healthy subjects. Antimicrob Agents Chemother 2009; 53(9):3720–3725.
99. Ginsberg AM, Laurenzi MW, Rouse DJ, et al. Assessment of the effects of the nitroimidazo-oxazine PA-824 on renal function in healthy subjects. Antimicrob Agents Chemother 2009; 53(9):3726–3733.

15
The Future of Tuberculosis Vaccinology

JELLE THOLE
TuBerculosis Vaccine Initiative, Lelystad, The Netherlands
RUTH GRIFFIN and DOUGLAS YOUNG
CMMI, Department of Infectious Diseases and Microbiology, Imperial College London, London, U.K.

I. The TB Vaccine Challenge: To Improve on Bacille Calmette-Guérin

The outcome of infection by *Mycobacterium tuberculosis* is crucially dependent on the immune response of the host. Most infected individuals mount a response that is sufficient to prevent progression to disease but allow persistence of viable bacteria in the form of a latent infection. Ten percent of infected individuals develop clinical tuberculosis (TB) during their life, either as a result of failure to control the initial infection or due to reinfection or reactivation of latent infection (1). In immunocompromised individuals, the risk of developing tuberculosis increases to 5% to 10% annually. The development of secondary disease due to reinfection or reactivation of latent infection highlights a major challenge for TB vaccines. The hallmark of the adaptive immune system is its ability to learn from an initial infection how to mount a rapid and effective response when re-exposed to the same pathogen. Classically, vaccination mimics the learning process associated with natural infection. Development of a secondary disease in individuals who had contained a primary infection with *M. tuberculosis* shows that the robust learning process seen for a disease like smallpox does not always occur for TB (1). Similarly, individuals who have been cured of TB remain susceptible to reinfection and further disease (2).

A. Benefits and Limitations of BCG

The bacille Calmette-Guérin (BCG) vaccine—a strain of *Mycobacterium bovis* attenuated by laboratory passage—follows the classical paradigm of attempting to reproduce the immunogenicity of natural infection in the absence of pathological sequelae. Evidence from a range of experimental animal models demonstrates that it is able to accomplish this goal. Vaccinated animals mount an accelerated immune response that restricts multiplication of *M. tuberculosis* in the early phase of infection, reduces pathology, and prolongs survival. From these experimental results, it would be predicted that BCG would have a protective effect at least against progression to primary TB in humans. Support for this is provided by clinical trials of neonatal BCG vaccination, which demonstrate a reduction of around two-thirds in the incidence of severe forms of childhood TB, particularly meningitis (3–5). However, vaccination has proved less effective in older age groups. Although trials in U.K. school children demonstrated 80% protection against primary

TB, the efficacy of this vaccine varies from 0% to 80% in different countries with a consistently low efficacy in many tropical regions of the world where the vaccine is most needed (6–10). A range of hypotheses have been put forward to account for the disparity in BCG effectiveness, including the methodology of administration and age at vaccination (11), variations in the efficacy of BCG substrains (12), variations in the pathogenesis of different strains of *M. tuberculosis* (13), and an influence of environmental non-TB mycobacteria on immunity (7,8). Exposure to environmental mycobacteria could limit the impact of BCG vaccination by inducing immunity that masks the effect of subsequent BCG vaccination (14,15), or by having a direct antagonistic influence on subsequent BCG vaccination (16,17). Alternatively, environmental mycobacteria may inhibit BCG multiplication and thereby curtail the vaccine-induced immune response before it is fully developed (18,19). Whatever is the underlying mechanism, it is clear that BCG vaccination has failed to limit the incidence of the infectious forms of adult pulmonary TB in countries where TB is highly prevalent.

A more recent complication in the use of BCG in HIV prevalent countries was caused by the increased risk of development of disseminated BCG disease in HIV-infected children immunized at birth. This increased occurrence has led to the recommendation by the Global Advisory Committee on Vaccine Safety (GACVS) that children who are known to be HIV infected should no longer be immunized with BCG (20).

Despite these limitations, BCG represents an essential benchmark for scientists generating novel vaccines. Its efficacy against childhood disease makes BCG a key component of the Expanded Program on Immunization vaccination regimen; it has proven efficacy against the related mycobacterial disease of leprosy (21); and there is some evidence of a general benefit on infant mortality (22). Although limited evidence from U.K. trials suggest that the impact of BCG vaccination wanes over a period of 10 to 15 years, a 50-year follow-up of American Indians and Alaska natives who participated in a placebo-controlled BCG vaccine trial shows that it has lifelong benefits in some settings (23).

B. Future Vaccine Design

In view of the above limitations of BCG, several avenues for the designing of improved TB vaccines can be followed.

1. Firstly, such vaccines could be designed that prevent establishment of the initial infection upon exposure. Such vaccines should induce an effective response in the airway or lung—most likely at the mucosal lung surface—modulating interaction, uptake, and multiplication inside the initial host cells that encounter the bacterium. Though several approaches are underway to develop such (mucosal) vaccines, these are restricted by current limitations in understanding of the very first interactions between host and bacterium in the airway and lung, and the factors that determine whether exposure leads to infection. Mechanisms with the potential for vaccine-based intervention include induction of antibodies that enhance mucociliary clearance or antimicrobial responses during phagocytosis.

2. A second avenue is based on the design of vaccines that focus on reducing the risk of disease in infected individuals, either by preventing establishment of latent infection or by preventing progression to disease following reactivation or reinfection. Again, prospects for rational vaccine design are hindered by an incomplete understanding of the complex molecular and cellular processes

underlying these events. Several promising approaches are underway at pre-clinical and clinical stages. One way forward is to supplement the current BCG vaccine, for example, by augmenting responses to particular antigens or priming additional T cell subsets, either by improving BCG itself or by combining BCG with additional "booster" vaccines. Candidates following the first strategy include recombinant BCG engineered to enhance particular immune functions and novel attenuated *M. tuberculosis* strains with improved immunogenicity. Booster approaches include use of candidates based on selected *M. tuberculosis* antigens delivered using recombinant viral vectors or as purified proteins with adjuvant. These candidates could be used either to boost the response primed by initial BCG vaccination or to boost responses in individuals already exposed to *M. tuberculosis* itself. Potential alternative mechanisms that could be involved include disruption of receptor–ligand interactions involved in regulatory networks and immune exhaustion, or priming of alternative subsets of immune cells, for example, those stimulated by lipids.

3. A third avenue is to modulate the immune response in individuals already carrying *M. tuberculosis* in the form of latent infection or even active disease. Chronic infection is commonly associated with attenuation of immune effector mechanism as a result of immune exhaustion or establishment of regulatory T cell networks; vaccines could function by replenishing depleted responses or by modulating immune networks. Several vaccine developments are underway at preclinical and clinical stages that aim to impact on time, dose, and number of different drugs used in the current DOTS strategy. Current approaches are based on killed whole-cell mycobacterial preparations, but it is likely that in the future a number of the above approaches will be considered for therapeutic applications as well. An important consideration is that immune stimulation could adversely affect treatment efficacy by driving bacteria into drug-tolerant nonreplicating phenotypes.

II. New Vaccine Candidates: Genomics and Development of New TB Vaccines

Production of new TB vaccine candidates has been greatly facilitated by advances in mycobacterial genomics over the last decade (24). It is now possible to clone antigen-encoding genes from *M. tuberculosis* for use in DNA or protein production for subunit vaccines or for expression in a range of vaccine delivery systems. Novel genes can be introduced and expressed in BCG, and conversely individual genes can be modified or deleted in BCG or in *M. tuberculosis* itself. Several hundred new candidates have been generated and tested in experimental animal models, predominantly using standard protocols in central testing facilities supported by the U.S. National Institutes of Health and the European Union (25,26). Strategies for generating candidates have been based on engineering of live mycobacteria to produce attenuated variants of *M. tuberculosis* or recombinant BCG; or on targeting selected antigen subunits for delivery as DNA or proteins in adjuvant or as components of recombinant live vaccine vectors. Although most of these vaccines are based on protein components, some recent developments have also focused on the antigenic and adjuvant properties of the glycolipids present in the mycobacterial cell wall. In this section, we will focus on analysis of the different hypotheses and specific immunological profiles underpinning the development of 50 of these new vaccine candidates (27).

A. Live Mycobacterial Vaccines

Vaccines with Greater Resemblance to M. tuberculosis

BCG is an attenuated variant of *M. bovis*, and immunological differences between the vaccine and the pathogen may limit its efficacy. Thus, attempts have been made to attenuate *M. tuberculosis* and at the same time maintaining its immunogenic properties. The deletion of virulence associated genes (such as *lysA*, *panCD*, and RD1) and genes encoding two component systems (*phoP*) have all successfully led to the attenuation of *M. tuberculosis* (28,29–33). Most of these are unable to cause disease in normal mice, or are significantly less pathogenic than BCG in severe combined immunodeficient (SCID) mice. This offers the hope of a vaccine that could safely be used in areas such as equatorial Africa where HIV and *M. tuberculosis* coinfection are common (34). These vaccine candidates are currently all in the preclinical stage of development (Table 1). They vary in their protective efficacy, with some matching BCG in protection but surpassing BCG in terms of safety (30). Because *M. tuberculosis* as a vaccine vector is potentially hazardous, all derived candidates must contain at least two different mutations to reduce the risk of reversion and thus meet the safety regulatory requirements for such delivery systems (35).

Enhancing the Immunogenicity of BCG

Genome sequence comparisons have enabled us to precisely determine the genetic differences between BCG and *M. tuberculosis*. The first region of deletion to be discovered in BCG, called RD1, comprises genes encoding two important antigens ESAT6 and CFP10 (24,36–38). The restoration of RD1 in recombinant BCG improved the protective efficacy of this organism, but also raised concern with regard to its raised virulence in SCID mice as compared to BCG (Table 1) (39,40). More subtle BCG::RD1 mutants are currently being developed, retaining the improved protective efficacy whereas decreasing its virulence.

Another recombinant strain of BCG has been engineered to overexpress Ag85B (rBCG30, Table 1) and was found to have improved protective efficacy in a guinea pig model (41–43). A safer and more efficacious replication-limited variant of rBCG30 (rBCGMbtB30) has recently been designed for use in HIV-positive individuals (44).

Several attempts have been made to enhance the immunogenicity of BCG by engineering expression of mammalian cytokines by recombinant BCG, particularly to augment the protective Th1 response associated with macrophage activation (45). An alternative approach has been to enhance the ability of BCG to trigger CD8 T cells. Experiments in mice demonstrate an important role for these cells in protection against *M. tuberculosis* (46), and the existing BCG vaccine has very little ability to prime a CD8 response (47). To achieve this, Stefan Kaufmann and coworkers genetically modified BCG to express listeriolysin, a hydrolytic enzyme that damages the phagosomal membrane that encloses BCG within cells, making mycobacterial antigens more accessible for presentation to CD8 T cells (48). This strain was further engineered to eliminate mycobacterial urease activity, optimizing the pH for listeriolysin activity. The resultant strain, ΔureChly$^+$ rBCG promoted improved cross priming, culminating in improved T cell-mediated protection against *M. tuberculosis* (Table 1) (49). It is currently being evaluated in a phase I trial.

Table 1 Preclinical and Clinical Stage Live Attenuated Candidates

Product	Developer	Design	Planning phase I	Vaccine target[a]	Specific immunological profile
A. Preclinical stage					
1. rBCG ARMF	UCLA (Los Angeles, USA)	rBCG overexpressing Mtb30KD	2009	2	Improved BCG with strong response to 30 kDa
2. rBCGMtbB30	UCLA (Los Angeles, USA)	Limited replicating rBCG overexpressing Mtb30KD	2009	2	Improved BCG with strong response to 30 kDa
3. rBCGhIIFN-γ	UCLA (Los Angeles, USA)	rBCG overexpressing Mtb30KD and expressing IFN-γ	2009–2010	2	Improved BCG with strong response to 30 kDa and expressing active IFN-y
4. AERAS-407	AERAS (Rockville, USA)	rBCG::Pfo escaping vacuole and expressing common, latency and resuscitation antigens	2009	2	Improved BCG with better CD8 responses, improved cross-priming capacities, and additional responses to secreted, latency, and resuscitation antigens
5–8. mc2 6220/6221/6222/6231	Albert Einstein (New York, USA)	Attenuated auxotroph Mtb::ΔlysA and/or ΔpanCD	Late 2009	2	Similar responses to those induced by wt TB
9. mc2 5059	Albert Einstein (New York, USA)	Pro-apoptotic BCG::ΔpnuoG	Late 2009	2	BCG with improved Proapoptotic and Cross-priming capacities
10. MTB::ΔPhoP	University of Zaragoza (Zaragoza, Spain)	Attenuated *M. tuberculosis* :: ΔPhoP	Late 2009–2010	2	Similar responses to those induced by wt TB
11. HG856-BCG	Shanghai H&G Biotechnology (Shanghai, China)	BCG expressing chimeric ESAT6/AG85 Fusion protein	2010	3	Improved BCG with strong response to 30 kDa and AG85

12. PaBCG	Vander Bilt (Nashville, USA)	Proapoptotic BCG with reduced SOD, GlnaI, Thioredoxin, and thioredoxin reductase	TBD	2	Improved BCG with Proapoptotic and cross-priming capacities
13. BCG-RD1	Institute Pasteur, Paris	rBCG with RD1 region of Mtb	TBD	2	Improved BCG with TB specific antigens
14–16. BCG.ManLam BCG.PIM; BCG.GLP	NVI, Netherlands	BCG ::Δ ManLam BCG::Δ PIM BCG::ΔGLP	TBD	2	Improved BCG with genes encoding immunosuppressive lipid molecules removed
17. rBCG TB-Malaria	Universiti Sains Malaysia	Rec. BCG expressing multiple epitopes of *M. tuberculosis* fused to Malarial epitopes and antigens	TBD	2	Elicits T cell responses to *M. tuberculosis* epitopes and T and B cell responses against the malarial antigens and epitopes
18. rBCG T+B	Universiti Sains Malaysia	Rec. BCG expressing multiple T and B epitopes of *M. tuberculosis*	TBD	2	Elicits and T cell and antibody responses against the selected epitopes
19. rM.smegmatis T+B	Universiti Sains Malaysia	Rec. *M. smegmatis* expressing multiple T and B epitopes of *M. tuberculosis*	TBD	2	
B. Clinical Stage					
20. rBCG30	UCLA (Los Angeles, USA)	Recombinant BCG expressing High amounts of antigen 85B	Phase I	2	Improved BCG and strong response to 30 kDa
21. rBCG::Δ Ure::Hly	VPM (Hannover, Germany)/ MPIIB (Berlin, Germany)	rBCG expressing hemolysin of *Listeria monocytogenes*	Phase I	2	Improved BCG with stronger CD8 responses and cross-priming capacities

[a] 1, exposure stage, aiming to prevent establishment of initial infection. 2, infection stage, aiming to prevent disease development from initial, secondary or latent infection. 3, disease stage, therapeutic vaccines as adjunct to treatment with drugs.

Aeras have successfully expressed perfringolysin in BCG, which has the advantage of functioning at a higher pH than listeriolysin thereby negating the need for the elimination of urease activity. Aeras are using this recombinant strain to overexpress selected common, latency, and resuscitation antigens (Table 1). To further improve the immunogenicity, several other BCG constructs have been engineered, in which the expression of specific genes, such as *nuoG* and *sodA*, has been reduced or abrogated, leading to proapoptotic constructs with improved cross-priming abilities (Table 1).

Countering Immunosuppressive Effects of M. tuberculosis and BCG

The success of *M. tuberculosis* as a pathogen is dependent on its ability to survive host immune responses and it is likely that this has been accompanied by a selection of factors that subvert immunity. Therefore, in contrast to the conventional vaccine paradigm, the natural immune response to *M. tuberculosis* may be suboptimal, and the route to a more effective vaccine may be to remove these immunomodulatory components that suppress innate immune interactions and subsequent adaptive responses. An example of a potent *M. tuberculosis* inhibitor of innate immunity is superoxide dismutase (SOD). Diminished SOD production in a mutant of *M. tuberculosis* was associated with both increased early mononuclear infiltration and apoptosis at the infection site, leading to attenuation greater than that of BCG in the mouse model of *M. tuberculosis* infection (50). More recently, it has been demonstrated that subtle differences in the pattern of glycans and lipids present on the mycobacterial surface promote different innate and subsequent adaptive responses (51). Optimizing the orchestration of innate immune signaling could provide an important strategy for the development of improved vaccines. Several laboratories, including Bill Jacobs and coworkers at the Albert Einstein School of Medicine and Peter van der Ley and coworkers at the Netherlands Vaccine Institute have adopted this approach of preventing the expression of mycobacterial components that suppress the immune system. Several such *M. tuberculosis* and BCG candidates are being developed at preclinical stages (Table 1).

B.   Subunit Vaccines

Development of subunit vaccines involves selection of candidate antigens and appropriate delivery systems. Increasingly, the latter step is being viewed in the context of prime-boost systems using BCG either as primer or booster. Three hypotheses have been pursued for antigen selection.

Secreted Antigens

The protective efficacy of BCG depends on it being viable, and one of the characteristic features of viability is the ability to secrete antigens. It can be anticipated that antigens that are secreted from live mycobacteria will be immediately available for immune recognition well before intracellular antigens are released from lysed organisms, and may therefore be more appropriate targets for an early immune response (52). Peter Andersen and colleagues have pursued this hypothesis in an exhaustive screen of *M. tuberculosis* antigens that are released from bacteria growing in a defined culture medium (53). Based on a systematic evaluation of a large number of antigens, they have identified members of two protein families as showing encouraging potential for subunit vaccines. Firstly, the family comprising Ag85A and Ag85B, which are the most abundant protein components in culture filtrates and encode mycolyl transferase enzymes that are involved in the formation of the mycobacterial cell wall (54). Secondly, the family comprising the low molecular weight proteins, ESAT6 and CFP10, are encoded by adjacent genes in RD1 (hence deleted from BCG) (55) and form dimers (56,57). ESAT6, CFP10, and TB10.4 belong to a family of proteins that are exported by specialized secretion systems and are highly immunogenic. Several fusion proteins based on secreted proteins, such as Ag85B/ESAT6, and Ag85B/TB10.4 fusion protein subunit vaccines have been developed and are now being evaluated in phase I/phase IIa clinical trials (Table 2).

Antigens Expressed In Vivo
A limitation of the culture filtrate screen is that it only detects antigens expressed by the bacteria in vitro. It may be that an optimal vaccine should be customized to the antigen repertoire expressed in vivo. Antigens expressed by dormant bacteria in latently infected individuals represent one distinct repertoire of antigens not normally expressed in vitro. In particular, the DosR regulon has been implicated to encode an important set of proteins expressed during a hypoxia model of latency (58,59) and several DosR-associated antigens are now being considered in subunit vaccines or recombinant vaccines in a backbone of common, secreted antigens (Table 2). One possible candidate antigen is a member of the alpha-crystallin family of chaperone proteins that is expressed at high levels under hypoxic conditions (60). Similarly, antigens specifically expressed during resuscitation of the bacterium from its dormant stage have been identified (61,62), and again these are being built in as part of vectored or subunit vaccines with common and dormancy-associated antigens (Table 2).

Antigens Recognized by the Natural Immune Response
A strategy that circumvents potential differences between in vitro and in vivo expression is based on the hypothesis that the optimal antigens for subunit vaccines will be those that are recognized by T cells from tuberculin-positive individuals who have been exposed to infection but show no sign of clinical disease. Reed and colleagues carried out the most extensive systematic screen based on this hypothesis. They identified predominantly intracellular proteins such as Mtb32 and Mtb39, which were combined to generate a fusion protein Mtb72f, that is now being tested in phase I and II trials (Table 2) (63–67).

Adjuvanted Proteins
Delivery of purified proteins in appropriate adjuvants, provides a simple and effective strategy for vaccine production. Experiments in mouse and guinea pig models demonstrated that by selecting appropriate adjuvants it is possible to generate protective efficacy comparable to BCG using culture filtrate proteins and, in some cases, defined individual antigens or fusions. Although progress has been limited by the fact that few of the adjuvants approved for human use are effective in inducing T cell responses, promising data have been generated using Mtb72f and derived mutant M72 in the adjuvants AS02A and AS01B (68,69); and Ag85B/ESAT6 and Ag85B/TB10.4 in adjuvants IC31 (70–72) and CAF01 (73–75) (Table 2).

C. Expanding the T Cell Response for Improved Protection
Current adjuvant formulations predominantly induce CD4 T cell responses. Although a CD4 T cell response is the classic protective lymphocytic response against TB (76,77), there is mounting evidence that CD8 responses may be required in addition for optimal

Table 2 Preclinical and Clinical Stage Subunit Candidates

Product	Developer	Design	Planning phase I	Vaccine target[a]	Specific immunological profile
A. Preclinical Stage Subunit in adjuvant					
22. Nas L3/Htk BCG	Karolinska (Stockholm, Sweden)	Heat-killed BCG in NasL3 adjuvant	2009–2010	1, 2, 3	Local and systemic responses similar to BCG
23. H1/CAF01	SSI (Copenhagen, Denmark)	AG85B-ESAT6 in DDA/TDB adjuvant	2008	2	Strong Ag85b-ESAT6-Rv2660c CD4 IFN-γ and polyfunctional T cell reponses; Induction of memory T cells.
24. r30	UCLA (Los Angeles, USA)	Purified antigen 85B from *M. smegmatis*	2009	2	Effective responses to native 30 kDa
25. Nas L3/AM85B	Karolinska (Stockholm, Sweden)	ArabinoMannan from Mtb coupled to Ag85B in NasL3 adjuvant	2008/2009	2, 3	Local and systemic responses to 85 B
26. HBHA	Institute Pasteur Lille	Natively purified heparin binding hemagglutinin adhesin of *M. tuberculosis*	2009	1, 2	Strong CD4 and CD8 IFN-γ T cell responses and cytotoxic functions induced
27. HspC TB vaccine	Immunobiology	Heat shock protein antigen complexes	2009	2	Efficient antigen presentation via HSPs
28. hspDNA vaccine	Sequella/University of Cardiff	HSP65 DNA/Cpg	2009	3	Significant CD4 and CD8 T cells induced
29. HG856A	Shanghai H&G Biotechnology	Chimeric ESAT6/AG85a DNA vaccine—two copies of ESAT6 in AG85a gene	2009	3	Significant CD4 and CD8 T cells induced
30. TBVax	Epivax (Providence, USA)	Epitope-based DNA-prime/Peptide Boost delivered in liposomes and with CpG	2014	2	Significant CD4 and CD8 T cells induced

31–33. PP1; PP2; PP3	Colorado State University	Pool of selected proteins with boosting capacity of BCG	TBD	2	Strong boosting antigens
34, 35. F36; F727	Colorado State University	Correctly acylated Rv1411 and ESAT6	TBD	2, 3	Immune responses to native products
36. Ac2SGL	CNRS (Paris, France)	Diacylated sulfoglycolipid	TBD	2, 3	Induction of CD1 restricted responses
37. R32Kda-BCG	Bhagawan/Blue Peter (Hyderabad, India)	Purified r32 kDa antigen	TBD	2	Significant high level of IFN-γ responses induced
38. ID83	IDRI, Seattle	Adjuvanted subunit vaccines composed of three different proteins	TBD	2	
39. HG85A/B	Shanghai H&G Biotechnology (Shanghai, China)	Chimeric Ag85B Ag85A DNA vaccine	TBD	3	
Subunit delivered by vector					
40. AERAS-405	AERAS (Rockville, USA)	Shigella delivered dsRNA encoding many antigens	2008	2	CD4 and CD8 responses induced to latency and resuscitation antigens
41. HG856-SeV	Shanghai H&G Biotechnology (Shanghai, China)	Sendai virus expressing chimeric ESAT6/AG85 fusion protein	2010	3	Significant CD4 and CD8 response to 30 kDa and AG85
42. HVJ-Liposome/HSP65 DNA+IL12 DNA	Osaka University (Osaka, Japan)	Hemagglutinating virus Japan liposome delivered DNA of HSP65 and IL12	TBD	2	Significant CD4 and CD8 and TH1 responses induced
43. Streptomyces live vector	Finlay Institute (Habana, Cuba)	Rec. Streptomyces expressing multiple T and B epitopes of *M. tuberculosis*	TBD	2	Immunization elicits recognitions of proteins of mycobacteria

(Continued)

Table 2 Preclinical and Clinical Stage Subunit Candidates (*Continued*)

Product	Developer	Design	Planning phase I	Vaccine target [a]	Specific immunological profile
B. Clinical stage Subunit in adjuvant					
44. Hybrid1/IC31	SSI (Copenhagen, Denmark)	Subunit recombinant fusion Subunit of ag85B/ESAT6 in IC31 adjuvant	Phase IIa	2	Strong CD4 responses, including, IFN-γ and polyfunctional T cells. Induction of memory T cells.
45. M72/AS01b	GSKBIO (Rixensart, Belgium)	Subunit recombinant fusion of Rv1196/Rv0125 in ASO1b adjuvant	Phase IIa	2	Strong T cell responses in humans
46. HyVAC4/IC31 (AERAS 404)	SSI/AERAS/ Sanofi-Pasteur	Subunit recombinant fusion subunit of ag85B/TB10.4 in IC31 adjuvant	Phase I	2	Strong CD4 responses, including, IFN-γ and polyfunctional T cells. Induction of memory T cells.
47. Inactivated *M. vaccae*	SR pharma (London, UK)	Heat-inactivated bacterial suspension of *M. vaccae*	Phase III	2, 3	Immune response to common mycobacterial antigens
48. RUTI	BRI-Badalona (Badalona, Spain)	Fragmented Mtb cells	Phase I	3	Strong cellular and humoral responses
Subunit delivered by vector					
49. MVA85A	UOXF (Oxford, UK)	Modified vaccinia expressing antigen 85A	Phase IIb	2, 3	Strong CD4 and significant CD8 responses; Induces polyfunctional T cells to antigen 85A
50. Ad35ag85AB; TB10.4 (AERAS 402)	Crucell (Leiden, the Netherland)/ AERAS (Rockville, USA)	Replication deficient Adenovirus35 expressing AG 85A; 85B, and TB10.4	Phase I	2	Strong CD4 and CD8 responses induced

[a] 1, exposure stage, aiming to prevent establishment of initial infection. 2, infection stage, aiming to prevent disease development from initial, secondary or latent infection. 3, disease stage, therapeutic vaccines as adjunct to treatment with drugs.

vaccine efficacy (78–82). A series of studies have shown that the delivery of purified DNA encoding mycobacterial antigens, primes CD8 responses and confers a level of protection at least comparable to that obtained with adjuvanted protein vaccines in mice (83–85). One group has shown that DNA vaccination can induce a protective response capable of promoting bacterial clearance in mice that already have an established *M. tuberculosis* infection (86). However, this approach has not progressed to human trials as a result of the poor immunogenicity of current DNA vectors, the lack or reproducibility in different animal models, and concerns about the potential for induction of immunopathological responses.

An alternative strategy to induce CD8 T cells involves the delivery of antigens as components of recombinant viral vectors. This approach has been pursued using a recombinant smallpox vaccine system based on Modified Vaccinia Ankara expressing *M. tuberculosis* Ag85A (MVA85A) (Table 2) (87). The MVA construct confers protection comparable to BCG in mice and better than BCG in a guinea pig model (87,88). Interestingly, in spite of the rationale for choosing a viral vector, protection appears to be mediated by CD4 rather than CD8 T cells. As discussed below, this candidate has progressed into phase IIb trials, showing excellent immunogenicity and safety (Table 2). Recombinant adenoviral vectors are also being used as delivery systems for candidate antigens such as Ag85A (Table 1). Adenoviruses have advantages over MVA in the logistics of large-scale production. A replication-deficient Adenovirus35 expressing Ag85A, Ag85B, and TB10.4 has been shown to induce significant CD8 responses, and is currently being evaluated in a phase I trial (Table 2). In addition to conventional CD4 and CD8 T cells, several other T cell subsets have been implicated in the immune response to mycobacterial infection. These include T cells expressing a γδ receptor and CD1-restricted T cells capable of recognizing nonprotein antigens (89,90). The extent to which these T-cells are required for priming memory responses following vaccination and contributing to protection following challenge, is not known. One possibility is that they play a role in the interface between innate and adaptive responses, and that their modulation could provide a useful adjunct during conventional vaccination. A sulfoglycolipid antigen discovered by Germain Puzo and coworkers as a CD1-restricted antigen holds promise in this context and is currently being evaluated as a candidate subunit vaccine. The additional advantage of CD1-restricted antigens is that they also stimulate CD4 and CD8 negative T cell subsets and therefore may be of particular help in stimulating an immune response in HIV-infected individuals.

D. Enhancing the Efficacy of BCG in Prime-Boost Regimens

Although some of the candidates described above have performed better than BCG in particular animal models, it is their use in combination with BCG that holds the most promise. Prime-boost regimes—in which an immune response to an antigen is established by delivery in one vaccine vector and then augmented by delivery in an alternative vector—have shown considerable promise in HIV and malaria vaccinology. The TB subunit candidates entering into clinical trials are all anticipated to be used in prime-boost combinations with BCG.

III. Clinical Trials

The vaccine candidates discussed earlier were generated as part of a very extensive program of research in experimental animal models during the 1990s. It was then time that the TB vaccine research moved into human trials, but there were limitations in experience and infrastructure to take this forward. The only trials previously carried out were focused on assessing heat-killed *Mycobacterium vaccae* as an adjunct to chemotherapy (Table 1) (91–95). The need to develop vaccine trial expertise was recognized by the Sequella Foundation (subsequently, the Aeras Global TB Vaccine Foundation), who obtained funding from the Bill & Melinda Gates Foundation to set up a comparative trial of different delivery systems for BCG at a site near Cape Town. For the first Global Plan of the Stop TB Partnership, the New Vaccines Working Group set the goal of initiating clinical trials of five novel vaccine candidates by 2005. Eight candidates are currently being tested in clinical trials and over 10 more are scheduled to be tested, starting in 2008 (Tables 1 and 2). The goal set by the Working Group for the second Global Plan is to have a safe, effective, and licensed vaccine available at reasonable cost by 2015. An extensive network of clinical trials will be required to meet this goal.

A. Phase I and IIa Immunogenicity and Safety Trials

The first stage of moving a candidate from preclinical development to clinical trials is to produce the vaccine to Good Manufacturing Practice (GMP) with detailed toxicology and tissue distribution studies performed in small animals. Having carried out these preclinical studies, the vaccine is tested in small groups of individuals (around 20 per arm) in phase I studies and in larger groups with up to 300 individuals per arm in phase IIa trials. Whereas phase I studies provide initial data on safety and (often) immunogenicity, phase IIa trials generate more extensive immunogenicity and safety data and provide an opportunity to test vaccine lot consistency, dosing, and safety and immunogenicity in various age groups. For vaccines intended for neonates, safety is evaluated initially in adults, followed by age de-escalating trials until safety is demonstrated in the target group. On average, it is anticipated this will involve around six permutations with approximately 30 individuals in each arm of the study. Investigation of immunogenicity in groups with varying exposure to environmental mycobacteria represents one important factor highlighted by previous BCG trials.

MVA85A was the first candidate TB subunit vaccine to enter human trials since BCG over 80 years ago (Table 1). Helen McShane and colleagues began testing their vaccine in September 2002, and have since generated encouraging safety and immunogenicity data in a series of different phase I and IIa trials, both in the United Kingdom and in two TB-endemic sites in Africa. These workers showed that BCG prime followed by an MVA85A boost is more effective at raising an immune response compared to MVA85A or BCG alone. A small efficacy (phase IIb) trial in infants is scheduled to start in early 2009 (87,88,96–100). Another promising virally vectored vaccine—based on a replication deficient Adenovirus35 expressing Ag 85A, 85B, and TB10.4—has been evaluated in 2008 in a phase I trial with encouraging safety data and exceptionally strong CD8 immune responses (101).

Two subunit vaccines have been evaluated in phase I and initial phase IIa trials in US and Europe; Mtb72F in AS02A formulation ("bridged" to 72M in AS01B) and Ag85B-ESAT6 (H1) in IC31 adjuvant. Both 72M and H1 show promising safety and immunogenicity and now enter phase I/II studies in endemic countries. A third vaccine, Ag85B-TB10.4 (Hyvac4) in IC31, has entered a phase I trial in 2008 in Europe. This vaccine is similar to H1 but ESAT6 has been replaced by TB10.4, aiming to avoid the use of the diagnostically relevant ESTA6 molecule for vaccine purposes.

Finally, two live vaccines that might replace BCG are now in phase I trials—rBCG30 (41–43) and rBCG::Hly. Careful assessment in a systematic series of phase I trials is essential to establish vaccine safety. In addition to safety in uninfected healthy individuals, it is crucial to evaluate stringently the safety of the vaccine in individuals with latent TB infection and that it is safe in HIV-immunocompromised subjects, particularly for live vaccines.

Immunogenicity Markers

It would be enormously beneficial to assess vaccine efficacy by some simple immunological measurement. Considerable effort has been invested in discerning those immune responses that could be considered as "correlates" of protection (i.e., responses that are associated with protective immunity even though they may not have a direct causal link with protection) or as "surrogates" of protection (i.e., responses that are directly involved in protective mechanisms). At present we do not have any validated correlates or surrogates. To truly validate such biomarkers it is necessary to reliably identify distinct protected and unprotected populations, and it can be argued that having a vaccine with proven efficacy will be a prerequisite for such validation.

Tuberculin status is not a reliable predictor of disease susceptibility (102). Measuring T cell repertoire also has limitations. Though it is known that a vaccine is unlikely to confer protection if it fails to induce a population of T cells that produce interferon-γ (IFN-γ) in response to mycobacterial antigens (49,103), simple measurement of the magnitude of the IFN-γ response does not correlate with efficacy (104). In fact, the magnitude of the IFN-γ response following infection provides a correlate of disease progression (105–107). A potential method for evaluating vaccine efficacy in the context of T cell activity may involve assay of T cell homing to the lung (108). This technology was originally developed for testing the efficacy of HIV vaccines, where T cell homing to the gut (the main infection site in primates) is measured as a correlate of immune protection. Alternatively, surface markers on antigen-specific cells (particularly those associated with memory phenotypes) may prove informative, and assays that directly assess functional antimycobacterial activity may also have a role. In the absence of an established correlate or surrogate measures for TB vaccines, it will be important to maximize identification of immunological markers during phase II studies.

C. Phase IIb and III Efficacy Trials

Ultimately, the efficacy of new TB vaccines will have to be assessed by measuring their ability to protect against disease in phase III trials. Progression from phase II to phase III trials represents a major commitment of funding and human resources, with cohorts expanding from around 300 to around 30,000 individuals to obtain a statistically robust trial size. However, too much effort, time, and money on obtaining such statistically robust figures on vaccine efficacy may impede progress in vaccine development. An alternative strategy is to have an escalating phase IIb study, in which the vaccine is delivered to an increasingly expanded cohort, with immunogenicity and disease incidence measures used as "Go/NoGo" criteria for moving toward a final statistically robust trial size. A pilot-scale phase IIb efficacy trial involving several thousands of infants is currently being scheduled for MVA85A to start in early 2009 in Cape Town, South Africa.

Two different scenarios can be proposed for phase III trials. In the first, the new candidate would be delivered to a neonatal cohort together with, or shortly after, routine BCG vaccination. Incident disease would be monitored over the next three to four years. Such a trial could be added on to the current Cape Town trial of BCG delivery systems. This trial would test the ability of the new vaccine to improve on BCG-induced protection against primary TB in children; a prolonged follow-up would be required in order to determine whether improved efficacy at this stage was associated with reduced incidence of disease in later life.

In the second trial design, the new vaccine would be delivered to a teenage cohort who had received BCG vaccination at birth. It would be anticipated that this population would include individuals for whom BCG was their only mycobacterial exposure, as well as individuals whose immune system had already been primed by *M. tuberculosis* and who may be harboring latent infection. The two groups could be distinguished by immunological tests (e.g., using RD1 antigens) and a decision could be made whether to employ universal vaccination or to select the *M. tuberculosis*-naïve subgroup (as was done for BCG trials). If the trial is conducted in a high-incidence area, the naïve subgroup may represent only a small portion of the population. Again, incident cases would be monitored over a three- to four-year period, corresponding to the peak incidence of young adult TB. This scenario has the attraction of directly targeting adult pulmonary TB. The vaccine would, however, have to be successful in redirecting an immune response in individuals already primed by previous exposure to mycobacteria. In South Africa, studies on the vaccination of over 8000 adolescents with previous exposure to *M. tuberculosis*, are underway (sponsored by Aeras) to evaluate efficacy against acquisition of new infection and re-activation from latent infection. A similar scale study is due to commence in India, which will further aid in determining sample sizes required for the evaluation of vaccine efficacy.

D.   Phase IV Trials

These trials are postlicensure studies that use the infrastructure of the country in which the vaccine is being administered to monitor safety and determine the efficacy of the vaccine in epidemiological studies.

E.   Timelines and Logistics

Given the uncertainties surrounding mechanisms of immunity and protection, it is important that multiple vaccine candidates are evaluated and in parallel to successfully achieve the goal of a licensed vaccine by 2015 (Fig. 1).

A realistic plan is to bring 20 candidates into phase I trials over this period, with the assumption that around half will progress to phase II, leading to four full phase III trials. Candidates currently entered into clinical trials are expected to complete phase I and II by 2009–2012, with the first phase III trials to be completed by 2013 (Table 1,2; Fig. 1).

Although vaccine development can be represented as a simple linear pipeline, the reality is more likely to involve into an iterative learning process, in which early candidates may fail but nonetheless providing crucial immunological insights that feed back into refinement of subsequent generations of improved candidates and biomarkers for assessing vaccine efficacy.

This is an ambitious but feasible program. It will require substantial funding, estimated at around US $1 billion in additional resources. However, the payoff would

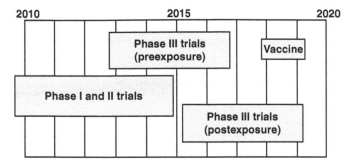

Figure 1   Projected Timeline for TB Vaccine Development.

be a truly powerful new tool that would allow not only disease control but also potential elimination of TB by 2050.

References

1. Smith PG, Ross AR. Epidemiology of tuberculosis. In: Bloom BR, ed. Tuberculosis: Pathogenesis, Protection, and Control. Washington, D.C.: American Society of Microbiology, 1994.
2. van Rie A, Warren R, et al. Exogenous reinfection as a cause of recurrent tuberculosis after curative treatment. N Engl J Med 1999; 341(16):1174–1179.
3. al-Kassimi FA, al-Hajjaj MS, al-Orainey IO, et al. Does the protective effect of neonatal BCG correlate with vaccine-induced tuberculin reaction? Am J Respir Crit Care Med 1995; 152(5)(Pt 1):1575–1578.
4. Colditz GA, Berkey CS, Mosteller F, et al. The efficacy of bacillus Calmette–Guerin vaccination of newborns and infants in the prevention of tuberculosis: Meta-analyses of the published literature. Pediatrics 1995; 96(1)(Pt 1):29–35.
5. Miceli I, de Kantor IN, Colaiacova D, et al. Evaluation of the effectiveness of BCG vaccination using the case-control method in Buenos Aires, Argentina. Int J Epidemiol 1988; 17(3): 629–634.
6. Bloom BR, Fine PEM. The BCG Experience: Implications for Future Vaccines Against Tuberculosis. Washington, D.C.: American Society for Microbiology, 1994.
7. Fine PE. The BCG story: Lessons from the past and implications for the future. Rev Infect Dis 1989; 11(suppl. 2):S353–S359.
8. Fine PE. Variation in protection by BCG: Implications of and for heterologous immunity. Lancet 1995; 346(8986):1339–1345.
9. Smith DW, Wiegeshaus EH, Edwards ML. The protective effects of BCG vaccination against tuberculosis. In: Bendinelli M, Friedman H, eds. *Mycobacterium tuberculosis*. New York, NY: Plenum Publishing Corporation, 1988:341–370.
10. ten Dam HG. Research on BCG vaccination. Adv Tuberc Res 1984; 21:79–106.
11. Tripathy SP. The case for BCG. Ann Natl Acad Med Sci 1983; 19(1):11–21.
12. Lagranderie MR, Balazuc AM, Deriaud E, et al. Comparison of immune responses of mice immunized with five different *Mycobacterium bovis* BCG vaccine strains. Infect Immun 1996; 64(1):1–9.
13. Chan J, Kaufmann SHE. In: Bloom, ed. Immune Mechanisms of Protection, Pathogenesis and Control. *Tuberculosis: pathogenesis, protection and control.* Washington, D.C.: B. R. American Society of Microbiology, 1994.

14. Palmer CE, Long MW. Effects of infection with atypical mycobacteria on BCG vaccination and tuberculosis. Am Rev Respir Dis 1966; 94(4):553–568.
15. Weiszfeiler JG, Karasseva V. Mixed mycobacterial infections. Rev Infect Dis 1981; 3(5):1081–1083.
16. Rook GA, Bahr GM, Stanford JL. The effect of two distinct forms of cell-mediated response to mycobacteria on the protective efficacy of BCG. Tubercle 1981; 62(1):63–68.
17. Stanford JL, Shield MJ, Rook GA. How environmental mycobacteria may predetermine the protective efficacy of BCG. Tubercle 1981; 62(1):55–62.
18. Brandt L, Feino Cunha J, Weinreich Olsen A, et al. Failure of the *Mycobacterium bovis* BCG vaccine: Some species of environmental mycobacteria block multiplication of BCG and induction of protective immunity to tuberculosis. Infect Immun 2002; 70(2):672–678.
19. Fine PE, Vynnycky E. The effect of heterologous immunity upon the apparent efficacy of (e.g., BCG) vaccines. Vaccine 1998; 16(20):1923–1928.
20. Revised BCG vaccination guidelines for infants at risk for HIV infection. Wkly Epidemiol Rec 2007; 82 (21):193–196.
21. Fine PE, Rodrigues LC. Modern vaccines. Mycobacterial diseases. Lancet 1990; 335(8696):1016–1020.
22. Kristensen I, Aaby P, Jensen H. Routine vaccinations and child survival: Follow up study in Guinea Bissau, West Africa. Br Med J 2000; 321(7274):1435–1438.
23. Aronson NE, Santosham M, Comstock GW, et al. Long-term efficacy of BCG vaccine in American Indians and Alaska Natives: A 60-year follow-up study. JAMA 2004; 291(17):2127–2128.
24. Cole ST, Brosch R, Parkhill J, et al. Deciphering the biology of *Mycobacterium tuberculosis* from the complete genome sequence. Nature 1998; 393(6685): 537–544.
25. Izzo A, Brandt L, Lasco T, et al. NIH pre-clinical screening program: Overview and current status. Tuberculosis (Edinb) 2005; 85(1–2):25–28.
26. Williams A, James BW, Bacon J, et al. An assay to compare the infectivity of *Mycobacterium tuberculosis* isolates based on aerosol infection of guinea pigs and assessment of bacteriology. Tuberculosis (Edinb) 2005; 85(3):177–184.
27. TB vaccines Pipeline; STOP TB Partnership; Working Group on New TB vaccines; September 2008.
28. Perez E, Samper S, Bordas Y, et al. An essential role for phoP in *Mycobacterium tuberculosis* virulence. Mol Microbiol 2001; 41(1):179–187.
29. Hondalus MK, Bardarov S, Russell R, et al. Attenuation of and protection induced by a leucine auxotroph of *Mycobacterium tuberculosis*. Infect Immun 2000; 68(5):2888–2898.
30. Smith DA, Parish T, Stoker NG, et al. Characterization of auxotrophic mutants of *Mycobacterium tuberculosis* and their potential as vaccine candidates. Infect Immun 2001; 69(2):1142–1150.
31. Sambandamurthy VK, Derrick Sc, Hsu T, Chen B, Larsen MH, Jalapathy KV, Chen M, Kim J, Porcelli SA, Chan J, Morris SL, Jacobs WR Jr. *Mycobacterium tuberculosis* DeltaRD1 DeltapanCD: a safe and limited replicating mutant strain that protects immunocompetent and immunocompromised mice against experimental tuberculosis. Vaccine. 2006; 24(37–39):6309–6320.
32. Waters WR, Palmer MV, Nonnecke BJ, et al. Failure of a *Mycobacterium tuberculosis* DeltaRD1 DeltapanCD double deletion mutant in a neonatal calf aerosol *M. bovis* challenge model: Comparisons to responses elicited by *M. bovis* bacilli Calmette Guerin. Vaccine 2007; 25(45):7832–7840.
33. Gonzalo-Asensio J, Mostowy S, Harders-Westerveen J, et al. A missing piece in the inricate puzzle of *Mycobacterium tuberculosis* virulence. PloS One 2008; 3(10):e3496.
34. Campos JM, Simonetti JP, Pone MV, et al. Disseminated bacillus Calmette–Guerin infection in HIV-infected children: Case report and review. Pediatr AIDS HIV Infect 1996; 7(6): 429–432.

35. Kamath AT, Fruth U, Brennan MJ, et al; AERAS Global TB Vaccine Foundation, World Health Organization. New live mycobacterial vaccines: The Geneva consensus on essential steps towards clinical development. Vaccine 2005; 23(29):3753–3761.

36. Brosch R, Gordon SV, Marmiesse M, et al. A new evolutionary scenario for the *Mycobacterium tuberculosis* complex. Proc Natl Acad Sci U S A 2002; 99(6):3684–3689.

37. Majlessi L, Brodin P, Brosch R, et al. Influence of ESAT-6 secretion system 1 (RD1) of *Mycobacterium tuberculosis* on the interaction between mycobacteria and the host immune system. J Immunol 2005: 174:3570–3579.

38. Brodin P, Majlessi L, Marsollier L, et al. Dissection of ESAT-6 system 1 of *Mycobacterium tuberculosis* and impact on immunogenicity and virulence. Infect Immun 2006; 74:88–98.

39. Demangel C, Brodin P, Cockle PJ, et al. Cell envelope protein PPE68 contributes to *Mycobacterium tuberculosis* RD1 immunogenicity independently of a 10-kilodalton culture filtrate protein and ESAT-6. Infect Immun 2004; 72(4):2170–2176.

40. Pym AS, Brodin P, Majlessi L, et al. Recombinant BCG exporting ESAT-6 confers enhanced protection against tuberculosis. Nat Med 2003; 9(5):533–539.

41. Horwitz MA, Harth G. A new vaccine against tuberculosis affords greater survival after challenge than the current vaccine in the guinea pig model of pulmonary tuberculosis. Infect Immun 2003; 71(4):1672–1679.

42. Horwitz MA, Harth G, Dillon BJ, et al. Recombinant bacillus Calmette–Guerin (BCG) vaccines expressing the *Mycobacterium tuberculosis* 30-kDa major secretory protein induce greater protective immunity against tuberculosis than conventional BCG vaccines in a highly susceptible animal model. Proc Natl Acad Sci U S A 2000; 97(25):13853–13858.

43. Hoft DF, Blazevic A, Abate G, et al. A new recombinant bacille Calmette-Guérin vaccine safely induces significantly enhanced tuberculosis-specific immunity in human volunteers. J Infect Dis 2008; Sep 22. [Epub ahead of print.]

44. Tullius MV, Harth G, Maslesa-Galic S, et al. A Replication-Limited Recombinant *Mycobacterium bovis* BCG vaccine against tuberculosis designed for human immunodeficiency virus-positive persons is safer and more efficacious than BCG. Infect Immun 2008; 76(11):5200–5214.

45. Murray PJ, Aldovini A, Young RA. Manipulation and potentiation of antimycobacterial immunity using recombinant bacille Calmette–Guerin strains that secrete cytokines. Proc Natl Acad Sci U S A 1996; 93(2):934–939.

46. Sousa AO, Mazzaccaro RJ, Russell RG, et al. Relative contributions of distinct MHC class I-dependent cell populations in protection to tuberculosis infection in mice. Proc Natl Acad Sci U S A 2000; 97(8):4204–4208.

47. Flynn JL, Goldstein MM, Triebold KJ, et al. Major histocompatibility complex class I-restricted T cells are required for resistance to *Mycobacterium tuberculosis* infection. Proc Natl Acad Sci U S A 1992; 89(24):12013–12017.

48. Hess J, Miko D, Catic A, et al. *Mycobacterium bovis* bacille Calmette-Guerin strains secreting listeriolysin of *Listeria monocytogenes*. Proc Natl Acad Sci U S A 1998; 95(9):5299–5304.

49. Grode L, Seiler P, Baumann S, et al. Increased vaccine efficacy against tuberculosis of recombinant *Mycobacterium bovis* bacille Calmette–Guerin mutants that secrete listeriolysin. J Clin Investig 2005; 115(9):2472–2479.

50. Edwards KM, Cynamon MH, Voladri RKR. Iron-cofactored superoxide dismutase inhibits host responses to *Mycobacterium tuberculosis*. Am J Respir Crit Care Med 2001; 164:2213–2219.

51. Reed MB, Domenech P, Manca C, et al. A glycolipid of hypervirulent tuberculosis strains that inhibits the innate immune response. Nature 2004; 431d(7004):84–87.

52. Andersen P. Effective vaccination of mice against *Mycobacterium tuberculosis* infection with a soluble mixture of secreted mycobacterial proteins. Infect Immun 1994; 62(6): 2536–2544.

53. Andersen P, Askgaard D, Ljungqvist L, et al. Proteins released from *Mycobacterium tuberculosis* during growth. Infect Immun 1991; 59(6):1905–1910.
54. Content J, de la Cuvellerie A, de Wit L, et al. The genes coding for the antigen 85 complexes of *Mycobacterium tuberculosis* and *Mycobacterium bovis* BCG are members of a gene family: Cloning, sequence determination, and genomic organization of the gene coding for antigen 85-C of *M. tuberculosis*. Infect Immun 1991; 59(9):3205–3212.
55. Berthet FX, Rasmussen PB, Rosenkrands I, et al. A *Mycobacterium tuberculosis* operon encoding ESAT-6 and a novel low-molecular-mass culture filtrate protein (CFP-10). Microbiology 1998; 144(Pt 11):3195–3203.
56. Louise R, Skjot V, Agger EM, et al. Antigen discovery and tuberculosis vaccine development in the post-genomic era. Scand J Infect Dis 2001; 33(9):643–647.
57. Alderson MR, Bement T, Day CH, et al. Expression cloning of an immunodominant family of *Mycobacterium tuberculosis* antigens using human CD4(+) T cells. J Exp Med 2000; 191(3):551–560.
58. Voskuil MI, Schnappinger D, Visconti KC, et al. Inhibition of respiration by nitric oxide induces a *Mycobacterium tuberculosis* dormancy program. J Exp Med 2003; 198(5):705–713.
59. Roupie V, Romano M, Zhang L, et al. Immunogenicity of eight dormancy regulon-encoded preoteins of *Mycobacterium tuberculosis* in DNA-vaccinated and tuberculosis-infected mice. Infect Immun 2007; 75(2):941–949.
60. Sherman DR, Voskuil M, Schnappinger D, et al. Regulation of the *Mycobacterium tuberculosis* hypoxic response gene encoding alpha-crystallin. Proc Natl Acad Sci U S A 2001; 98(13):7534–7539.
61. Yeremeev VV, Kondratieva TK, Rubakova EI, et al. Proteins of the Rpf family: Immune cell reactivity and vaccination efficacy against tuberculosis in mice. Infect Immun 2003; 71(8):4789–4794.
62. Mollenkopf HJ, Grode L, Mattow J, et al. Application of mycobacterial proteomics to vaccine design: Improved protection by *Mycobacterium bovis* BCG prime-Rv3407 DNA boost vaccination against tuberculosis. Infect Immun 2004; 72(11):6471–6479.
63. Dillon DC, Alderson MR, Day CH, et al. Molecular characterisation and human T-cell responses to a member of a novel *Mycobacterium tuberculosis* mtb39 gene family. Infect Immun 1999; 67(6):2941–2950.
64. Skeiky YA, Alderson MR, Ovendale PJ, et al. Differential immune responses and protective efficacy induced by components of a tuberculosis polyprotein vaccine, Mtb72F, delivered as naked DNA or recombinant protein. J Immunol 2004; 172(12):7618–7628.
65. Brandt L, Skeiky YA, Alderson MR, et al. The protective effect of the *Mycobacterium bovis* BCG vaccine is increased by coadministration with the *Mycobacterium tuberculosis* 72-kilodalton fusion polyprotein Mtb72F in M. tuberculosis-infected guineapigs. Infect Immun 2004; 72(11):6622–6632.
66. Irwin SM, Izzo AA, Dow SW, et al. Tracking antigen-specific CD8 T lymphocytes in the lungs of mice vaccinated with the Mtb72F polyprotein. Infect Immun 2005; 73(9):5809–5816.
67. Tsenova L, Harbacheuski R, Moreira AL, et al. Evaluation of the Mtb72F polyprotein vaccine in a rabbit model of tuberculous meningitis. Infect Immun 2006; 74(4):2392–2401.
68. Reed SG, Alderson MR, Dalemans W, et al. Prospects for a better vaccine against tuberculosis [Review]. Tuberculosis (Edinb) 2003; 83(1–3):213–219.
69. Garcon N, Chomez P, Van mechelen M. GlaxoSmithKline Adjuvant Systems in vaccines: Concepts, achievements and perspectives. Exp Rev Vaccines 2007; 6(5)723–739.
70. Agger EM, Rosenkrands I, Olsen AW, et al. Protective immunity to tuberculosis with Ag85B-ESAT-6 in a synthetic cationic adjuvant system IC31. Vaccine 2006; 24(26):5452–5460.
71. Kamath AT, Valenti MP, Rochat AF, et al. Protective anti-mycobacterial T cell responses through exquisite in vivo activation of vaccine-targeted dentritic cells. Eur J Immunol 2008; 38(5):1247–1256.

72. Lingnau K, Riedl K, von Gabain A. IC31 and IC30, novel types of vaccine adjuvant based on peptide delivery systems. Expert Rev Vaccines 2007; 6(5):741–746.

73. Christensen D, Foged C, Rosenkrands I, et al. Trehalose preserves DDA/TDB liposones and their adjuvant effect during freeze-drying. Biochim Biophys Acta 2007; 1768(9):2120–2129.

74. Christensen D, Kirby D, Foged C, et al. Alpha,alpha'-rehalose 6,6'-debehenate inn non-phospholipid-based liposomes enables direct interaction with trehalose, offering stability during freeeze-drying. Biochim Biophys Acta 2008; 1778(5):1365–1373.

75. Agger EM, Rosenkrands I, Hansen J, et al. Cationic liposomes formulated with synthetic mycobacterial cordfactor (CAF01): A versatile adjuvant for vaccines with different immuno-logical requirements. PLoS One 2008; 3(9): e3116.

76. Munk ME, Emoto M. Functions of T-cell subsets and cytokines in mycobacterial infections. Eur Respir J Suppl 1995; 20:668s–675s.

77. Chackerian AA, Perera TV, Behar SM. Gamma interferon-producing CD4+ T lymphocytes in the lung correlate with resistance to infection with *Mycobacterium tuberculosis*. Infect Immun 2001; 69(4):2666–2674.

78. van Pinxteren LA, Cassidy JP, Smedegaard BH, et al. Control of latent *Mycobacterium tuberculosis* infection is dependent on CD8 T cells. Eur J Immunol 2000; 30(12):3689–3698.

79. Canaday DH, Wilkinson RJ, Li Q. CD4(+) and CD8(+) T cells kill intracellular *Mycobacterium tuberculosis* by a perforin and Fas/Fas ligand-independent mechanism. J Immunol 2001; 167(5):2734–2742.

80. Serbina NV, Flynn JL. CD8(+) T cells participate in the memory immune response to *Mycobacterium tuberculosis*. Infect Immun 2001; 69(7):4320–4328.

81. Stenger S. Cytolytic T cells in the immune response to *Mycobacterium tuberculosis*. Scand J Infect Dis 2001; 33(7):483–487.

82. Turner J, D'Souza CD, Pearl JE, et al. CD8- and CD95/95L-dependent mechanisms of resistance in mice with chronic pulmonary tuberculosis. Am J Respir Cell Mol Biol 2001; 24(2):203–209.

83. Fonseca DP, Benaissa-Trouw B, van Engelen M, et al. Induction of cell-mediated immunity against *Mycobacterium tuberculosis* using DNA vaccines encoding cytotoxic and helper T-cell epitopes of the 38-kilodalton protein. Infect Immun 2001; 69(8):4839–4845.

84. Vordermeier HM, Zhu X, Harris DP. Induction of CD8+ CTL recognizing mycobacterial peptides. Scand J Immunol 1997; 45(5):521–526.

85. Zhu X, Venkataprasad N, Thangaraj HS, et al. Functions and specificity of T cells following nucleic acid vaccination of mice against *Mycobacterium tuberculosis* infection. J Immunol 1997; 158(12):5921–5926.

86. Lowrie DB, Tascon RE, Bonato VL, et al. Therapy of tuberculosis in mice by DNA vaccina-tion. Nature 1999; 400(6741):269–271.

87. McShane H, Pathan AA, Sander CR. Recombinant modified vaccinia virus Ankara express-ing antigen 85A boosts BCG-primed and naturally acquired antimycobacterial immunity in humans. Nat Med 2004; 10(11):1240–1244.

88. McShane H, Pathan AA, Sander CR, et al. Boosting BCG with MVA85A: The first candi-date subunit vaccine for tuberculosis in clinical trials. Tuberculosis (Edinb) 2005; 85(1–2): 47–52.

89. Kaufmann SH. Gamma/delta and other unconventional T lymphocytes: What do they see and what do they do? Proc Natl Acad Sci U S A 1996; 93(6):2272–2279.

90. Moody DB, Ulrichs T, Muhlecker W, et al. CD1c-mediated T-cell recognition of isoprenoid glycolipids in *Mycobacterium tuberculosis* infection. Nature 2000; 404(6780):884–888.

91. Stanford JL, De las Aguas J, Turres P, et al. Studies on the effects of a potential immunother-apeutic agent in leprosy patients. Health Coop Pap 1987; 7:201–206.

92. Poziak A, Stanford JL, Johnson NMcl, et al. Preliminary studies of immunotherapy of tuberculosis in man. Proceedings of the International Tuberculosis Congress, Singapore. Bull Int Union Against Tuberc Lung Dis 1987; 62:39–40.

93. Bahr GM, Shaaban MA, Gabriel M, et al. Improved immunotherapy for pulmonary tuberculosis with improved Mycobacterium vaccae. Tubercle 1990; 71:259–266.
94. Stanford JL, Bahr GM, Bypass O, et al. A modern approach to the immunotherapy of tuberculosis. Bull Int Union Against Tuberc Lung Dis 1990; 65:27–29.
95. Durban Immunotherapy Trial Group. Immunotherapy with *Mycobacterium vaccae* in patients with newly diagnosed pulmonary tuberculosis: A randomised controlled trial. Lancet 1999; 354:116–119.
96. Ibanga HB, Brookes RH, Hill PC, et al. Early clinical trials with a new tuberculosis vaccine, MVA85A, in tuberculosis-endemic countries: Issues in study design [Review]. Lancet Infect Dis 2006; 6(8):522–528.
97. Beveridge NE, Price DA, Casazza JP, et al. Immunisation with BCG and recombinant MVA85A induces long-lasting, polyfunctional Mycobacterium tuberculosis-specific CD4+memory T lymphocyte populations. Eur J Immunol 2007; 37(11):3089–3100.
98. Pathan AA, Sander CR, Fletcher HA, et al. Boosting BCG with recombinant modified vaccinia ankara expressing antigen 85A: Different boosting intervals and implication for efficacy trials. PLoS ONE. 2007; 2(10):e1052.
99. Hawkridge T, Scriba TJ, Gelderbloem S, et al. Safety and immunogenecity of a new tuberculosis vaccine, MVA85A, in healthy adults in South Africa. J Infect Dis 2008; 198(4):544–552.
100. Brookes RH, Hill PC, Owiafe PK, et al. Safety and immunogenecity of the candidate tuberculosis vaccine MVA85A in West Africa. PLoS ONE 2008; 3(8):e2921.
101. Radosevic K, Wieland CW, Rodriquez A, et al. Protective immune responses to a recombinant adenovirus type 35 tuberculosis vaccine in two mouse strains: CD4 and CD8 T-cell epitope mapping and role of gamme interferon. Infect Immun 2007; 75(8):4105–4115.
102. Fine PE, Sterne JA, Ponnighaus JM, et al. Delayed-type hypersensitivity, mycobacterial vaccines and protective immunity. Lancet 1994; 344(8932):1245–1249.
103. Cooper AM, Dalton DK, Stewart TA, et al. Disseminated tuberculosis in interferon gamma gene-disrupted mice. J Exp Med 1993; 178(6):2243–2247.
104. Agger EM, Andersen P. Tuberculosis subunit vaccine development: On the role of interferon-gamma. Vaccine 2001; 19(17–19):2298–2302.
105. Vordermeier HM, Chambers MA, Cockle PJ, et al. Correlation of ESAT-6-specific gamma interferon production with pathology in cattle following *Mycobacterium bovis* BCG vaccination against experimental bovine tuberculosis. Infect Immun 2002; 70(6):3026–3032.
106. McMurray DN. A coordinated strategy for evaluating new vaccines for human and animal tuberculosis. Tuberculosis (Edinb) 2001; 81(1–2):141–146.
107. Beveridge NE, Fletcher HA, Hughes J, et al. A comparison of IFNgamme detection methods used in tuberculosis vaccine trials. Tuberculosis (Edinb) 2008; 88(6):631–640
108. Forbes EK, Sander C, Ronan EO, et al. Multifunctional, high-level cytokine-producing Th1 cells in the lung, but not spleen, correlate with protection against *Mycobacterium tuberculosis* aerosol challenge in mice. J Immunol 2008; 181(7):4955–4964.

Index